IMMUNOTHERAPY OF CANCER

CANCER DRUG DISCOVERY AND DEVELOPMENT

BEVERLY A. TEICHER, SERIES EDITOR

IMMUNOTHERAPY OF CANCER

Edited by

MARY L. DISIS, MD

University of Washington School of Medicine
Seattle, WA

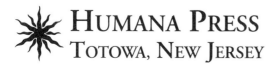

HUMANA PRESS
TOTOWA, NEW JERSEY

© 2006 Humana Press Inc.
999 Riverview Drive, Suite 208
Totowa, New Jersey 07512

www.humanapress.com

Production Editor: Amy Thau

Cover design by Patricia F. Cleary

This publication is printed on acid-free paper. ∞
ANSI Z39.48-1984 (American National Standards Institute)
Permanence of Paper for Printed Library Materials

For additional copies, pricing for bulk purchases, and/or information about other Humana titles, contact Humana at the above address or at any of the following numbers: Tel.:973-256-1699; Fax: 973-256-8341; Email: orders@humanapr.com; or visit our Website: http://humanapress.com

Printed in the United States of America.   10 9 8 7 6 5 4 3 2 1
eISBN: 1-59745-011-1
Library of Congress Cataloging-in-Publication Data
Immunotherapy of cancer / edited by Mary L. Disis.
     p. cm. -- (Cancer drug discovery and development)
Includes bibliographical references and index.
ISBN 1-58829-564-8 (alk. paper)
1. Cancer--Immunotherapy. 2. Antineoplastic agents--Design. I. Disis,
Mary L. II. Series.
RC271.I45I466 2006
616.99'4061--dc22
                    2005017065

PREFACE

Tumor immunology is a scientific discipline that is driven by clinical translation. For many decades, scientists both at the bench and at the bedside have struggled with determining the role immunity may play in tumor eradication, if any. For many years, the major question driving the field was whether human tumors were immunogenic. Over the last decade, literally thousands of immunogenic proteins related to tumors have been identified, resulting in a host of new targets for immunomodulation.

Successful active immunization against cancer has long been a goal of tumor immunologists. Generating a native endogenous immune response against cancer offers many advantages as compared with more standard anticancer therapies. Stimulating a cellular immune response would allow cancer cells to potentially be eradicated at multiple metastatic sites since competent T-cells can "home" to antigen. Successful vaccination would generate immunological memory, allowing the eradication of tumors at times of disease relapse, which may take place years after primary therapy. The identification of specific tumor antigens has fueled the development of a variety of vaccine technologies aimed at increasing the magnitude of the tumor-specific immune response. Furthermore, technologies have been developed to quantitatively and reproducibly measure tumor immunity. Immunological monitoring techniques have evolved from novel laboratory tools to robust clinical assays capable of estimating the potency of immune-based therapies.

Vaccines for protection against infectious agents have been one of the most successful interventions in medicine. However, few vaccines are utilized to treat ongoing established infections. Similarly, cancer vaccines have had little success in eradicating growing cancers. The last several years have led to the development of a variety of clinical strategies that may prove more effective in established disease states. Adoptive T-cell therapy, donor lymphocyte infusion after transplant, or infusions of novel cytokines may all boost tumor-specific T-cell immunity above the level that can be achieved with vaccination alone. Indeed, stimulating the "graft-vs-leukemia effect" with donor lymphocyte infusion in subjects who have relapsed after allogeneic transplants for hematopoietic malignancy has become a standard of care and a life-saving measure. Thus, immune-based strategies can be developed both to prevent relapse in minimal residual disease states, as well as to treat existing cancers.

The last decade of research in tumor immunology has seen the adoption of a multitude of immune-based therapies into the standard practice of oncology. Monoclonal antibodies targeting tumor antigens have revolutionized cancer treatment for patients with lymphoma, breast cancer, and other solid tumors. Antibody therapy has now been shown to have both biological, as well as immunological, effects. Antibodies targeting growth factor receptors will bind to inhibit cell signaling and limit unregulated growth. However, the binding of a monoclonal antibody may also activate immune system cells to respond to antigens expressed by tumors, thus stimulating endogenous immunity.

Finally, the role of the tumor microenvironment is critical in modulating and shaping the tumor-specific immune response. Advances in recent years have pointed to the most important mechanisms limiting the immune response in cancer patients, and these environmental influences can be modulated in vivo with novel reagents. Thus, treatments are directed both at initiating and expanding a cancer-specific immune response, as well as reigning in the environment from preventing the function of immune effectors. Clearly, combination immune-based approaches may be more potent than any strategy used in isolation.

Immunotherapy of Cancer provides a comprehensive overview of both the science and clinical translation of tumor immunology. Each chapter is designed to give the reader the scientific basis behind the novel therapy and outline basic theory, as well as practical treatment applications. Tremendous scientific advances in basic and molecular immunology have resulted in explosive growth both in our understanding of how cancer is recognized by the immune system, as well as in our ability to control and modulate that recognition. *Immunotherapy of Cancer* provides the springboard for applying the most important findings in tumor immunology to any basic laboratory program or clinical oncology practice.

Mary L. Disis, MD

CONTENTS

CONTRIBUTORS

BOND ALMAND, MD • *Tumor Vaccine Group, Department of Oncology, University of Washington School of Medicine, Seattle, WA*

STEPHEN M. ANSELL, MD, PhD • *Division of Hematology Research, Mayo Clinic, Rochester, MN*

CARLOS L. ARTEAGA, MD • *Departments of Medicine and Cancer Biology and Breast Cancer Program, Vanderbilt-Ingram Comprehensive Cancer Center, Vanderbilt University School of Medicine, Nashville, TN*

MOHAMED AWAD, MD • *Center for Surgery Research, Cleveland Clinic Foundation, Cleveland, OH*

HELGA BERNHARD, MD • *Department of Hematology/Oncology, Klinikum Rechts der Isar, Technical University Munich (TUM), Munich, Germany; Clinical Cooperation Group Vaccinology, GSF–National Research Center for Environment and Health, Neuherberg, Germany; and Technical University Munich, Munich, Germany*

MALAYA BHATTACHARYA-CHATTERJEE, PhD • *The Vontz Center for Molecular Studies, University of Cincinnati, Cincinnati, OH*

MICHAEL R. BISHOP, MD • *NIH/NCI/CCR Experimental Transplantation and Immunology Branch, Bethesda, MD*

ERNEST C. BORDEN, MD • *Taussig Cancer Center, Cleveland Clinic Foundation, Cleveland, OH*

HOSSEIN BORGHAEI, DO • *Division of Medical Sciences, Department of Medical Oncology, Fox Chase Cancer Center, Philadelphia, PA*

DIRK H. BUSCH, MD • *Department of Microbiology/ Immunology, Klinikum Rechts der Isar, Technical University Munich (TUM), Munich, Germany; Clinical Cooperation Group Vaccinology, GSF–National Research Center for Environment and Health, Neuherberg, Germany; and Technical University Munich, Munich, Germany*

MICHAEL A. CALIGIURI, MD • *Division of Hematology and Oncology, and Comprehensive Cancer Center, College of Medicine and Public Health, Ohio State University, Columbus, OH*

MICHAEL CAMPOLI, BS • *Department of Immunology, Roswell Park Cancer Institute, Buffalo, NY*

ESTEBAN CELIS, MD, PhD • *Department of Pediatrics and Tumor Immunotherapy Program of the Stanley S. Scott Cancer Center, Louisiana State University School of Medicine, New Orleans, LA*

SUNIL K. CHATTERJEE, PhD • *Division of Hematology/Oncology, Department of Internal Medicine, and The Barrett Cancer Center, University of Cincinnati Medical Center, Cincinnati, OH*

JOSEPH I. CLARK, MD • *Division of Hematology/Oncology, Cardinal Bernardin Cancer Center, Loyola University Chicago Stritch School of Medicine, Chicago, IL*

PETER A. COHEN, MD • *Center for Surgery Research, Cleveland Clinic Foundation, Cleveland, OH*

JOSE-RAMON CONEJO-GARCIA, MD, PhD • *Center for Research on Women's Health and Reproduction, and Abramson Cancer Research Institute, University of Pennsylvania School of Medicine, Philadelphia, PA*

HEINKE CONRAD, BS • *Department of Hematology/Oncology, Technical University of Munich, Munich, Germany*

GEORGE COUKOS, MD, PhD • *Center for Research on Women's Health and Reproduction, and Abramson Cancer Research Institute, University of Pennsylvania School of Medicine, Philadelphia, PA*

TYLER J. CURIEL, MD, MPH • *The Henderson Professor of Medicine, Chief, Section of Hematology and Medical Oncology, Department of Medicine, Tulane Medical School, New Orleans, LA*

JIE DAI, MD • *Center for Immunotherapy of Cancer and Infectious Diseases, University of Connecticut Health Center, Farmington, CT*

EDUARDO DAVILA, MD, PhD • *Department of Pediatrics and Tumor Immunotherapy Program of the Stanley S. Scott Cancer Center, Louisiana State University School of Medicine, New Orleans, LA*

EVELYNA DERHOVANESSIAN, DIPL BIOL • *Section for Transplantation Immunology, Centre for Medical Research, University of Tübingen Medical School, Tübingen, Germany*

MARY L. DISIS, MD • *Tumor Vaccine Group, Department of Oncology, University of Washington School of Medicine, Seattle, WA*

JULIE Y. DJEU, PhD • *Immunology Program, H. Lee Moffitt Cancer Center and Research Institute, Tampa, FL*

LEISHA A. EMENS, MD, PhD • *Department of Oncology, The Johns Hopkins University School of Medicine, Sidney Kimmel Comprehensive Cancer Center, Baltimore, MD*

SHERIF S. FARAG, MD, PhD • *Division of Hematology and Oncology, and Comprehensive Cancer Center, Ohio State University, College of Medicine and Public Health, Columbus, OH*

SOLDANO FERRONE, MD, PhD • *Department of Immunology, Roswell Park Cancer Institute, Buffalo, NY*

THOMAS FLAD, PhD • *Section for Transplantation Immunology, Centre for Medical Research, University of Tübingen Medical School, Tübingen, Germany*

KENNETH A. FOON, MD • *Division of Hematology/Oncology, Department of Internal Medicine, and The Barrett Cancer Center, University of Cincinnati Medical Center, Cincinnati, OH*

TERRY J. FRY, MD • *Pediatric Oncology Branch, National Cancer Institute, Bethesda, MD*

DMITRY GABRILOVICH, MD, PhD • *Department of Interdisciplinary Oncology, University of South Florida, and the H. Lee Moffitt Cancer Center, Tampa, FL*

KERSTIN GEBHARD • *Department of Hematology/Oncology, Technical University of Munich and Clinical Cooperation Group Vaccinology, GSF–National Research Center for Environment and Health, Neuherberg, Germany; and Technical University Munich, Munich, Germany*

SUSAN GROSHEN, PhD • *Department of Preventive Medicine, University of Southern California, Keck School of Medicine, and the Norris Comprehensive Cancer Center, Los Angeles, CA*

NANCY M. HARDY, MD • *NIH/NCI/CCR Experimental Transplantation and Immunology Branch, Bethesda, MD*

LISA M. HARLAN, PhD • *Immunology Program, H. Lee Moffitt Cancer Center and Research Institute, Tampa, FL*

ELIZABETH M. JAFFEE, MD • *Departments of Oncology, Immunology, Pathology, and Pharmacology, The Johns Hopkins University School of Medicine, Sidney Kimmel Comprehensive Cancer Center, Baltimore, MD*

HOWARD L. KAUFMAN, MD • *Departments of Surgery and Pathology, College of Physicians and Surgeons, Columbia University, New York, NY*

THORSTEN KLAMP, PhD• *Department of Internal Medicine III, Johannes Guttenberg University, Mainz, Germany*

ASHLEY KNIGHTS, MSC • *Section for Transplantation Immunology, Centre for Medical Research, University of Tübingen Medical School, Tübingen, Germany*

KEITH L. KNUTSON, PhD • *Department of Immunology, Mayo Clinic College of Medicine, Rochester, MN*

MICHAEL KOSLOWSKI, MD • *Department of Internal Medicine III, Johannes Guttenberg University, Mainz, Germany*

SEBASTIAN KREITER, MD • *Department of Internal Medicine III, Johannes Guttenberg University, Mainz, Germany*

HEESUN KWAK, PhD • *Departments of Surgery and Pathology, College of Physicians and Surgeons, Columbia University, New York, NY*

DOUGLAS W. LEAMAN, PhD • *Department of Biological Sciences, University of Toledo, Toledo, OH*

ZIHAI LI, MD, PhD • *Center for Immunotherapy of Cancer and Infectious Diseases, University of Connecticut Health Center, Farmington, CT*

CRYSTAL L. MACKALL, MD • *Pediatric Oncology Branch, National Cancer Institute, Bethesda, MD*

HOLDEN T. MAECKER, PhD • *BD Biosciences, Immunocytometry Systems, San Jose, CA*

DAVID A. MANKOFF, MD, PhD • *Division of Nuclear Medicine, University of Washington School of Medicine, Seattle, WA*

KIM A. MARGOLIN, MD • *Professor of Medicine, City of Hope National Medical Center, Los Angeles, CA*

FRANCESCO M. MARINCOLA, MD • *Immunogenetics Section, Department of Transfusion Medicine, Clinical Center, National Institutes of Health, Bethesda, MD*

GABRIELLA MARINCOLA, BS • *Immunogenetics Section, Department of Transfusion Medicine, Clinical Center, National Institutes of Health, Bethesda, MD*

STEPHANIE MCARDLE, PhD • *The School of Biomedical and Natural Sciences, The Nottingham Trent University, Nottingham, United Kingdom*

NOWEEDA MIRZA, PhD • *Department of Interdisciplinary Oncology, and the H. Lee Moffitt Cancer Center, University of South Florida, Tampa, FL*

LUDMILA MÜLLER, PhD • *Section for Transplantation Immunology, Centre for Medical Research, University of Tübingen Medical School, Tübingen, Germany*

JULIA NEUDORFER • *Department of Hematology/Oncology, Technical University of Munich and Clinical Cooperation Group Vaccinology, GSF–National Research Center for Environment and Health, Neuherberg, Germany; and Technical University of Munich, Munich, Germany*

MICHAEL I. NISHIMURA, PhD • *Department of Surgery, Pritzker School of Medicine at the University of Chicago, Chicago, IL*

GRAHAM PAWELEC, PhD • *Section for Transplantation Immunology, Centre for Medical Research, University of Tübingen Medical School, Tübingen, Germany*

CHRISTIAN PESCHEL, MD • *Department of Hematology/Oncology, Technical University of Munich, Munich, Germany*

GINA R. PETRONI, PhD • *Division of Biostatistics and Epidemiology and the University of Virginia Cancer Center, The University of Virginia Health System, Charlottesville, VA*

ROBERT REES, PhD • *The School of Biomedical and Natural Sciences, The Nottingham Trent University, Nottingham, United Kingdom*

R. TODD REILLY, PhD • *Department of Oncology, The Johns Hopkins University School of Medicine, Sidney Kimmel Comprehensive Cancer Center, Baltimore, MD*

MATTHEW K. ROBINSON, PhD • *Division of Medical Sciences, Department of Medical Oncology, Fox Chase Cancer Center, Philadelphia, PA*

NITIN ROHATGI, MD • *Division of Hematology/Oncology, Department of Internal Medicine, and The Barrett Cancer Center, University of Cincinnati Medical Center, Cincinnati, OH*

SHAUN ROSEBECK, BS • *Department of Biological Sciences, University of Toledo, Toledo, OH*

JEFFREY J. ROSZKOWSKI, MS • *Department of Surgery, Pritzker School of Medicine at the University of Chicago, Chicago, IL*

DORINDA ROUCH, MD • *Departments of Medicine and Cancer Biology and Breast Cancer Program, Vanderbilt-Ingram Comprehensive Cancer Center, Vanderbilt University School of Medicine, Nashville, TN*

ASIM SAHA, PhD • *Division of Hematology/Oncology, Department of Internal Medicine, and The Barrett Cancer Center, University of Cincinnati Medical Center, Cincinnati, OH*

UGUR SAHIN, MD • *Department of Internal Medicine III, Johannes Guttenberg University, Mainz, Germany*

SUYU SHU, PhD • *Center for Surgery Research, Cleveland Clinic Foundation, Cleveland, OH*

RAKESH SHUKLA, PhD • *Division of Hematology/Oncology, Department of Internal Medicine, and The Barrett Cancer Center, University of Cincinnati Medical Center, Cincinnati, OH*

CRISTINA I. TRUICA, MD • *Departments of Medicine and Cancer Biology and Breast Cancer Program, Vanderbilt-Ingram Comprehensive Cancer Center, Vanderbilt University School of Medicine, Nashville, TN*

ÖZLEM TÜRECI, MD • *Department of Internal Medicine III, Johannes Guttenberg University, Mainz, Germany*

GEORGE A. VIELHAUER, PhD • *Tumor Vaccine Group, Department of Oncology, University of Washington School of Medicine, Seattle, WA*

LOUIS M. WEINER, MD • *Division of Medical Sciences, Department of Medical Oncololgy, Fox Chase Cancer Center, Philadelphia, PA*

THOMAS E. WITZIG, MD • *Division of Hematology Research, Mayo Clinic, Rochester, MN*

WEIPING ZOU, MD, PhD • *Section of Hematology and Medical Oncology, Department of Medicine, Tulane Medical School, New Orleans, LA*

1

Discovery of Target Molecules for Cancer Immunotherapy by Genetic and Bioinformatic Approaches

*Özlem Türeci, Thorsten Klamp,
Michael Koslowski, Sebastian Kreiter,
and Ugur Sahin*

SUMMARY

It has been a long-standing vision of scientists studying tumor immunology to use the immune system's effectors for the therapy of cancer by directing them against target molecules expressed selectively on tumor cells. Different genetic approaches for discovery of such target candidates have been developed over the last 15 yr and are being pursued. The classical approaches apply expression cloning using either cancer-reactive T-lymphocytes or autoantibodies in crude patient sera as probes to identify target molecules of spontaneous immune responses. Recent concepts utilizing high-density microarray analysis, subtractive library approaches, or *in silico* cloning aim at the identification of genes with cancer cell-associated expression and subsequently address the immunogenicity of such molecules with reverse immunology. This chapter summarizes the peculiarities of these approaches, reflects on rationale criteria for selection of vaccine candidates, and discusses how integrated discovery and validation strategies may assist in the delivery of suitable targets.

Key Words: Cancer immunotherapy; target discovery; immunogenicity; autoantigens; tumor.

1. USING IMMUNE EFFECTORS FROM CANCER PATIENTS AS PROBES FOR IDENTIFICATION OF CANCER VACCINE TARGETS

A vaccine antigen has to fulfill at least two fundamental requirements:

1. Immunogenicity, i.e., a robust antigen-specific immune response can be induced in tumor-bearing hosts (for the purpose of therapeutic vaccination) or healthy individuals (for prophylactic vaccination).
2. Selectivity, i.e., the respective antigen or at least a deduced immunogenic epitope is present mainly or exclusively on tumor cells.

From: *Cancer Drug Discovery and Development: Immunotherapy of Cancer*
Edited by: M. L. Disis © Humana Press Inc., Totowa, NJ

Tumor antigens eliciting spontaneous immune responses in the tumor-bearing host comply at least with the first requirement. Consequently, first-generation tumor antigens were discovered by systematically deciphering the molecular targets of spontaneous anti-tumor immune responses in cancer patients.

1.1. Identification of Tumor-Associated Antigens by T-Cell Expression Cloning

Modern tumor immunology began with the observation that specific immunization of inbred mice with tumors induced by chemical carcinogens results in rejection of subsequently transplanted tumors. The most important lessons deduced from these tumor transplantation studies were:

1. Pre-exposure with syngeneic tumor cells, but not nontransformed cells, protects animals from subsequent challenge with lethal amounts of tumor cells, pointing toward the presence of tumor-specific antigens *(1,2)*.
2. Preimmunization with the majority of the carcinogen-induced tumors provides protection only against the individual tumor *(3)*, whereas some tumors provide also protection against other tumors *(4)*, pointing toward the presence of either individual or shared tumor antigens.
3. Depletion of T-lymphocytes in preimmunized mice abrogates protection from lethal tumor challenge *(5,6)*, establishing T-lymphocytes as the major mediators of antitumor immunity in these models.

The technical basis for human cellular tumor immunology was provided by the discovery of interleukin 2 *(7,8)* and by the establishment of conditions for ex vivo culture of T-lymphocytes *(9)*, enabling the expansion and long-term culture of cytotoxic T-cells with antitumor specificity *(10–13)*. The existence of tumor-specific antigens in humans was unequivocally demonstrated in 1991, when Boon and colleagues succeeded in the identification of human melanoma antigen MZ2-E, encoded by the melanoma-associated antigen 1 *(MAGE-1)* gene *(14)*. The technique they pioneered employed in vivo sensitized tumor-reactive cytotoxic T-lymphocytes (CTLs) originating from tumor-infiltrating lymphocytes or peripheral blood mononuclear cells (PBMCs) of cancer patients. In a first step, these T-cells are expanded in vitro with irradiated autologous tumor cell cultures to obtain stable CTL clones with lytic activity restricted exclusively to cancer cells *(15)*. To isolate the gene coding for the relevant tumor antigen, the CTL clones are restimulated with major histocompatibility complex (MHC) class I-matched antigen-negative surrogate cells *(12)* that are transfected with pooled clones from autologous tumor-cell derived genomic or cDNA expression libraries. The ability of transfectants to stimulate these CTLs is measured by using cytokine release or cell-mediated cytotoxicity assays *(14)*. Finally, the molecular nature of the antigens is determined after monoclonalization by sequencing of the inserts. To identify the minimal antigenic peptide of the tumor antigen recognized by the T-cell receptor (TCR) of a specific CTL clone, histocompatibility leukocyte antigen (HLA)-matched target cells lacking the antigen are transfected with gene fragments or loaded with synthetic peptides corresponding to the tumor antigen *(16)*. This elegant genetic approach and its variants are still being broadly applied. Such an approach has identified several shared tumor antigens, among them members of the *MAGE*, *GAGE*, and *BAGE* antigen gene families, as well as individual antigens derived from mutated genes *(17–19)*. Modifications of this strategy were extended in order to identify MHC class II-restricted tumor antigen epitopes recognized by CD4[+] T-helper cells *(20–22)*, which are pivotal in the initiation and maintenance of antitumor immunity *(23)*. The same principle, to screen with tumor-reactive T-lymphocytes for the recognized antigens, is also pursued by the so-called biochemical approach *(24,25)*, which uses CTL clones as probes on fractionated peptide pools eluted from the surface MHC molecules of CTL-sensitive tumor cells *(26)*.

The T-cell-based antigen-discovery approaches depend highly on the availability of tumor-specific T-cells. The major bottleneck for these approaches is to establish stable tumor cell lines from autologous or at least HLA-matched cancer tissues, which are mandatory for repetitive stimulation and expansion of the CTL clones and lines. With melanoma and renal cell carcinoma being exceptions, the establishment of tumor cell lines and T-cell clones remains a difficult task for most solid cancers and is a critical limitation for the broad application of these methods. Consequently, the majority of tumor antigens discovered by these strategies were derived from so-called "immunogenic" malignancies, such as melanoma and renal cancer.

1.2. Serological Analysis of Tumor-Associated Antigens by Recombinant cDNA Expression Cloning

Even though tumor rejection has been attributed to CTLs, it is common knowledge that antitumor immune recognition is a concerted immunological action. A large body of evidence points to a coordinated recruitment of CD4[+] and CD8[+] T- and B-cell responses to the same tumor antigen and suggests that once immune recognition of an antigen is elicited, it is not restricted to merely one effector type *(27)*. In fact, prevalence of high-titer immunoglobulin (Ig)G antibodies may implicate a high probability of at least cognate T-cell help for B-cell isotype switching and probably also of concomitant CTL induction. Furthermore, it is frequently argued that the T-cell repertoire of cancer patients is deleted for many relevant CTL precursors. However, it is quite unlikely that a concomitant antibody response toward antigens (in particular, intracellular antigens), to which respective CTLs have been deleted, would also be erased *(28)*. Thus, specific antibodies may be the persisting hallmark of a substantial tumor/immune system encounter and may help to trace back to deleted CTL specificities. Based on these rationales, we designed a systematic and unbiased strategy, termed serological analysis of tumor antigens by recombinant cDNA expression cloning (SEREX), using the autoantibody repertoire of cancer patients *(29)*.

For SEREX, cDNA expression libraries are constructed from fresh tumor specimens, packaged into λ-phage vectors, and expressed recombinantly in *Escherichia coli*. Recombinant proteins generated during the lytic infection of bacteria are transferred onto nitrocellulose filters. These are incubated with diluted and extensively preabsorbed serum of the patient from whom the tumor specimen was derived (autologous cloning). Clones reactive with high-titered IgG antibodies are visualized using an enzyme-conjugated secondary antibody specific for human IgG. Positive clones are subcloned to monoclonality, thus allowing the direct molecular characterization *(30)*.

The SEREX approach has several unique features. There is no need for established tumor cell lines and precharacterized CTL clones. The use of fresh tumor specimens prevents in vitro artifacts associated with tumor cell culture. Screening for high-titered IgG autoantibodies biases for immune responses supported by cognate T-cell help.

The broad and coordinated use of SEREX by many other laboratories has resulted in the identification of a multitude of autoantigens, including antigens with selective expression in cancer cells *(27,31–33)*, also among them are those already identified by T-cell expression cloning, such as NY-Eso-I and *MAGE* family members. Most of these antigens are deposited in the Cancer Immunome Database, which harbors clone entries representing more than 2000 different autoantigens (www2.licr.org/CancerImmunomeDB *[34]*). This database is the first comprehensive collection providing an authentic snapshot and comprehensive picture of the entire human adult IgG repertoire, shaped along the life of cancer patients.

In contrast to T-cell-based expression cloning, where the screening probe is a monospecific CTL with precharacterized tumor-associated lytic pattern, SEREX makes use of polyclonal human sera representing the entire repertoire of IgG autoantibodies. Consequently, the large panel of identified autoantigens has to be deconvoluted to determine the tumor-associated ones among them. For this purpose, autoantigens reactive exclusively with the sera of cancer patients but not with sera of appropriate controls (including healthy individuals) are tracked down by differential serology *(35)*. Such studies have revealed that a substantial number of antigens identified by SEREX are recognized at comparable titers by sera of healthy individuals *(36,37)* and do not seem to depend on the neoplasm. Recently, we reported that infection-associated autoimmunity contributes significantly to such noncancer-related autoantibodies *(38)*.

For several autoantigens originally discovered by SEREX and displaying a seroreactivity restricted to cancer patients, strong concomitant T-helper-cell and CTL responses have been subsequently observed in cancer patients. One example is NY-ESO-1, discovered by SEREX immunoscreening *(39)*, and shown to elicit high-titer IgG in cancer patients but not healthy controls *(40)*. Subsequently, several groups reported that epitopes derived from this antigen are recognized in the context of MHC class I *(41–45)*, as well as MHC class II molecules *(46,47)* by tumor-specific T-cell clones isolated from cancer patients. Moreover, NY-ESO-1 proved to be an immune target eliciting simultaneously both antibody and T-cell responses in the same patients *(48)*. NY-ESO-1 is currently being evaluated as a cancer vaccine in several clinical phase I/IIa trials *(49)*. Similar data were obtained for SSX2/HOM-Mel-40 *(50–54)*. This retrospectively supported our starting assumption that the detour via seroresponses may lead to tumor antigens eliciting robust T-cell responses *(27,29,55)*.

2. USING GENE EXPRESSION PROFILING FOR THE IDENTIFICATION OF VACCINE CANDIDATES

The extensive use of cDNA expression cloning with immune effectors resulted in the identification of a number of tumor-associated antigens. Whereas all of these are by definition immunogenic, not all of them comply with the second of the required characteristics of a target suitable for vaccination, namely with selective expression in cancer cells as compared with normal cells. Complementary discovery technologies for vaccine candidates were inaugurated using differential expression in cancer as search criterion.

2.1. Subtractive Library Methods: Discovery of Cancer Genes by Physical Enrichment of Differentially Expressed Clones

The generation of cDNA libraries enriched for genes selectively expressed or overexpressed in cancer allows an unbiased discovery of cancer vaccine candidates. For this purpose, a number of relatively robust methods have been established in the last 15 yr *(56–60)*. What these techniques have in common is that they are based on annealing a driver population of nucleic acids, which represents transcripts from control tissues/cells, under stringent hybridization conditions to a tester population, which further represents transcripts from tissues/cells of interest. First-generation subtractive methods aimed at the physical removal of driver/tester heterodimers by labeling and immobilization of the driver population *(59)*. Recent methods, such as suppressive subtractive hybridization *(57)* or cDNA representational difference analysis *(61)*, rely on the selective inhibition of amplification of such heterodimers. The clones obtained from such libraries are subjected to sequencing, and their expression patterns are analyzed by reverse transcriptase-polymerase chain reaction (RT-PCR). Several cancer/germline genes, including *LAGE-1 (62)*, *MAGE-E1 (63)*, and sarcoma antigen *(64)*, have been identified by subtractive approaches. Because the proportion of "real hits" may be too small in such libraries, it is advisable to use a second filter for the selection of clones. To this aim, several groups combined subtractive libraries with microarray analysis *(56)* to determine rapidly the identity and expression patterns of the respective clones. Moreover, this method, called "subtractive microarray," removes much of the noise and low-differential signal intensities found in normal nonsubtractive microarray approaches. Subtractive cDNA expression libraries have also been combined with immunoscreening approaches, an example being SEREX analyses of libraries enriched for germ-cell-specific genes, resulting in the identification of several cancer/germline antigens *(65,66)*.

2.2. DNA Microarray Analysis: Discovery of Vaccine Candidates by Genome-Wide Expression Analysis

The unveiling of the human genome and the development of high-density gene arrays harboring several thousands of genes has revolutionized the way to conduct gene expression profiling. Two different kinds of microarray formats exist: either cDNA sequences prepared by reverse transcription, or oligonucleotide sequences representing small but highly specific segments of a target gene are anchored to known locations on a solid surface *(67,68)*. Commercial vendors provide whole-genome scale arrays of both formats. Depending on the system, RNA or cDNA obtained from tissues is hybridized on these slides to measure the expression level of each gene. The truly revolutionary aspect of microarray analysis lies in the fact that, within a given cell population, the expression of tens of thousands of genes, and ultimately the entire genome, can be assayed simultaneously. This capability, when coupled with powerful data analysis software, allows rapid comparison of gene expression between different cell populations. In the cancer field, microarrays allow discovery of genes differentially expressed in malignant cells as compared with the normal counterpart *(69,70)*. With regard to the identification of vaccine candidates, the following issues have to be considered. A direct "matched-pair" comparison of expression profile of tumor samples and corresponding normal tissues usually results in the identification of several hundreds of differentially expressed genes. The vast majority of these are "pseudohits," resulting from altered cellular composition of tumor and normal tissue (e.g., by contaminating lymphocytes and macrophages in tumor or presence of additional cell types in the normal tissue), altered proportions of cells in different phases of cell cycle, or activation of secondary transcriptional programs (e.g., transcriptional responses to inflammation, hypoxia, or other environmental stress signals). One option to determine authentically cancer cell-related genes is the application of laser microdissection on tumor and normal tissue sections to get rid of contaminating cellular sources. Only low amounts of RNA can be extracted from tissue harvested by microdissection, and preamplification before hybridization is required. The additional steps involved (preparation of tissue sections, staining/fixation protocols, microscopic analysis, microdissection, preamplification) are labor-intensive and increase the methodical variance. Therefore, we established a computational simulation of tissue microdissection integrated in DNA microarray analysis *(71)*. The key principle of our strategy is to generate a relational database of expression profiles for multiple normal and neoplastic bulk tissue samples, as well as contaminating cell types, and to apply Boolean operators (AND, OR, BUTNOT) for database mining to search for genes with expression patterns of interest. In this regard, we used the BUTNOT operator to eliminate gene signatures of contaminating cells within conventionally dissected tissue specimens, and identified several new markers for colon cancer and non-small-cell lung cancer.

It is an attractive strategy for cancer vaccine development to combine transcriptome analysis with methods for rapid deduction of MHC binding epitopes. Two related approaches have been proposed for this purpose. Both approaches apply microarray analyses to reveal genes that are specifically expressed or upregulated in cancer tissues. Feeding these candidate genes into prediction software to scan for MHC class II- *(72)* or MHC class I- binding epitopes *(73,74)* delivers a large set of potential HLA ligands within a matter of days. The next step is to directly combine transcriptome information from DNA microarray analysis with data obtained from biochemical characterization of peptides eluted from MHC molecules to identify processed and presented epitopes of overexpressed genes *(75)*.

2.3. In Silico *Cloning:*
Discovery of Cancer Genes by Data Mining

The enormous amount of biological information generated by large-scale genome sequencing efforts over the past years and stored in public databases has triggered a paradigm shift in biomedical research that fundamentally changed the way in which new knowledge can be achieved. In the early 1990s, when the first nucleotide and protein sequences became accessible in the public domain, these small data sets were mainly used for validation purposes and for comparison of experimentally achieved results with published data. Today, in contrast, a vast and still-growing abundance of sequence data is being filed in hundreds of public databases, of which to maintain a current and comprehensive view is nearly impossible for scientists.

However, the public warehouses of data derived from high-throughput research in the fields of proteomics, genomics, and transcriptomics enable the skilled scientist to design novel, innovative experimental approaches using data-mining strategies for the identification of differentially expressed genes that might qualify as vaccine candidates for immunotherapy of cancer. The Web hosts a large number of relevant public information resources:

1. Bibliographic databases:
   a. PubMed: www.ncbi.nlm.nih.gov/entrez/query.fcgi?db=PubMed.
2. Sequence databases:
   a. GenBank: www.ncbi.nlm.nih.gov/Genbank/index.html.
   b. European Molecular Biology Laboratory: www.ebi.ac.uk/embl.
   c. DNA Database of Japan: www.ddbj.nig.ac.jp.
   d. National Center for Biotechnology Information Reference Sequence: www.ncbi.nlm.nih.gov/RefSeq.
   e. Swiss-Prot: www.expasy.org/sprot.

3. Genetic mapping databases:
    a. LocusLink: www.ncbi.nlm.nih.gov/LocusLink/.
    b. GDB (Human Genome Database): www.gdb.org.
4. Gene information databases:
    a. Online Mendelian Inheritance in Man: www.ncbi.nlm.nih.gov/entrez/query.fcgi?db= OMIM.
    b. GeneCards: www.bioinfo.weizmann.ac.il/cards/index.shtml.
5. Microarray expression databases:
    a. Stanford Microarray Database: http://genome-www5.stanford.edu.

Many of these have evolved from mere data and sequence repositories to highly specialized and organized data management systems equipped with functional retrieval systems, enabling the exhaustive exploitation of the information relevant to scientists from different fields.

Data obtained by high-volume sequencing ventures, such as expressed sequence tag (EST) and serial analysis of gene expression (SAGE) projects, is particularly attractive for the *in silico* identification of differentially expressed genes. Because each of the transcribed sequence fragments is annotated with its tissue source, these databases can be considered as containing expression information on thousands of known, as well as hitherto unknown, genes across a diversity of normal and tumor tissues. Strategies for distilling targets from such large EST and SAGE collections rely primarily on treating sequence pools derived from the same tissue source, such as virtual cDNA libraries and digitally simulating procedures comparable to subtractive hybridization or differential display.

Digital differential display, originally invented for the analysis of SAGE data, *(76)* is an example for such an approach. It is a sequence hit-counting method that enables the user to determine the fold differences between the libraries being compared, using statistical methods to infer the quantitative amounts of transcript levels. At the current stage, SAGE data have the drawback that the publicly accessible databases are not representational enough and do not comprehensively cover a sufficient number of different human tissues. The amount of publicly available EST data, i.e., libraries and sequences, exceeds substantially SAGE expression data. The EST database (www.ncbi.nlm.nih.gov/projects/ dbEST) is a division of GenBank that contains sequence data and other information on "single-pass" cDNA sequences (ESTs). As of mid-2000, the EST database contained 1.7 million human EST records. Since then, this number has grown to more than 5.4 million sequences represented in more than 8300 libraries from more than 60 different tissues and cell lines, representing one of the fastest growing data repositories in the public domain. This huge amount of data allows for the identification of differentially expressed genes with high efficiency. However, the statistical analysis of transcripts levels in different organs is hampered because of the usage of different protocols for the generation of libraries (normalized vs nonnormalized vs subtracted). Therefore, experimental validation of the computationally achieved results is essential. Studies for the identification of gene products with selective expression in tumor cells can be performed either using raw and unfiltered EST data *(77–79)* or by using data sets with reduced complexity *(80,81)*. To this aim, ESTs are either organized using gene-centered algorithms, where sequences are clustered along the coding sequences annotated on genomic DNA (UniGene: www. ncbi.nlm.nih.gov/entrez/query.fcgi?db=unigene), or ESTs are aligned to obtain consensus sequences representing single transcripts, so that alternatively spliced products are grouped separately (The Institute for Genomic Resources Gene Indices: www.tigr.org/tdb/

tgi/). Recently, we reported the *in silico* cloning of novel cancer/germline genes by combining data mining with electronic and experimental expression analyses. Based on the notion of ectopic activation of germ cell-specific genes in tumors, we assumed that novel cancer/germline genes would be identified merely by investigating as many germ cell-specific genes in tumor tissues as possible *(82)*. First, a list of candidate genes was generated by mining the National Center for Biotechnology Information Reference Sequence database for genes annotated to be specifically expressed in germ cells. Electronic expression analyses of these genes by electronic Northern blot led to the exclusion of half of the genes because of matching ESTs from healthy adult somatic tissues. RT-PCR expression analysis in a large set of normal tissues further reduced the number of candidate sequences, because germ cell-specificity could not be confirmed for most of the genes. Analyzing the remaining germ cell-specific genes in a comprehensive set of tumors and tumor cell lines finally resulted in the identification of six novel cancer/germline genes. In a follow up study, we were able to determine class predictors that quickly and efficiently allow the discrimination of putative cancer/germline genes from strictly germ cell-specific genes *(55)*. Compilation of these class predictors within an appropriate data mining script will allow an even more-targeted and tailor-made prediction and identification of new cancer/germline genes. For lactate dehydrogenase C, one of the novel cancer/germline genes, we found splice variants exclusively expressed in cancer cells. The identification of tumor-specific splice variants is of particular interest, because they are a potential source for neo-epitopes. However, integrated information on alternatively spliced transcripts and their respective expression is still missing. Information, mainly based on EST data is scattered throughout multiple databases (e.g., AceView: www.ncbi.nlm.nih.gov/IEB/Research/Acembly; AltSplice: www.ebi.ac.uk/asd/altsplice; and Extended Alternatively Spliced EST Database: http://eased.bioinf.mdc-berlin.de). Genome-wide searches for the detection of tumor-related splice variants depend on the implementation of tailor-made data-mining strategies *(83,84)*.

3. CATEGORIZATION OF VACCINE CANDIDATES

The pool of tumor antigens discovered by the described technologies and the number of novel epitopes deduced from them is large and still growing *(19)*. Based on the molecular properties, the identified tumor antigens and gene products with selective expression in cancer can be classified in different categories.

3.1. Cancer/Germline Genes

Somatic cells that are germ cell-specific normally restricted to early stages of gametogenesis and transcriptionally repressed in normal adults are aberrantly reactivated in a broad range of cancers *(32)*. The transcription of these genes in normal somatic tissues is suppressed by complete methylation of cytosine–phosphate–guanine islands in their promoters *(85)* and activation in cancer correlates with hypomethylation *(55,86)*. Typically, these genes are not tumor type-specific, but each of them is expressed in varying frequencies in a broad range of cancers entities *(87)*. Examples are MAGE, B-melanoma antigen, and SSX gene family members; NY-ESO-1/L-antigen 1; and *SCP-1*.

3.2. Tissue- or Cell-Type-Specific Genes

Expression of highly selective differentiation antigens is confined to certain specialized normal cell types and neoplastic cells of the same lineage. Examples are melanocyte antigens including melan-A/melanoma antigen recognized by T-cell 1, gp100, tyrosinase, tyrosinase-related protein 1, and tyrosinase-related protein 2, which show maintained expression in malignant melanoma and elicit immune responses in the respective patients *(88,89)*. Other examples are differentiation antigens of prostate (e.g., prostate-specific antigen and prostate acid phosphatase); thyroid specific antigens as thyreoglobulin *(90)* or calcitonin *(91)*; breast differentiation markers like mammaglobin or NY-BR-1 *(92)*; and differentiation markers of colon mucosa as A33 *(93)* or carcinoembryonic antigen *(94)*, the latter misleadingly termed as an embryonic antigen.

3.3. Tumor-Specific Splice Variants

It has been tentatively estimated that the human genome harbors 30,000–40,000 genes. However, the number of different transcripts is much higher because of the diversity of splicing events. Extrapolating the prevalence of splice variants for known genes and our own observations from data mining combined with multiplex RT-PCR analysis, we estimated that more than 600,000 splice variants exist. Despite this huge number, only a few tumor-associated splice variants have been described so far, among them variants of lactate dehydrogenase C and malignant melanoma-associated 1a and 1b *(82,95–97)*. Systematic screening technologies are being developed to exploit this still neglected source for tumor specific epitopes.

3.4. Genes Overexpressed in Cancer

Genomic amplification or transcriptional dysregulation may result in overexpression of ubiquitous genes in cancer. HER2/*neu (98)*, epidermal growth factor receptor, *survivin (99–101)*, Wilms' tumor 1 *(102–104)*, and a large number of oncogenes *(105)* belong to this category of tumor antigens.

3.5. Mutated Gene Products

Somatic mutations in the coding sequence of genes may lead to novel tumor-specific epitopes. Examples are immunogenic mutations of *CDK4 (106)*, β-*catenin (107)*, and *caspase 8 (108)*.

3.6. Antigens Resulting From Posttranslational Alterations

Tumor-associated posttranslational effects may lead to immunogenicity of proteins. This not only includes altered posttranslational sequence editing (e.g., tyrosinase *[109]*), differential glycosylation (e.g., mucin 1 *[110]*), but also dysregulated stability or degradation (e.g., p53 *[111]*) and altered subcellular localization (e.g., CDC27 *[112]*). Technological advances may assist in expansion of this heterogeneous group of antigens. One example is highly sensitive mass spectroscopy techniques *(113,114)*, enabling the identification of tumor-associated alterations of the phosphorylation status of MHC-bound peptides.

3.7. Antigens Encoded by Viral Genes

A significant fraction of human cancers has a clear association with virus infection, and the respective viral oncogenes may be considered tumor antigens. This includes, for example, *E6* and *E7* oncogenes of the human papilloma virus in cervical cancer or Epstein-Barr virus proteins in nasopharyngeal carcinoma and lymphoma *(115,116)*.

4. VALIDATION OF DISCOVERED GENE PRODUCTS AND EVALUATION AS TARGETS FOR CANCER VACCINATION

As the comprehension of the complex mechanisms underlying tumor immunity, auto-immunity, tolerance, and tumor-immune escape has advanced substantially in recent years, a clear understanding of rational criteria to be met by an appropriate cancer vaccine target has emerged. Moreover, the state of the art regarding preclinical and clinical development of approved immunotherapeutics, i.e., in the field of monoclonal antibody thera-peutics, should be factored in when evaluating cancer vaccine candidates. According to pharmaceutical standards, a novel drug application is validated if phase II or phase III clin-ical trials demonstrate its clinical efficacy in a statistically significant manner. Consider-ing the long and cost-intensive preclinical and clinical development taking at least 5–8 yr, surrogate parameters are required for selection of the best gene products from the huge number of molecularly defined candidates worth being funneled into the preclinical and clinical development process.

4.1. Theoretical Considerations on Immunogenicity

A number of factors affect the degree to which a vaccine candidate will be immunoge-nic. These include the frequency and avidity of precursor T-cells capable of recognizing antigenic peptides and the HLA-binding affinity of the recognized epitopes. Technically speaking, higher-avidity T-cells recognizing epitopes binding with high affinity to MHC molecules are more sensitive in detection and more effective in the elimination of target cells expressing critical amounts of antigens, as compared with those with lower-avidity TCR-recognizing, weak MHC-binding epitopes. However, because of mechanisms of central and peripheral immune tolerance, autoreactive T-cells with high avidity toward self-antigens are preferentially incapacitated (117,118). They are deleted either intrathy-mically or in peripheral lymphoid tissue or they become anergic. Accordingly, the amount of expression of the antigen in the thymus and normal peripheral tissues has an impact on the capability to induce immune responses. Viral oncogenes and mutated genes are not affected by deletional or nondeletional tolerance mechanisms and would be ideal vaccine targets. However, only a small number of rare cancer types have a viral etiopathogenesis (119), and a minority of frequently occurring mutations seems to be immunologically rec-ognized. The low prevalence of these types of vaccine candidates across patient popu-lations overweighs their potential advantage of strict tumor specificity and altered self, hampering the development of therapeutic cancer vaccines for broad clinical use.

With regard to the degree of tumor cell selectivity, the second best candidates are can-cer/germline genes and highly tissue-specific differentiation genes. According to recent reports, expression of at least some of these lineage-specific genes may be promoted in medullary thymic epithelial cells (MTECs) by the transcriptional regulator AIRE (120). However, deduction of high likelihood of failure to break tolerance against a self-antigen from its expression in MTECs would be a misconception of the complexity of tolerance mechanisms. It, for example, does not take into consideration whether antigen-specific CD4+ cells are tolerized in addition to CTLs. Notably, the cancer/germline gene NY-Eso-1 has been detected in MTECs, but is one of the most immunogenic self-antigens in mela-noma patients against which endogenous CTL and T-helper cells are found frequently. In addition, it has to be emphasized that negative selection, rather than leading to an exhaus-tive elimination or irreversible anergization of all autoreactive T-cells, is a quantitative process, reducing the number of high-avidity T-cell precursors. Because, in particular, TCR binding to high-affinity peptides is affected, it could make sense to consider low-affinity binders as MHC ligands (at least for highly overexpressed genes) because of the higher chance to address high-avidity T-cells *(121)*. In this regard, a major technical challenge for vaccine development is to choose appropriate strategies for selection of epitopes and establish immunization protocols, allowing the stimulation and expansion of high-avidity T-cells present at very low frequencies in bulk lymphocyte populations. This means each antigen, epitope, and vaccine composition has to be tested experimentally for its immunogenicity.

The value of a pre-existing endogenous immune response against a target candidate in cancer patients (as it is per definition the case for tumor antigens discovered by cDNA expression cloning with immune effectors) for predicting its immunotherapeutic potential is still a matter of debate. It is conceivable that tumor-associated gene products that appear "immunologically ignored" in patients with manifest tumors (e.g., because of ignorance or deletion/anergy of the respective clones at an early stage of disease) might be superior in a therapeutic setting. Redirecting immunity to tumor-associated structures not spontaneously attacked might result in more-efficient clinical outcomes.

4.2. Considerations on Technical Strategies to Determine Immunogenicity

The general technical strategy for testing the immunogenicity of a vaccine candidate is to use antigen-expressing tumor cells or pulsed antigen-presenting cells for stimulation of autologous or HLA-matched bulk lymphocyte populations obtained from tumor patients (e.g., tumor-infiltrating lymphocytes, or PBMCs) or healthy donors (PBMCs). T-lymphocyte populations expanded during culture are tested for their specificity by using readouts such as cytokine secretion, proliferation, cytotoxic response, or tetramer binding. For this purpose, a broad armentarium of "reverse immunology" tools has emerged in the last decade *(122)*. These include tools for epitope prediction *(72,123–125)* protocols for culturing, antigen loading and maturation of dendritic cells *(126,127)*, recombinant viral expression vectors suitable for infection of dendritic cells *(94,128,129)*, assays for detection, and isolation of single-antigen-reactive T-cells including cytokine secretion assays *(130,131)* and tetramer staining *(132)*. The critical quality control when using the reverse immunology approaches is to show unequivocally that T-lymphocytes expanded with these approaches display an epitope-dependent activity, and that epitopes derived from the vaccine candidates are naturally processed and presented on the surface of tumor cells, eliciting recognition and effector mechanisms by the respective T-cells. Many issues cannot be addressed in the above-described in vitro systems, and the availability of preclinical animal models would be desirable. To mimic the human situation in the mouse, transgenic mice strains were established, including animals transgenic for HLA class I and HLA class II molecules *(133)*. To avoid the use of a neoantigen, studies in these systems have to be carried out with the mouse orthologue of the vaccine candidate. Thus, the xenogenicity of such mouse systems cannot be compensated. The translation of data derived from them to human clinical trials is compromised, because the likelihood is low that the vaccine candidate under investigation has exactly the same tissue distribution in mouse and man, is similarly processed, gives rise to epitopes of comparable immunogenicity, has the same profile of tolerance for CD4$^+$ and CD8$^+$ T-cells, and so on. However, the HLA transgenic mouse system has proved to be highly efficient in facilitating epitope discovery *(134,135)*.

4.3. Considerations on the Expression Pattern of Tumor Antigens

Because there is the potential risk of inducing harmful autoimmunity against nonmalignant tissues expressing the self-antigen by the therapeutically intended successful activation of self-reactive T-cells, expression of a vaccine candidate should be selective for cancer cells (136). The vaccine candidate should be restricted to dispensable organs, in which immunopathology would not precipitate clinically intolerable toxicity. Expression of the vaccine candidate in tumor cells should be considerably higher than in the highest-expressing indispensable healthy cell type.

Moreover, there are several features affecting the clinical applicability and the effectiveness of targeted therapeutics in general and which apply for cancer vaccines. First, stable expression of the vaccine candidate already in early stages of neoplastic transformation, and its prevalence in both primary lesions as well as metastasis is required. Second, the majority of cells in a given tumor should express the target antigen. Third, a potential target should be comprehensive in its expression across the patient population. Pantumoral antigens as represented by cancer/germline genes, which are not restricted to one cancer type but found in the majority of entities, are particularly attractive.

Consequently, validation of vaccine candidates should include diligent analysis of distribution in healthy tissues and antigen typing in a statistically relevant number of tumor biopsy specimens. In addition to quantitative transcript profiling, vaccine candidates have to be evaluated on a protein level, for which immunohistochemistry (IHC) is still the gold standard. New developments in IHC technology have increased sensitivity and allowed the rapid analysis of a large set of samples by using tissue microarrays (137) for higher throughput. The generation of effective monoclonal or polyclonal antibodies specifically reactive against a new vaccine candidate and establishment of individual IHC protocols remains a major hurdle in achieving this goal, and makes IHC a rate-limiting step in the validation process. Correlation of tumor profiling with clinical and histopathological data allows assessment of the tumor stages and patient populations amenable for trials using the respective potential target.

With melanoma being an exception, there are still only a limited number of valuable vaccine candidates for the majority of solid cancers with high prevalence, e.g., colorectal, breast, lung, pancreatic, renal, and prostate cancer. For the majority of currently available vaccine candidates, there is limited data correlating expression with disease stage. Moreover, the majority of vaccine candidates are not comprehensively expressed across the patient population in a given cancer type. In addition, most of the tumor antigens expressed in cancer are not homogenously detected within all cells of an individual tumor (138,139). This observation further emphasizes the need for expanding the pool of candidate targets.

4.4. Biological Significance of Vaccine Candidates for the Tumor Phenotype

It has been observed in clinical vaccine trials that targeting nonessential melanoma antigens identified by classic tumor antigen-discovery approaches may be associated with outgrowth of antigen-loss tumor cell variants (140–143). These observations, regardless whether antitumor immunity is the driving force for antigen loss, clearly point out the necessity to reduce the risk of such immune escape by targeting gene products seminal for maintenance of the malignant phenotype and for cancer cell survival. Notably, this does not mean essentially that such genes have to be oncogenic on their own.

Thus, parts of the validation process have to tackle the biological significance and the dispensability of the target candidate in tumor cells. For many of the gene products of interest, functional data already available in the public domain and in peer-reviewed journals may assist in hypothesis building with regard to the potential functional role of the respective gene in cancer cells. Moreover, novel technologies of functional genomics may be exploited. The use of small interfering RNA technology allows the knockdown of specific transcripts and thereby simulates loss of function of a gene of interest *(144)*. In an analogy, gain of function of a gene can be mimicked by its heterologous expression in transfectants. The consecutive effects of such gene-specific modifications can be assessed in assays measuring proliferation, survival, and cell cycle activity to determine genes with pivotal relevance in the integrity of the cancer cell. Most importantly, the cell culture systems in which such effects are assessed should reflect the cellular state of the human cancer type to be addressed. For example, a gene might contribute only to preservation of the malignant phenotype in cells with AKT kinase hyperactivation or with loss of function of a particular tumor suppressor. If considering vaccination as part of a multimodal therapeutic approach, genes critically involved in prognostically unfavorable cell functions as metastasis may be considered as good targets as well, even if they are not stably or homogenously expressed.

5. PERSPECTIVES

Extensive exploitation of classical identification techniques for tumor-associated antigens together with advanced genomic-discovery approaches unraveling unique tumor markers are providing a still-growing pool of potential cancer vaccine targets. Because the appropriate vaccine candidates are the Rosetta stone of successful cancer vaccination, the ultimate aim is to accomplish a detailed mapping of the "cancer immunome." However, in an analogy to the completion of the human genome draft, which has not revolutionized our understanding of cellular physiology and pathology, the availability of a comprehensive pool of immunogenic epitopes will not catapult antigen-specific vaccination into the circle of approved standard therapy regimens. Clearly, the interplay of a diversity of factors has impact on the outcome of therapeutic vaccination. Many of these factors are not directly related to the characteristics of the target itself but depend on the vaccine formula, the vaccination protocol, the type of adjuvant, and so forth. Although until recently, immunotherapies have yielded limited success, they have been educative with regard to critical parameters for the design of cancer vaccines. This and the remarkable technological progress made over the past decade allow systematic identification of the most appropriate vaccine candidates out of the many provided by the discovery approaches. There are several steps involved in the generation of antitumor immune responses. First, there must be efficient uptake of antigen by professional antigen-presenting cells, followed by antigen processing and migration to draining lymph nodes. Antigen presentation, leading to induction and expansion of appropriate helper and cytotoxic T-cells unaffected by tolerance mechanisms and bearing the cognate receptor, is necessary. These effector cells must reach distant tumor sites, recognize, and lyse the tumors. A persistent memory pool of effectors is mandatory to challenge tumors bearing the same antigen that might grow out over time. Ultimately, an adaptive response should be generated to control antigen-escape variants. The potency of the response, once induced, must be increased to the magnitude of that as found in infectious disease settings. A break anywhere in this sequence can give rise to disease progression. In fact, specific immune responses to tumor antigens in vitro can be detected in patients undergoing various immunotherapies, but do not trans-late to a desired clinical response.

A major step forward in understanding and improving vaccine efficacy in cancer immunotherapy is the combination of clinical studies with appropriate, well-timed, and accurate immunological monitoring. The objective should be to reevaluate all variables in the entire procedure of cancer vaccination, starting with knowledge-based selection of the target candidate and most likely proceeding in iterative cycles, which will eventually lead to successful and therapeutically efficient induction of sustained and robust immune responses.

REFERENCES

1. Gross L. Intradermal immunization of C3H mice against a sarcoma that originated in an animal of the same line. *Cancer Res* 1943; 3:326–333.
2. Klein G, Sjorgen HO, Klein E, et al. Demonstration of resistance against methylcholanthrene-induced sarcomas in the primary autochthonous host. *Cancer Res* 1960; 20:1561–1572.
3. Prehn RT, Main JM. Immunity to methylcholanthrene-induced sarcomas. *J Natl Cancer Inst* 1957; 18: 769–778.
4. Donawho C, Kripke ML. Immunogenicity and cross-reactivity of syngeneic murine melanomas. *Cancer Commun* 1990; 2:101–107.
5. Rouse BT, Rollinghoff M, Warner NL. Anti-theta serum-induced suppression of the cellular transfer of tumour-specific immunity to a syngeneic plasma cell tumour. *Nat New Biol* 1972; 238:116–117.
6. Rouse BT, Rollinghoff M, Warner NL. Tumor immunity to murine plasma cell tumors. II. Essential role of T lymphocytes in immune response. *Eur J Immunol* 1973; 3:218–224.
7. Morgan DA, Ruscetti FW, Gallo R. Selective in vitro growth of T lymphocytes from normal human bone marrows. *Science* 1976; 193:1007–1008.
8. Taniguchi T, Matsui H, Fujita T, et al. Structure and expression of a cloned cDNA for human interleukin-2. *Nature* 1983; 302:305–310.
9. Gillis S, Smith KA. Long-term culture of tumour-specific cytotoxic T cells. Nature 1977; 268:154–156.
10. Livingston PO, Shiku H, Bean MA, et al. Cell-mediated cytotoxicity for cultured autologous melanoma cells. *Int J Cancer* 1979; 24:34–44.
11. Wolfel T, Klehmann E, Muller C, et al. Lysis of human melanoma cells by autologous cytolytic T-cell clones. Identification of human histocompatibility leukocyte antigen A2 as a restriction element for three different antigens. *J Exp Med* 1989; 170:797–810.
12. Van den Eynde EB, Hainaut P, Herin M, et al. Presence on a human melanoma of multiple antigens recognized by autologous CTL. *Int J Cancer* 1989; 44:634–640.
13. Topalian SL, Solomon D, Rosenberg SA. Tumor-specific cytolysis by lymphocytes infiltrating human melanomas. *J Immunol* 1989; 142:3714–3725.
14. van der Bruggen BP, Traversari C, Chomez P, et al. A gene encoding an antigen recognized by cytolytic T lymphocytes on a human melanoma. *Science* 1991; 254:1643–1647.
15. Herin M, Lemoine C, Weynants P, et al. Production of stable cytolytic T-cell clones directed against autologous human melanoma. *Int J Cancer* 1987; 39:390–396.
16. Traversari C, van der Bruggen BP, Luescher IF, et al. A nonapeptide encoded by human gene MAGE-1 is recognized on HLA-A1 by cytolytic T lymphocytes directed against tumor antigen MZ2-E. *J Exp Med* 1992; 176:1453–1457.
17. Van den Eynde BJ, van der Bruggen BP. T-cell defined tumor antigens. *Curr Opin Immunol* 1997; 9: 684–693.
18. van der Bruggen BP, Zhang Y, Chaux P, et al. Tumor-specific shared antigenic peptides recognized by human T cells. *Immunol Rev* 2002; 188:51–64.
19. Novellino L, Castelli C, Parmiani G. A listing of human tumor antigens recognized by T cells: March 2004 update. *Cancer Immunol Immunother* 2004; 54:187–207.
20. Wang RF, Appella E, Kawakami Y, et al. Identification of TRP-2 as a human tumor antigen recognized by cytotoxic T lymphocytes. *J Exp Med* 1996; 184:2207–2216.

21. Wang RF, Wang X, Atwood AC, et al. Cloning genes encoding MHC class II-restricted antigens: mutated CDC27 as a tumor antigen. *Science* 1999; 284:1351–1354.

22. Chiari R, Hames G, Stroobant V, et al. Identification of a tumor-specific shared antigen derived from an Eph receptor and presented to CD4 T cells on HLA class II molecules. *Cancer Res* 2000; 60:4855–4863.

23. Toes RE, Ossendorp F, Offringa R, Melief CJ. CD4 T cells and their role in antitumor immune responses. *J Exp Med* 1999; 189:753–756.

24. Falk K, Rotzschke O, Rammensee HG. Cellular peptide composition governed by major histocompatibility complex class I molecules. *Nature* 1990; 348:248–251.

25. Rotzschke O, Falk K, Deres K, et al. Isolation and analysis of naturally processed viral peptides as recognized by cytotoxic T cells. *Nature* 1990; 348:252–254.

26. Cox AL, Skipper J, Chen Y, et al. Identification of a peptide recognized by five melanoma-specific human cytotoxic T-cell lines. *Science* 1994; 264:716–719.

27. Sahin U, Tureci O, Pfreundschuh M. Serological identification of human tumor antigens. *Curr Opin Immunol* 1997; 9:709–716.

28. Hartley SB, Cooke MP, Fulcher DA, et al. Elimination of self-reactive B lymphocytes proceeds in two stages: arrested development and cell death. *Cell* 1993; 72:325–335.

29. Sahin U, Tureci O, Schmitt H, et al. Human neoplasms elicit multiple specific immune responses in the autologous host. *Proc Natl Acad Sci USA* 1995; 92:11,810–11,813.

30. Tureci O, Usener D, Schneider S, Sahin U. Identification of tumor-associated autoantigens with SEREX. *Methods Mol Med* 2004; 109:137–154.

31. Tureci O, Sahin U, Pfreundschuh M. Serological analysis of human tumor antigens: molecular definition and implications. *Mol Med Today* 1997; 3:342–349.

32. Scanlan MJ, Simpson AJ, Old LJ. The cancer/testis genes: review, standardization, and commentary. *Cancer Immun* 2004; 4:1.

33. Old LJ, Chen YT. New paths in human cancer serology. *J Exp Med* 1998; 187:1163–1167.

34. Jongeneel V. Towards a cancer immunome database. *Cancer Immun* 2001; 1:3.

35. Krause P, Tureci O, Micke P, et al. SeroGRID: an improved method for the rapid selection of antigens with disease related immunogenicity. *J Immunol Methods* 2003; 283:261–267.

36. Scanlan MJ, Gout I, Gordon CM, et al. Humoral immunity to human breast cancer: antigen definition and quantitative analysis of mRNA expression. *Cancer Immun* 2001; 1:4.

37. Scanlan MJ, Welt S, Gordon CM, et al. Cancer-related serological recognition of human colon cancer: identification of potential diagnostic and immunotherapeutic targets. *Cancer Res* 2002; 62:4041–4047.

38. Ludewig B, Krebs P, Metters H, et al. Molecular characterization of virus-induced autoantibody responses. *J Exp Med* 2004; 200:637–646.

39. Chen YT, Scanlan MJ, Sahin U, et al. A testicular antigen aberrantly expressed in human cancers detected by autologous antibody screening. *Proc Natl Acad Sci USA* 1997; 94:1914–1918.

40. Stockert E, Jager E, Chen YT, et al. A survey of the humoral immune response of cancer patients to a panel of human tumor antigens. *J Exp Med* 1998; 187:1349–1354.

41. Zeng G, Aldridge ME, Wang Y, et al. Dominant B cell epitope from NY-ESO-1 recognized by sera from a wide spectrum of cancer patients: implications as a potential biomarker. *Int J Cancer* 2004; 4:268–273.

42. Valmori D, Dutoit V, Lienard D, et al. Naturally occurring human lymphocyte antigen-A2 restricted CD8$^+$ T-cell response to the cancer testis antigen NY-ESO-1 in melanoma patients. *Cancer Res* 2000; 60:4499–4506.

43. Jager E, Chen YT, Drijfhout JW, et al. Simultaneous humoral and cellular immune response against cancer-testis antigen NY-ESO-, definition of human histocompatibility leukocyte antigen (HLA)-A2-binding peptide epitopes. *J Exp Med* 1998; 187:265–270.

44. Aarnoudse CA, van den Doel PB, Heemskerk B, Schrier PI. Interleukin-2-induced, melanoma-specific T cells recognize CAMEL, an unexpected translation product of LAGE-1. *Int J Cancer* 1999; 82:442–448.

45. Benlalam H, Linard B, Guilloux Y, et al. Identification of five new HLA-B*3501-restricted epitopes derived from common melanoma-associated antigens, spontaneously recognized by tumor-infiltrating lymphocytes. *J Immunol* 2003; 171:6283–6289.

46. Jager E, Jager D, Karbach J, et al. Identification of NY-ESO-1 epitopes presented by human histocompatibility antigen (HLA)-DRB4*0101-0103 and recognized by CD4(+) T lymphocytes of patients with NY-ESO-1-expressing melanoma. *J Exp Med* 2000; 191:625–630.

47. Zeng G, Touloukian CE, Wang X, et al. Identification of CD4$^+$ T cell epitopes from NY-ESO-1 presented by HLA-DR molecules. *J Immunol* 2000; 165:1153–1159.

48. Jager E, Chen YT, Drijfhout JW, et al. Simultaneous humoral and cellular immune response against cancer-testis antigen NY-ESO-, definition of human histocompatibility leukocyte antigen (HLA)-A2-binding peptide epitopes. *J Exp Med* 1998; 187:265–270.

49. Davis ID, Chen W, Jackson H, et al. Recombinant NY-ESO-1 protein with ISCOMATRIX adjuvant induces broad integrated antibody and CD4($^+$) and CD8($^+$) T cell responses in humans. *Proc Natl Acad Sci USA* 2004; 101:10,697–10,702.

50. Ayyoub M, Hesdorffer CS, Metthez G, et al. Identification of an SSX-2 epitope presented by dendritic cells to circulating autologous CD4$^+$ T cells. *J Immunol* 2004; 172:7206–7211.

51. Ayyoub M, Hesdorffer CS, Montes M, et al. An immunodominant SSX-2-derived epitope recognized by CD4$^+$ T cells in association with HLA-DR. *J Clin Invest* 2004; 113:1225–1233.

52. Sato Y, Nabeta Y, Tsukahara T, et al. Detection and induction of CTLs specific for SYT-SSX-derived peptides in HLA-A24($^+$) patients with synovial sarcoma. *J Immunol* 2002; 169:1611–1618.

53. Ayyoub M, Stevanovic S, Sahin U, et al. Proteasome-assisted identification of a SSX-2-derived epitope recognized by tumor-reactive CTL infiltrating metastatic melanoma. *J Immunol* 2002; 168:1717–1722.

54. Tureci O, Sahin U, Schobert I, et al. The *SSX-2* gene, which is involved in the t(X;18) translocation of synovial sarcomas, codes for the human tumor antigen HOM-MEL-40. *Cancer Res* 1996; 56:4766–4772.

55. Koslowski M, Bell C, Seitz G, et al. Frequent nonrandom activation of germ-line genes in human cancer. *Cancer Res* 2004; 64:5988–5993.

56. van den Berg N, Crampton BG, Hein I, et al. High-throughput screening of suppression subtractive hybridization cDNA libraries using DNA microarray analysis. *Biotechniques* 2004; 37:818–824.

57. Diatchenko L, Lau YF, Campbell AP, et al. Suppression subtractive hybridization: a method for generating differentially regulated or tissue-specific cDNA probes and libraries. *Proc Natl Acad Sci USA* 1996; 93:6025–6030.

58. Herfort MR, Garber AT. Simple and efficient subtractive hybridization screening. *Biotechniques* 1991; 11:598, 600, 602–598, 600, 604.

59. Rubenstein JL, Brice AE, Ciaranello RD, et al. Subtractive hybridization system using single-stranded phagemids with directional inserts. *Nucleic Acids Res* 1990; 18:4833–4842.

60. Timblin C, Battey J, Kuehl WM. Application for PCR technology to subtractive cDNA cloning: identification of genes expressed specifically in murine plasmacytoma cells. *Nucleic Acids Res* 1990; 18: 1587–1593.

61. Hubank M, Schatz DG. Identifying differences in mRNA expression by representational difference analysis of cDNA. *Nucleic Acids Res* 1994; 22:5640–5648.

62. Lethe B, Lucas S, Michaux L, et al. LAGE-1, a new gene with tumor specificity. *Int J Cancer* 1998; 76:903–908.

63. Gure AO, Stockert E, Arden KC, et al. CT10: a new cancer-testis (CT) antigen homologous to CT7 and the MAGE family, identified by representational-difference analysis. *Int J Cancer* 2000; 85:726–732.

64. Martelange V, De Smet C, De Plaen E, et al. Identification on a human sarcoma of two new genes with tumor-specific expression. *Cancer Res* 2000; 60:3848–3855.

65. Tureci O, Sahin U, Koslowski M, et al. A novel tumour associated leucine zipper protein targeting to sites of gene transcription and splicing. *Oncogene* 2002; 21:3879–3888.

66. Tureci O, Sahin U, Zwick C, et al. Identification of a meiosis-specific protein as a member of the class of cancer/testis antigens. *Proc Natl Acad Sci USA* 1998; 95:5211–5216.

67. Lipshutz RJ, Fodor SP, Gingeras TR, Lockhart DJ. High density synthetic oligonucleotide arrays. *Nat Genet* 1999; 21:20–44.

68. Schena M. Genome analysis with gene expression microarrays. *Bioessays* 1996; 18:427–431.

69. Han H, Bearss DJ, Browne LW, et al. Identification of differentially expressed genes in pancreatic cancer cells using cDNA microarray. *Cancer Res* 2002; 62:2890–2896.

70. Jiang Y, Harlocker SL, Molesh DA, et al. Discovery of differentially expressed genes in human breast cancer using subtracted cDNA libraries and cDNA microarrays. *Oncogene* 2002; 21:2270–2282.

71. Tureci O, Ding J, Hilton H, et al. Computational dissection of tissue contamination for identification of colon cancer-specific expression profiles. *FASEB J* 2003; 17:376–385.

72. Sturniolo T, Bono E, Ding J, et al. Generation of tissue-specific and promiscuous HLA ligand databases using DNA microarrays and virtual HLA class II matrices. *Nat Biotechnol* 1999; 17:555–561.

73. Rammensee HG, Weinschenk T, Gouttefangeas C, Stevanovic S. Towards patient-specific tumor antigen selection for vaccination. *Immunol Rev* 2002; 188:164–176.

74. Buus S, Claesson MH. Identifying multiple tumor-specific epitopes from large-scale screening for over-expressed mRNA. *Curr Opin Immunol* 2004; 16:137–142.

75. Weinschenk T, Gouttefangeas C, Schirle M, et al. Integrated functional genomics approach for the design of patient-individual antitumor vaccines. *Cancer Res* 2002; 62:5818–5827.

76. Lal A, Lash AE, Altschul SF, et al. A public database for gene expression in human cancers. *Cancer Res* 1999; 59:5403–5407.

77. Vasmatzis G, Essand M, Brinkmann U, et al. Discovery of three genes specifically expressed in human prostate by expressed sequence tag database analysis. *Proc Natl Acad Sci USA* 1998; 95:300–304.

78. Bera TK, Lee S, Salvatore G, et al. MRP8, a new member of ABC transporter superfamily, identified by EST database mining and gene prediction program, is highly expressed in breast cancer. *Mol Med* 2001; 7:509–516.

79. Iavarone C, Wolfgang C, Kumar V, et al. PAGE4 is a cytoplasmic protein that is expressed in normal prostate and in prostate cancers. *Mol Cancer Ther* 2002; 1:329–335.

80. Scanlan MJ, Gordon CM, Williamson B, et al. Identification of cancer/testis genes by database mining and mRNA expression analysis. *Int J Cancer* 2002; 98:485–492.

81. Dong XY, Su YR, Qian XP, et al. (2003) Identification of two novel CT antigens and their capacity to elicit antibody response in hepatocellular carcinoma patients. *Br J Cancer* 2003; 89:291–297.

82. Koslowski M, Tureci O, Bell C, et al. Multiple splice variants of lactate dehydrogenase C selectively expressed in human cancer. *Cancer Res* 2002; 62:6750–6755.

83. Xu Q, Lee C. Discovery of novel splice forms and functional analysis of cancer-specific alternative splicing in human expressed sequences. *Nucleic Acids Res* 2003; 31:5635–5643.

84. Hui L, Zhang X, Wu X, Lin Z, Wang Q, Li Y, Hu G. Identification of alternatively spliced mRNA variants related to cancers by genome-wide ESTs alignment. *Oncogene* 2004; 23:3013–3023.

85. De Smet C, Lurquin C, Lethe B, et al. DNA methylation is the primary silencing mechanism for a set of germ line- and tumor-specific genes with a CpG-rich promoter. *Mol Cell Biol* 1999; 19:7327–7335.

86. De Smet C, De Backer O, Faraoni I, et al. The activation of human gene MAGE-1 in tumor cells is correlated with genome-wide demethylation. *Proc Natl Acad Sci USA* 1996; 93:7149–7153.

87. Sahin U, Tureci O, Chen YT, et al. Expression of multiple cancer/testis (CT) antigens in breast cancer and melanoma: basis for polyvalent CT vaccine strategies. *Int J Cancer* 1998; 78:387–389.

88. Ramirez-Montagut T, Turk MJ, Wolchok JD, et al. Immunity to melanoma: unraveling the relation of tumor immunity and autoimmunity. *Oncogene* 2003; 22:3180–3187.

89. Zarour H, De Smet C, Lehmann F, et al. The majority of autologous cytolytic T-lymphocyte clones derived from peripheral blood lymphocytes of a melanoma patient recognize an antigenic peptide derived from gene Pmel17/gp100. *J Invest Dermatol* 1996; 107:63–67.

90. Morishita M, Uchimaru K, Sato K, et al. Thyroglobulin-pulsed human monocyte-derived dendritic cells induce CD4+ T cell activation. *Int J Mol Med* 2004; 13:33–39.

91. Schott M, Feldkamp J, Klucken M, et al. Calcitonin-specific antitumor immunity in medullary thyroid carcinoma following dendritic cell vaccination. *Cancer Immunol Immunother* 2002; 51:663–668.

92. Jager D, Unkelbach M, Frei C, et al. Identification of tumor-restricted antigens NY-BR-1, SCP-1, and a new cancer/testis-like antigen NW-BR-3 by serological screening of a testicular library with breast cancer serum. *Cancer Immun* 2002; 2:5.

93. Heath JK, White SJ, Johnstone CN, et al. The human A33 antigen is a transmembrane glycoprotein and a novel member of the immunoglobulin superfamily. *Proc Natl Acad Sci USA* 1997; 94:469–474.

94. Tsang KY, Zaremba S, Nieroda CA, et al. Generation of human cytotoxic T cells specific for human carcinoembryonic antigen epitopes from patients immunized with recombinant vaccinia-CEA vaccine. *J Natl Cancer Inst* 1995; 87:982–990.

95. Brinkman BM. Splice variants as cancer biomarkers. *Clin Biochem* 2004; 37:584–594.

96. de Wit NJ, Weidle UH, Ruiter DJ, van Muijen GN. Expression profiling of MMA-1a and splice variant MMA-1b: new cancer/testis antigens identified in human melanoma. *Int J Cancer* 2002; 98:547–553.

97. Sanchez Lockhart M, Hajos SE, Basilio FM, et al. Splice variant expression of CD44 in patients with breast and ovarian cancer. *Oncol Rep* 2001; 8:145–151.

98. Fisk B, Blevins TL, Wharton JT, Ioannides CG. Identification of an immunodominant peptide of HER-2/*neu* protooncogene recognized by ovarian tumor-specific cytotoxic T lymphocyte lines. *J Exp Med* 1995; 181:2109–2117.

99. Hirohashi Y, Torigoe T, Maeda A, et al. An HLA-A24-restricted cytotoxic T lymphocyte epitope of a tumor-associated protein, survivin. *Clin Cancer Res* 2002; 8:1731–1739.

100. Andersen MH, Pedersen LO, Becker JC, Straten PT. Identification of a cytotoxic T lymphocyte response to the apoptosis inhibitor protein survivin in cancer patients. *Cancer Res* 2001; 61:869–872.

101. Schmitz M, Diestelkoetter P, Weigle B, et al. Generation of survivin-specific CD8[+] T effector cells by dendritic cells pulsed with protein or selected peptides. *Cancer Res* 2000; 60:4845–4849.

102. Bellantuono I, Gao L, Parry S, et al. Two distinct HLA-A0201-presented epitopes of the Wilms' tumor antigen 1 can function as targets for leukemia-reactive CTL. *Blood* 2002; 100:3835–3837.

103. Oka Y, Elisseeva OA, Tsuboi A, et al. Human cytotoxic T-lymphocyte responses specific for peptides of the wild-type Wilms' tumor gene (WT1) product. *Immunogenetics* 2000; 51:99–107.

104. Tamaki H, Ogawa H, Inoue K, et al. Increased expression of the Wilms tumor gene (WT1) at relapse in acute leukemia. *Blood* 1996; 88:4396–4398.

105. Disis ML, Cheever MA. Oncogenic proteins as tumor antigens. *Curr Opin Immunol* 1996; 8:637–642.

106. Wolfel T, Hauer M, Schneider J, et al. A p16INK4a-insensitive CDK4 mutant targeted by cytolytic T lymphocytes in a human melanoma. *Science* 1995; 269:1281–1284.

107. Robbins PF, El Gamil M, Li YF, et al. A mutated beta-catenin gene encodes a melanoma-specific antigen recognized by tumor infiltrating lymphocytes. *J Exp Med* 1996; 183:1185–1192.

108. Mandruzzato S, Brasseur F, Andry G, et al. A CASP-8 mutation recognized by cytolytic T lymphocytes on a human head and neck carcinoma. *J Exp Med* 1997; 186:785–793.

109. Skipper JC, Hendrickson RC, Gulden PH, et al. An HLA-A2-restricted tyrosinase antigen on melanoma cells results from posttranslational modification and suggests a novel pathway for processing of membrane proteins. *J Exp Med* 1996; 183:527–534.

110. Finn OJ, Jerome KR, Henderson RA, et al. MUC-1 epithelial tumor mucin-based immunity and cancer vaccines. *Immunol Rev* 1995; 145:61–89.

111. Zwaveling S, Vierboom MP, Ferreira Mota SC, et al. Antitumor efficacy of wild-type p53-specific CD4(+) T-helper cells. *Cancer Res* 2002; 62:6187–6193.

112. Wang RF, Wang X, Rosenberg SA. Identification of a novel major histocompatibility complex class II-restricted tumor antigen resulting from a chromosomal rearrangement recognized by CD4(+) T cells. *J Exp Med* 1999; 189:1659–1668.

113. Zarling AL, Ficarro SB, White FM, et al. Phosphorylated peptides are naturally processed and presented by major histocompatibility complex class I molecules in vivo. *J Exp Med* 2000; 192:1755–1762.

114. Ficarro SB, McCleland ML, Stukenberg PT, et al. Phosphoproteome analysis by mass spectrometry and its application to *Saccharomyces cerevisiae*. *Nat Biotechnol* 2002; 20:301–305.

115. Galloway DA. Papillomavirus vaccines in clinical trials. *Lancet Infect Dis* 2003; 3:469–475.

116. Israel BF, Kenney SC. Virally targeted therapies for EBV-associated malignancies. *Oncogene* 2003; 22:5122–5130.

117. Sherman LA, Morgan DJ, Nugent CT, et al. Self-tolerance and the composition of T cell repertoire. *Immunol Res* 2000; 21:305–313.

118. Ohashi PS. Immunology. Exposing thy self. *Science* 2002; 298:1348–1349.

119. Ressing ME, Sette A, Brandt RM, et al. Human CTL epitopes encoded by human papillomavirus type 16 E6 and E7 identified through in vivo and in vitro immunogenicity studies of HLA-A*0201-binding peptides. *J Immunol* 1995; 154:5934–5943.

120. Gotter J, Brors B, Hergenhahn M, et al. Medullary epithelial cells of the human thymus express a highly diverse selection of tissue-specific genes colocalized in chromosomal clusters. *J Exp Med* 2004; 199: 155–166.

121. Gross DA, Graff-Dubois S, Opolon P, et al. High vaccination efficiency of low-affinity epitopes in antitumor immunotherapy. *J Clin Invest* 2004; 113:425–433.

122. Sette A, Keogh E, Ishioka G, et al. Epitope identification and vaccine design for cancer immunotherapy. *Curr Opin Investig Drugs* 2002; 3:132–139.

123. Rammensee HG, Friede T, Stevanoviic S. MHC ligands and peptide motifs: first listing. *Immunogenetics* 1995; 41:178–228.

124. Buus S. Description and prediction of peptide-MHC binding: the "human MHC project." *Curr Opin Immunol* 1999; 11:209–213.

125. Parker KC, Bednarek MA, Coligan JE. Scheme for ranking potential HLA-A2 binding peptides based on independent binding of individual peptide side-chains. *J Immunol* 1994; 152:163–175.

126. Bender A, Sapp M, Schuler G, et al. Improved methods for the generation of dendritic cells from nonproliferating progenitors in human blood. *J Immunol Methods* 1996; 196:121–135.

127. Sallusto F, Lanzavecchia A. Efficient presentation of soluble antigen by cultured human dendritic cells is maintained by granulocyte/macrophage colony-stimulating factor plus interleukin 4 and downregulated by tumor necrosis factor alpha. *J Exp Med* 1994; 179:1109–1118.

128. Toes RE, Hoeben RC, van der Voort EI, et al. Protective anti-tumor immunity induced by vaccination with recombinant adenoviruses encoding multiple tumor-associated cytotoxic T lymphocyte epitopes in a string-of-beads fashion. *Proc Natl Acad Sci USA* 1997; 94:14,660–14,665.

129. Brossart P, Goldrath AW, Butz EA, et al. Virus-mediated delivery of antigenic epitopes into dendritic cells as a means to induce CTL. *J Immunol* 1997; 158:3270–326.

130. Miyahira Y, Murata K, Rodriguez D, et al. Quantification of antigen specific CD8+ T cells using an ELISPOT assay. *J Immunol Methods* 1995; 181:45–54.

131. Fujihashi K, McGhee JR, Beagley KW, et al. Cytokine-specific ELISPOT assay. Single cell analysis of IL-2, IL-4 and IL-6 producing cells. *J Immunol Methods* 1993; 160:181–189.

132. Altman JD, Moss PA, Goulder PJ, et al. Phenotypic analysis of antigen-specific T lymphocytes. *Science* 1996; 274:94–96.

133. Pajot A, Michel ML, Fazilleau N, et al. A mouse model of human adaptive immune functions: HLA-A2.1-/HLA-DR1-transgenic H-2 class I-/class II-knockout mice. *Eur J Immunol* 2004; 34:3060–3069.

134. Theobald M, Biggs J, Dittmer D, et al. Targeting p53 as a general tumor antigen. *Proc Natl Acad Sci USA* 1995; 92:11,993–11,997.

135. Visseren MJ, van der Burg SH, van der Voort EI, et al. Identification of HLA-A*0201-restricted CTL epitopes encoded by the tumor-specific MAGE-2 gene product. *Int J Cancer* 1997; 73:125–130.

136. Houghton AN, Guevara-Patino JA. Immune recognition of self in immunity against cancer. *J Clin Invest* 2004; 114:468–471.

137. Kononen J, Bubendorf L, Kallioniemi A, et al. Tissue microarrays for high-throughput molecular profiling of tumor specimens. *Nat Med* 1998; 4:844–847.

138. Jungbluth AA, Chen YT, Stockert E, et al. Immunohistochemical analysis of NY-ESO-1 antigen expression in normal and malignant human tissues. *Int J Cancer* 2001; 92:856–860.

139. Dhodapkar MV, Osman K, Teruya-Feldstein J, et al. Expression of cancer/testis (CT) antigens MAGE-A1, MAGE-A3, MAGE-A4, CT-7, and NY-ESO-1 in malignant gammopathies is heterogeneous and correlates with site, stage and risk status of disease. *Cancer Immun* 2003; 3:9.

140. Riker A, Cormier J, Panelli M, et al. Immune selection after antigen-specific immunotherapy of melanoma. *Surgery* 1999; 126:112–120.

141. Thurner B, Haendle I, Roder C, et al. Vaccination with mage-3A1 peptide-pulsed mature, monocyte-derived dendritic cells expands specific cytotoxic T cells and induces regression of some metastases in advanced stage IV melanoma. *J Exp Med* 1999; 190:1669–1678.

142. Yee C, Thompson JA, Byrd D, et al. Adoptive T cell therapy using antigen-specific CD8+ T cell clones for the treatment of patients with metastatic melanoma: in vivo persistence, migration, and antitumor effect of transferred T cells. *Proc Natl Acad Sci USA* 2002; 99:16,168–16,173.

143. Jager E, Ringhoffer M, Karbach J, et al. Inverse relationship of melanocyte differentiation antigen expression in melanoma tissues and CD8+ cytotoxic-T-cell responses: evidence for immunoselection of antigen-loss variants in vivo. *Int J Cancer* 1996; 66:470–476.

144. Elbashir SM, Harborth J, Lendeckel W, et al. Duplexes of 21-nucleotide RNAs mediate RNA interference in cultured mammalian cells. *Nature* 2001; 411:494–498.

2

Current Strategies for the Identification of Immunogenic Epitopes of Tumor Antigens

Ludmila Müller, Stephanie McArdle, Evelyna Derhovanessian, Thomas Flad, Ashley Knights, Robert Rees, and Graham Pawelec

SUMMARY

Peptide-based cancer immunotherapy relies on the identification of epitopes recognized by T-lymphocytes. Because of the high degree of polymorphism of human leukocyte antigens and issues of tumor escape from the immune response, the availability of a wide choice of diverse epitopes is essential for the therapist. There are a number of different approaches for identifying new class I- and class II-restricted target antigens appropriate for immunotherapy and as discussed in this volume, several of these are complimentary. The strategy of "reverse immunology," which is presented in this chapter, is applied for prediction of tumor-associated antigens by *in silico* screening sequences of selected proteins for peptides with high binding affinity to different human leukocyte antigen molecules. Subsequently, these peptides are synthesized and tested experimentally. Here, we outline some of the most prominent current algorithms and methods for assessing the immunogenicity of the predicted peptides in vitro and in vivo. We also describe the complimentary approach of isolating major histocompatibility complex-associated peptides from target cells followed by sequencing using reverse phase high-pressure liquid chromatography fractionation and mass spectrometric analysis. We conclude by discussing some of the potential advantages and disadvantages of these methods and problems associated with their application.

Key Words: Tumor immunology; immunoinformatics; T-cell sensitization; reverse immunology; tumor antigens; transgenic mouse model; immunoaffinity chromatography; mass spectrometry.

1. INTRODUCTION

The idea of the immune system recognizing and responding to tumors goes back to the end of 19th century, when rare spontaneous tumor regression events were observed after infectious episodes. The modern era of tumor immunology began decades later. The concept of immunosurveillance of cancer was put forth in 1970 by Burnet *(1)*. This idea was

From: *Cancer Drug Discovery and Development: Immunotherapy of Cancer*
Edited by: M. L. Disis © Humana Press Inc., Totowa, NJ

later to be discredited because of several observations that the incidence of tumor development was not significantly higher in athymic nude mice compared with wild-type mice *(2)* or in immunodeficient individuals compared with immune competent hosts *(3)*. It was accepted that tumors are not different from normal tissue for the immune system, i.e., they do not express any tumor antigens *(4)*. The turning point was in 1982 when van Pel and Boon *(5)* showed that protective immunity could be established against nonimmunogenic tumors when the immune system is properly activated. They explained the inability of the immune system to fight cancer as an inability of the tumors to activate the immune system, rather than lack of tumor-rejection antigens. It is now widely accepted that the immune system indeed can be manipulated to specifically recognize and eliminate tumor cells as demonstrated in animal models and illustrated in some clinical trials (reviewed in refs. *6* and *7*).

Since the molecular cloning of melanoma-associated antigen, the first identified human tumor antigen recognized by cytotoxic T-cells in 1991 *(8)*, and identification of the first tumor-specific CD8$^+$ T-cell epitope from the same antigen 1 yr later *(9)*, molecular identification and characterization of novel tumor-associated antigens (TAAs) has evolved rapidly. With the identification of the first human leukocyte antigen (HLA) class II-restricted epitope in 1994 *(10)*, much attention has also been paid to the role of CD4$^+$ T-cells in antitumor immunity.

Despite the fact that a large number of T-cell defined TAA epitopes are now identified, the majority are class I-restricted and are limited to few HLA alleles, widely expressed in the Caucasian population. Moreover, there has been a strong focus on melanoma, and few TAA epitopes have been identified in other tumors. To overcome such limitations, the search for new TAAs from histologically different tumors and containing peptide epitopes restricted to less-frequent HLA alleles remains of crucial importance. With the human genome sequenced, novel proteins have been identified, some of which may be potential targets for induction of an immune response against cancer.

2. CLASSIFICATION OF KNOWN TUMOR ANTIGENS

Tumor antigens can be divided in two major groups: those unique to an individual tumor and those shared between different tumors. *Unique antigens* commonly result from a mutation in the coding region of a ubiquitously expressed gene. They can arise through different mechanisms, such as point or frameshift mutations, which have been described in a wide range of malignancies like melanoma (for examples, *see* refs. *[11]*, renal cell carcinoma *[12,13]*, lung *[14]*, colorectal *[15]*, head and neck *[16]*, and bladder cancer *[17]*). Another mechanism, often observed in different kinds of leukemia, involves translocation of chromosomes, which results in fusion of distant genes and the synthesis of a novel fusion protein that may contain new T-cell epitopes, usually spanning the fusion junction *(18)*.

Various HLA class I and HLA class II epitopes have already been reported that arise from these mutated gene products (*[19]*; www.cancerimmunity.org). Such tumor-specific antigens could play an important role in the natural antitumor immune response of individual patients. An immune response to these antigens seems to be associated with a good prognosis *(20–22)*. However, most of them cannot be widely used as immunotherapeutic targets, because they are not shared by tumors from different patients.

Shared tumor antigens are present on many independent tumors and can be divided, in turn, into three groups according to their expression pattern (www.cancerimmunity.org):

1. *Cancer-germline* or *cancer-testis (CT) antigens* arise from reactivation of genes that are normally silent in adult tissue and become activated in different tumor histotypes *(23)*. Their expression on normal tissue is limited to placental trophoblasts and testicular germ cells. Because these cells lack major histocompatibility complex (MHC) class I and class II molecules, no epitopes of these antigens should be expressed on the surface of these tissues. These antigens can therefore be regarded as tumor-specific or tumor-associated antigens. More than 20 different CT antigens have been shown to be expressed in bladder, breast, colon, non-small cell lung, prostate, and renal cancers, as well as melanoma. In contrast, esophageal, gastric, head and neck, and ovarian cancers, as well as leukemia/lymphoma, hepatocellular carcinoma, and sarcoma, appear to be moderate expressors of CT antigens, with the expression of 10–20 CT antigen families *(24)*. With 44 gene families already identified, 19 of which encode an immunogenic gene product, this group of antigens is the largest and best-characterized group of TAA. Because of their immunogenicity and restricted expression, CT antigens seem to be ideal for use as cancer vaccines. These TAA have indeed been one of the main components of the antitumor vaccines tested in the clinic during the last decade.

2. *Differentiation antigens.* The expression of this group of antigens is restricted to the tumor itself and the normal tissue from which the tumor arose. So far, most TAA of this type have been reported in melanoma and normal melanocytes *(25)*. Many of these melanocyte lineage-related proteins are involved in the biosynthesis of melanin. Other differentiation antigens have also been reported in prostate *(26,27)* and gut carcinoma *(28)*. Because the expression of these antigens is not restricted to tumor tissue, their use as targets for cancer immunotherapy may result in autoimmunity toward the corresponding normal tissue. Nevertheless, this group of tumor-associated antigens has been, and is, commonly used in current cancer vaccination trials, often together with CT antigens.

3. *Overexpressed antigens* are expressed in a wide variety of normal tissues and overexpressed in tumors. Genes encoding widely expressed TAA have been detected in histologically different types of tumors, as well as in many normal tissues, generally with lower expression levels. It is difficult to make predictions regarding the safety of targeting these overexpressed antigens with tumor vaccines. Because a minimal amount of peptide is required for cytotoxic T-lymphocyte (CTL) recognition, the low level of expression of these genes in normal tissues may result in an inadequate amount of epitope presentation on the surface of these normal cells and render the latter resistant to CTL recognition. Among the most interesting TAAs of this group are the antiapoptotic proteins (livin, survivin), human telomerase reverse transcriptase, and tumor suppressor proteins (e.g., p53).

3. REVERSE IMMUNOLOGY APPROACH AS A STRATEGY FOR IDENTIFICATION OF TAA

3.1. Epitope Selection

The "reverse immunology" approach for antigen discovery implies the use of *in silico*, or computer-aided, prediction of antigenic determinants from tumor antigens that the investigator believes may represent an attractive target for immune therapy, for example, if an antigen is only expressed in tumor tissue or if it is expressed in a wide array of tumor types. Following selection of the target antigen and the prediction of potential T-cell epitopes, these are then synthesized and screened for their immunogenicity and their natural processing and presentation in the context of MHC, either in in vitro assays or with in vivo models. This method has largely replaced the technique involving the production of a panel of overlapping peptides that span the whole of the target protein; a method that is costly in terms of both the quantity of synthetic peptides required and the amount of time required to screen the peptide library. The reverse immunological method, in theory, should reduce both the cost of investigation, as well as the workload required to identify novel T-cell epitopes.

T-cell epitopes derived from the target protein and presented in the context of MHC are usually between 9 and 20 amino acids in length, depending on whether they are restricted to MHC class I or class II molecules. For a peptide to be presented in the context of an MHC molecule, the protein must first undergo a number of steps that will result in the transport and cleavage of this peptide. These steps vary considerably, depending on the origin of the protein. Intracellular proteins, such as those resulting from viral infection or oncogenic transformation, are processed by the cell in a way that leads to presentation by the MHC class I molecule, present on essentially all normal nucleated cells. Extracellular proteins such as those internalized or engulfed by antigen-presenting cells (APCs) are processed in a manner resulting in MHC class II presentation. More is known currently about the mechanisms of class I processing than class II; however, the whole story for both pathways is probably far from complete. To complicate matters further, nonclassical pathways of MHC processing are also involved and may represent an overlap between these two pathways; these have been reviewed elsewhere *(29)*.

The number of computer-aided tools available for the prediction of T-cell epitopes reflects somewhat the current level of understanding of antigen processing, and hence, the tools for CTL epitope prediction outnumber those for T-helper (Th) epitope prediction. Furthermore, the current array of "immunoinformatic" tools for CTL prediction only represents a few of the known processes important for epitope generation. Briefly, this involves the degradation of proteins within the cytoplasm to peptide fragments by proteases and the proteasome, where a selection of peptide fragments is then transported via transporter associated with antigen processing (TAP) proteins to the endoplasmic reticulum (ER), where newly synthesized MHC molecules are located. Within the ER, peptides undergo further N-terminal trimming before their subsequent loading into the empty MHC-binding groove ready for transport to the cell surface. Despite this complexity, computer algorithms representing two of these steps, peptide–MHC interactions, and more recently, proteasomal degradation, have enabled the successful identification of many T-cell epitopes in recent years.

3.1.1. Prediction of MHC–Peptide Binding

The first of these prediction tools, and the major criteria used to date for initial selection of epitopes, was based on the discovery that MHC molecules of one type would bind peptides with similar structural characteristics, or "motifs" *(30)*. Such fundamental discoveries have led to the ability to use computer-based algorithms to screen protein sequences for peptides of defined lengths that should bind to an MHC molecule of the investigator's interest. These algorithms fall into several categories based on the rules that govern the programs. The simplest of these approaches are based on anchor-motif patterns, where the information that determines if a peptide is going to bind into the groove is simply determined by the presence or absence of key anchor residues in positions known to be favorable for interactions with the particular MHC-binding cleft of interest. These algorithms tend to have low prediction accuracy, as they do not take into account the other amino acids within the peptide and their potential interactions with the MHC pocket. For example, if a peptide were to have the small and hydrophobic anchor residues in positions 2 and 9 required for a favorable binding, but also a large bulky amino acid that would interfere with binding at another site, this would not be taken into account. Therefore, models that consider every amino acid within a peptide and assign it a positive or negative value, depending on the characteristics of the MHC groove with which it will interact, give much greater accuracy. These algorithms are based on matrices and are known as motif-matrices or quantitative matrices; an example of one of the most commonly used is SYFPEITHI (*[31]*; www.syfpeithi.de). This algorithm is an evidence-based motif matrix, as the data used within the algorithm are derived from knowledge of actual natural MHC ligands and can predict both class I and class II epitopes. A similar tool called BIMAS (http://bimas.cit.nih.gov/) generates results expressed as estimated peptide dissociation values. Another matrix-based prediction tool is TEPITOPE (*[32]*; www.vaccinome. com), where matrices are constructed, again, based on the interaction of every amino acid within the MHC binding cleft. However, rather than determining this empirically for each HLA allele, TEPITOPE combines these data with HLA sequence variation data to form virtual matrices. This program is restricted to only MHC class II predictions, though allowing for the prediction of highly promiscuous peptides within one search. Another method utilizes the power of artificial neural networks. These are self-training systems that will predict results with very high accuracy, although only after initial training with a large data set, and therefore, their major disadvantage is in the required amount of training data. Examples for this method of epitope selection are such programs as PREDICT (http://sdmc.lit.org.sg:8080/predict/) and nHLAPred (http://www.imtech.res.in/raghava/nhlapred/).

3.1.2. Proteasomal Cleavage Prediction

Although a peptide's ability to bind MHC is the overwhelming factor in terms of whether the epitope can be presented to a T-cell and hence, the primary selection criterion, one must also consider whether this peptide is likely to be available to the empty MHC molecule for binding in the first place. The degradation of proteins into TAP-transportable fragments for transport into the ER is carried out by the proteasome, which is charged with the task of recycling proteins that either are no longer needed within the cell or are damaged; these are then broken down into short peptide subunits before subsequent degradation into their single-amino acid components by other peptidases. A proportion of these peptides are rescued from recycling by their uptake into the ER by TAP. Current data support the hypothesis that for a peptide to bind MHC class I, the C terminus of the peptide must be correctly cleaved within the proteasome, and the remaining N-terminal amino acids that need to be removed to produce the peptide of 8–10 amino acids result from cleavage within the ER by aminopeptidases. To further strengthen the interaction between the proteasome and its role in providing peptides for class I MHC presentation, the immune effector molecule interferon (IFN)-γ can result in the modulation of the proteins comprising the proteasome and an additional regulator protein, resulting in an "immunoproteasome" that generates different peptide fragments to that of its constitutive relative. The immunoproteasome is currently believed to be responsible for the generation of the majority of CTL epitopes (*33,34*); however, this is still a point of debate.

Once a list of MHC class I-binding peptides has been produced using one of the aforementioned prediction tools, investigators can refine this to include only those that are likely to result from the correct proteasomal cleavage. Furthermore, for defining CTL epitopes, only peptides that will have either the exact length peptide produced within the proteasome or the correctly cleaved C-terminal with flanking N-terminal residues are included. Several computational tools have been developed that are based on proteasomal in vitro cleavage data. All of these tools, including PaProC (*[35]*; www.paproc.de), NetChop (*[36]*; [http://www.cbs.dtu.dk/services/NetChop/), and FragPredict (*[37]*; www.mpiib-berlin.mpg.de/MAPPP/), will allow the user to predict cleavages based on the human 20S proteasome. The PaProC server now also allows users to select whether they wish to predict cleavage using the constitutive human proteasome or base predictions on the immunoproteasome *(33)*. This is a valuable tool, as there are currently data suggesting that some tumor epitopes would only be produced by the immunoproteasome, such as the melanoma-associated antigen 3 (MAGE-3) epitope identified by Schultz et al. *(38)*. Moreover, whereas Dissemond et al. showed that the presence of components of the immunoproproteasome in spontaneously regressing tumors were associated with the presence of tumor-infiltrating lymphocytes *(39)*, Meidenbauer et al. demonstrated that a lack of immunoproteasome components was responsible for a tumor-specific CTL's inability to lyse autologous tumor *(40)*. This suggests that the loss of immunoproteasome components by tumors may act as an immune escape mechanism. Consequently, as the jury is still out on the exact role of the immunoproteasome and its interactions in tumor immunology, selection of epitopes produced by both types of proteasome and their subsequent testing either in vitro or in vivo should shed more light on which epitopes are more suitable for inclusion in immunotherapeutic protocols.

Two publicly available tools, MAPPP (*[41]*; www.mpiib-berlin.mpg.de/MAPPP/) and RANKPEP (*[42,43]*; http://mif.dfci.harvard.edu/Tools/rankpep.html) offer the ability to combine both the prediction of MHC-binding peptides and screen these for proteasomal cleavage leading to the generation of the correct C-terminal motif, within one search. Combining both of these parameters should result in an increase in accuracy and the significance of the predicted epitopes. However, any model is only as good as the data used to generate it, and as these models are currently based on restricted data sets from either limited in vitro studies or lists of natural T-cell epitopes that are currently known, the accuracy of the results will certainly still be improved. A comparison of three of these methods has been compiled by Saxova and colleagues *(44)*, who assessed the ability of these programs to predict the correct cleavage of known natural MHC class I ligands. Values ranging from 40 to 80% accuracy were determined using this model, and this value was described as the sensitivity. However, a specificity value for each method was also determined, and this represents the likelihood of the program to predict an epitope that would contain a cleavage site within the peptide with a higher probability than the C-terminal cleavage. The three programs compared varied in both of these values, and generally, the programs with the higher sensitivity had the lower specificity, although updated versions of some of the models are now available.

3.1.3. Problems Associated With *In Silico* Prediction

Although many epitopes have now been defined using reverse-immunology prediction, and several of these have been implemented in vaccine protocols, the methodology is not without drawbacks. The epitopes that are selected with this method tend only to be high-affinity epitopes, as the aim of the prediction software is to select the top few percentages of strong binding peptides. However, often many of these high-affinity peptides on lengthy testing in vitro do not demonstrate immunogenicity. As many tumor antigens fall into the category of overexpressed self-antigens, and some of these, such as human telomerase reverse transcriptase, are interesting candidates because of their wide expression-pattern in tumors, there is a desire to evade the tolerance that CTLs naturally have high-affinity peptides from these self-antigens. One method is to target the low-affinity "cryptic epitopes" contained within these antigens—those that are normally neglected during epitope prediction. Another disadvantage of the method that has been recently highlighted is that some peptides presented in the context of MHC are not necessarily derived from classical proteasomal cleavage. It has been demonstrated that peptide splice variants, short MHC-restricted peptides composed of two non-contiguous sections of the same protein, are produced within the proteasome (45,46). It is currently not known what proportion of the peptides displayed by MHC result from such peptide-splicing events, and their general importance in tumor recognition by T-cells is unclear. Moreover, peptide splicing can be included among several other posttranslational modifications that can occur to a potential T-cell epitope and that we are currently unable to model *in silico*.

3.1.4. UTILIZATION OF EPITOPE PREDICTION TOOLS

Questions regarding which antigens should be targeted for use in tumor vaccine protocols—how many epitopes should be used, and whether these should comprise MHC class I epitopes alone or in combination with class II motifs to engage T-cell help—are the subject of many ongoing studies and have been covered in numerous review articles (47,48). However, several clinical trials that have focused on using single MHC class I epitopes to induce an antitumoral CTL response have been disappointing. The reasons for this may be multiple, but one factor that is likely to have contributed to the poor outcome is the lack of T-cell help provided by CD4 T-cells. Several studies are currently aimed at using multiepitope vaccines (49), including Th epitopes (50), combinations of both multivalent vaccines and Th epitopes (51), and class II-restricted epitopes that contain class I motifs (52), among others, to circumvent some of the shortcomings. We have recently applied the combination of MHC peptide binding predictions with proteasome processing algorithms to select several peptides from the novel cancer/germline antigen HAGE. One of these peptides, a class II-binding 15-mer selected because it contains a class I-binding 9-mer with a correctly predicted C-terminal cleavage, demonstrates immunogenicity in both human in vitro assays and in transgenic mouse models. Furthermore, sensitization with dendritic cells (DCs) pulsed with the 15-mer results in both CD8 and CD4 T-cells specific for the class I and class II motifs, respectively (Knights et al., unpublished data).

3.2. Screening Immunogenicity of Predicted T-Cell Epitopes

3.2.1. IN VITRO

Once peptides are identified using one or a combination of the database searches, they can then be synthesized and further assessed for their ability to bind to the appropriate HLA allele, using, for example, T2 cells. This HLA stabilization assay can be used in conjunction with other assays to assess peptide binding. After the respective candidate peptides are synthesized, their immunogenicity can be examined using different approaches of reverse immunology. The synthetic peptides can be used for T-cell sensitization experiments in vitro or for immunization of transgenic mice in vivo. The source of T-lymphocytes for priming of naïve T-cells or restimulation of precursor T-cells in vitro might be the peripheral blood of tumor patients or healthy donors. The peptide-specific T-cell lines or T-cell clones that are obtained then have to be tested for tumor-cell recognition. The main obstacle in using patient-derived T-lymphocytes for activation experiments is that the majority does not respond or responds very weakly to tumor antigens. Different strategies are required to overcome the difficulties of nonresponsiveness by providing an optimal activation environment in vitro. On the other hand, most TAA represent self-proteins and as result of tolerance, are poorly immunogenic. Immunomodulation with cytokines may break tolerance and allow tumor antigen-reactive T-cells to recognize their respective tumor antigen or to activate naïve T-lymphocytes *de novo*. Many cytokines have demonstrated immunomodulatory activities in this context. As reported for breast cancer, melanoma, renal cancer, and neuroblastoma, a combination of interleukin (IL)-2 and IL-12 in vitro may strongly enhance the development of tumor-specific CD8[+] CTL and prevent overgrowth of nonspecific, less-effective lymphokine-activated killer cells (reviewed in ref. 53). In our priming experiments, we have also used IL-12, because it has been reported that regulation of IFN-γ production in stimulated peripheral blood mononuclear cell (PBMC) cultures requires direct involvement of IL-12. Such cytokine modulation of the priming conditions gave rise to antigen-specific, granulocyte/macrophage colony-stimulating factor (GM-CSF)- and IFN-γ-secreting cells. Synergistic effects of IL-4 with IL-12 on IFN-γ production by DC have also been reported *(54,55)*. IL-12 is known to promote a potent cellular immune response in which tumor-specific CTL and Th cells are induced to secrete Th1 cytokines *(56–58)*. Consistently, part of the modulatory activities of several other well-recognized Th1- and Th2-driving factors, such as IFN-γ, IL-4, IL-10, prostaglandin E2, and IFN-α, is mediated by regulating either the production of IL-12, or the responsiveness to this cytokine *(59)*. In cytokine-modified mixed lymphocyte-tumor cell cultures, we have developed culture conditions for the expansion of CD4 and CD8 effector cells from PBMCs of chronic myeloid leukemia (CML) patients by the addition of GM-CSF, IL-4, and in some cultures, IL-7 and IL-12. Our data showed enhanced T-cell responses in IL-12-supplemented mixed lymphocyte-tumor cell, particularly secretion of IFN-γ *(60)*.

APCs play an essential role in the generation of tumor-specific immune responses. The most potent of them, the DCs, are capable of activating both antigen-specific cytotoxic and Th cells. Consequently, it is now accepted that for the optimal implementation of an immunotherapeutic approach to cancer therapy, both CD8 cytotoxic cells and CD4 helper cells, predominantly the Th1 polarization, should be targeted. Numerous investigations have involved the use of DCs as APCs in an attempt to stimulate both primary and secondary immune responses, even to poorly immunogenic tumor antigens. We have shown that using monocyte-derived DCs for peptide presentation, in addition to B-cell receptor (bcr)/Abelson leukemia virus (abl), in CML the reciprocal abl/bcr fusion products may also be immunogenic, and that certain breakpoint peptides contain both MHC class I- and II-binding peptides that stimulate CD4 helper cells, as well as CD8 CTLs. The latter respond not only to peptide but also to primary CML tumor cells, indicating that these TAAs are indeed expressed on the cell surface and could represent novel targets for immunotherapy *(61,62)*.

DCs can be easily generated from the monocytic fraction of peripheral blood by culture in GM-CSF and IL-4, followed by maturation, for example, with tumor necrosis factor α. According to a consensus protocol established by the European Union Concerted Action on Peptide Sensitization Consortium (an EU-sponsored collaboration, active 1999–2001, *see* http://www.medizin.uni-tuebingen.de/eucaps/), in addition to this cytokine as a maturation signal, we also use polyriboinosinic-polyribocytidylic acid (poly I:C), a synthetic molecule composed of double-stranded RNA (to induce maturation) for generating DCs in serum-free medium. We tested the validity of the inclusion of this factor *(63)*, and phenotypic analysis of these cells revealed that exclusion of poly I:C resulted in DCs with a lower expression of HLA-DR, CD86, and CD1a, with little to no expression of CD83 when compared with cells matured in the presence of poly I:C. Another group has also previously described the use of this molecule to induce stable maturation of DCs and described DCs with a phenotype consisting of high levels of HLA-DR, CD86, and CD83 surface expression, as well as functional characteristics comparable to DC generated in monocyte-conditioned medium *(64)*. It is therefore likely that inclusion of this factor will be beneficial for functional DC generation.

Autologous irradiated PBMCs loaded with an appropriate peptide could also be used in priming experiments, as well as for rechallenge of activated T-cells. To provide an enhanced population of APCs, some protocols recommend the use of the plastic adherent fraction of autologous PBMCs. However, following several attempts to restimulate cells in this manner, this protocol in our hands led to the repeatedly observed induction of apoptosis, even despite the addition of both IL-7 and IL-12 during the restimulation stage, known for their ability not only to drive cells toward a Th1 polarization, but also for their T-cell growth factor and antiapoptotic properties. An attractive tool applied recently for activation and expansion of peptide-specific T-lymphocytes *in vitro,* helping to overcome many of the obstacles associated with limitations in current approaches, is artificial APCs, known as aAPCs *(65,66)*. These artificial cells have several distinct advantages over cellular APCs, including DCs: they can be prepared and stored for long-term use without loss of activity and, remarkably, they can be adopted easily using different HLA complexes for different HLA-specific responses *(67)*. The aAPC system allows the exact control of the MHC density, enabling selective elicitation of high- or low-avidity antigen-specific CTL responses with high efficiency from healthy individuals *(66)*.

Once T-cell lines or T-cell clones are established, they need to be screened for their specificity. A number of sophisticated technologies are available to quantify peptide-specific and tumor-cell-specific activity of generated T-cells, even at the single-cell level. The most common techniques to validate their specificity include the enzyme-linked immunospot assay, which is based on the detection of cytokine secretion in response to antigen-specific restimulations, and standard ^{51}Cr release or lactate dehydrogenase release assays, both of which determine the capability to kill peptide-pulsed target cells in a peptide-specific manner. Another attractive method described recently for identification of antigen-specific CD8$^+$ T-cells with cytolytic activity is a flow cytometric assay for degranulation, a novel technique which measures the exposure of CD107, present in the membrane of cytotoxic granules, at the cell surface as a result of degranulation—a necessary precursor of cytolysis *(68)*. During the process of cell killing by release of cytotoxic mediators, such as perforin and granzymes, CD107a becomes transiently mobilized to the cell surface, allowing rapid identification and isolation of antigen-specific cytolytic T-cells *(69)*. We used this method in our experiments on defining the immunogenicity of HAGE antigen- and heme oxygenase 1-derived peptides for screening specificity of the generated T-cells. The most important characteristic of this test is that it provides information on not only the frequency and phenotype of the T-cells in question, but also their functional status.

Such tests as cytokine-secretion assays, intracellular cytokine analysis, HLA tetramer, and multimer staining have been thoroughly validated and established recently as methods to quantify the induction of antigen-specific T-cells. Thus, recent developments in this field now allow combinations of technologies not only to enumerate antigen-specific T-cell responses, but in parallel, to define the phenotype and functionality of the detected T-cells (reviewed in ref. *70*).

Once peptide specificity of the generated T-cells is verified, the critical step is to demonstrate the recognition of HLA-matched tumor cell lines or patients' tumor cells. It is also important to show if the peptide epitopes, which were previously identified by means of prediction algorithm methods, are naturally processed and presented on tumor cells. Peptides could be identified by elution from tumor cells using methods described herein, or tumor recognition by the generated T-cells could be screened by using tumor cells expressing, or not expressing, the antigen of interest and coexpressing (or not) the required MHC restriction element. A tool enabling investigators to locate tumor cell lines bearing particular selected combinations of HLA alleles, TAA, cytokine secretion, accessory molecule expression, and so on, is now available for on-line searching at http://www.ebi.ac.uk/ipd/estdab. This EU-supported research infrastructure (*see* http://www.medizin.uni-tuebingen.de/estdab/) provides these certified tumor cell lines to qualified investigators (so far limited to melanoma lines).

3.2.2. IN VIVO

The immunogenicity of the predicted peptides can also be tested in vivo using mice transgenic for different HLA antigens. For the most part, HLA-A*0201, HLA-DRB*0101, and DRB*0401 transgenic mice have been used for this purpose, because these are the most common class I and II alleles, respectively, in European and North American Caucasian populations.

3.2.2.1. HLA-A2 Transgenic Mouse Model, HHD II. The HHD II mouse provides a good animal model for the study of HLA-A2-restricted CTL responses in vivo *(71,72)*. These animals express a single MHC class I molecule consisting of the human HLA-A2.1 a1 and a2 domains, the murine H-2Dba3, transmembrane, and cytoplasmic class I heavy chain regions, covalently linked to human b2-microglobulin, allowing for HLA-A2-restricted antigen presentation *(72)*. The HHD II mice have been used extensively for the identification of HLA-A2.1-restricted CTL responses and may be superior to the "conventional" HLA-A*0201/Kb transgenic mouse model *(71,73)*. We have shown that these animals respond to human p53 peptides by mounting HLA-A2-restricted responses to epitopes previously defined in humans, and that they are indeed superior to the HLA-A*0201/Kb transgenic mouse model (Fig. 1). We also identified a novel HLA-A2 prostatic acid phosphatase-derived peptide using this model. (The peptides used are shown in Table 1.) At 1 wk post-immunization, cytotoxicity was assessed using RMAS cells transfected with the HHD II gene (*RMAS-A2*) as targets, and IFN release monitored. Prostatic acid phosphatase- and p53-derived peptide immunization resulted in CTLs capable of specifically killing relevant peptide-pulsed RMAS-A2+, in an HLA-A2-restricted manner

Fig. 1. (*Opposite page*) Mean cytotoxic T-lymphocyte (CTL) activity of splenocytes cultured in vitro following immunization with peptide. At 1 wk postimmunization, the CTL activity of splenocytes cultured for 5 d in vitro with the peptide was assessed using RMAS/A2 transfected cells pulsed with peptides (relevant PAP135, irrelevant GP100) for (**A**) C57 human leukocyte antigen (HLA)-A2.1 and (**B**) HHD II transgenic mice transgenic mice. (**Note:** Results presented are representative results ± SEM.) * Denotes significance compared with irrelevant. (**C**) To confirm that the cytotoxic responses observed following immunization with PAP135 are restricted to HLA-A2.1, a blocking

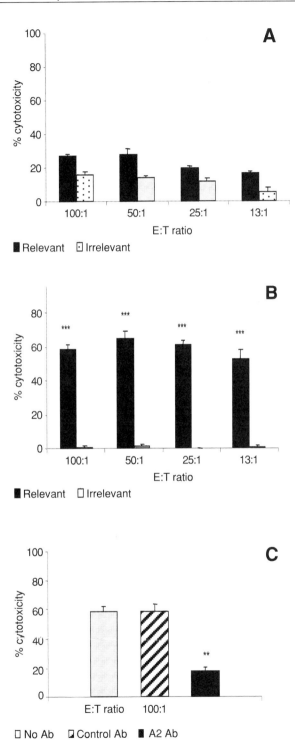

Fig. 1. *(continued)* antibody specific for A2.1 was used in the chromium release assay to block any A2.1 mediated responses. Results demonstrate that the addition of 3 μg of the A2 antibody was sufficient to reduce target cell cytotoxicity from 59% (control and untreated) to 18% (A2), a significant reduction of CTL activity by 41%.

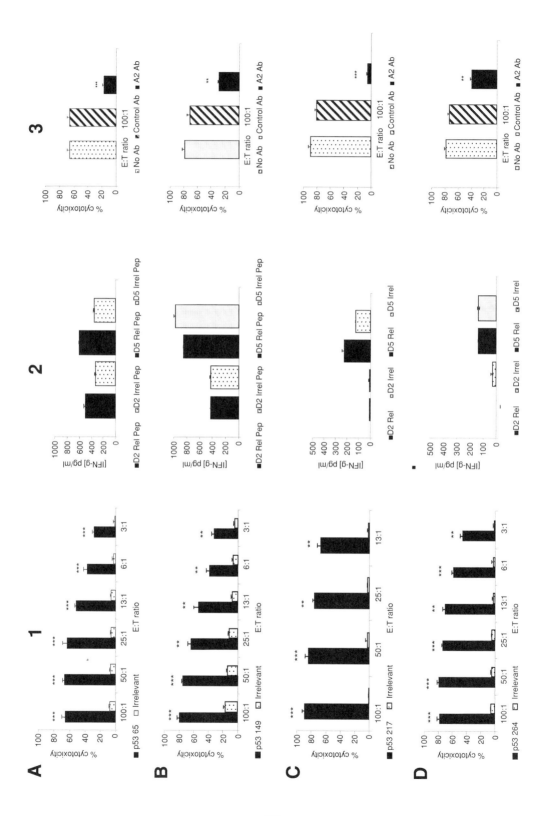

Table 1

Peptides Used for Experiments, Synthesized at Alta Bioscience (Birmingham, UK)
and Dissolved in 100% Dimethyl Sulfoxide at a Concentration of 10 mg/mL

Protein	Peptide region	Sequence	SYFPEITHI scoring
p53	264–272	LLGRNSFEV	24
	65–63	RMPEAAPPV	21
	149–147	STPPPGTRV	19
	217–225	VVPYEPPEV	17
Prostatic acid phosphatase	135–143	ILLWQPIPV	24

Table 2

Summary of Peptide Immunization in HHD II Mice

Peptide used for immunization	Strain	Cytotoxicity: responders/no. immunized	Ab block: responders/ no. immunized	Specific IFN-γ: responders/no. immunized
p53 65	HHD II	2/3	2/3	1/3[a]
p53 149	HHD II	3/3	3/3	0/3
p53 217	HHD II	4/6	3/3	1/3
p53 264	HHD II	3/6	2/3	0/3

[a]Negative animal in the cytotoxicity assay was negative for IFN-γ production as measured by enzyme-linked immunosorbent assay.Ab, antibody; IFN-γ, interferon-γ.

(Figs. 1 and 2). A difference of almost 40% of killing was obtained in the HHD II mice compared with the conventional HLA-A*0201/Kb transgenic mice (Fig. 1). This was usually accompanied by a strong IFN-γ production (Figs. 1 and 2; Table 2).

Several in vitro stimulations are, however, needed to obtain murine CD8+ T-cells capable of killing human cancer cells *(74)*. This is probably because of the fact that, unless CD8+ T-cells generated are of very high avidity for the peptide, the recognition of the target cells by CD8+ cells requires not only contact between the MHC/peptide and T-cell receptor, but also between the CD8+ chain and the α3 loop of the MHC class I molecule from the same species. Still, using the HHD II mice as a screening model, it has been possible to assess the effect of various modifications within the peptide sequence, as well

Fig. 2. *(Opposite page)* Summary for p53 peptide-immunized splenocytes. Cytotoxicity responses of cytotoxic T-lymphocytes (CTL) generated from HHD II splenocytes immunized with 100 μg of relevant class I peptide and 140 μg of class II helper peptide in phosphate-buffered saline in a 1:1 ratio with incomplete Freud's adjuvant. At 1 wk post immunization, the CTL activity of splenocytes cultured for 5 d in vitro with lipopolysaccharide blasts pulsed with 100 μg/mL of relevant or irrelevant peptide was assessed by standard chromium release assay using RMAS-A2 cells pulsed with peptide as the targets. **(1)** Mean cytotoxicity T-lymphocytes (CTL) activity of splenocytes cultured in vitro after DNA immunization, against RMAS-A2 cells pulsed with relevant (black bars) p53 peptide-65 **(A)**, 149 **(B)**, 217 **(C)**, or 264 **(D)**, or pulsed with irrelevant PAP135 peptide (open bars). **(2)** Effect of human leukocyte antigen (HLA)-A2.1 blocking antibody on HHD II-immunized splenocyte cytotoxicity. Three microliters per well of either blocking antibody or isotype control was added to some wells set aside in the chromium release assay. **(3)** Supernatants collected on day 2 (D2) and day 5 (D5) of in vitro culture were assayed for interferon-γ concentration by enzyme-linked immunosorbent assay, values expressed as pg/mL. ***Denotes significance in **(A1)**, **(B1)**, **(C1)**, and **(D1)** compared with irrelevant peptide, in **(A3)**, **(B3)**, **(C3)**, and **(D3)** compared with isotype control/without antibodies.

as the immunogenicity of different fractions of peptides eluted from tumor cells (75,76). CTLs generated with some altered peptides have been shown to not only recognize and kill target cells pulsed with modified peptide, but also to recognize and kill target cells pulsed with the wild-type sequence (75). Moreover, HHD II mice have proven to be a very useful model to study, assess, and compare the efficiency of different vaccine forms, such as naked plasmid DNA encoding either multi-epitopes, containing class I and class II, or whole-protein sequences either as single agents or in a prime-boost regimen (77,78). CTL activities of splenocytes from HHD II mice, immunized three times with gold-labeled DNA encoding the entire human mutated p53 protein at position 273 at weekly intervals and stimulated once in vitro with peptide 65, 149, 264 and 217, could be generated against RMAS/A2 cells pulsed with the same peptides, with the exception of RMAS/A2 cells pulsed with the 264 peptide that were not killed (Fig. 3). These results are in accordance with previous published work where peptide 264 was reported not to be produced from p53 protein mutated at position 273 (79).

We provide the above concrete examples in a little more detail in order to illustrate that it is therefore possible to use HHD mice not only to identify immunogenic peptides, but also, and more importantly, to test whether they are endogenously processed. Thus, the HHD II mouse provides an ideal model for the identification of novel immunogenic peptide but can also be used for preclinical evaluation of vaccine constructs as potential immunogens in vivo (see Figs. 1–3). Some investigators, however, have reported that the peptide repertoire resulting from the endogenous processing of human papilloma virus-derived proteins by HHD II mice differs from humans, and that caution is required when interpreting data obtained using these mice. In any event, results from HHD II mice will always need verification using in vitro cultures from healthy donors and cancer patients.

3.2.2.2. HLA-DR4 and HLA-DR1 Transgenic Mouse Models.

HLA-DR1$^{+/+}$/IA$^{+/+}$ and HLA-DR4$^{+/+}$/IE$^{0/0}$ transgenic mice provide good models of the human CD4$^+$ T-cell immune response (80) and can be used for the identification of MHC class II peptides. Analogous to class I above, MHC class II peptides derived from tumor-associated proteins, such as p53, can be synthesized and used to immunize DR4 and DR1 transgenic mice. We have employed this approach for the identification of a novel p53 class II peptide (81). Mice were immunized twice with peptides in incomplete Freund's adjuvant, and 7 d after the last immunization, splenocytes were stimulated in vitro with the same peptide. Seven days later, CD4$^+$ T-cells were tested for their ability to respond specifically to peptide-pulsed DCs, tumor lysate-pulsed DCs, or tumor cells directly. We were able to show specific DR-restricted proliferation and cytokine production by splenocytes derived from p53 peptide-immunized animals. Moreover, mature DCs prepulsed with lysate of p53 overexpressing tumors were also recognized. This work was then translated into the human system using HLA-DR4/DR1 PBMCs from healthy donors, with similar results (81). Furthermore, in the same way that HHD II mice have proven superior to the conventional A2/Kb transgenic mice (see Subheading 3.2.2.1), Pajot et al. have recently demonstrated the superiority of HLA-DR1$^{+/+}$/IAβ$^{0/0}$ transgenic mice (82) over HLA-DR1$^{+/+}$/IAβ$^{+/+}$ mice for this purpose.

3.2.2.3. Double Transgenics.

Many groups are now looking into the generation of mice transgenic for both human class I and class II molecules and knockouts of the murine class I and class II molecules. Some groups have been able to generate mice transgenic for class I molecules as well as a tumor antigen (83). Both of these models will prove extremely useful in the investigation of the role of CD4$^+$ T-cells in the generation of CTLs and

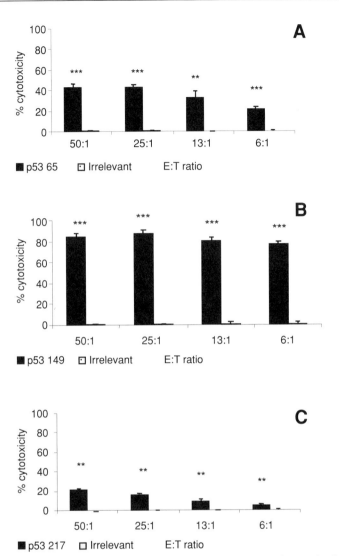

Fig. 3. Cytotoxic T-lymphocyte (CTL) activity of splenocytes derived from mice immunized with naked DNA coding for the entire human mutated p53 protein and stimulated in vitro once with p53 peptides. CTL activity of splenocytes from HHD II mice immunized three time using gold-labeled DNA encoding the entire p53 protein at weekly intervals. Each gold "bullet" contained 3 μg of DNA, prepared in advance, administered intraperitoneally with a gene gun using compressed helium. CTL activity was measured 5 d after in vitro restimulation with peptide p53 65, 149, and 217— **(A)**, **(B)**, and **(C)**, respectively—by chromium release assay using RMAS/A2 cells pulsed with peptide as target cells. Representative traces, $n = 4$ for each peptide. ***/**Denotes significance when compared with irrelevant peptide pulsed target cell killing.

their antitumoral effect. These mice will also allow the study of tolerance toward a particular tumor antigen and how to understand the antigen's effect(s).

3.3. Direct Isolation and Analysis of MHC-Associated Peptides

As discussed above, reverse immunology approaches are a powerful means for the definition of unmodified, high-affinity MHC-binding peptides as potential T-cell epitopes.

However, MHC peptides with low MHC receptor-binding affinities or those carrying posttranslational modifications can hardly be predicted with this approach. Among posttranslational modifications of MHC peptides, phosphorylation *(84)*, glycosylation *(85, 86)*, deamidation of asparagine to aspartic acid *(87)*, and deimination of arginine to citrulline *(88)* are known examples. Just recently, a novel posttranslational modification of MHC peptides was described: the generation of antigenic peptides by slicing and splicing of noncontiguous protein fragments via the proteasome *(45,46)*. All these modification possibilities lead to a tremendous diversity of MHC ligands. Therefore, the arduous approach of direct biochemical isolation for identifying potential T-cell epitopes remains an indispensable tool. As sources for the isolation of MHC peptides, either cell lines or native tumor material (solid tissue or blood from leukemia patients) can be used. The advantage of using cell lines is their nearly unlimited expansion capability in vitro, which allows higher yields of isolated peptides and makes the subsequent sequence analysis simpler. However, after many culture passages, it is not clear how representative the MHC peptide repertoire of a cell line is compared with the originating tumor. Where it is feasible, direct analysis of uncultured material is preferable. Two main methods based on either immunoaffinity chromatography or acid stripping of cell surfaces are normally used for the isolation of MHC peptides.

3.3.1. Isolation by Immunoaffinity Chromatography

The immunoaffinity chromatography method for the isolation of MHC complexes was already described in the late 1970s *(89)* and is based on the solubilization of the MHC complexes and their subsequent specific isolation by immobilized monoclonal antibodies (MAbs). Most of the yet known MHC peptides were isolated by this method or modifications thereof. A comprehensive list of peptides with their associated MHC alleles can be found in the SYFPEITHI database (www.syfpeithi.de). Because of the central importance of this technique, we describe our own approach in detail.

The source material for this isolation approach is normally frozen tissue, blood cells, or pellets from cultured cell lines. Requirements for providing good amounts of peptides for sequence analysis are about 10^9 cells; however, with improvements made in mass spectrometry (MS), this amount is continuously decreasing. This is very important for the analysis of native tumor tissue samples, where often only very small samples are available after surgical excision. Solid tissue is first mechanically crushed, e.g., using a ceramic mortar filled with liquid nitrogen. As soon as the material is thawed for the lysing process, cellular proteases must be blocked by protease inhibitors to avoid any cleavage of the MHC receptor complexes, which could lead to their loss. Apart from protease inhibitors, the lysis buffer normally contains between 0.5 and 2% of a detergent to solubilize the MHC receptor complexes by covering the insoluble lipophilic transmembrane regions. During the whole lysing process, it has to be ensured that the pH value is held constant between 7.0 and 8.0, because lower pH values cause release of the MHC peptides from their receptors, leading to their loss. The lysis is performed for several hours by gentle stirring of the tissue with lysis buffer. After centrifugation and filtering, the lysate is passed over MHC-specific MAbs immobilized on sepharose beads either by covalent chemical bonds or on protein A or G sepharose beads by specific noncovalent interaction with the antibody Fc part. The antibody specificity can be either for a certain single MHC receptor type (e.g., HLA-A2) or for many different types in parallel. The two most frequently used MAbs to isolate human MHC complexes (HLA complexes) are the pan-HLA class I (i.e., all types of HLA-A, -B, and -C) antibody W6/32 *(90)* and the pan-HLA-DR antibody L243 *(91)*. Technically, the binding step can be performed by cycling the lysate over antibody columns with peristaltic pumps or in batch mode by coincubating the lysate with the antibody and protein G sepharose beads in one tube. After the binding of the MHC complexes, the beads are washed with high-pressure liquid chromatography (HPLC)-grade water to remove all detergent from the lysis buffer, which interferes with subsequent mass spectrometric analysis. The release of the MHC complexes from the antibodies is normally accomplished by treatment with acid, typically trifluoroacetic acid, at pH 3.0, which causes the breakage of all noncovalent bonds. In addition to the released MHC peptides, the eluate therefore also contains MHC proteins (i.e., MHC class I: α-chain and β2-microglobulin, MHC class II: α- and β-chain) and the antibody itself (if not covalently immobilized). The peptides can be separated from the proteins by ultrafiltration using a membrane with a molecular cutoff of 10 kDa. The flowthrough containing the MHC peptide pool is lyophilized before fractionation and sequence analysis.

The disadvantages of this approach are the requirement for large amounts of MHC-specific antibodies (10–30 mg per isolation), the complexity of the protocol, and the impossibility of distinguishing between intracellular MHC complexes and those from MHC actually expressed at the cell surface. The unequivocal advantage is the high purity of the MHC peptide isolate.

3.3.2. ISOLATION BY ACID ELUTION OF CELL SURFACES

The acid elution method was first described in 1993 *(92)* and is based on the release of MHC class I peptides from the cell surface by a short (15–300 s) acid treatment at pH 3.3 with a mixed citrate–phosphate buffer. This method is not used as frequently as the immunoaffinity chromatography, but it has been successfully employed, e.g., to identify T-cell epitopes from melanoma cells *(93)* and an immunogenic peptide deriving from the bcr–abl fusion protein *(94)*.

As a source of material for this isolation approach, trypsinized adherent cells can be used, as well as suspension cells. These cells are accessible for the acid treatment, in contrast to solid tumor tissue, where protocols for this approach still have to be established. The crucial requirement of the method, but also its main advantage, is that the cells remain intact during the acid treatment. Cell damage would cause the release of proteases generating peptide fragments from highly abundant cell proteins and of cytoplasmic peptides and proteins. After elution, the peptides are mostly concentrated on cation exchange or reversed-phase cartridges before they are further analyzed. The apparent advantages of this method are its simplicity, cost-effectiveness, and the outlook to obtain mainly cell surface MHC peptides, which are the relevant ones for T-cell recognition. The big disadvantage is that the acid treatment is a rather unspecific method of isolation, cell damage during the process can hardly be avoided, and therefore, the resulting MHC peptides are always contaminated by non-MHC peptides and proteins (e.g., proteolytic fragments, cytoplasmic peptides, peptides from other peptide receptors).

3.3.3. FRACTIONATION AND SEQUENCE ANALYSIS OF ISOLATED MHC PEPTIDES

The sequence analysis of MHC peptide pools is a colossal challenge. On the one hand, the peptide pools are highly complex and estimated to consist of tens of thousands of different peptides even from only one cell type *(95)*. On the other hand, the yield of peptides after isolation is low: from only several picomoles of the most dominant peptides

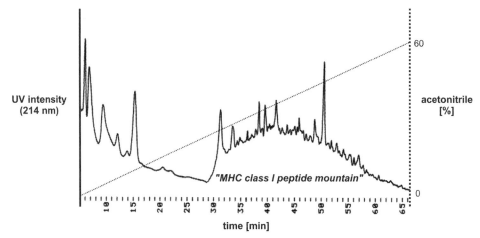

UV intensity (214 nm)

acetonitrile [%]

"MHC class I peptide mountain"

60

0

time [min]

Fig. 4. Typical reversed-phase high-pressure liquid chromatography ultraviolet chromatogram of the fractionation of a major histocompatibility complex (MHC) class I peptide pool isolated by immuno-affinity chromatography with the monoclonal antibody W6/32. The MHC peptides are eluting from 30 to 65 min, giving the characteristic mountain shape.

to less than a few attomoles of less abundant peptides. Additionally, the physicochemical properties of the different peptides are rather similar (more so for MHC class I peptides with a typical length of 8–10 amino acids than for class II peptides with different lengths of approx 9–30 amino acids), which makes their purification difficult. Purification is most commonly performed by liquid chromatography, particularly by reversed-phase (RP)-HPLC, where the peptides are separated according to their lipophilicity. Ultraviolet chromatograms of such fractionations recorded at 214 nm (absorption maximum of the peptide bond) typically appear in the shape of a mountain (Fig. 4). The reason for this is that before a peptide completely elutes from the column (which would cause the respective peak to reach the baseline) another, slightly more lipophilic peptide coelutes. To improve the separation of MHC peptide pools, multidimensional liquid chromatography approaches are applicable. These are already standard in proteomics analyses *(96)*, e.g., of tryptic pool digests of cell lysates or serum. Once the peptides are fractionated, the sequence analysis is the next difficult task. At the beginning of the 1990s, MHC peptides were frequently sequenced by automated Edman degradation *(97)*, which is based on the stepwise chemical degradation of a peptide from the N terminus by phenylisothiocyanate and the identification of the cleaved amino acids by HPLC. The sensitivity of the method is in the low picomole range, so that only high-abundant MHC peptides can be identified. If several peptides are mixed, which frequently occurs in MHC peptide fractions, the data interpretation is very difficult or impossible because of an overlap of degraded amino acids. Since the first time that MS was used for the characterization of MHC class I *(98)* and class II *(99)* associated peptides in 1992, there has been rapid development in MS technology, driven not only by immunological questions, but also especially by proteomics projects. The basis of MS is an accurate determination of molecular masses of analyte molecules. For sequence analyses, peptides are fragmented (MS/MS) by collision-induced dissociation through a collision gas (e.g., argon) or by postsource decay, induced after ionization of the analyte by an ultraviolet laser. The mass spectra of the fragment ions generated are used to deduce the peptide sequence. Even peptides from complex mixtures can be sequenced by MS because of the capability of modern instruments to select single precursor molecules for fragmentation (precursor selection). State-of-the-art MS instruments provide a sensitivity for MHC peptides in the subfemtomole range with a mass accuracy of lower than 5 ppm *(100)*. MS can today be regarded as the gold standard for the analysis of MHC peptides. To sequence a maximum number of peptides from one isolation, the peptides can be directly transferred to a mass spectrometer from the RP-HPLC system for fragmentation analyses (online liquid chromatography-MS/MS). With this technique, hundreds of peptide fragment spectra can be recorded in one run. However, sequence data interpretation is still the bottleneck in the identification of the peptides. Several computer algorithms are available to automatically deduce peptide sequences from peptide fragment spectra (e.g., SEQUEST¨: http://fields.scripps.edu/sequest/), but as yet, no one algorithm is providing high enough confidence to accept the suggested sequences without checking output by hand, which is highly time-consuming. To obtain the highest reliability of a sequence, the postulated peptide can be synthesized and fragmented and the spectra of the original and the synthetic peptide compared like a fingerprint *(101)*.

4. CONCLUDING REMARKS AND PERSPECTIVE

Although the results on identification of tumor-associated antigens are very encouraging, there is still a requirement for more T-cell epitopes to enable at least the most frequent tumors and the most common HLA-phenotypes to be covered by vaccines providing optimal targets for specific and effective immune intervention in cancer. Despite the enormous progress made in the last decade toward discovery of novel tumor antigens, new strategies are still needed. A novel method for their identification is the comparative expression profiling of a tumor and the corresponding autologous normal tissue at mRNA or DNA level by DNA microarray technology *(102–104)*. It is worth noting that some of the widely expressed/overexpressed TAAs were discovered by DNA microarray technologies, combined with new immunological tools such as reverse immunology and tetramer staining *(105)*. Another promising approach for the differential analysis of MHC peptides from cancerous tissue and the benign tissue counterpart was described recently *(106)*. The basis of the method is the labeling of peptides from the benign tissue with a light, and the peptides from the cancer tissue with a heavy, stable isotope tag or vice versa. The difference of the tags consists of an exchange of four hydrogen atoms (H_4, light) by four deuterium atoms (D_4, heavy), which can easily be distinguished ($\Delta 4$ Da) by MS. Importantly, the light- and heavy-labeled corresponding peptides retain the same physicochemical properties, namely, that they coelute from the RP-HPLC and appear as ion pairs with a mass difference of 4 Da. The intensities of the respective pairs can be used for the relative quantification of MHC peptides being present in both normal and cancer tissue. Despite the fact that several hundred peptides can now be identified from the isolation of a single tumor tissue because of recent hardware and methodological improvements, we are still far from the clarification of the entire MHC peptide repertoire, on demand from each individual tumor.

ACKNOWLEDGMENTS

This work was supported by the EU Project OISTER, project number QLG1-CT-2002-00668, EU Project ENACT (FP6 503306), and by the Margarete von Wrangell-Habilitationprogramm of MWK Baden-Württemberg.

REFERENCES

1. Burnet FM. The concept of immunological surveillance. *Prog Exp Tumor Res* 1970; 13:1–27.
2. Rygaard J, Povlsen CO. The mouse mutant nude does not develop spontaneous tumours. An argument against immunological surveillance. *Acta Pathol Microbiol Scand (B) Microbiol Immunol* 1974; 82: 99–106.
3. Gatti RA, Good RA. Occurrence of malignancy in immunodeficiency diseases. A literature review. *Cancer* 1971; 28:89–98.
4. Hewitt HB, Blake ER, Walder AS. A critique of the evidence for active host defence against cancer, based on personal studies of 27 murine tumours of spontaneous origin. *Br J Cancer* 1976; 33:241–259.
5. Van Pel A, Boon T. Protection against a nonimmunogenic mouse leukemia by an immunogenic variant obtained by mutagenesis. *Proc Natl Acad Sci USA* 1982; 79:4718–4722.
6. Jager E, Jager D, Knuth A. Clinical cancer vaccine trials. *Curr Opin Immunol* 2002; 14:178–182.
7. Parmiani G. Vaccine therapy of cancer. *Suppl Tumori* 2002; 1(Suppl):S28.
8. van der Bruggen P, Traversari C, Chomez P, et al. A gene encoding an antigen recognized by cytolytic T lymphocytes on a human melanoma. *Science* 1991; 254:1643–1647.
9. Traversari C, van der Bruggen P, Luescher IF, et al. A nonapeptide encoded by human gene MAGE-1 is recognized on HLA-A1 by cytolytic T lymphocytes directed against tumor antigen MZ2-E. *J Exp Med* 1992; 176:1453–1457.
10. Topalian SL, Rivoltini L, Mancini M, et al. Human CD4+ T cells specifically recognize a shared melanoma-associated antigen encoded by the tyrosinase gene. *Proc Natl Acad Sci USA* 1994; 91:9461–9465.
11. Chiari R, Foury F, De Plaen E, Baurain JF, Thonnard J, Coulie PG. Two antigens recognized by autologous cytolytic T lymphocytes on a melanoma result from a single point mutation in an essential housekeeping gene. *Cancer Res* 1999; 59:5785–5792.
12. Brandle D, Brasseur F, Weynants P, Boon T, Van den EB. A mutated HLA-A2 molecule recognized by autologous cytotoxic T lymphocytes on a human renal cell carcinoma. *J Exp Med* 1996; 183:2501–2508.
13. Gaudin C, Kremer F, Angevin E, Scott V, Triebel F. A *hsp70-2* mutation recognized by CTL on a human renal cell carcinoma. *J Immunol* 1999; 162:1730–1738.
14. Echchakir H, Mami-Chouaib F, Vergnon I, et al. A point mutation in the alpha-actinin-4 gene generates an antigenic peptide recognized by autologous cytolytic T lymphocytes on a human lung carcinoma. *Cancer Res* 2001; 61:4078–4083.
15. Maccalli C, Li YF, El Gamil M, Rosenberg SA, Robbins PF. Identification of a colorectal tumor-associated antigen (COA-1) recognized by CD4(+) T lymphocytes. *Cancer Res* 2003; 63:6735–6743.
16. Mandruzzato S, Brasseur F, Andry G, Boon T, van der Bruggen P. A CASP-8 mutation recognized by cytolytic T lymphocytes on a human head and neck carcinoma. *J Exp Med* 1997; 186:785–793.
17. Gueguen M, Patard JJ, Gaugler B, et al. An antigen recognized by autologous CTLs on a human bladder carcinoma. *J Immunol* 1998; 160:6188–6194.
18. Klein G. Dysregulation of lymphocyte proliferation by chromosomal translocations and sequential genetic changes. *Bioessays* 2000; 22:414–422.
19. Novellino L, Castelli C, Parmiani G. A listing of human tumor antigens recognized by T cells: March 2004 update. *Cancer Immunol Immunother* 2004; 54:187–207.
20. Baurain JF, Colau D, van Baren N, et al. High frequency of autologous anti-melanoma CTL directed against an antigen generated by a point mutation in a new helicase gene. *J Immunol* 2000; 164:6057–6066.
21. Karanikas V, Colau D, Baurain JF, et al. High frequency of cytolytic T lymphocytes directed against a tumor-specific mutated antigen detectable with HLA tetramers in the blood of a lung carcinoma patient with long survival. *Cancer Res* 2001; 61:3718–3724.
22. Novellino L, Renkvist N, Rini F, et al. Identification of a mutated receptor-like protein tyrosine phosphatase kappa as a novel, class II HLA-restricted melanoma antigen. *J Immunol* 2003; 170:6363–6370.
23. De Smet C, Lurquin C, Lethe B, Martelange V, Boon T. DNA methylation is the primary silencing mechanism for a set of germ line- and tumor-specific genes with a CpG-rich promoter. *Mol Cell Biol* 1999; 19:7327–7335.
24. Scanlan MJ, Simpson AJ, Old LJ. The cancer/testis genes: review, standardization, and commentary. *Cancer Immun* 2004; 4:1.
25. Anichini A, Maccalli C, Mortarini R, et al. Melanoma cells and normal melanocytes share antigens recognized by HLA-A2-restricted cytotoxic T cell clones from melanoma patients. *J Exp Med* 1993; 177:989–998.

26. Nelson PS, Gan L, Ferguson C, et al. Molecular cloning and characterization of prostase, an androgen-regulated serine protease with prostate-restricted expression. *Proc Natl Acad Sci USA* 1999; 96:3114–3119.

27. Stephenson SA, Verity K, Ashworth LK, Clements JA. Localization of a new prostate-specific antigen-related serine protease gene, KLK4, is evidence for an expanded human kallikrein gene family cluster on chromosome 19q13.3-13.4. *J Biol Chem* 1999; 274:23,210–23,214.

28. Tsang KY, Zaremba S, Nieroda CA, Zhu MZ, Hamilton JM, Schlom J. Generation of human cytotoxic T cells specific for human carcinoembryonic antigen epitopes from patients immunized with recombinant vaccinia-CEA vaccine. *J Natl Cancer Inst* 1995; 87:982–990.

29. Gromme M, Neefjes J. Antigen degradation or presentation by MHC class I molecules via classical and non-classical pathways. *Mol Immunol* 2002; 39:181–202.

30. Falk K, Rotzschke O, Stevanovic S, Jung G, Rammensee HG. Allele-specific motifs revealed by sequencing of self-peptides eluted from MHC molecules. *Nature* 1991; 351:290–296.

31. Rammensee H, Bachmann J, Emmerich NP, Bachor OA, Stevanovic S. SYFPEITHI: database for MHC ligands and peptide motifs. *Immunogenetics* 1999; 50:213–219.

32. Sturniolo T, Bono E, Ding J, et al. Generation of tissue-specific and promiscuous HLA ligand databases using DNA microarrays and virtual HLA class II matrices. *Nat Biotechnol* 1999; 17:555–561.

33. Toes RE, Nussbaum AK, Degermann S, et al. Discrete cleavage motifs of constitutive and immunoproteasomes revealed by quantitative analysis of cleavage products. *J Exp Med* 2001; 194:1–12.

34. Nussbaum AK, Kuttler C, Tenzer S, Schild H. Using the World Wide Web for predicting CTL epitopes. *Curr Opin Immunol* 2003; 15:69–74.

35. Nussbaum AK, Kuttler C, Hadeler KP, Rammensee HG, Schild H. PAProC: a prediction algorithm for proteasomal cleavages available on the WWW. *Immunogenetics* 2001; 53:87–94.

36. Kesmir C, Nussbaum AK, Schild H, Detours V, Brunak S. Prediction of proteasome cleavage motifs by neural networks. *Protein Eng* 2002; 15:287–296.

37. Holzhutter HG, Frommel C, Kloetzel PM. A theoretical approach towards the identification of cleavage-determining amino acid motifs of the 20 S proteasome. *J Mol Biol* 1999; 286:1251–1265.

38. Schultz ES, Chapiro J, Lurquin C, et al. The production of a new MAGE-3 peptide presented to cytolytic T lymphocytes by HLA-B40 requires the immunoproteasome. *J Exp Med* 2002; 195:391–399.

39. Dissemond J, Goette P, Moers J, et al. Immunoproteasome subunits LMP2 and LMP7 downregulation in primary malignant melanoma lesions: association with lack of spontaneous regression. *Melanoma Res* 2003; 13:371–377.

40. Meidenbauer N, Zippelius A, Pittet MJ, et al. High frequency of functionally active Melan-a-specific T cells in a patient with progressive immunoproteasome-deficient melanoma. *Cancer Res* 2004; 64:6319–6326.

41. Hakenberg J, Nussbaum AK, Schild H, et al. MAPPP: MHC class I antigenic peptide processing prediction. *Appl Bioinformatics* 2003; 2:155–158.

42. Reche PA, Glutting JP, Reinherz EL. Prediction of MHC class I binding peptides using profile motifs. *Hum Immunol* 2002; 63:701–709.

43. Reche PA, Glutting JP, Zhang H, Reinherz EL. Enhancement to the RANKPEP resource for the prediction of peptide binding to MHC molecules using profiles. *Immunogenetics* 2004; 56:405–419.

44. Saxova P, Buus S, Brunak S, Kesmir C. Predicting proteasomal cleavage sites: a comparison of available methods. *Int Immunol* 2003; 15:781–787.

45. Hanada K, Yewdell JW, Yang JC. Immune recognition of a human renal cancer antigen through post-translational protein splicing. *Nature* 2004; 427:252–256.

46. Vigneron N, Stroobant V, Chapiro J, et al. An antigenic peptide produced by peptide splicing in the proteasome. *Science* 2004; 304:587–590.

47. Gilboa E. The promise of cancer vaccines. *Nat Rev Cancer* 2004; 4:401–411.

48. Berzofsky JA, Terabe M, Oh S, et al. Progress on new vaccine strategies for the immunotherapy and prevention of cancer. *J Clin Invest* 2004; 113:1515–1525.

49. Akiyama Y, Maruyama K, Nara N, et al. Cytotoxic T cell induction against human malignant melanoma cells using HLA-A24-restricted melanoma peptide cocktail. *Anticancer Res* 2004; 24:571–577.

50. Müller L, Knights A, Pawelec G. Synthetic peptides derived from the Wilms' tumor 1 protein sensitize human T lymphocytes to recognize chronic myelogenous leukemia cells. *Hematol J* 2003; 4:57–66.

51. Cathcart K, Pinilla-Ibarz J, Korontsvit T, et al. A multivalent bcr-abl fusion peptide vaccination trial in patients with chronic myeloid leukemia. *Blood* 2004; 103:1037–1042.

52. Zeng G, Li Y, El Gamil M, et al. Generation of NY-ESO-1-specific CD4+ and CD8+ T cells by a single peptide with dual MHC class I and class II specificities: a new strategy for vaccine design. *Cancer Res* 2002; 62:3630–3635.

53. Pawelec G, Rees RC, Kiessling R, et al. Cells and cytokines in immunotherapy and gene therapy of cancer. *Crit Rev Oncog* 1999; 10:83–127.

54. Fukao T, Matsuda S, Koyasu S. Synergistic effects of IL-4 and IL-18 on IL-12-dependent IFN-gamma production by dendritic cells. *J Immunol* 2000; 164:64–71.

55. Müller L, Pawelec G. Chronic phase CML patients possess T cells capable of recognising autologous tumour cells. *Leuk Lymphoma* 2002; 43:943–951.

56. Kang WK, Park C, Yoon HL, et al. Interleukin 12 gene therapy of cancer by peritumoral injection of transduced autologous fibroblasts: outcome of a phase I study. *Hum Gene Ther* 2001; 12:671–684.

57. Melero I, Mazzolini G, Narvaiza I, Qian C, Chen L, Prieto J. IL-12 gene therapy for cancer: in synergy with other immunotherapies. *Trends Immunol* 2001; 22:113–115.

58. Paul S, Regulier E, Poitevin Y, Hormann H, Acres RB. The combination of a chemokine, cytokine and TCR-based T cell stimulus for effective gene therapy of cancer. *Cancer Immunol Immunother* 2002; 51:645–654.

59. Kalinski P, Schuitemaker JH, Hilkens CM, Wierenga EA, Kapsenberg ML. Final maturation of dendritic cells is associated with impaired responsiveness to IFN-gamma and to bacterial IL-12 inducers: decreased ability of mature dendritic cells to produce IL-12 during the interaction with Th cells. *J Immunol* 1999; 162:3231–3236.

60. Müller L, Provenzani C, Pawelec G. Generation of chronic myelogenous leukemia-specific T cells in cytokine-modified autologous mixed lymphocyte/tumor cell cultures. *J Immunother* 2001; 24:482–492.

61. Wagner WM, Ouyang Q, Pawelec G. Peptides spanning the fusion region of Abl/Bcr are immunogenic and sensitize CD8(+) T lymphocytes to recognize native chronic myelogenous leukemia. *Leukemia* 2002; 16:2341–2343.

62. Wagner WM, Ouyang Q, Pawelec G. The *abl/bcr* gene product as a novel leukemia-specific antigen: peptides spanning the fusion region of abl/bcr can be recognized by both CD4+ and CD8+ T lymphocytes. *Cancer Immunol Immunother* 2003; 52:89–96.

63. Knights AJ, Zaniou A, Rees RC, Pawelec G, Müller L. Prediction of an HLA-DR-binding peptide derived from Wilms' tumour 1 protein and demonstration of in vitro immunogenicity of WT1(124-138)-pulsed dendritic cells generated according to an optimised protocol. *Cancer Immunol Immunother* 2002; 51:271–281.

64. Verdijk RM, Mutis T, Esendam B, et al. Polyriboinosinic polyribocytidylic acid (poly[I:C]) induces stable maturation of functionally active human dendritic cells. *J Immunol* 1999; 163:57–61.

65. Oelke M, Maus MV, Didiano D, June CH, Mackensen A, Schneck JP. Ex vivo induction and expansion of antigen-specific cytotoxic T cells by HLA-Ig-coated artificial antigen-presenting cells. *Nat Med* 2003; 9:619–624.

66. Walter S, Herrgen L, Schoor O, et al. Cutting edge: predetermined avidity of human CD8 T cells expanded on calibrated MHC/anti-CD28-coated microspheres. *J Immunol* 2003; 171:4974–4978.

67. Oelke M, Schneck JP. HLA-Ig-based artificial antigen-presenting cells: setting the terms of engagement. *Clin Immunol* 2004; 110:243–251.

68. Betts MR, Brenchley JM, Price DA, et al. Sensitive and viable identification of antigen-specific CD8+ T cells by a flow cytometric assay for degranulation. *J Immunol Methods* 2003; 281:65–78.

69. Rubio V, Stuge TB, Singh N, et al. Ex vivo identification, isolation and analysis of tumor-cytolytic T cells. *Nat Med* 2003; 9:1377–1382.

70. Britten CM, Müller L, Knights A, Pawelec G. Cancer Immunotherapy 2004: Mainz, Germany, 6–7 May 2004. *Cancer Immunol Immunother* 2004; 53:1153–1158.

71. Firat H, Cochet M, Rohrlich PS, et al. Comparative analysis of the CD8(+) T cell repertoires of H-2 class I wild-type/HLA-A2.1 and H-2 class I knockout/HLA-A2.1 transgenic mice. *Int Immunol* 2002; 14: 925–934.

72. Pascolo S, Bervas N, Ure JM, Smith AG, Lemonnier FA, Perarnau B. HLA-A2.1-restricted education and cytolytic activity of CD8(+) T lymphocytes from beta2 microglobulin (beta2m) HLA-A2.1 monochain transgenic H-2Db beta2m double knockout mice. *J Exp Med* 1997; 185:2043–2051.

73. Ramage JM, Metheringham R, Moss R, Spendlove I, Rees R, Durrant LG. Comparison of the immune response to a self antigen after DNA immunisation of HLA*A201/H-2Kb and HHD transgenic mice. *Vaccine* 2004; 22:1728–1731.

74. Pascolo S, Schirle M, Guckel B, et al. A MAGE-A1 HLA-A A*0201 epitope identified by mass spectrometry. *Cancer Res* 2001; 61:4072–4077.

75. Corbet S, Nielsen HV, Vinner L, et al. Optimization and immune recognition of multiple novel conserved HLA-A2, human immunodeficiency virus type 1-specific CTL epitopes. *J Gen Virol* 2003; 84:2409–2421.

76. Gritzapis AD, Sotiriadou NN, Papamichail M, Baxevanis CN. Generation of human tumor-specific CTLs in HLA-A2.1-transgenic mice using unfractionated peptides from eluates of human primary breast and ovarian tumors. *Cancer Immunol Immunother* 2004; 53:1027–1040.

77. Shi TD, Wu YZ, Jia ZC, Zhou W, Zou LY. Therapeutic polypeptides based on HBcAg(18-27) CTL epitope can induce antigen-specific CD(8)(+) CTL-mediated cytotoxicity in HLA-A2 transgenic mice. *World J Gastroenterol* 2004; 10:1222–1226.

78. Himoudi N, Abraham JD, Fournillier A, et al. Comparative vaccine studies in HLA-A2.1-transgenic mice reveal a clustered organization of epitopes presented in hepatitis C virus natural infection. *J Virol* 2002; 76:12,735–12,746.

79. Theobald M, Ruppert T, Kuckelkorn U, et al. The sequence alteration associated with a mutational hotspot in p53 protects cells from lysis by cytotoxic T lymphocytes specific for a flanking peptide epitope. *J Exp Med* 1998; 188:1017–1028.

80. Sonderstrup G, Cope AP, Patel S, et al. HLA class II transgenic mice: models of the human CD4+ T-cell immune response. *Immunol Rev* 1999; 172:335–343.

81. Rojas JM, McArdle SE, Horton RB, et al. Peptide immunisation of HLA-DR-transgenic mice permits the identification of a novel HLA-DRbeta1*. *Cancer Immunol Immunother* 2004; 54:243–253.

82. Pajot A, Pancre V, Fazilleau N, et al. Comparison of HLA-DR1-restricted T cell response induced in HLA-DR1 transgenic mice deficient for murine MHC class II and HLA-DR1 transgenic mice expressing endogenous murine MHC class II molecules. *Int Immunol* 2004; 16:1275–1282.

83. Zhou H, Luo Y, Mizutani M, et al. A novel transgenic mouse model for immunological evaluation of carcinoembryonic antigen-based DNA minigene vaccines. *J Clin Invest* 2004; 113:1792–1798.

84. Zarling AL, Ficarro SB, White FM, Shabanowitz J, Hunt DF, Engelhard VH. Phosphorylated peptides are naturally processed and presented by major histocompatibility complex class I molecules in vivo. *J Exp Med* 2000; 192:1755–1762.

85. Haurum JS, Hoier IB, Arsequell G, et al. Presentation of cytosolic glycosylated peptides by human class I major histocompatibility complex molecules in vivo. *J Exp Med* 1999; 190:145–150.

86. Van den Steen PE, Proost P, Brand DD, Kang AH, Van Damme J, Opdenakker G. Generation of glycosylated remnant epitopes from human collagen type II by gelatinase B. *Biochemistry* 2004; 43:10,809–10,816.

87. Skipper JC, Hendrickson RC, Gulden PH, et al. An HLA-A2-restricted tyrosinase antigen on melanoma cells results from posttranslational modification and suggests a novel pathway for processing of membrane proteins. *J Exp Med* 1996; 183:527–534.

88. Hill JA, Southwood S, Sette A, Jevnikar AM, Bell DA, Cairns E. Cutting edge: the conversion of arginine to citrulline allows for a high-affinity peptide interaction with the rheumatoid arthritis-associated HLA-DRB1*0401 MHC class II molecule. *J Immunol* 2003; 171:538–541.

89. Parham P. Purification of immunologically active HLA-A and -B antigens by a series of monoclonal antibody columns. *J Biol Chem* 1979; 254:8709–8712.

90. Parham P, Barnstable CJ, Bodmer WF. Use of a monoclonal antibody (W6/32) in structural studies of HLA-A,B,C, antigens. *J Immunol* 1979; 123:342–349.

91. Shackelford DA, Lampson LA, Strominger JL. Separation of three class II antigens from a homozygous human B cell line. *J Immunol* 1983; 130:289–296.

92. Storkus WJ, Zeh HJ III, Salter RD, Lotze MT. Identification of T-cell epitopes: rapid isolation of class I-presented peptides from viable cells by mild acid elution. *J Immunother* 1993; 14:94–103.

93. Castelli C, Storkus WJ, Maeurer MJ, et al. Mass spectrometric identification of a naturally processed melanoma peptide recognized by CD8+ cytotoxic T lymphocytes. *J Exp Med* 1995; 181:363–368.

94. Clark RE, Dodi IA, Hill SC, et al. Direct evidence that leukemic cells present HLA-associated immunogenic peptides derived from the BCR-ABL b3a2 fusion protein. *Blood* 2001; 98:2887–2893.

95. Cox AL, Skipper J, Chen Y, et al. Identification of a peptide recognized by five melanoma-specific human cytotoxic T cell lines. *Science* 1994; 264:716–719.

96. McDonald WH, Yates JR III. Shotgun proteomics and biomarker discovery. *Dis Markers* 2002; 18:99–105.

97. Stevanovic S, Jung G. Multiple sequence analysis: pool sequencing of synthetic and natural peptide libraries. *Anal Biochem* 1993; 212:212–220.

98. Hunt DF, Henderson RA, Shabanowitz J, et al. Characterization of peptides bound to the class I MHC molecule HLA-A2.1 by mass spectrometry. *Science* 1992; 255:1261–1263.

99. Chicz RM, Urban RG, Lane WS, et al. Predominant naturally processed peptides bound to HLA-DR1 are derived from MHC-related molecules and are heterogeneous in size. *Nature* 1992; 358:764–768.

100. Spengler B. De novo sequencing, peptide composition analysis, and composition-based sequencing: a new strategy employing accurate mass determination by Fourier transform ion cyclotron resonance mass spectrometry. *J Am Soc Mass Spectrom* 2004; 15:703–714.

101. Flad T, Spengler B, Kalbacher H, et al. Direct identification of major histocompatibility complex class I-bound tumor-associated peptide antigens of a renal carcinoma cell line by a novel mass spectrometric method. *Cancer Res* 1998; 58:5803–5811.

102. De Groot AS, Sbai H, Aubin CS, McMurry J, Martin W. Immuno-informatics: mining genomes for vaccine components. *Immunol Cell Biol* 2002; 80:255–269.

103. Schena M, Shalon D, Davis RW, Brown PO. Quantitative monitoring of gene expression patterns with a complementary DNA microarray. *Science* 1995; 270:467–470.

104. Boer JM, Huber WK, Sultmann H, et al. Identification and classification of differentially expressed genes in renal cell carcinoma by expression profiling on a global human 31,500-element cDNA array. *Genome Res* 2001; 11:1861–1870.

105. Weinschenk T, Gouttefangeas C, Schirle M, Integrated functional genomics approach for the design of patient-individual antitumor vaccines. *Cancer Res* 2002; 62:5818–5827.

106. Lemmel C, Weik S, Eberle U, et al. Differential quantitative analysis of MHC ligands by mass spectrometry using stable isotope labeling. *Nat Biotechnol* 2004; 22:450–454.

3 Current and Future Role of Natural-Killer Cells in Cancer Immunotherapy

Lisa M. Harlan and Julie Y. Djeu

SUMMARY

Natural-killer (NK) cells are a class of lymphocytes distinct in their ability to identify and kill transformed self-cells without priming. Recognition is via receptors that bind unique but common surface molecules induced on these cells. These properties characterize NK cells as unique effectors for use in immunotherapy. Discussed here are past and current experiments and clinical trials geared toward enhancing NK cell cytotoxicity in three general ways:

1. Modification of the NK cell to activate or enhance cytolytic activity.
2. Modification of the tumor to make it more readily identified and more immunogenic.
3. Modification of other immune cells to affect indirectly NK cell activity or to elicit a cooperative effect with both an innate and adaptive immune response.

Key Words: NK cells; cancer; immunotherapy; inhibitory receptors; activating receptors; cytokines; KIR mismatch; allogeneic BMT; tumor modification; dendritic cells; T-cells.

1. IMMUNOTHERAPY

Traditional therapies for cancer have included surgery, radiotherapy, chemotherapy, or all of the above. However, in recent years, numerous means for manipulation of the immune system have been developed as strategies for cancer treatment. These are collectively called *immunotherapy*, which is designed to produce immunity to a specific cancer.

The idea of the immune system being used in cancer treatment is credited to William B. Coley *(1)*. Coley noted that some of his patients with sarcoma had spontaneous regression of their tumors, and this correlated with a bacterial infection. Coley then used the bacteria to infect cancer patients and in some cases, complete tumor regression was achieved. Recently, the role of the immune system in the disease of cancer was further defined as "immunoediting" *(2)*. As described, cancer immunoediting is a process of three phases: elimination (immunosurveillance), equilibrium, and escape. The basic premise of this concept is that the immune system uses a multifaceted approach to fight cancer, involving both adaptive and innate immunity, and requires a constant process of

From: *Cancer Drug Discovery and Development: Immunotherapy of Cancer*
Edited by: M. L. Disis © Humana Press Inc., Totowa, NJ

maintenance to rid the body of transformed cells. However, there are times when the transformed cells are able to withstand the surveillance and maintenance and begin to grow in an uncontrolled manner.

The immune system and its components are now being investigated as tools for immunotherapy. T-cells (both helper CD4[+] and cytotoxic CD8[+] cells), natural-killer (NK) cells, dendritic cells (DCs), antibodies, vaccines using the whole tumor or common tumor antigens, and immune response mediators, such as cytokines, are being investigated as mechanisms to stimulate the immune response against a cancer. This chapter will focus on how NK cells are being used in immunotherapy.

2. NK CELLS

2.1. Biology

NK cells are a class of lymphocytes distinct from T- and B-cells that constitute about 10% of peripheral blood lymphocytes in healthy individuals (3). NK cells, like T- and B-cells, express receptors specific for target cells. However, unlike T- and B-cells, these receptors are not encoded by genes that undergo recombination (4). In humans, two major NK cell populations have been identified based on the surface density of CD56, the most commonly used surface marker to identify NK cells in a population. CD56[dim] CD16[+] NK cells are thought to be the terminally differentiated cytotoxic effector cells, whereas CD56[bright] CD16[-] NK cells regulate other cells through cytokine release. The major role of NK cells is recognition of self-proteins that have been upregulated in transformed cells ("induced self-recognition") or recognition of self-proteins that have been downregulated in transformed cells ("missing self-recognition") (4). The primary pathway that NK cells use to lyse a target cell is through the intimate, directed release of cytolytic granules containing perforin and granzymes. However, fatty acid synthase (Fas)–Fas ligand inter- actions, tumor necrosis factor (TNF)-related apoptosis-inducing ligand, and membrane TNF-α are also mechanisms used by NK cells to induce cytotoxicity. NK cells also can mediate an adaptive immune response through secretion of cytokines, such as interferon (IFN)-γ, which directs a T-helper (Th)1 response. Finally, NK cells express CD16, a low- affinity Fc receptor for immunoglobulin G, thus allowing NK cells to participate in anti- body-dependent cell-mediated cytotoxicity (5).

2.2. NK Cell Receptors

NK cells express two types of surface receptors, inhibitory and activating, that regulate NK cell activity. Studies in mice and man have revealed some differences between the two species; however, all inhibitory receptors are specific for class I major histocompatibility complex (MHC)/human leukocyte antigen (HLA) molecules and, on engagement, block NK cell cytotoxicity, i.e., if the NK cell perceives sufficient MHC/HLA density, the NK cell possessing the relevant inhibitory receptor will refrain from attacking the target cell. In mice, Ly49 receptors, which are C-type lectin-like molecules, bind D[d] as well as other classical class I MHC molecules. In humans, killer immunoglobulin-like receptors (KIRs) interact with HLA class I-A, -B, -C, and -G to work as inhibitory receptors. The hetero- dimeric receptor CD94/NKG2A, expressed in both mice and man, interacts with HLA class I-E. The inhibitory receptor ILT2/LIR1, expressed weakly in NK cells, recognizes a broad range of HLA class I molecules (3,4). Engagement of these molecules will transmit inhibitory signals through immunoreceptor tyrosine-based inhibition motifs present in the cytoplasmic portion of the molecule. These motifs bind *src* homology domain 2-containing tyrosine phosphatase 1 that is recruited to interrupt signal transduction leading to tumor lysis. These receptor–ligand interactions thus protect normal, self-cells from NK cell cytotoxicity, whereas cells with low or absent MHC class I expression will be lysed.

Cell lysis also may be affected when the NK cell receives an activating signal through the interaction of activating receptors on NK cells with their ligands on potential target cells. Activating receptors that recognize class I molecules are homologous to inhibitory receptors in the extracellular and transmembrane domains, but lack the immunoreceptor tyrosine-based inhibition motif-containing cytoplasmic domain. They include Ly49D and H (mice), KIR2DS and KIR3DS (man), and NKG2C (mice and man) *(4,6)*. Other activating receptors that do not recognize class I molecules include natural cytotoxicity receptors and NKG2D *(6)*. There are three types of natural cytotoxicity receptors: NKp46, NKp44, and NKp30. NKp46 and NKp30 are expressed on both activated and resting NK cells, whereas NKp44 is expressed only on activated NK cells. The ligands for these receptors have not been identified. NKG2D is a C-type lectin molecule expressed on NK cells, CD8$^+$ T-cells, and γδ T-cells. Several ligands for NKG2D have been identified, including MHC class I chain (MIC)-related A, MICB, and UL-16-binding protein molecules, of which there are five. Engagement of any of these receptors results in activation of the NK cell. The choice of pathway leading to activation is dependent on which molecule is triggered. NKp44 and KIR2DS associate with an adaptor protein, DAP12, whereas NKp30 and NKp46 associate with either the CD3 ζ-chain or FcRγ. Each of these adaptor proteins transmits signals through immunoreceptor tyrosine-based activation motifs present in their cytoplasmic domains and signals via Syk or Zap-70 *(7,8)*. In contrast, NKG2D is associated with the adaptor protein, DAP10. DAP10 activates PI3 kinase through the presence of an YxxM motif *(9)*. The presence of both inhibitory and activating receptors on NK cells allows for efficient surveillance and killing of transformed self-cells. Thus, tumor cell killing is based on an equilibrium representing the balance between the ability of the tumor cell to deliver inhibitory signals to the NK cell and the ability of the tumor to elaborate activating receptors that target the NK cell.

2.3. NK Cells, Cancer, and Immunotherapy

In addition to tumor lysis in vitro, NK cells have been demonstrated to have a role in tumor cell growth and metastasis in vivo. In mice, transplanted tumor growth and metastasis are much more severe when NK cells are depleted. NK cell depletion also reduces tumor specific cytotoxic T-lymphocyte activity *(10)*. Additionally, studies have demonstrated that perforin-deficient mice are more sensitive and develop more tumors when exposed to the carcinogen methylcholanthrene, compared with normal mice. Depletion of the CD8$^+$ T-cells had no effect on the incidence or kinetics of the developing tumors *(11–14)*. As an apparent escape mechanism, renal cell carcinoma, B-cell lymphoma, cervical, breast, rectal, and melanomas represent only a few of the cancers that downregulate MHC class I on the surface of their tumor cells *(15–18)*. This downregulation results in NK cell-mediated tumor lysis because of the lack of the ligand to trigger an inhibitory signal, leaving the presence of an activating signal.

The adoptive transfer of NK cells has been successful at demonstrating antitumor activity toward solid tumors and is associated with a decrease in graft-vs-host disease (GVHD).

Adoptively transferred donor T-cells typically target malignant cells but also target self, resulting in GVHD. However, alloreactive NK cells, through the mismatch of HLA class I ligands, can condition recipients enough to allow safe infusion of T-cells for immune reconstitution and reduce the infection-related morbidity and mortality that are associated with extensive graft T-cell depletion *(19,20)*. These studies and others demonstrate that NK cells are required for prevention of tumor growth and are worthwhile effectors to explore for potential use in immunotherapy.

3. NK CELL IMMUNOTHERAPY

In general, there appear to be three different avenues for enhancing the usefulness of NK cells in cancer immunotherapy:

1. Modification of the NK cell to activate or enhance cytolytic activity.
2. Modification of the tumor to make it more readily identified and more immunogenic.
3. Modification of other immune cells in order to affect indirectly NK cell activity or to elicit a cooperative effect with both an innate and adaptive immune response. Promising leads in animal models have culminated in a multitude of clinical trials, and significant progress has been made. As lessons are learned, new approaches are being developed and tested in mice before bringing them to the clinic. The following sections focus on how NK cells have been utilized as an immunotherapeutic means to treat cancer, and we discuss in some detail what the future holds.

3.1. Modulation of NK Cell Activity

NK cells are thought to be constitutively active in that they do not require specific antigen priming; however, they do require a signal from an activating receptor to acquire effector capabilities. NK cell activation can occur through several additional pathways beyond the engagement of activating receptors. These include responses to cytokines and chemokines, CD40–CD40 ligand interactions, and interactions with tumor cells.

3.1.1. CYTOKINES/CHEMOKINES

In man, the earliest clinical immunotherapy studies using NK cells began as a result of therapeutic approaches using interleukin (IL)-2. Repeated in vivo administration of recombinant IL-2 or in vitro incubation of NK cells with IL-2 was found to enhance NK cell cytotoxicity *(21–24)*. However, the toxicity seen in patients associated with IL-2 was less than desirable and prompted scientists to return to the bench and begin further studies in both mice and man with other cytokines including IFN-α *(25)*, IL-12 *(26)*, IL-18 *(27)*, IL-21 *(28)*, and IL-15 *(29)*.

Some of the in vitro studies using human cells determined IL-2 to be required exclusively for NK expansion and cytotoxicity *(30)*. However, the requirement of IL-15 for NK cell development was discovered in mice, in that IL-15$^{-/-}$ mice lack NK cells *(31)*. Most human studies done with cytokines have been in vitro; however, they are slowly moving to the clinic. Patients with stable hairy cell leukemia (HCL) treated with either IFN-α or IL-2 exhibited NK activity *(32)*. Additionally, HCL continuous cell lines, otherwise resistant to NK cell-mediated cytotoxicity, were somewhat sensitive to killing with IFN-α-treated NK cells *(33)*. NK cells activated in the presence of IL-12 express high CD56 levels and have heightened effector functions such as proliferation and IFN-γ secretion *(34)*. In the clinic, administration of recombinant human IL-12 resulted in an increase in NK cell number and augmented cytolytic activity *(35)*.

Studies using mice have shed light on the potential of other cytokines to enhance NK cell activity. IL-18 is an important factor in IFN-γ gene activation and therefore a potential factor to activate NK cells and induce IFN-γ secretion. Furthermore, administration of IL-18 stimulates T- and NK cell antitumor activity, and this effect was decreased in mice depleted of NK cells *(27)*. Another cytokine implicated in NK cell function is IL-21, in that IL-21$^{-/-}$ mice have impaired NK cell function. Additionally, in mice bearing subcutaneous tumors, systemic administration of plasmid DNA encoding murine IL-21 significantly inhibited tumor growth and prolonged survival without severe toxicity effects. The antitumor activity mediated by IL-21 was abolished following NK cell depletion *(28)*.

Overall, these studies demonstrate the ability of various cytokines used individually to enhance NK cell activity. However, in vivo, the tumor and NK cell microenvironment is likely a mixture of cytokines and chemokines produced by not only inflammatory cells, but also by the tumor cells. Furthermore, introduction of one cytokine in excess into the local environment will undoubtedly exert regulatory effects on synthesis of other cytokines, exacerbating an imbalance. Therefore, it is vital to understand fully the combined effects of these cytokines on NK cell activity.

Combination therapies aim to enhance the individual cytokine antitumor activities for a more effective treatment. In vitro activation of NK cells with the combination of IL-2 and IL-12 resulted in significant lysis of otherwise NK-resistant tumor cell lines *(26)*. These studies have been translated into the clinic to offer more efficient treatment options for patients. Similar to studies using each cytokine alone, NK activity in peripheral blood samples from HCL patients was increased after stimulation by IL-2 and IFN-β *(36)*. It also was determined that the combination of IL-2 and IFN-α increased the number of NK cells, and this correlated with a positive treatment response in advanced tumor patients *(37)*. Compared with either cytokine alone, IL-2 and IL-12 were determined to have synergistic effects on IFN-γ production and enhancement of NK cell activity in cutaneous T-cell lymphoma patients *(38)*. Additionally, both IL-2 and IL-12 have synergistic effects with rituximab, a chimeric murine/human monoclonal antibody to CD20. Early phase clinical trials indicate that the combinations appear to be effective in B-cell non-Hodgkin's lymphoma *(39,40)*. IL-2 also has been combined with trastuzumab (a humanized murine monoclonal antibody to HER-2), and in this instance, resulted in enhanced NK cell killing (via antibody-dependent cell-mediated cytotoxicity) of breast cancer targets *(41)*. Another immunotherapeutic approach is combining IL-2 and ex vivo heat shock protein 70 peptide-activated peripheral blood lymphocytes. This treatment resulted in not only an increase in NK cell numbers but also an enhanced cytotoxicity against heat shock protein 70 membrane-positive colon carcinoma cells *(42)*.

Combination studies in mice also show potential to translate to clinical studies. Individually, IL-12 can enhance NK cell proliferation and cytolytic activity, whereas engagement of 4-1BB on antigen-presenting cells (APCs) promotes Th1 development and induces and sustains cytolytic activity. The potential that these treatments could offer together was demonstrated through the transfer of the *IL-12* gene into mice inoculated with melanoma along with anti-4-1BB treatment. This combination synergistically induced a reduction in tumor growth, and this was attributed to both NK cells and CD8$^+$ T-cells in that depletion of either cell population before treatment abolished the efficacy of the combination *(43)*. The combination therapy approaches makes it possible to enhance NK cell activity and makes it feasible to use lower dose treatments and thus decrease the toxicity associated with higher dose treatments.

Chemokines (chemoattractant cytokines) are small molecules that have been established in recent years as a primary guidance system for immune cell homing. Cells elaborating appropriate chemokine receptors home to specific lymph nodes or to sites of inflammation, as well as several other relevant sites. In addition, chemokines can have direct modulatory effects on specific cells, as stimulation of chemokine receptors causes changes in gene expression, as well as migratory effects. Thus, chemokines play several important roles in modulating an immune response and making the immune response more efficient. Studies of the effects of various chemokines remain at the bench and much is yet to be understood. However, the chemokines CCL2, CCL3, CCL4, CCL5, CCL7, CCL8, CXCL10, and CX3CL1 have been shown to enhance cytotoxic granule release in resting NK cells (reviewed in ref. *44*). It is thought that this is because of induction of increased expression of an adhesion molecule and therefore enhanced NK cell: target-cell contact. Studies in mice have demonstrated that some chemokines can enhance NK cell activity. CX3CL1 (fractalkine) was demonstrated to have a role in NK cell lysis of YAC-1 cells in vivo *(45)*. Radiolabeled YAC-1 cells, when intravenously injected into C57BL/6 mice, localized to the lungs and were found to have been cleared by NK cells. However, pretreatment of mice with a blocking antibody to CX3CL1 or CX3CR1 resulted in decreased target-cell clearance. Furthermore, inoculation of mice with the 3LL lung carcinoma cell gene modified with fractalkine increased NK cell activity, and depletion of NK cells resulted in decreased tumor growth inhibition *(46)*. At the very least, chemokines could potentially serve as potent antitumor effectors through the chemoattraction of NK cells to the tumor sites, followed by activation of the NK cells. Because all functions of all chemokines remain undiscovered, these molecules will undoubtedly have additional benefits to the fight with cancer.

3.1.2. OTHER MEANS OF NK CELL ACTIVATION

Studies in both mice and man have shown there are alternative ways to active NK cells beyond activating receptors or cytokines and chemokines. NK cells express CD40 ligand, a co-stimulatory molecule that interacts with CD40 expressed on DCs, B-cells, monocytes, and tumor cells. In man, NK cells can be activated because of CD40–CD40 ligand interactions *(47)*. Further studies in mice have determined that treatment of tumor-bearing mice with anti-CD40 results in antitumor and antimetastatic effects. However, when NK cells are depleted, this activity is abrogated *(48)*. These data also demonstrated that the tumor cells were CD40-negative and proposed the NK cell activation was because of cytokine secretion from anti-CD40-stimulated DCs. Other murine studies have demonstrated that overexpression of oncogenes in NK cells could provide yet another avenue of NK cell expansion and long-term survival. T- and NK cells had increased expression of Fas ligand and higher levels of IFN-γ after Myb-related protein B was overexpressed in lymphoid tissues *(49)*. NK cells expressing Fas ligand could interact with tumors expressing Fas and induce apoptosis in the tumor cells. Translating the murine studies to man could be another way to enhance the efficacy of immunotherapy.

Furthermore, NK cells treated with thalidomide, a glutamic acid derivative with anti-inflammatory and immunomodulating properties, showed significantly increased lytic activity. It is hypothesized that thalidomide mediates its antimultiple myeloma effect, in part by modulating NK cell number and activity *(50)*.

Although still in their infancy, each of these studies demonstrates a unique way to activate NK cells and enhance effector function. These studies predict a scope of therapeutic approaches that will eventually be sufficiently broad to access a large number of tumor types and situations.

3.1.3. ENHANCEMENT OF NK CELL–TUMOR CELL INTERACTIONS

In addition to activating the NK cells, getting the NK cells to the tumor is an important aspect for an effective immunotherapy. Targeting the NK cell to the tumor by adoptive transfer and bringing them into close proximity increases the chance of tumor cell lysis. In mice, the antitumor effect of systemic delivery of NK cells and γδ T-cells indicate that both can prevent the subcutaneous growth of autologous melanoma *(51)*. The donor NK cells were detected at the tumor site, and they maintained their inhibitory effect on tumor growth after treatment was stopped. In man, NK cells transfused into patients disperse throughout the body, showing preference for the liver, spleen, and bone marrow. Donor NK cells are detectable at 3 d, but cleared from the blood by 7 d. In addition, 50% of metastases tested indicated an accumulation of NK cells *(52)*.

One way to better target NK cells to the tumor is through the modification of the NK cell. This approach is supported by in vitro studies using NK cell lines, and in vivo studies in the murine produce promising results. The human NK cell line YT was modified by transfection with the cDNA of the human asialoglycoprotein receptor, which recognizes carbohydrates containing terminal galactosyl residues, found on tumor cells. Cytolytic activity toward a number of tumor lines was increased using these genetically modified NK cells *(53)*. Furthermore, an NK cell line modified to express a tumor specific chimeric immunoglobulin T-cell receptor, inhibited tumor growth in vivo after adoptive transfer into nonobese diabetic/severe combined immunodeficient mice *(54)*.

NK cell lines, such as NK-92, are effective at killing a number of tumor targets, both in vitro and in vivo, including chronic myeloid lymphoma, acute myeloid leukemia (AML), and acute lymphoblastic leukemia *(55)*. NK-92 transfected with IL-15 cDNA proliferated at a higher rate and performed better in long-term cultures. In addition, NK-92 cells transfected with IL-15 demonstrated a higher level of cytotoxicity against a broad range of target tumor cells, correlating with an increase in perforin, Fas ligand, and IFN-γ secretion *(56)*. In addition, NK-92 cells stably transfected with the chemokine stem cell factor experienced increased cell proliferation and stronger cytotoxicity *(57)*. Similar to the case with IL-15, the NK-92 cells transfected with stem cell factor had an increase in perforin and Fas ligand. Thus, gene-modified NK cell lines show significant promise for adoptive cellular immunotherapy.

Bispecific monoclonal antibody development provides yet another way to target NK cells and enhance cytotoxicity, and it is currently being used in human studies. These antibodies are designed to recognize two different cell surface proteins and can be used to generate and stabilize effector–target cell interaction. HRS-3/A9 is an anti-CD16/CD30 bispecific monoclonal antibody with one arm that will bind to CD30, (a protein expressed on the majority of Hodgkin and Reed-Sternberg cells), and the other arm capable of binding to the NK surface protein CD16, simultaneously activating the NK cell *(58)*. Similarly, anti-CD30 antibody/IL-2 fusion protein, binds to CD30 and the IL-2 receptor and stimulates proliferation of preactivated T-cells and induces resting NK cells to lyse lymphoma cells *(59)*.

Advances in adoptive cell immunotherapy have been made in the treatment of some cancers, including squamous cell carcinoma of the head and neck and melanoma *(60–62)*. However, for NK cells to be most useful in immunotherapy, activation and homing will continue to be important events to understand.

3.1.4. KIR Incompatibility and Allogeneic Bone Marrow Transplantation

More recent data suggest that immunotherapeutic strategies using KIR-incompatible allogeneic NK cells in bone marrow transplantation (BMT) can be of benefit. Several studies in both mice and man provide evidence that these cells can mediate antileukemic effects against AML and solid tumors, such as renal cell carcinoma and melanoma *(63,64)*. In addition, use of either autologous or allogeneic NK cells will result in a good graft-vs-leukemia effect with little graft-vs-host effect *(64,65)*. Ruggeri et al. demonstrated that alloreactive NK cells demonstrate graft-vs-leukemia and prevent GVHD by eliminating the recipients APCs in AML. Again, the idea of combining therapies prevailed in the clinic and resulted in the finding that human NK cell cytotoxicity toward human leukemia cells with KIR mismatch increased with the number of receptor–ligand mismatch pairs or pre-stimulation with IL-12 and IL-18 *(66)*.

Allogeneic BMT is also being used for the treatment of cancer. However, there are some serious obstacles limiting the efficacy of BMT, including GVHD, tumor relapse, and the inherent dangers associated with immunosuppressed patients. Therefore, most of this work is still being done in mice. However, as mentioned above, adoptive immunotherapy of NK cells following an allogeneic BMT has been shown to be successful at preventing GVHD and mediating graft-vs-tumor effects. One way to augment this activity is to block the interaction of inhibitory receptors and their ligands. Blockade of LY49C using F(ab)$'_2$ fragments of the 5E6 monoclonal antibody resulted in increased cytotoxicity and decreased tumor cell growth *(67,68)*. It is proposed that a mechanism by which NK cells prevent GVHD and promote graft-vs-tumor effects is through the immunosuppressive cytokine transforming growth factor (TGF)-β *(69)*. This is based on data that anti-TGF-β completely abrogated the protective effects of NK cells on GVHD in mice following BMT.

3.2. Modification of the Tumor Cell

Transformed cells have the ability to modify their own functions, including rate of division and cell surface composition. Tumors have evolved in numerous ways to evade the immune response, including the downregulation of activating ligands and the secretion of immunosuppressive mediators. Therefore, modification of a transformed cell to allow an efficient immune response is another way to increase the efficacy of immunotherapy.

3.2.1. Cytokines/Chemokines

Systemic cytokine therapy has often been associated with clinical toxicity. This is because of the multiple properties of cytokines on cells other than NK cells. Genetic modification of a tumor cell to express a cytokine or chemokine has two advantages. First, localization of a cytokine or chemokine at the tumor site potentially affects only the necessary cells. Second, it is an efficient way to attract immune cells to the tumor site. So far, these studies have been conducted only in mice, but they show promise for yet another strategy in cancer immunotherapy.

Numerous studies have been conducted with cytokine-transformed tumor cells, indicating the potential for this strategy *(70)*. Some of the earlier studies, using IL-2 and IFN-γ, indicated that NK cells played a role in rejection of these cytokine-transformed tumors *(71, 72)*. Studies also done in mice demonstrate that coexpression of B7.1 (the activating counter receptor for CD28 on T-cells) and IFN-γ in MCA106 fibrosarcoma tumor cells induces antitumor immunity, owing in part to NK cells and in part to CD8$^+$ and CD4$^+$ T-cells *(73)*. Additionally, it has been demonstrated that IL-10 expression in a tumor cell line leads to enhanced NK cell activity *(74)*. Further studies demonstrated that following injection into nude mice, the growth of human pancreatic cancer cells retrovirally transduced with murine IL-21, and IL-23 was retarded compared with that of parent tumors. Following depletion of NK cells, the growth retardation was abrogated *(75)*. Studies with chemokines, such as CKβ-11, have also demonstrated similar effects. A murine breast cancer cell line was retrovirally transduced with CKβ-11 and injected into mice. Not only did these mice not have tumor growth, but CKβ-11 also mediated rejection of the tumor in an NK cell-dependent manner, in that depletion of NK cells significantly reduced the CKβ-11 antitumor activity *(76)*. Each of these studies shows the potential use of localized cytokines or chemokines to not only reduce tumor growth, but also enhance the immune response to the tumor.

3.2.2. NK-RECOGNIZABLE LIGANDS

Expression of NKG2D ligands by tumor cells is one way NK cells are activated. However, work in mice has revealed that some tumors do not express these ligands. The B16-BL6 melanoma cell line is one such tumor line, yet when transfected with the NKG2D retinoic acid early inducible gene *(RAE)*-1 ligand or H60 ligand, the tumor was rejected by syngeneic B6 mice *(77)*. Similarly, the MHC class I-positive tumor cell line RMA normally is resistant to NK cell lysis. However, when RMA cells were transfected with the NKG2D ligand, RAE-1, the tumor was rejected *(78)*. Despite being positive or negative for MHC class I, tumors bearing NKG2D ligands are susceptible to NK cell lysis and present yet another option in gene-mediated immunotherapy.

Interestingly, it has been demonstrated in man that tumors have the ability to shed ligands such as MICA/B, thus evading potential NK cell activity *(79)*. The shedding of these ligands has been correlated with a decrease in NK cell activity, possibly through the downregulation of NKG2D on the surface of the NK cell. This was shown to be treatable however, when treatment of cells with IL-2 or IL-15 in vitro upregulated surface NKG2D expression, and cytotoxicity was enhanced *(80)*. Others have demonstrated that high serum levels of soluble MICA correlate with advanced stages of cancer. However, in the presence of a matrix metalloproteinase inhibitor, levels of soluble MICA were reduced *(81)*. An increase in MICA surface expression on the tumor cell would allow an interaction with NKG2D, thus triggering a NK cell response, and approaches to modulate expression of these types of receptors are an exciting area of research. The information available from both murine and human studies has shed light on the importance of regulating NK recognizable ligand expression.

3.2.3. BLOCKING NK INHIBITORY SUBSTANCES PRODUCED BY TUMORS

TGF-β is an immunosuppressive molecule produced by many nucleated cell types and present in platelets. TGF-β is also known to be produced by tumor cells. Not only does TGF-β inhibit cytotoxic T-lymphocyte development and cytotoxic activity, but it also inhibits cell proliferation and APC activity (reviewed in ref. *82*). Additionally, and seemingly in contrast, TGF-β promotes proliferation, differentiation, angiogenesis, and metastasis of tumor cells. In humans, it has been demonstrated that one mechanism by which TGF-β promotes tumor growth is through the negative modulation of NK cell activity via downregulation of the activating receptor, NKG2D *(83)*. This information supported further studies with TGF-β in mice. Here, it has been demonstrated that depletion of γδ T-cells enhances NK cell activity. Antibody-blocking studies demonstrated that the inhibitory effect of the γδ T-cells was partially mediated by IL-10 and TGF-β *(84)*. Several methods are currently under development in mice to neutralize the immunosuppressive effects of TGF-β. TGF-β antisense oligonucleotides reduce tumor growth and enhance their tumorigenicity *(85)*. Systemic administration of TGF-β neutralizing antibodies suppressed the growth of a human breast cancer cell line in athymic mice and simultaneously increased NK cell activity. In NK cell deficient mice, this effect was not observed *(86)*. Thus, blocking TGF-β could lend itself to be an effective means to enhance NK cell immunotherapy.

3.3. Modification of Other Immune Cells

Activation of NK cells can result in the secretion of cytokines including IFN-γ, TNF-α, and granulocyte/macrophage colony-stimulating factor. The secretion of these cytokines can influence responses by other immune cells, such as DCs and T-cells *(87)*. IFN-γ can polarize the T-cell response to Th1 (favoring cell-mediated immunity), whereas granulocyte/macrophage colony-stimulating factor can influence the maturation of DCs. In turn, activated T-cells and DCs can secrete cytokines, such as IL-2 and IL-12, respectively, that result in NK cell activation *(88)*. Because of the very complex crosstalk between the innate and adaptive immunity, this regulatory loop eventually will be used as an advantage in immunotherapy.

3.3.1. DCs and T-Cells

DCs are recognized for their ability to serve as APCs, with an ability to activate T-cells and sustain the immune response. DCs primed to tumor-associated antigens have become an interesting variation to vaccination against a cancer, and introduction of tumor-derived mRNA into DCs to generate a more tumor-directed antigen presentation has attracted a lot of interest lately. DCs are also able to activate NK cells. In mice, DCs not primed to any tumor antigen, induced protection against tumor lung metastasis resulting from injection of a syngeneic colon or lung carcinoma. The protection was abrogated following NK cell depletion *(13)*. As mentioned, DCs can regulate NK cell function through the release of IL-12. In vitro, coculture of DCs with fixed tumor cells results in the secretion of IL-12. Following coculture of the IL-12-secreting DCs with NK cells, there was an increase in NK cell cytolytic activity *(89)*. It has also been demonstrated in mice that NKG2D-triggered NK cell cytotoxicity results in specific secondary tumor immunity *(90)*. RMA-S tumors expressing the murine NKG2D ligand, RAE-1β, triggered NK cell cytotoxicity, and when both CD4+ and CD8+ T-cells were depleted, this resulted in the mice failing to respond to secondary RMA tumor challenge. Therefore, the activation of NK cells will not only result in cytotoxic activity toward the tumor, but activated NK cells also can recruit dendritic cells and T-cells for a more comprehensive, and therefore more effective, immune response. These exciting results have translated to human studies in a number of diseases *(91)*.

4. FUTURE OF NK CELL USE IN IMMUNOTHERAPY

The goal of immunotherapy is to activate a part of the immune system that is otherwise not responding to a tumor. The primary objective of the work discussed herein was to identify specific approaches and the specific components of the immune system most appropriate to elicit the maximally efficient response to each tumor. The future of immunotherapy is complex, and a number of circumstances will need to be considered. The patient, tumor type, stage of disease, and previous treatment ultimately will have great influence on the efficacy of any immunotherapy regimen. NK cells must be able to home in on the tumor and recruit effective help. Defining how NK cells find their target in vivo will be an important area of study in optimizing NK cell immunotherapy. Understanding tumor microenvironment, NK cell migration, NK cell interaction with the extracellular matrix, and NK interactions with DCs will be critical *(92)*. Modulating the tumor environment so that NK cells can more specifically identify and lyse the tumors will be another important avenue of development. Realizing the potential interactions with other cells of the immune system is necessary as well. In relation to translational science, most of these studies are still at the bench, some have translated to the bedside, and some of those have returned to the bench. Ultimately, the combination of a number of the studies mentioned in this chapter could lead to the most effective treatment for the widest variety of tumors.

REFERENCES

1. Coley WB. The treatment of malignant tumors by repeated inoculations of erysipelas. With a report of ten original cases. 1893. *Clin Orthop* 1991; 262:3–11.
2. Dunn GP, Old LJ, Schreiber RD. The immunobiology of cancer immunosurveillance and immunoediting. *Immunity* 2004; 21:137–148.
3. Raulet DH. Natural killer cells. In: Paul WE, ed. *Fundamental Immunology*. Philadelphia: Lippincott-Raven. 1999: pp. 365–391.
4. Raulet DH. Interplay of natural killer cells and their receptors with the adaptive immune response. *Nat Immunol* 2004; 5:996–1002.
5. Lanier LL, Le AM, Phillips JH, Warner NL, Babcock GF. Subpopulations of human natural killer cells defined by expression of the Leu-7 (HNK-1) and Leu-11 (NK-15) antigens. *J Immunol* 1983; 131:1789–1796.
6. Wu J, Lanier LL. Natural killer cells and cancer. *Adv Cancer Res* 2003; 90:127–156.
7. Jiang K, Zhong B, Gilvary DL, et al. Syk regulation of phosphoinositide 3-kinase-dependent NK cell function. *J Immunol* 2002; 168:3155–3164.
8. Djeu JY, Jiang K, Wei S. A view to a kill: signals triggering cytotoxicity. *Clin Cancer Res* 2002; 8:636–640.
9. Jiang K, Zhong B, Gilvary DL, et al. Pivotal role of phosphoinositide-3 kinase in regulation of cytotoxicity in natural killer cells. *Nat Immunol* 2000; 1:419–425.
10. Geldhof AB, Van Ginderachter JA, Liu Y, Noel W, Raes G, De Baetselier P. Antagonistic effect of NK cells on alternatively activated monocytes: a contribution of NK cells to CTL generation. *Blood* 2002; 100:4049–4058.
11. Smyth MJ, Crowe NY, Godfrey DI. NK cells and NKT cells collaborate in host protection from methyl-cholanthrene-induced fibrosarcoma. *Int Immunol* 2001; 13:459–463.
12. Crowe NY, Smyth MJ, Godfrey DI. A critical role for natural killer T cells in immunosurveillance of methylcholanthrene-induced sarcomas. *J Exp Med* 2002; 196:119–127.
13. van den Broeke LT, Daschbach E, Thomas EK, Andringa G, Berzofsky JA. Dendritic cell-induced activation of adaptive and innate antitumor immunity. *J Immunol* 2003; 171:5842–5852.
14. Kagi D, Ledermann B, Burki K, et al. Cytotoxicity mediated by T cells and natural killer cells is greatly impaired in perforin-deficient mice. *Nature* 1994; 369:31–37.
15. Redondo M, Garcia J, Villar E, et al. Major histocompatibility complex status in breast carcinogenesis and relationship to apoptosis. *Hum Pathol* 2003; 34:1283–1289.
16. Agrawal S, Kishore MC. MHC class I gene expression and regulation. J Hematother *Stem Cell Res* 2000; 9:795–812.
17. Atkins D, Ferrone S, Schmahl GE, Storkel S, Seliger B. Down-regulation of HLA class I antigen processing molecules: an immune escape mechanism of renal cell carcinoma? *J Urol* 2004; 171(Pt 1):885–889.
18. Vitale M, Rezzani R, Rodella L, et al. HLA class I antigen and transporter associated with antigen processing (TAP1 and TAP2) down-regulation in high-grade primary breast carcinoma lesions. *Cancer Res* 1998; 58:737–742.
19. Parham P, McQueen KL. Alloreactive killer cells: hindrance and help for haematopoietic transplants. *Nat Rev Immunol* 2003; 3:108–122.
20. Ruggeri L, Capanni M, Martelli MF, Velardi A. Cellular therapy: exploiting NK cell alloreactivity in transplantation. *Curr Opin Hematol* 2001; 8:355–359.

21. Grimm EA, Mazumder A, Zhang HZ, Rosenberg SA. Lymphokine-activated killer cell phenomenon. Lysis of natural killer-resistant fresh solid tumor cells by interleukin 2-activated autologous human peripheral blood lymphocytes. *J Exp Med* 1982; 155:1823–1841.

22. Grimm EA, Jacobs SK, Lanza LA, Melin G, Roth JA, Wilson DJ. Interleukin 2-activated cytotoxic lymphocytes in cancer therapy. *Symp Fundam Cancer Res* 1986; 38:209–219.

23. Phillips JH, Lanier LL. Dissection of the lymphokine-activated killer phenomenon. Relative contribution of peripheral blood natural killer cells and T lymphocytes to cytolysis. *J Exp Med* 1986; 164:814–825.

24. Rosenberg SA, Lotze MT, Muul LM, et al. Observations on the systemic administration of autologous lymphokine-activated killer cells and recombinant interleukin-2 to patients with metastatic cancer. *N Engl J Med* 1985; 313:1485–1492.

25. Ahlberg R, MacNamara B, Andersson M, et al. Stimulation of T-cell cytokine production and NK cell function by IL-2, IFN-alpha and histamine treatment during remission of non-Hodgkin's lymphoma. *Hematol J* 2003; 4:336–341.

26. Lehmann C, Zeis M, Uharek L. Activation of natural killer cells with interleukin 2 (IL-2) and IL-12 increases perforin binding and subsequent lysis of tumour cells. *Br J Haematol* 2001; 114:660–665.

27. Xiang J, Chen Z, Huang H, Moyana T. Regression of engineered myeloma cells secreting interferon-gamma-inducing factor is mediated by both CD4(+)/CD8(+) T and natural killer cells. *Leuk Res* 2001; 25:909–915.

28. Wang G, Tschoi M, Spolski R, et al. In vivo antitumor activity of interleukin 21 mediated by natural killer cells. *Cancer Res* 2003; 63:9016–9022.

29. Lum JJ, Schnepple DJ, Nie Z, et al. Differential effects of interleukin-7 and interleukin-15 on NK cell anti-human immunodeficiency virus activity. *J Virol* 2004; 78:6033–6042.

30. Peng BG, Liang LJ, He Q, Huang JF, Lu MD. Expansion and activation of natural killer cells from PBMC for immunotherapy of hepatocellular carcinoma. *World J Gastroenterol* 2004; 10:2119–2123.

31. Kennedy MK, Glaccum M, Brown SN, et al. Reversible defects in natural killer and memory CD8 T cell lineages in interleukin 15-deficient mice. *J Exp Med* 2000; 191:771–780.

32. Bigda J, Mysliwska J, Baran W, Hellmann A, Mysliwski A. Interleukin 2- and interferon alpha induced natural killer cell activity as a marker of progression in hairy cell leukemia. *Leuk Lymphoma* 1993; 9: 371–376.

33. Reiter Z, Ozes ON, Blatt LM, Taylor MW. Cytokine and natural killing regulation of growth of a hairy cell leukemia-like cell line: the role of interferon-alpha and interleukin-2. *J Immunother* 1992; 11:40–49.

34. Loza MJ, Perussia B. The IL-12 signature: NK cell terminal CD56+ high stage and effector functions. *J Immunol* 2004; 172:88–96.

35. Robertson MJ, Cameron C, Atkins MB, et al. Immunological effects of interleukin 12 administered by bolus intravenous injection to patients with cancer. *Clin Cancer Res* 1999; 5:9–16.

36. Liberati AM, De Angelis V, Fizzotti M, et al. Natural-killer-stimulatory effect of combined low-dose interleukin-2 and interferon beta in hairy-cell leukemia patients. *Cancer Immunol Immunother* 1994; 38:323–331.

37. Atzpodien J, Kirchner H, Korfer A, et al. Expansion of peripheral blood natural killer cells correlates with clinical outcome in cancer patients receiving recombinant subcutaneous interleukin-2 and interferon-alpha-2. *Tumour Biol* 1993; 14:354–359.

38. Zaki MH, Wysocka M, Everetts SE, et al. Synergistic enhancement of cell-mediated immunity by interleukin-12 plus interleukin-2: basis for therapy of cutaneous T cell lymphoma. *J Invest Dermatol* 2002; 118:366–371.

39. Ansell SM. Adding cytokines to monoclonal antibody therapy: does the concurrent administration of interleukin-12 add to the efficacy of rituximab in B-cell non-hodgkin lymphoma? *Leuk Lymphoma* 2003; 44:1309–1315.

40. Gluck WL, Hurst D, Yuen A, et al. Phase I studies of interleukin (IL)-2 and rituximab in B-cell non-Hodgkin's lymphoma: IL-2 mediated natural killer cell expansion correlations with clinical response. *Clin Cancer Res* 2004; 10:2253–2264.

41. Repka T, Chiorean EG, Gay J, et al. Trastuzumab and interleukin-2 in HER2-positive metastatic breast cancer: a pilot study. *Clin Cancer Res* 2003; 9:2440–2446.

42. Krause SW, Gastpar R, Andreesen R, et al. Treatment of colon and lung cancer patients with ex vivo heat shock protein 70-peptide-activated, autologous natural killer cells: a clinical phase I trial. *Clin Cancer Res* 2004; 10:3699–3707.

43. Xu D, Gu P, Pan PY, Li Q, Sato AI, Chen SH. NK and CD8+ T cell-mediated eradication of poorly immunogenic B16-F10 melanoma by the combined action of IL-12 gene therapy and 4-1BB costimulation. *Int J Cancer* 2004; 109:499–506.

44. Robertson MJ. Role of chemokines in the biology of natural killer cells. *J Leukoc Biol* 2002; 71:173–183.

45. Robinson LA, Nataraj C, Thomas DW, et al. The chemokine CX3CL1 regulates NK cell activity in vivo. *Cell Immunol* 2003; 225:122–130.

46. Guo J, Chen T, Wang B, et al. Chemoattraction, adhesion and activation of natural killer cells are involved in the antitumor immune response induced by fractalkine/CX3CL1. *Immunol Lett* 2003; 89:1–7.

47. Amakata Y, Fujiyama Y, Andoh A, Hodohara K, Bamba T. Mechanism of NK cell activation induced by coculture with dendritic cells derived from peripheral blood monocytes. *Clin Exp Immunol* 2001; 124: 214–222.

48. Turner JG, Rakhmilevich AL, Burdelya L, et al. Anti-CD40 antibody induces antitumor and antimetastatic effects: the role of NK cells. *J Immunol* 2001; 166:89–94.

49. Powzaniuk MA, Trotta R, Loza MJ, et al. B-Myb overexpression results in activation and increased Fas/Fas ligand-mediated cytotoxicity of T and NK cells. *J Immunol* 2001; 167:242–249.

50. Davies FE, Raje N, Hideshima T, et al. Thalidomide and immunomodulatory derivatives augment natural killer cell cytotoxicity in multiple myeloma. *Blood* 2001; 98:210–216.

51. Lozupone F, Pende D, Burgio VL, et al. Effect of human natural killer and gammadelta T cells on the growth of human autologous melanoma xenografts in SCID mice. *Cancer Res* 2004; 64:378–385.

52. Brand JM, Meller B, Von Hof K, et al. Kinetics and organ distribution of allogeneic natural killer lymphocytes transfused into patients suffering from renal cell carcinoma. *Stem Cell Dev* 2004; 13:307–314.

53. Schirrmann T, Pecher G. Tumor-specific targeting of a cell line with natural killer cell activity by asialoglycoprotein receptor gene transfer. *Cancer Immunol Immunother* 2001; 50:549–556.

54. Schirrmann T, Pecher G. Human natural killer cell line modified with a chimeric immunoglobulin T-cell receptor gene leads to tumor growth inhibition in vivo. *Cancer Gene Ther* 2002; 9:390–398.

55. Yan Y, Steinherz P, Klingemann HG, et al. Antileukemia activity of a natural killer cell line against human leukemias. *Clin Cancer Res* 1998; 4:2859–2868.

56. Zhang J, Sun R, Wei H, Tian Z. Characterization of interleukin-15 gene-modified human natural killer cells: implications for adoptive cellular immunotherapy. *Haematologica* 2004; 89:338–347.

57. Zhang J, Sun R, Wei H, Tian Z. Characterization of stem cell factor gene-modified human natural killer cell line, NK-92 cells: implication in NK cell-based adoptive cellular immunotherapy. *Oncol Rep* 2004; 11:1097–1106.

58. Hartmann F, Renner C, Jung W, et al. Anti-CD16/CD30 bispecific antibody treatment for Hodgkin's disease: role of infusion schedule and costimulation with cytokines. *Clin Cancer Res* 2001; 7:1873–1881.

59. Heuser C, Guhlke S, Matthies A, et al. Anti-CD30-scFv-Fc-IL-2 antibody-cytokine fusion protein that induces resting NK cells to highly efficient cytolysis of Hodgkin's lymphoma derived tumour cells. *Int J Cancer* 2004; 110:386–394.

60. Hoffmann TK, Bier H, Whiteside TL. Targeting the immune system: novel therapeutic approaches in squamous cell carcinoma of the head and neck. *Cancer Immunol Immunother* 2004; 53:1055–1067.

61. Dudley ME, Rosenberg SA. Adoptive-cell-transfer therapy for the treatment of patients with cancer. *Nat Rev Cancer* 2003; 3:666–675.

62. Rosenberg SA. Progress in human tumour immunology and immunotherapy. *Nature* 2001; 411:380–384.

63. Igarashi T, Wynberg J, Srinivasan R, et al. Enhanced cytotoxicity of allogeneic NK cells with killer immunoglobulin-like receptor ligand incompatibility against melanoma and renal cell carcinoma cells. *Blood* 2004; 104:170–177.

64. Ruggeri L, Capanni M, Urbani E, et al. Effectiveness of donor natural killer cell alloreactivity in mismatched hematopoietic transplants. *Science* 2002; 295:2097–2100.

65. Velardi A, Ruggeri L, Moretta A, Moretta L. NK cells: a lesson from mismatched hematopoietic transplantation. *Trends Immunol* 2002; 23:438–444.

66. Leung W, Iyengar R, Turner V, et al. Determinants of antileukemia effects of allogeneic NK cells. *J Immunol* 2004; 172:644–650.

67. Koh CY, Blazar BR, George T, et al. Augmentation of antitumor effects by NK cell inhibitory receptor blockade in vitro and in vivo. *Blood* 2001; 97:3132–3237.

68. Koh CY, Raziuddin A, Welniak LA, Blazar BR, Bennett M, Murphy WJ. NK inhibitory-receptor blockade for purging of leukemia: effects on hematopoietic reconstitution. *Biol Blood Marrow Transplant* 2002; 8:17–25.

69. Asai O, Longo DL, Tian ZG, et al. Suppression of graft-versus-host disease and amplification of graft-versus-tumor effects by activated natural killer cells after allogeneic bone marrow transplantation. *J Clin Invest* 1998; 101:1835–1842.

70. Rosenthal FM, Zier KS, Gansbacher B. Human tumor vaccines and genetic engineering of tumors with cytokine and histocompatibility genes to enhance immunogenicity. *Curr Opin Oncol* 1994; 6:611–615.

71. Rosenthal FM, Cronin K, Bannerji R, Golde DW, Gansbacher B. Augmentation of antitumor immunity by tumor cells transduced with a retroviral vector carrying the interleukin-2 and interferon-gamma cDNAs. *Blood* 1994; 83:1289–1298.

72. Bannerji R, Arroyo CD, Cordon-Cardo C, Gilboa E. The role of IL-2 secreted from genetically modified tumor cells in the establishment of antitumor immunity. *J Immunol* 1994; 152:2324–2332.

73. Yang S, Vervaert CE, Seigler HF, Darrow TL. Tumor cells cotransduced with B7.1 and gamma-IFN induce effective rejection of established parental tumor. *Gene Ther* 1999; 6:253–262.

74. Kundu N, Fulton AM. Interleukin-10 inhibits tumor metastasis, downregulates MHC class I, and enhances NK lysis. *Cell Immunol* 1997; 180:55–61.

75. Ugai S, Shimozato O, Yu L, et al. Transduction of the IL-21 and IL-23 genes in human pancreatic carcinoma cells produces natural killer cell-dependent and -independent antitumor effects. *Cancer Gene Ther* 2003; 10:771–778.

76. Braun SE, Chen K, Foster RG, et al. The CC chemokine CK beta-11/MIP-3 beta/ELC/Exodus 3 mediates tumor rejection of murine breast cancer cells through NK cells. *J Immunol* 2000; 164:4025–4031.

77. Diefenbach A, Jensen ER, Jamieson AM, Raulet DH. Rae1 and H60 ligands of the NKG2D receptor stimulate tumour immunity. *Nature* 2001; 413:165–171.

78. Cerwenka A, Baron JL, Lanier LL. Ectopic expression of retinoic acid early inducible-1 gene (RAE-1) permits natural killer cell-mediated rejection of a MHC class I-bearing tumor in vivo. *Proc Natl Acad Sci USA* 2001; 98:11,521–11,526.

79. Groh V, Wu J, Yee C, Spies T. Tumour-derived soluble MIC ligands impair expression of NKG2D and T-cell activation. *Nature* 2002; 419:734–738.

80. Wu JD, Higgins LM, Steinle A, Cosman D, Haugk K, Plymate SR. Prevalent expression of the immunostimulatory MHC class I chain-related molecule is counteracted by shedding in prostate cancer. *J Clin Invest* 2004; 114:560–568.

81. Salih HR, Rammensee HG, Steinle A. Cutting edge: down-regulation of MICA on human tumors by proteolytic shedding. *J Immunol* 2002; 169:4098–4102.

82. de Visser KE, Kast WM. Effects of TGF-beta on the immune system: implications for cancer immunotherapy. *Leukemia* 1999; 13:1188–1199.

83. Lee JC, Lee KM, Kim DW, Heo DS. Elevated TGF-beta1 secretion and down-modulation of NKG2D underlies impaired NK cytotoxicity in cancer patients. *J Immunol* 2004; 172:7335–7340.

84. Seo N, Tokura Y, Takigawa M, Egawa K. Depletion of IL-10- and TGF-beta-producing regulatory gamma delta T cells by administering a daunomycin-conjugated specific monoclonal antibody in early tumor lesions augments the activity of CTLs and NK cells. *J Immunol* 1999; 163:242–249.

85. Marzo AL, Fitzpatrick DR, Robinson BW, Scott B. Antisense oligonucleotides specific for transforming growth factor beta2 inhibit the growth of malignant mesothelioma both in vitro and in vivo. *Cancer Res* 1997; 57:3200–3207.

86. Arteaga CL, Hurd SD, Winnier AR, Johnson MD, Fendly BM, Forbes JT. Anti-transforming growth factor (TGF)-beta antibodies inhibit breast cancer cell tumorigenicity and increase mouse spleen natural killer cell activity. Implications for a possible role of tumor cell/host TGF-beta interactions in human breast cancer progression. *J Clin Invest* 1993; 92:2569–2576.

87. Mailliard RB, Son YI, Redlinger R, et al. Dendritic cells mediate NK cell help for Th1 and CTL responses: two-signal requirement for the induction of NK cell helper function. *J Immunol* 2003; 171:2366–2373.

88. Moretta L, Ferlazzo G, Mingari MC, Melioli G, Moretta A. Human natural killer cell function and their interactions with dendritic cells. *Vaccine* 2003; 21(Suppl 2):S38–S42.

89. Alli RS, Khar A. Interleukin-12 secreted by mature dendritic cells mediates activation of NK cell function. *FEBS Lett* 2004; 559:71–76.

90. Westwood JA, Kelly JM, Tanner JE, Kershaw MH, Smyth MJ, Hayakawa Y. Cutting edge: novel priming of tumor-specific immunity by NKG2D-triggered NK cell-mediated tumor rejection and Th1-independent CD4+ T cell pathway. *J Immunol* 2004; 172:757–761.

91. Akbar SM, Murakami H, Horiike N, Onji M. Dendritic cell-based therapies in the bench and the bedsides. *Curr Drug Targets Inflamm Allergy* 2004; 3:305–310.

92. Albertsson PA, Basse PH, Hokland M, et al. NK cells and the tumour microenvironment: implications for NK-cell function and anti-tumour activity. *Trends Immunol* 2003; 24:603–609.

4

The Role of Immune Monitoring in Evaluating Cancer Immunotherapy

Holden T. Maecker

SUMMARY

Just as cancer vaccines have evolved tremendously over the past decades, so too have the methods used to monitor the immune responses that they are intended to induce. In this chapter, current cellular immune monitoring methods will be reviewed briefly in an effort to compare and contrast their utility. These methods include cytotoxicity and proliferation assays (radioactive and nonradioactive), cytokine assays (bulk and single-cell assays), and major histocompatibility complex–peptide multimer staining. Furthermore, the role that these assays can play in evaluating a cancer vaccine will be examined critically. It is likely that modern immune monitoring assays can be useful for comparing the immunogenicity of different vaccine approaches, even across clinical trials, but only if they are sufficiently standardized. Whether such assays will eventually be able to predict clinical efficacy of a vaccine remains to be determined.

Key Words: Intracellular cytokine: T-cell; immune function; in vitro; cellular immunity.

1. DESCRIPTION OF ASSAYS

1.1. Historical Perspective

In the 1950s, it was first demonstrated that mice could be rendered immune to a syngeneic tumor via pre-exposure to killed tumor cells *(1)*. Experiments in the following decades suggested the widely generalized conclusion that, whereas tumor-specific antibodies might be sufficient for protection against leukemias, cellular immunity was responsible for immunity to most tumors *(2,3)*. However, viable methods for inducing cellular immune responses in humans have only recently been brought to bear *(4,5)*. These include the use of antigen-pulsed dendritic cells or vaccines containing adjuvants such as cytosine/phosphate/guanine-rich oligodeoxynucleotides. Even these modalities may not prove sufficient to induce protective responses against the majority of human tumors, but some modest successes have spurred the initiation of many new clinical trials in a variety of solid tumor settings *(6–11)*.

Along with the difficulty of inducing strong cellular immune responses has been the difficulty of assaying for those responses *(12,13)*. Early assays, used successfully in mouse models, included proliferation assays based on ^{3}H-thymidine incorporation, and cytotoxicity assays based on ^{51}Cr release. The former was taken largely as an indicator of antigen-

From: *Cancer Drug Discovery and Development: Immunotherapy of Cancer*
Edited by: M. L. Disis © Humana Press Inc., Totowa, NJ

specific CD4 T-cell activity *(14)*, whereas the latter was presumed to be a measure of antigen-specific CD8 T-cell function *(15)*. However, in addition to being labor-intensive and difficult to perform reproducibly, these assays were not particularly quantitative. Absolute comparisons between labs, or even between experiments, were difficult to make. Moreover, because the assays were read out from bulk cultures, it was impossible to be sure which phenotype of cells was responsible for the observed activity.

1.2. Modern Assays of Cellular Immunity

Single-cell assays, detected via imaging or flow cytometry, have revolutionized the cellular immune monitoring field *(16,17)*, just as new vaccine modalities have reinvigorated the field of tumor immunotherapy. These assays include enzyme-linked immunospot (ELISPOT) *(18)* and cytokine flow cytometry (CFC) *(19)* as measures of cytokine-producing cells, CD107 expression as a measure of degranulation *(20)*, major histocompatibility complex (MHC)–peptide tetramer staining as a measure of epitope-specific T-cells *(21)*, and proliferative assays based on bromodeoxyuridine (BrdU) *(22)* or carboxyfluorescein succinimidyl ester (CFSE) labeling *(23)*. These assays all bring much-needed quantitation to cellular immune monitoring, as they have the ability to count a true number of antigen-specific or antigen-responsive cells. Methods based on flow cytometry as a readout (CFC, CD107, tetramers, and BrdU/CFSE) have the additional ability to simultaneously phenotype the cells of interest, determining not only their T-cell subset (CD4 or CD8) but also their expression of any number of memory/effector or activation markers.

1.2.1. ENZYME-LINKED IMMUNOSPOT ASSAYS

ELISPOT assays are based on the capture of secreted cytokines by cells plated on filter-bottom, multiwell plates *(18)*. The plates are first coated with a cytokine-capture antibody, and, after incubation with stimulated cells for 24–48 h, are then treated with an enzyme-labeled detector antibody. Colored spots indicative of cytokine-secreting cells are visualized by addition of a substrate. The spots are counted, either manually using a dissecting microscope or by an automated plate reader, and the results reported as spot-forming cells (SFCs) per X input peripheral blood mononuclear cells ([PBMCs]; usually 10^6 PBMCs).

Two major attributes of ELISPOT are responsible for its popularity: the ability to work in 96-well plates and use automated readers results in reasonably high throughput, and the assay can be quite sensitive, thanks to generally low backgrounds of cytokine-secreting cells. Most laboratories would consider 20 SFCs per 10^6 PBMCs as a positive result, given a background of 0–5 SFCs per 10^6 PBMCs. This results in a sensitivity of 1/50,000, which is difficult to achieve by other methodologies.

1.2.2. CYTOKINE FLOW CYTOMETRY

CFC is a general term for the flow cytometric detection of cytokines, with the most common methodology being intracellular cytokine staining ([ICS] Fig. 1A *[24,25]*). These assays use shorter stimulation times than ELISPOT (most commonly 6 h), and can be done using either whole blood *(26)* or PBMCs *(19)*. The cells are fixed, permeabilized, and then subjected to staining for intracellular (and cell surface) markers. For surface-staining antibodies whose binding is sensitive to fixation and permeabilization, a staining step can be added before fixation.

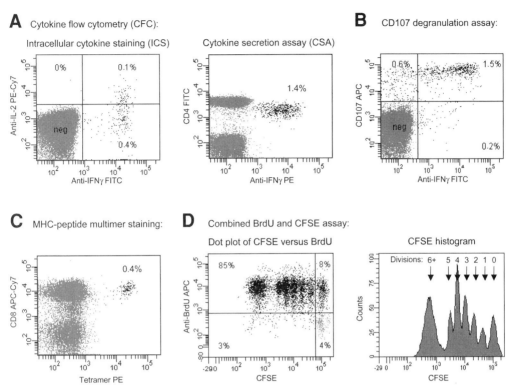

Fig. 1. Examples of data from single-cell flow cytometric assays. **(A)** Cytokine flow cytometry can be performed by intracellular cytokine staining (left panel, in this example using peripheral blood mononuclear cells [PBMCs] stimulated with a peptide mixture corresponding to cytomegalovirus pp65+IE-1 proteins, and showing interferon [IFN]-γ vs interleukin-2 staining from CD3⁺CD4⁺ lymphocytes). When enrichment or further manipulation of live antigen-specific cells is desired, a cytokine secretion assay can be performed (right panel, PBMCs stimulated with pp65 protein and showing IFN-γ vs CD4 staining from CD3⁺ lymphocytes). **(B)** CD107 staining as a measure of degranulation is shown in this example using PBMCs stimulated with a pp65 peptide mixture. Staining for IFN-γ vs CD107 is shown for CD3⁺CD8⁺ lymphocytes. **(C)** Major histocompatibility complex–peptide multimer staining was performed in this example using PBMCs stained with a human leukocyte antigen-A0201 tetramer loaded with cytomegalovirus pp65$_{495–503}$ peptide. CD8 vs tetramer staining is shown for CD3⁺ lymphocytes. **(D)** Combined bromodeoxyuridine (BrdU) and carboxyfluorescein succinimidyl ester (CFSE) labeling was performed in this example using PBMCs stimulated with staphylococcal enterotoxin B for 5 d, with BrdU present for the last 6 h of stimulation. CFSE vs BrdU staining is shown for CD3⁺CD8⁺ lymphocytes (left panel). A histogram of CFSE staining for the same population is shown in the right panel, with peaks labeled according to the number of cell divisions. (All data are from the IFCS 2004 course at BD Biosciences, October 19–22, 2004, http://www.ifcs2004.org/, except panel B, which is courtesy of Maria Suni, BD Biosciences, San Jose, CA.)

Other variations of CFC include the cytokine secretion assay (*see* Fig. 1A *[27]*), in which bifunctional antibodies are used to label leukocytes and make them act as surface capture sites for secreted cytokine. Under the right conditions of incubation time and cell concentration, cytokines secreted by stimulated cells will tend to be captured by the same cells, allowing for quantitation by flow cytometry and/or enrichment by magnetic particle labeling. The cytokine secretion assay, although technically more demanding than ICS, has the advantage of allowing for sorting and enrichment of live cytokine-producing cells.

The major attribute of CFC driving its increasing popularity is its multiparametric nature. By reading out not only CD4 and/or CD8 T-cell subset markers, but also multiple cytokines and memory/effector markers, CFC has the potential to functionally characterize the responding cells beyond the capabilities of any other assays. In addition, the relatively short turnaround time and compatibility with multiwell plates makes it possible to consider CFC as a monitoring assay, even for relatively large clinical trials.

1.2.3. CD107 DEGRANULATION ASSAY

A relatively new methodology, CD107 degranulation assays rely on the exocytosis of granule proteins CD107a and CD107b (also known as lysomal-associated membrane protein 1 and lysomal-associated membrane protein 2, respectively) from the membrane of cytotoxic granules to the cell membrane on engagement of a cytotoxic cell with its target (see Fig. 1B; [20]). This transient cell-surface expression of CD107 proteins is most efficiently detected by addition of fluorescent-labeled antibodies to CD107 during an incubation period of 4–6 h.

Like CFC, CD107 assays provide a multiparametric readout of antigen-specific cell function. Because they can easily be combined with intracellular cytokine detection, they can essentially be considered part of the CFC assay family, adding degranulation as a functional readout in addition to cytokines. However, it should be noted that technical conditions of stimulation, such as the use and concentration of monensin vs brefeldin A as a protein trafficking inhibitor, will affect differentially the readout of CD107 and certain cytokines. Thus, it is important when doing such combined assays that the results be compared with single CFC and CD107 assays done under optimal conditions to avoid a biased readout because of compromises made in the combined assay conditions.

1.2.4. MHC–PEPTIDE MULTIMER STAINING

Perhaps the simplest of the cellular immune monitoring assays is based on the binding of multimeric MHC–peptide complexes to T-cells that display cognate T-cell receptor specificity (see Fig. 1C; [21]). By fluorescent labeling of the MHC–peptide complexes, it is possible to create a multiparametric flow cytometry assay. Whereas multimerization of the MHC–peptide complex is required for avid binding, dimers (28), tetramers (21), and pentamers (http://www.proimmune.com/) have all been used successfully.

A salient feature of these assays is their functional independence (which allows readout of all cells of a given specificity). By combining these assays with CFC, for example, it is possible to detect what fraction of epitope-specific cells has a given function like cytokine production. As mentioned earlier, combined assays should first be validated against single multimer or CFC assays to avoid bias in the combined readout.

1.2.5. PROLIFERATION ASSAYS BASED ON BrdU INCORPORATION OR CFSE LABELING

Recently, a resurgence of interest in proliferation assays by flow cytometry has occurred, in part because of the technical development of assays based on BrdU (22) and CFSE labeling (23), and in part because of findings in the HIV field that the proliferative potential of antigen-specific CD8 T-cells may predict clinical outcome (29,30).

Whereas the two assays are fundamentally different, both measure in vitro proliferation of stimulated cells, usually in 2–7 d, but it can be even longer. CFSE assays require the prelabeling of cells with the cytophilic dye, CFSE, which remains bound to intracytoplasmic proteins. With each cell division, the amount of CFSE fluorescence is essentially halved, allowing one to count the number of divisions that a set of cells has undergone. In practice, this can become difficult, particularly beyond three or four divisions, unless labeling conditions are ideal. The readout of CFSE by flow cytometry can be combined with other markers, including cytokines (if the cells are restimulated in the presence of a secretion inhibitor for the terminal part of the incubation). It should be noted, however, that phenotypic and functional markers detected at the end of a lengthy stimulation period may or may not be indicative of the expression of those markers by the precursor cells immediately ex vivo.

BrdU incorporation is, in one sense, a simpler assay, in that it does not require prelabeling of cells. BrdU is simply added at some point in the culture period and becomes incorporated into DNA by dividing cells. It is detected by anti-BrdU antibodies, which are generally used along with fixation, permeabilization, and DNase treatment of the cells, to allow the antibody access to BrdU incorporated into the cell's DNA. BrdU incorporation does not lend itself to counting of cell divisions as does CFSE, although it is arguably more sensitive, in that it can detect cells that have synthesized DNA but have not yet divided (*see* Fig. 1D).

The main advantage of both of these methods is that they allow for a single-cell, multiparametric readout of proliferative potential, which is impossible by any other methodology. It should be realized that this is tempered by the loss of quantitation associated with longer stimulation periods, as one cannot accurately account for apoptosis of stimulated cells. However, these assays can be used as an independent readout, in addition to shortterm assays, such as CFC, to assess proliferative capacity in a semiquantitative manner.

2. COMPARISON OF ASSAYS

Numerous studies have compared subsets of the above assays to each other and to traditional bulk assays, such as ^{3}H-thymidine incorporation and ^{51}Cr release *(31–37)*. Such comparisons can be biased by the technical conditions used, especially because there is no universal agreement on optimally standardized versions of most of these assays. Despite this caveat, some generalizations can be drawn with regard to sensitivity, background, turnaround time, readout, and automation compatibility of the various assays (Table 1).

2.1. Quantitative Aspects

2.1.1. DEFINING AND MEASURING SENSITIVITY

Assay sensitivity has been a contentious topic on several levels. First, what is meant by sensitivity? Second, how should sensitivity be measured? Third, what is the required sensitivity of a method to be useful for cancer vaccine monitoring?

The answer to the first question may seem obvious. Sensitivity can be defined as the lowest limit of detection of a positive signal above background. Thus, ELISPOT assays, which can easily detect one positive event in 50,000 or even lower *(38)*, have the lowest limit of detection of any of the assays previously discussed. However, head-to-head comparisons of ELISPOT and CFC have generally concluded that CFC assays detect a higher frequency of positive cells in clinical samples *(31–34,37)*. How is this possible? A clue may be found in the backgrounds of the two assays: CFC generally has backgrounds in the range of 0.01–0.05% *(39)*, whereas ELISPOT backgrounds tend to be much lower, approx 1–5 per 10^6 PBMCs *(40–42)*. Assuming that much of the background is true cytokine-producing cells, this suggests that ELISPOT actually has a lower efficiency of detection than

Table 1
Assay Comparisons

Feature	ELISPOT	CFC	CD107	MHC–peptide multimers	BrdU or CFSE
Typical limit of detection	1:50,000 PBMC	0.05% of CD4 or 0.12% of CD8 T-cells	0.2% of CD8 T-cells	0.02% of CD8 T-cells	0.2% of CD4 or CD8 T-cells
Typical background	<1:200,000	0.01% of CD4, 0.03% of CD8 T-cells	0.05% of CD8 T-cells	0.005% of CD8 T-cells	0.05% of CD4 or CD 8 T-cells
Detection efficiency	Low	High	High	High	High
Turnaround time	2 d	10 h	10 h	3 h	3–7 d
Information content	Low	High	High	High, but epitope restricted	High, but semi-quantitative
Automation potential	Medium	Medium	Medium	High	Low

ELISPOT, enzyme-linked immunospot; CFC, cytokine flow cytometry; MHC, major histocompatibility complex; BrdU, bromodeoxyuridine; CFSE, carboxyfluorescein succinimidyl ester.

CFC. This could be because CFC detects cells that only express cytokine transiently and do not build up enough secreted cytokine to be seen by ELISPOT. What is not clear is whether the reduced detection efficiency of ELISPOT is fully offset by the reduced background; in part, this depends on what criteria for positivity over background are applied.

This leads to the second question of how to measure sensitivity. A general methodology might be as follows. First, identify a donor that has a known positive response and another that has a known negative response. Next, perform serial dilutions of the positive donor's cells into the cells of the negative donor, and then perform the assays in question. The limit of detection of each assay is taken as the lowest point at which a positive response can be determined as statistically different from negative (defined by the response from the negative donor alone). The efficiency of detection can be taken as the ratio of the response from a given assay to the response from a "gold standard" assay at that response level. The efficiency of detection may vary, of course, with response magnitude. Whereas the limit of detection is what is most traditionally referred to as sensitivity, both limit of detection and detection efficiency impact the utility of the assay.

Having defined sensitivity and how it might best be measured, we can then also ask the question: What level of sensitivity is required for monitoring of cancer vaccines? This is the most difficult question, because there is, as of yet, no correlation of a particular cellular immune response with protection by a cancer vaccine in humans. There is thus no way to determine what level of cellular immune response would need to be measured to have clinical utility. There are data in mice suggesting that the magnitude of an interferon (IFN)-γ response can predict clearance of tumor from vaccinated mice on challenge *(43)*. However, this study used reverse transcriptase-polymerase chain reaction to measure IFN-γ production, so translating magnitudes to those found by methods more commonly used in human clinical trials is difficult. Some relevant information may be gleaned from cellular responses to infectious diseases. Chronic viral diseases, such as cytomegalovirus and HIV, tend to induce strong cellular immune responses, well above 0.1% as measured by IFN-γ CFC (*[19,39,44–47]*; although responses to HIV decline with antiviral therapy or with progressive disease). Theoretical calculations have suggested that similar or even higher levels of cellular responses would be required for prophylactic vaccines in HIV *(48)*. If this were true, we might assume that cancer vaccines will also need to induce high-level responses, above the limit of detection of all the assays mentioned in this chapter. This leads to a conundrum, because current cancer vaccines have generally not induced such strong responses in the majority of vaccinees. Thus, there is a tendency to choose the assay with the lowest limit of detection to look for any indication of a cellular response, even if that response might not be clinically relevant.

2.1.2. Quantitative Comparisons Among Assays

With these ideas in mind, it is clear that meaningful quantitative comparisons among different assays are rare. Whiteside et al. compared ELISPOT, CFC, and tetramer assays in the setting of a multi-epitope melanoma vaccine *(36)*. Although responses to the vaccine were few and weak, the highest number of peptide-specific CD8+ T-cells could be detected by tetramer, followed by CFC, and then ELISPOT assays. Stronger responses were seen in a study by Walker et al. to a melanoma peptide vaccine *(49)*. These authors compared tetramer and CFC responses in 33 patients and found excellent correlation. However, several patients showed discordance between the two assays, in which tetramer staining was consistently higher than IFN-γ CFC. This was attributed to the postvaccination development of anergic cells, which had specificity for the cognate MHC–peptide complex but could not produce cytokines.

Comparisons between assays in infectious disease settings are more numerous *(31–35,37)*. These studies generally concur with the conclusions above, namely that the efficiency of detection of tetramer assays is higher than that of CFC or ELISPOT (likely because of the occurrence of nonfunctional cells), and that the efficiency of detection of CFC is the same or higher than that of ELISPOT. CD107 degranulation tends to correlate with CFC *(20,50,51)*, although there are differences in stimulation thresholds for each assay, and there can be significant populations of CD107+/IFN-γ− and (less frequently) CD107−/IFN-γ+ populations of antigen-specific cells. Some studies have suggested potential cutoffs for positivity in CFC or ELISPOT based on studies of HIV- or cytomegalovirus-seropositive vs -seronegative donors *(37,39,52)*. Whereas these are in general agreement, there are variations dependent on antigen and sample type that suggest no universal cutoff can be applied to all assays of a given type.

2.1.3. Maximizing Results for a Given Assay

As a caveat to comparisons such as those listed earlier, one should realize that there are procedural variables that can affect the detection limit, background, and detection efficiency of any assay. These would in turn affect the comparison of that assay to other methods. Some of these variables will be unique to each assay, but others are common among several assays. These include sample type, stimulation efficiency, processing variables, number of events collected, and sample carryover artifacts.

The most common sample type used in clinical trials is cryopreserved PBMCs. As such, the method of cryopreservation can play a large role in the functional response obtained

Table 2
Number of Events to Collect to Discriminate Low Responses From Background

Background (%)	Lowest positive (%)	Number of events to collect	
		90% Power, p < 0.05	99% Power, p < 0.005
0.01	0.02	260,000	720,000
0.01	0.05	32,000	90,000
0.01	0.10	12,000	32,000
0.02	0.05	67,000	190,000
0.02	0.10	16,000	45,000
0.03	0.05	170,000	480,000
0.03	0.10	23,000	63,000
0.04	0.10	33,000	93,000
0.05	0.10	52,000	140,000
0.06	0.10	86,000	240,000
0.07	0.10	160,000	450,000
0.08	0.20	17,000	46,000
0.10	0.20	26,000	72,000

after thawing *(53,54)*. Even under the best circumstances, the response in cryopreserved PBMCs may be compromised compared with the response in fresh PBMC *(54a)*. However, this difference is minimized when peptide antigens are used as opposed to whole proteins *(55)*. Fresh whole blood and PBMCs are generally thought to be comparable *(26)*, although there is some evidence for superior results in PBMCs *(56)*.

Stimulation efficiency is a consideration for all functional assays. It is dependent on such variables as the type of stimulus (peptide, protein, etc. *[55]*), stimulation vessel (tube or well geometry and type of plastic), stimulation time *(57)*, stimulus concentration *(50)*, and presence of exogenous costimulatory antibodies (e.g., CD28 and CD49d; *[58]*).

Processing variables known to affect results include such things as the type and concentration of substrate used in ELISPOT assays, the type and concentration of secretion inhibitor used in CFC *(59)* and CD107 assays *(20)*, the use of EDTA to remove adherent cells in CFC, the method (including time and temperature) of cell permeabilization in ICS assays, and the addition of MHC–peptide multimers before or after stimulation.

The number of events collected in flow cytometry, or the number of input cells in ELISPOT, is directly proportional to the ability to discriminate low-positive responses from background. This can be determined by a power calculation (*[60]*; Table 2). For example, discrimination of a response of 0.05% from a background of 0.02% would require collection of 67,000 relevant events (CD4 or CD8 T-cells, for example), in order to attain 90% power and $p < 0.05$. On the other hand, a response of 0.1% can be distinguished from a background of 0.02% with collection of just 16,000 relevant events, for the same power and p value.

A related question centers around the precision of a measurement for a given number of events collected. Statistics can also be used to determine a confidence interval around the difference between two proportions, i.e., the difference between the percentage of positive cells in a test sample and the percentage of positive cells in a negative control. This confidence interval is entirely dependent on the number of events in each sample file

Table 3
Example of Confidence Interval Calculations
to Determine Whether Two Cytokine Flow Cytometry Results Are Significantly Different

Background (%)	Response (%)	Net response (%)	95% Confidence interval	Overlap?
For 25,000 relevant events per sample:				
0.01	0.11	0.10	0.057–0.143	Yes
0.01	0.20	0.19	0.133–0.247	
For 35,000 relevant events per sample:				
0.01	0.11	0.10	0.064–0.136	No
0.01	0.20	0.19	0.142–0.238	

(Table 3). Thus, the number of cells analyzed per sample will directly affect the observed sensitivity and precision of the assay.

Flow cytometry assays are subject to "carryover," or detection of events originating from a previous sample during the collection of a later sample. Such carryover can be partly instrument-dependent, but can also be dependent on procedural variables. For example, thorough backflushing of the fluidic system and/or running of a blank tube between samples can reduce the potential for carryover. In addition, placement of strong positive control samples at the end, rather than the beginning, of an experimental run, can reduce carryover artifacts.

The variability in protocols commonly in place in different laboratories means that factors, such as those listed in this section, can and do affect the results of the assays in question. Until these assays are standardized better, quantitative comparisons between different assays will be subject to differential results based on these kinds of variables.

2.2. Qualitative Aspects

In addition to the quantitative aspects of limit of detection, background, and detection efficiency, there are qualitative aspects that are easier to compare between the various cellular assays (see Table 1). Let us briefly consider these from the standpoint of their applicability to clinical trial immune monitoring.

First, there is assay turnaround time. This encompasses both incubation and sample handling time. One could argue that minimization of both is desirable: short incubation times increase accuracy by reducing the incidence of apoptosis and/or proliferative expansion, and short sample handling times increase throughput and reduce the chances of error. Tetramer assays, being the simplest in terms of protocol, have the shortest turnaround time, followed by CFC and CD107 assays, then ELISPOT and proliferation assays.

A second consideration is the information content of the assays. ELISPOT is limited to one, or at most, two parameters, whereas flow cytometry-based assays can assess many more parameters at once. MHC–peptide multimers have a different limitation in information content, in that they are restricted to detection of a single epitope, which is not likely to be representative of the response to a larger antigen (61,62). Moreover, because they are phenotypic assays, they cannot be used to assess cell function except in combination with assays like CFC.

A final consideration is that of automation capability. Simple assays, such as MHC–peptide multimer staining, may not require significant automation to be scalable to large clinical trials, but more complex assays will. Fortunately, all of the flow-cytometry based assays, and ELISPOT as well, are compatible with multiwell plate formats. Optimization of CFC in 96-well plates has recently been published (63,64). Further automation, in the form of sample-handling robotics, is also possible, although significantly more difficult to achieve (65).

3. EXAMPLES FROM CLINICAL TRIALS

In this section, we will consider selected examples of clinical trial results in which the cellular immune monitoring assays discussed earlier generated detectable ex vivo responses, and the lessons that these studies have taught.

3.1. Melanoma

Human melanomas are particularly antigenic tumors, such that CD8$^+$ T-cells specific for melanoma-associated antigens (melanoma antigen recognized by T-cells 1 or tyrosinase) could sometimes be detected without any prior vaccination (66). However, these T-cells, measured by MHC–peptide tetramers, were frequently nonfunctional for cytokine production.

Following vaccination with gp100-derived peptides, cytokine-producing T-cells could be readily detected by tetramer and CFC assays in a number of clinical trials (36,49,67–69). The responses in these studies ranged from 0.1 to 3.5% of CD8$^+$ T-cells and could be detected in the vast majority of patients in one study (49). These represent probably the highest and most consistent cellular immune responses reported in any tumor vaccine setting. However, discordance between tetramer staining and IFN-γ production have been noted (49,69), suggesting that some of the responses induced are nonfunctional. In addition, the fraction of tetramer-positive cells that could degranulate in response to antigen as displayed on tumor target cells was generally low in postvaccine samples (51). Furthermore, tetramer and CFC responses have not usually correlated with clinical regressions in these studies (67,68). These findings suggest that the quality of cellular responses elicited to date with melanoma vaccines may be insufficient to induce consistent clinical remissions.

3.2. Other Tumors

Most other solid tumors appear to be less immunogenic than melanomas, given the number of tumor-specific antigens that have been isolated. In addition, most vaccine trials have been conducted in patients with late-stage disease, in which the immune system already is likely to be suppressed significantly. Pretreatment of patients with radiation and chemotherapy also impairs cellular immune responses. As such, T-cell responses, when reported in cancer vaccine trials, have tended to be detected in a minority of patients, and then only with assays involving prolonged in vitro culture.

However, some clinical trials using modern vaccination approaches have shown frequent cellular responses using single-cell ex vivo assays. For example, peptide-pulsed dendritic cells have been used to induce cellular responses in breast and ovarian cancer patients (70). IFN-γ CFC responses of 0.5–2% of CD8$^+$ T-cells were detected in this study after three vaccinations. The peptides used encoded epitopes of Her-2/*neu* or mucin (MUC)-1 precursor tumor antigens. Responses detectable by ex vivo tetramer staining were also seen in colorectal cancer patients with carcinoembryonic antigen peptide-specific tetramers (71).

MUC-1, like some of the melanoma-associated antigens, has been demonstrated to be the target of natural cellular immunity, in the absence of vaccination. MUC-1-specific CFC responses were frequently demonstrated in patients with a variety of solid tumors by Karanikas et al. *(72)*. These responses were usually increased by MUC-1-specific vaccination.

Myeloma represents a disease in which patients tend to be heavily pretreated with chemotherapy, so cellular immune responses are likely to be difficult to detect. As such, ex vivo CFC responses to tumor idiotype or keyhole limpet hemocyanin were only occasionally identified in myeloma patients vaccinated with an idiotype–keyhole limpet hemocyanin vaccine *(73)*. It may also be argued that the protective response in this setting was more likely to be humoral, rather than cellular immunity, as has been demonstrated for follicular lymphoma idiotype vaccination *(74)*.

The ability to observe ex vivo cellular responses without prolonged expansion in culture suggests that cancer vaccines are becoming more immunogenic. In one study, ELISPOT responses to a melanoma-associated antigen 3 peptide (but not to four other antigenic peptides) were significantly correlated with reduced disease recurrence *(75)*. However, other studies with melanoma vaccines suggest no direct correlation of magnitude of tetramer or CFC response with clinical outcome *(67,68)*. This has led to the notion that multiple functions may need to be measured. For example, Rubio et al. measured cytotoxicity in response to physiological antigen *(51)*, a kind of measure of functional avidity. Memory/effector phenotyping of the responding T-cells has also been done *(49)*. Other investigators in the melanoma field have focused on the presence of regulatory T-cells in sentinel lymph nodes *(76)* or postvaccination in blood *(77)*. To this list, one might also add measurement of multiple cytokines, including regulatory cytokines, such as transforming growth factor-β and interleukin-10, and measurement of proliferative potential. From such broad-ranging parameters, a more complete picture of the cellular response evoked by vaccination may eventually allow the definition of a true immunological surrogate of clinical efficacy.

4. CONCLUSIONS

Modern assays of cellular immunity allow the detection of rare populations of antigen-specific T-cells on a single-cell basis, frequently with the ability to phenotype those cells using multiple parameters. Whereas quantitative comparisons have been made between assays, with some agreement in results, a lack of standardization of these assays still pervades the field. Only with standardized (hopefully, optimally standardized) assays can comparisons between different trials and different vaccine approaches be realized. This would be a timely occurrence, given the development of more immunogenic cancer vaccines in recent years, such that direct ex vivo detection of cellular responses is now common. However, it is also clear that the mere detection of a response to vaccination will not likely correlate with immune protection. Multiple functional analyses, perhaps accompanied with phenotypic markers of differentiation or enumeration of regulatory T-cells, will probably be required to develop a correlate of immune protection in malignant diseases.

REFERENCES

1. Prehn RT, Main JM. Immunity to methylcholanthrene-induced sarcomas. *J Natl Cancer Inst* 1957; 18: 769–778.
2. Old LJ, Boyse EA. Antigenic properties of experimental leukemias. I. Serological studies in vitro with spontaneous and radiation-induced leukemias. *J Natl Cancer Inst* 1963; 31:977–995.

3. Rouse BT, Rollinghoff M, Warner NL. Anti-theta serum-induced suppression of the cellular transfer of tumour-specific immunity to a syngeneic plasma cell tumour. *Nat New Biol* 1972; 238:116–117.

4. Finn OJ. Cancer vaccines: between the idea and the reality. *Nat Rev Immunol* 2003; 3:630–641.

5. Gilboa E. The promise of cancer vaccines. *Nat Rev Cancer* 2004; 4:401–411.

6. Crum CP, Rivera MN. Vaccines for cervical cancer. *Cancer J* 2003; 9:368–376.

7. Hernando JJ, Park TW, Kuhn WC. Dendritic cell-based vaccines in breast and gynaecologic cancer. *Anticancer Res* 2003; 23:4293–4303.

8. Ko BK, Kawano K, Murray JL, et al. Clinical studies of vaccines targeting breast cancer. *Clin Cancer Res* 2003; 9:3222–3234.

9. Hege KM, Carbone DP. Lung cancer vaccines and gene therapy. *Lung Cancer* 2003; 41(Suppl 1):S103–S113.

10. Basak SK, Kiertscher SM, Harui A, Roth MD. Modifying adenoviral vectors for use as gene-based cancer vaccines. *Viral Immunol* 2004; 17:82–196.

11. Castelli C, Rivoltini L, Rini F, et al. (2004). Heat shock proteins: biological functions and clinical application as personalized vaccines for human cancer. *Cancer Immunol Immunother* 2004; 53:27–233.

12. Mosca PJ, Hobeika AC, Clay TM, Morse MA, Lyerly HK. Direct detection of cellular immune responses to cancer vaccines. *Surgery* 2001; 129:248–254.

13. Coulie, PG, van der Bruggen P. T-cell responses of vaccinated cancer patients. *Curr Opin Immunol* 2003; 15:131–137.

14. Gehrz RC, Knorr SO. Characterization of the role of mononuclear cell subpopulations in the in vitro lymphocyte proliferation assay. *Clin Exp Immunol* 1979; 37:551–557.

15. McCoy JL, Herberman RB, Rosenberg EB, Donnelly FC, Levine PH, Alford C. 51 Chromium-release assay for cell-mediated cytotoxicity of human leukemia and lymphoid tissue-culture cells. *Natl Cancer Inst Monogr* 1973; 37:59–67.

16. Maecker HT, Maino VC, Picker LJ. Immunofluorescence analysis of T-cell responses in health and disease. *J Clin Immunol* 2000; 20:391–399.

17. Slansky JE. Antigen-specific T cells: analyses of the needles in the haystack. *PLoS Biol* 2003; 1:E78.

18. Czerkinsky C, Andersson G, Ekre HP, Nilsson LA, Klareskog L, Ouchterlony O. Reverse ELISPOT assay for clonal analysis of cytokine production. I. Enumeration of gamma-interferon-secreting cells. *J Immunol Methods* 1988; 110:29–36.

19. Waldrop SL, Pitcher CJ, Peterson DM, Maino VC, Picker LJ. Determination of antigen-specific memory/effector CD4+ T cell frequencies by flow cytometry: evidence for a novel, antigen-specific homeostatic mechanism in HIV-associated immunodeficiency. *J Clin Invest* 1997; 99:1739–1750.

20. Betts MR, Brenchley JM, Price DA, et al. Sensitive and viable identification of antigen-specific CD8+ T cells by a flow cytometric assay for degranulation. *J Immunol Methods* 2003; 281:65–78.

21. Altman JD, Moss PAH, Goulder PJR, et al. Phenotypic analysis of antigen-specific T lymphocytes. *Science* 1996; 274:94–96.

22. Mehta BA, Maino VC. Simultaneous detection of DNA synthesis and cytokine production in staphylococcal enterotoxin B-activated CD4+ T lymphocytes by flow cytometry. *J Immunol Methods* 1997; 208:49–59.

23. Fulcher D, Wong S. Carboxyfluorescein succinimidyl ester-based proliferative assays for assessment of T cell function in the diagnostic laboratory. *Immunol Cell Biol* 1999; 77:559–564.

24. Jung T, Schauer U, Heusser C, Neumann C, Rieger C. Detection of intracellular cytokines by flow cytometry. *J Immunol Methods* 1993; 159:197–207.

25. Prussin C, Metcalfe DD. Detection of intracytoplasmic cytokine using flow cytometry and directly conjugated anti-cytokine antibodies. *J Immunol Methods* 1995; 188:117–128.

26. Suni MA, Picker LJ, Maino VC. Detection of antigen-specific T cell cytokine expression in whole blood by flow cytometry. *J Immunol Methods* 1998; 212:89–98.

27. Brosterhus H, Brings S, Leyendeckers H, et al. Enrichment and detection of live antigen-specific CD4(+) and CD8(+) T cells based on cytokine secretion. *Eur J Immunol* 1999; 29:4053–4059.

28. Greten TF, Slansky JE, Kubota R, et al. Direct visualization of antigen-specific T cells: HTLV-1 Tax11-19-specific CD8(+) T cells are activated in peripheral blood and accumulate in cerebrospinal fluid from HAM/TSP patients. *Proc Natl Acad Sci USA* 1998; 95:7568–7573.

29. Migueles SA, Laborico AC, Shupert WL, et al. HIV-specific CD8(+) T cell proliferation is coupled to perforin expression and is maintained in nonprogressors. *Nat Immunol* 2002; 3:1061–1068.

30. Iyasere C, Tilton JC, Johnson AJ, et al. Diminished proliferation of human immunodeficiency virus-specific CD4+ T cells is associated with diminished interleukin-2 (IL-2) production and is recovered by exogenous IL-2. *J Virol* 2003; 77:10,900–10,909.

31. Kuzushima K, Hoshino Y, Fujii K, et al. Rapid determination of Epstein-Barr virus-specific CD8+ T-cell frequencies by flow cytometry. *Blood* 1999; 94:3094–3100.

32. Moretto WJ, Drohan LA, Nixon DF. Rapid quantification of SIV-specific CD8 T cell responses with recombinant vaccinia virus ELISPOT or cytokine flow cytometry. *AIDS* 2000; 14:2625–2627.

33. Asemissen AM, Nagorsen D, Keilholz U, et al. Flow cytometric determination of intracellular or secreted IFNgamma for the quantification of antigen reactive T cells. *J Immunol Methods* 2001; 251:101–108.

34. Pahar B, Li J, Rourke T, Miller CJ, McChesney MB. Detection of antigen-specific T cell interferon gamma expression by ELISPOT and cytokine flow cytometry assays in rhesus macaques. *J Immunol Methods* 2003; 282:103–115.

35. Sun Y, Iglesias E, Samri A, et al. A systematic comparison of methods to measure HIV-1 specific CD8 T cells. *J Immunol Methods* 2003; 272:23–34.

36. Whiteside TL, Zhao Y, Tsukishiro T, Elder EM, Gooding W, Baar J. Enzyme-linked immunospot, cytokine flow cytometry, and tetramers in the detection of T-cell responses to a dendritic cell-based multipeptide vaccine in patients with melanoma. *Clin Cancer Res* 2003; 9:641–649.

37. Karlsson AC, Martin JN, Younger SR, et al. Comparison of the ELISPOT and cytokine flow cytometry assays for the enumeration of antigen-specific T cells. *J Immunol Methods* 2003; 283:141–153.

38. Helms T, Boehm BO, Asaad RJ, Trezza RP, Lehmann PV, Tary-Lehmann M. Direct visualization of cytokine-producing recall antigen-specific CD4 memory T cells in healthy individuals and HIV patients. *J Immunol* 2000; 164:3723–3732.

39. Dunn HS, Haney DJ, Ghanekar SA, Stepick-Biek P, Lewis DB, Maecker HT. Dynamics of CD4 and CD8 T cell responses to cytomegalovirus in healthy human donors. *J Infect Dis* 2002; 186:15–22.

40. Smith JG, Liu X, Kaufhold RM, Clair J, Caulfield MJ. Development and validation of a gamma interferon ELISPOT assay for quantitation of cellular immune responses to varicella-zoster virus. *Clin Diagn Lab Immunol* 2001; 8:871–879.

41. Mwau M, McMichael AJ, Hanke T. Design and validation of an enzyme-linked immunospot assay for use in clinical trials of candidate HIV vaccines. *AIDS Res Hum Retroviruses* 2002; 18:611–618.

42. Lathey J. Preliminary steps toward validating a clinical bioassay: case study of the ELISpot assay. *Biopharm Intl* 2003; March:42–50.

43. Perez-Diez A, Spiess PJ, Restifo NP, Matzinger P, Marincola FM. Intensity of the vaccine-elicited immune response determines tumor clearance. *J Immunol* 2002; 168:338–347.

44. Kern F, Surel IP, Faulhaber N, et al. Target structures of the CD8(+)-T-cell response to human cytomegalovirus: the 72-kilodalton major immediate-early protein revisited. *J Virol* 1999; 73:8179–8184.

45. Kern F, Bunde T, Faulhaber N, et al. Cytomegalovirus (CMV) phosphoprotein 65 makes a large contribution to shaping the T cell repertoire in CMV-exposed individuals. *J Infect Dis* 2002; 185:1709–1716.

46. Gea-Banacloche JC, Migueles SA, Martino L, et al. Maintenance of large numbers of virus-specific CD8+ T cells in HIV- infected progressors and long-term nonprogressors. *J Immunol* 2000; 165:1082–1092.

47. Pitcher CJ, Quittner C, Peterson DM, et al. HIV-1-specific CD4+ T cells are detectable in most individuals with active HIV-1 infection, but decline with prolonged viral suppression. *Nat Med* 1999; 5:518–525.

48. Altes HK, Price DA, Jansen VA. Effector cytotoxic T lymphocyte numbers induced by vaccination should exceed levels in chronic infection for protection from HIV. *Vaccine* 2001; 20:3–6.

49. Walker EB, Haley D, Miller W, et al. gp100(209-2M) peptide immunization of HLA-A2+ stage I-III melanoma patients induces significant increase in antigen-specific effector and long-term memory CD8+ T cells. *Clin Cancer Res* 2004; 10:668–680.

50. Betts MR, Price DA, Brenchley JM, et al. The functional profile of primary human antiviral CD8+ T cell effector activity is dictated by cognate peptide concentration. *J Immunol* 2004; 172:6407–6417.

51. Rubio V, Stuge TB, Singh N, et al. Ex vivo identification, isolation and analysis of tumor-cytolytic T cells. *Nat Med* 2003; 9:1377–1382.

52. Trigona WL, Clair JH, Persaud N, et al. Intracellular staining for HIV-specific IFN-gamma production: statistical analyses establish reproducibility and criteria for distinguishing positive responses. *J Interferon Cytokine Res* 2003; 23:369–377.

53. Weinberg A, Wohl DA, Brown DG, et al. Effect of cryopreservation on measurement of cytomegalovirus-specific cellular immune responses in HIV-infected patients. *J Acquir Immune Defic Syndr* 2000; 25:109–114.

54. Costantini, A, Mancini S, Giuliodoro S, et al. Effects of cryopreservation on lymphocyte immunophenotype and function. *J Immunol Methods* 2003; 278:145–155.

54a. Maecker HT, Moon J, Bhatia S, et al. Impact of cryopreservation on tetramer, cytokine flow cytometry, and ELISPOT. *BMC Immunol* 2005; 6:17.

55. Maecker HT, Dunn HS, Suni MA, et al. Use of overlapping peptide mixtures as antigens for cytokine flow cytometry. *J Immunol Methods* 2001; 255:27–40.

56. Hoffmeister B, Bunde T, Rudawsky IM, Volk HD, Kern F. Detection of antigen-specific T cells by cytokine flow cytometry: the use of whole blood may underestimate frequencies. *Eur J Immunol* 2003; 33:3484–3492.

57. Nomura LE, Walker JM, Maecker HT. Optimization of whole blood antigen-specific cytokine assays for CD4+ T cells. *Cytometry* 2000; 40:60–68.

58. Waldrop SL, Davis KA, Maino VC, Picker LJ. Normal human CD4+ memory T cells display broad heterogeneity in their activation threshold for cytokine synthesis. *J Immunol* 1998; 161:5284–5295.

59. Nylander S, Kalies I, Brefeldin A, but not monensin, completely blocks CD69 expression on mouse lymphocytes: efficacy of inhibitors of protein secretion in protocols for intracellular cytokine staining by flow cytometry. *J Immunol Methods* 1999; 224:69–76.

60. Motulsky H. *Intuitive Biostatistics*. Oxford: Oxford University Press. 1995.

61. Betts MR, Casazza JP, Patterson BA, et al. Putative immunodominant human immunodeficiency virus-specific CD8(+) T- cell responses cannot be predicted by major histocompatibility complex class I haplotype. *J Virol* 2000; 74:9144–9151.

62. Ferrari G, Neal W, Ottinger J, et al. Absence of immunodominant anti-Gag p17 (SL9) responses among Gag CTL-positive, HIV-uninfected vaccine recipients expressing the HLA-A*0201 allele. *J Immunol* 2004; 173:2126–2133.

63. Suni MA, Dunn HS, Orr PL, et al. Performance of plate-based cytokine flow cytometry with automated data analysis. *BMC Immunology* 2003; 4:9.

64. Maecker HT. Cytokine flow cytometry. In: Hawley TS, Hawley RG, eds. *Flow Cytometry Protocols, 2nd Edition*. Totowa: Humana Press. 2004: pp. 95–107.

65. Dunne JF, Maecker HT. Automation of cytokine flow cytometry assays. *J Assoc Lab Automation* 2004; 9:5–9.

66. Lee PP, Yee C, Savage PA, et al. Characterization of circulating T cells specific for tumor-associated antigens in melanoma patients. *Nat Med* 1999; 5:677–685.

67. Lee KH, Wang E, Nielsen MB, et al. Increased vaccine-specific T cell frequency after peptide-based vaccination correlates with increased susceptibility to in vitro stimulation but does not lead to tumor regression. *J Immunol* 1999; 163:6292–6300.

68. Nielsen MB, Monsurro V, Migueles SA, et al. Status of activation of circulating vaccine-elicited CD8+ T cells. *J Immunol* 2000; 165:2287–2296.

69. Smith JW II, Walker EB, Fox BA, et al. Adjuvant immunization of HLA-A2-positive melanoma patients with a modified gp100 peptide induces peptide-specific CD8+ T-cell responses. *J Clin Oncol* 2003; 21: 1562–1573.

70. Brossart P, Wirths S, Stuhler G, Reichardt VL, Kanz L, Brugger W. Induction of cytotoxic T-lymphocyte responses in vivo after vaccinations with peptide-pulsed dendritic cells. *Blood* 2000; 96:3102–3108.

71. Fong L, Hou Y, Rivas A, et al. Altered peptide ligand vaccination with Flt3 ligand expanded dendritic cells for tumor immunotherapy. *Proc Natl Acad Sci USA* 2001; 98:8809–8814.

72. Karanikas V, Lodding J, Maino VC, McKenzie IF. Flow cytometric measurement of intracellular cytokines detects immune responses in MUC1 immunotherapy. *Clin Cancer Res* 2000; 6:829–837.

73. Maecker HT, Auffermann-Gretzinger S, Nomura LE, Liso A, Czerwinski DK, Levy R. Detection of CD4 T-cell responses to a tumor vaccine by cytokine flow cytometry. *Clin Cancer Res* 2001; 7(Suppl 3): 902s–908s.

74. Weng WK, Czerwinski D, Timmerman J, Hsu FJ, Levy R. Clinical outcome of lymphoma patients after idiotype vaccination is correlated with humoral immune response and immunoglobulin G Fc receptor genotype. *J Clin Oncol* 2004; 22:4717–4724.

75. Reynolds SR, Zeleniuch-Jacquotte A, Shapiro RL, et al. Vaccine-induced CD8+ T-cell responses to MAGE-3 correlate with clinical outcome in patients with melanoma. *Clin Cancer Res* 2003; 9:657–662.

76. Viguier M, Lemaitre F, Verola O, et al. Foxp3 expressing CD4+CD25 (high) regulatory T cells are over-represented in human metastatic melanoma lymph nodes and inhibit the function of infiltrating T cells. *J Immunol* 2004; 173:1444–1453.

77. Chakraborty NG, Chattopadhyay S, Mehrotra S, Chhabra A, Mukherji B. Regulatory T-cell response and tumor vaccine-induced cytotoxic T lymphocytes in human melanoma. *Hum Immunol* 2004; 65:794–802.

5 Statistical Analysis of Immune Response Assays in Cancer Immunotherapy Trials

Susan Groshen

SUMMARY

The continued attention to immunotherapy as a promising and critical component in the development of novel cancer therapies has also stimulated the development of new assays to assess the effect of these novel biotherapies on the immune system. For these new immunotherapies, pilot trials are needed to establish proof of principal: that the therapy can affect the patient and produce a change in the immunological status that has the potential to translate to an antitumor effect. Unfortunately, the majority of immune response assays in cancer immunotherapy trials have not been "validated" in the clinical setting. The development and validation of an immune response assay can be considered as having four general phases:

1. To establish accuracy/precision or sensitivity/specificity, and consistency/reproducibility of assay (in the laboratory).
2. To establish that assay can be used in clinical setting and is correlated with other established assays of same aspect of immune status or immunological effect.
3. To characterize of the association between assay result and antitumor effect.
4. To validate the assay as a surrogate end point.

At each phase, careful statistical analyses of these measures of immune response will increase the understanding of the biological effects of the new therapies and will expedite the evaluation of immunotherapies the clinical setting.

Key Words: Statistical analysis of immune response; immune response; assay; ELISPOT; immunotherapies.

1. INTRODUCTION

The continued attention to immunotherapy in general, and cancer vaccines in particular, as a promising and critical component in the development of novel cancer therapies has also led to the search for, and development of, new assays to assess the effect of these novel biotherapies on the immune system. Whether immunotherapy emerges as a strategy for cancer cytotoxic treatment, for treatment resulting in a cytostatic effect, or as an adjuvant in the setting of minimal residual disease, or some combination thereof, will depend on the tumor type, the stage of disease, as well as the immunotherapy itself. Regardless, in

From: *Cancer Drug Discovery and Development: Immunotherapy of Cancer*
Edited by: M. L. Disis © Humana Press Inc., Totowa, NJ

Table 1
Types of Assays for Immune Monitoring in Cancer Vaccine Trial

Type of response	Potential assays
CD8 T-cell response	ELISPOT, CFC, tetramer, qRT-PCR, LDA
CD4 T-cell response	Antigen-specific T-cell proliferation and cell-mediated cytotoxicity assays (with LDA), ELISPOT, CFC
Antibody response	ELISA, ELISPOT for memory B-cells

ELISPOT, enzyme-linked immunospot assay; CFC, cytokine flow cytometry; tetramer, major histocompatibility complex-peptide tetramer analysis; qRT-PCR, quantitative reverse transcription-polymerase chain reaction assay; LDA, limiting dilution analysis; ELISA, enzyme-linked immunosorbent assay.

the early stages of development, before an immunotherapy is taken to formal testing in large scale trials for clinical efficacy with traditional end points such as tumor response, time to progression, or overall survival, it is important and economically rational to determine that the immunotherapy is producing the intended immunological effects. These pilot (some times called phase 2) trials are needed to establish proof of principal: that the therapy can effect the host (the patient) and produce a change in the immunologic status of the patient that has the potential to translate to an antitumor effect.

There has been a marked increase in the number of assays that can be used to evaluate overall immune status and immunological changes induced by therapy, and more will be developed. This is a rapidly evolving area of research and almost surely, the immunological assays used today will be replaced within the next 5 yr with more specific or more precise assays. In a review of methodology available for immune monitoring in cancer vaccine trials, responses to vaccine strategies were broadly grouped into three categories: CD8 T-cell responses, CD4 T-cell responses, and antibody responses (1). For each of these broad categories, many assays exist with many variations; Table 1 lists examples of commonly used assays. This table is not meant to be complete, but rather to highlight the fact that there are many options available. Some assays, such at the cytokine flow cytometry and the enzyme-linked immunospot (ELISPOT) assays are functional and will measure an antigen-specific T-cell response; others, such as the tetramer assay, will detect and quantify antigen-specific T-cell frequencies. In addition, many of these assays as listed represent a class of assays rather than a single assay. For example, in the ELISPOT assay, the antigen or antigens, to which the T-cells respond, must be specified; generally, interferon-γ release is measured, but the assay can be modified to visualize the release of other cytokines.

Thus, the selection of the subset of immune assays to be used for a clinical trial will require not only specification of the type of assay, but also the peptides or antigens to be used in the assay, based on the specific vaccine. An important recommendation was that more than one type of assay should be used to assess the response to the immunotherapy (1). Clearly, the selection of an appropriate, comprehensive panel of assays is critical to the evaluation of a new immunotherapy regimen or strategy.

2. DEVELOPMENT OF IMMUNE RESPONSE ASSAYS IN CLINICAL TRIALS

In this chapter, we use the term *immune response* to mean a change in the levels of an assay; and we use the phrases *immune response* and *change in the immune response assay*

Table 2
Phases of Development of Immune Response Assay

Phase 1: assay development	Establish accuracy/precision or sensitivity/specificity and consistency/reproducibility of assay
Phase 2: initial clinical testing; verify ability to measure immunological effects	In cohorts of patients or in clinical trials of relevant immunotherapies; establish that assay can be used in clinical setting and is correlated with other established assays of same aspect of immune status or immunological effect
Phase 3: characterization of the association between assay result and anti-tumor effect	In clinical trials, examine new immune response and compare to "standard" clinical end points in prospective cancer immunotherapy trials
Phase 4: validation as surrogate end point	In randomized trials, confirm that changes in the immune response assay correspond to clinical effect of immunotherapy

interchangeably. We use the phrase *immunological effect* of the therapy to designate the actual change to the immune status of which we are attempting to measure with an assay.

Unfortunately, the majority of immune response assays in cancer immunotherapy trials have not been "validated" in the clinical setting. That is, it is not clear what the antitumor implications of these changes in the assay levels are in humans; to date, studies have not been completed that establish formally an association between the immune response and clinical outcome. Several trials have observed that patients with larger immune responses tended to have more favorable outcomes, but these have been small trials and require confirmation in larger trials with sufficient patients to better characterize the relationships *(2–4)*.

The assays listed in Table 1 above yield quantitative results. In comparing a pretreatment assay result to a posttreatment result, we generally assume that larger changes imply a larger the immunological effect, which, in turn, implies a greater likelihood of antitumor effect and clinical benefit. Whereas this is a reasonable hypothesis, it has not yet been adequately evaluated in humans. In addition, we do not know for a specific assay whether the immune response/clinical benefit relationship is continuous (i.e., larger assay changes will result in greater clinical benefit), or whether there is a threshold effect (the change in assay result must exceed some level before a clinical benefit is likely or more likely). For example in response to a dendritic cell (DC) vaccine, *a priori*, we do not know whether an increase in the number of spots in an ELISPOT assay results in a decrease in tumor burden (if measurable disease is present) or a delay in time to recurrence (in the adjuvant setting). Moreover, if some relationship does exist, we do not know its nature—whether, for example, a 10-fold increase in the number of spots is sufficient to produce a response or is there a continuous dose (spot)–response curve that we can estimate. Ironically, we cannot evaluate the association between a change in an immunological marker and clinical effect until we observe these clinical benefits in a reasonably large number of patients.

Many articles have been written to describe the phases of marker development *(5,6)*. Using these as guidelines, we can think of the development of an immune response assay as having four general phases, as summarized in Table 2. Although development proceeds on a continuum, with work in one phase incorporated into other phases, it is helpful to think of the milestones that are needed in order to shift from one phase to another. Before moving to phase 2, the technical issues of measuring the immune response should be resolved. The assay should be accurate in the sense that measured levels are close, on average, to the true levels in experiments with seeded or other artificial samples; the assay should be sufficiently precise with acceptable experimental variability (coefficients of variation of less than 20% are desirable and less is better); the assay should be reproducible in the sense that different laboratories should be able to produce comparable results. The technical challenges of the assay must be resolved in order for an assay to be a candidate for use in clinical trials.

Before shifting from phase 2 to phase 3, it is necessary to know how the assay performs in humans: the patients on the trials of immunotherapy. Questions requiring answers are: Is the assay logistically feasible, i.e., can specimens be processed as required? Are the differences among patients, as measured by the new assay, correlated with differences in a related, established immunological assay? Is the assay measuring what it is intended to measure in humans? In phase 2 of development, data are collected to begin to characterize the association between the immune response and likelihood of clinical benefit, but the emphasis in this phase is to verify that the assay is measuring the intended immunological effect in patients.

In phase 3, the goal is to characterize the association between the assay and clinical benefit. At the end of phase 3, we should know whether there is a continuous "dose–response" relationship or whether achieving a change greater than some threshold value is required, and if so, what that threshold, or "cutpoint," might be; we should have data to suggest that the immune response is necessary, sufficient, or both, in order to achieve the desired antitumor/clinical effect. In phase 4, the hurdle for establishing the immune response as a surrogate end point for clinical outcome is high. The immune response must be strongly associated with clinical outcome and must reflect the effect of the immunotherapy treatment in the same way as the direct measure of clinical outcome (7). Whether or not an immune response meets the criteria to serve as a surrogate for a clinical end point, immune responses have the potential to serve as very informative intermediate markers that can be used in early clinical testing to guide the development of new immunotherapies.

Currently, the majority of immune response assays utilized in clinical trials of cancer immunotherapies are in phase 2 or phase 3 of development: the assays have been established and studies are now necessary to verify that the particular immune response is meaningful either as an indicator of immunological effect or in the sense that it is associated with clinical efficacy. In the majority of trials, measures of immune response will serve as intermediate markers; they will measure the immunological effect that is a necessary change if the therapy is to produce the intended clinical benefit.

3. STATISTICAL ANALYSIS OF IMMUNE RESPONSE ASSAYS IN CLINICAL TRIALS

Generally, in the first two phases of development, the evaluation and analysis of an immune response assay is descriptive. Standard descriptive statistical methods, with an emphasis on plotting data and graphical displays, are usually sufficient for presenting the characteristics of the assay as a measure of immunological change. Whereas some of the analyses during the third phase of development are also descriptive and involve standard, familiar methods, others are more challenging. For all studies, the results of the immune response assays used in the trial should be summarized quantitatively. Initially, all data should be plotted and histograms used to review the patterns of the observations; plots can be especially helpful for examining changes in the assay levels from before to after treatment.

Usually, for each patient at each evaluation time and for each assay used in the trial to assess immune response, multiple replicates (e.g., multiple wells on a microtiter plate) are analyzed. Calculating the average of the replicates and using the average for subsequent statistical analysis is usually a reasonable strategy, because we are primarily interested in the patient-to-patient variability: before treatment, after treatment, and the change. However, initially, for each assay, it is useful to plot the within-patient standard deviation (i.e., among the replicates within each patient and for each time separately) against the patient average (within each patient at each time). If a correlation between the standard deviation and the average is observed (that is, on average the standard deviations tend to get larger as the averages increase), then a transformation should be found that will eliminate this association. Often, the logarithm or the square root transformation will eliminate the correlation between the standard deviation and the average. Subsequent analyses will be more straightforward when the noise (unexplained variability of the assay) and the signal (the mean for each patient) are independent. Ideally, we would like the variability to be constant and differences over time or between arms in a trial to be reflected in the averages.

If no correlation exists between the within-patient standard deviation and average, or if a transformation can be identified which eliminates the correlation, then usually, this will render the data compatible with the assumptions of the normal distribution (a unimodel, symmetric distribution with relatively few extreme values); in this situation, means, standard deviations, *t*-tests or analysis of variance—all the usual parametric statistical methods—will be appropriate and optimal. If no transformation is found, then most likely the assay results will appear skewed, or otherwise not "normal"-like, and then nonparametric methods should be considered: medians instead of means, quartiles and ranges instead of standard deviations can be used to summarize the overall patterns. The Wilcoxon (paired) signed rank test instead of the paired *t*-test can assess whether there were overall net changes before and after treatment. The Wilcoxon test instead of the two-sample *t*-test and the Kruskall–Wallis test instead of an analysis of variance can be used to compare groups if the clinical trial has more than one arm. These are all familiar, standard statistical methods that are described in most beginning statistics textbooks. If assays are repeated more than once posttreatment, then more complicated methods of analysis incorporating the repeated measures feature can be used (*7–9*). Regardless of the specific methods used, the analyses and comparisons should reflect the design of the trial. Scatter plots and correlations should also be used evaluate the association between the different assays used in the trial. Because these trials usually involve a relatively small number of patients (i.e., <100) graphical displays are a most effective tool for presenting patterns (*10*).

Oftentimes, in addition to summarizing the magnitude of changes of the assay values before and after treatment, it is of interest to establish whether the posttreatment assay value is greater than the pretreatment value, and classifying the patient as being an "immune responder." Methods to assess a change from before to after treatment are discussed in Subheading 3.3.

3.1. Phase 3 of Immune Response Assay Development:
Analyses to Assess the Association Between the Immune Response
and Clinical Outcome

Methods to evaluate the association between a marker—in this case, the immune response assay posttreatment or the change from pretreatment—and clinical outcome have been discussed extensively (11–15). Although immune response assays are different from the classical marker in that the immune response is observed only after treatment and hence, cannot be measured without treatment, the statistical methods for assessing its usefulness for predicting outcome are the same. If the relationship between the immune response assay results and clinical outcome is continuous, e.g., if larger the immune responses (i.e., greater changes from baseline), the more likely are to correspond to greater clinical benefit, then regression methods can be used to characterize the association. If the outcome is time to recurrence or time to progression, then the Cox proportional hazards model may be an appropriate model for relating immune response to outcome; if the outcome is tumor response, dichotomized as responder vs nonresponders, then a logistic regression can be used. One attractive feature of these regression models is that they permit the simultaneous evaluation of several immune response assays. Because the trials in which these assays are based are often small or moderate in size, the number of patients will limit the number of assays that can be examined at a time (11,16). Nonetheless, the potential exists to consider more than one assay at a time.

If the relationship between the immune response assay is not continuous and there is a threshold effect, e.g., if immune responses less than some amount are associated with a very low likelihood of clinical benefit, and if responses greater than that amount are associated with a much higher probability of benefit, then different analytic approaches are required. Two commonly used methods involve the construction and evaluation of receiver operator characteristic (ROC) curves (17–22) and methods for selecting "optimal" cutpoints (23–28).

Both methods are best understood when we consider the measure of clinical outcome as dichotomous, with patients classified as having a favorable or unfavorable clinical outcome. The methodology extends to outcomes such as survival and time to recurrence, but these are less intuitive to describe. In an ROC curve analysis, as well as for selecting an optimal cutpoint, each observed value of the quantitative immune response (e.g., the ratio of the after treatment assay result divided by the before treatment assay result) is considered to be a potential cutpoint. For each potential cutpoint, patients are divided into a "low" group, if their immune responses are less than the cutpoint, or into a "high" group, if their immune responses are equal to or greater than the potential cutpoint. For each potential cutpoint, patients are classified according to the clinical outcome experienced (favorable vs unfavorable) and by their observed values of the immune responses (below the potential cutpoint vs equal to or greater than the cutpoint). A 2×2 table can be constructed to display this crossclassification for each potential cutpoint.

To produce an ROC curve, the sensitivity and specificity associated with each potential cutpoint is calculated. Assuming that a greater immune response indicates more immunotherapy activity, then sensitivity is calculated as the proportion of patients who had a favorable clinical outcome among those whose immune response value fell into the high group; specificity is calculated as the proportion of patients who had an unfavorable clinical outcome among those whose immune response value was observed to be less than the potential cutpoint and therefore fell into the low group. For each potential cutpoint, the sensitivity is plotted as a function of the one minus the specificity. The resulting plot, called the ROC curve, allows one to visualize the sensitivity and specificity for each potential cutpoint. The area under this ROC curve is used as a measure of the strength of the relationship between the immune response and the clinical outcome. An area under the curve of 1.0 would indicate a perfect relationship, with a unique cutpoint with 100% sensitivity and 100% specificity; an area under the curve of 0.50 would indicate no relationship at all.

In contrast, for the optimal cutpoint method, the χ-square test statistic is calculated to measure the strength of the association between each potential cutpoint and clinical outcome, based on the 2×2 table previously described. The cutpoint that gives rise to the largest test statistic (and therefore the smallest p value) is called the optimal cutpoint. A corrected p value that accounts for the fact that every observed immune response value was tested as a potential cutpoint in order to select the one associated with the smallest nominal p value can be obtained using resampling methods. Confidence intervals can be constructed which reduce the bias in the estimate of the association between immune response and clinical outcome at the selected optimal cutpoint *(30)*.

The ROC curve analysis has the advantage that a cutpoint can be selected to achieve a prespecified sensitivity or specificity (but not usually both); the optimal cutpoint method is very flexible and often results in cutpoints that are less extreme. Regardless of the model or method used to characterize the relationship between immune response and clinical outcome, the findings will require confirmation with data from an independent cohort of patients. Furthermore, it should be stressed that these relationships are specific to the type of immunotherapy and the type of immune response assay. It cannot be assumed that an association between ELISPOT results for CD8 T-cell reactivity to one peptide and response to a peptide-pulsed DC vaccine will be the same as the association between the same ELISPOT assay and a DC vaccine in which the DCs are pulsed with different peptides. In that sense, the immune response assays are potential predictive markers, i.e., they can be used to predict response, or failure to respond, to a specific therapy.

3.2. Phase 4 of Immune Response Assay Development: Validation as Surrogate End Point

Whereas it may often be reasonable to hypothesize that a type of immunological change —as measured by an immune response assay—is a necessary condition for a specific immunotherapy to be effective, it cannot be assumed that this immunological change is a sufficient condition. In addition, there may be other immunological (or nonimmunological) effects produced by the therapy that lead to clinical benefit but that are not reflected in the immune response under consideration. Thus, the ability of an immune response to serve as a surrogate end point, which can substitute for the clinical outcome, cannot be assumed and needs to be rigorously verified with data from clinical trials. Prentice described the conditions that need to be met in order for a biomarker to qualify as a surrogate end point in clinical trials *(7)*. These conditions are that:

1. The treatment has a significant effect on the surrogate end point.
2. The treatment has a significant effect on the true clinical (outcome) end point.
3. The surrogate end point has a significant effect on the true clinical end point.
4. The full effect of the treatment on the true end point is captured by the surrogate end point.

Table 3
Mean and Standard Deviation for Enzyme-Linked Immunospot
(ELISPOT) Responses at Each of the Four Experimental Conditions

	Exposure to:	
	Irrelevant peptide	*Specific peptide*
Baseline	I_{pre} and $sd(I_{pre})$	S_{pre} and $sd(S_{pre})$
Posttreatment	I_{post} and $sd(I_{post})$	S_{post} and $sd(S_{post})$

Given the challenges of verifying all four of these conditions, it is not likely that many immune response assays, although very useful as intermediate end points, will be validated as surrogate end points *(31,32)*.

3.3. Criteria for Classifying an Immune Response Change as an "Immunological Response"

As stated, at the current time, in the majority of clinical trials of cancer immunotherapy, there is limited information regarding the relationship between immune response and clinical outcome. In particular, there is no way of knowing when, or even whether, a change is large enough to translate into clinical effect. However, although we cannot state that a change of some specified magnitude will result in clinical benefit, we nonetheless hypothesize that if changes are not produced, then it is unlikely that the proposed immunotherapy will function as intended. Therefore, in addition to summarizing the magnitude of the immune responses observed, it is very helpful to identify those patients whose immune response assay results were large enough posttreatment, relative to the pretreatment value, that we are confident that immunotherapy had an effect on the immune status of that patient, i.e., the patient can be classified as a (immune) responder.

It is not obvious *a priori* what criteria to use to define an immune responder, and in this situation, computer simulations can be helpful for deciding which rules are sufficiently, but not overly rigorous for defining a responder, because baseline and control values will be available for all the immune response assays. That is, we can propose rules for comparing baseline with posttreatment, and/or control with posttreatment, and evaluate the statistical properties of these rules with simulations. The ELISPOT assay can be used to illustrate this point. To explain how simulations can be used, consider the simplified situation: for each patient on a cancer vaccine trial, blood will be drawn pretreatment and at 3 mo posttreatment. In a 96-well microtiter plate, the peripheral blood mononuclear cells (PBMCs), from both time points, will be stimulated in vitro with a vaccine-specific peptide and then exposed to the vaccine-specific peptide or an irrelevant peptide (as the negative control). The same number of PBMCs will be used in each well, and for this example, we will assume that the same number of wells will be used for each of the four experimental conditions defined by the time point (pre- vs posttreatment) and the peptide (test vs control). In each well, the number of spots is counted, indicating the number of peptide-reactive (interferon-γ-secreting) T-cells in the PBMC sample. For each of the four experimental conditions, the mean and standard deviation are calculated over all the corresponding wells (as displayed in Table 3).

Many rules have been proposed to classify a T-cell response posttreatment as positive and increased relative to the pretreatment values. Four such rules, using the notations in

Table 3, classify the posttreatment ELISPOT response as a clear increase over baseline if:

1. $S_{post} > S_{pre} + 3 \times sd(S_{pre})$ and $S_{post} > C$.
2. $S_{post} > 3 \times S_{pre}$ and $S_{post} > C$.
3. $S_{post} > 2 \times S_{pre} + 2 \times sd(S_{pre})$ and $S_{post} > C$.
4. $(S_{post} - I_{post}) > 2(S_{pre} - I_{pre}) + 2\,sd(S_{pre})$ and $(S_{post} - I_{post}) > I_{post} + 2 \times sd(I_{post})$ and $S_{post} > C$.

Here, C is minimum number of spots that should be present; often C is 10 or 20. Rule 1 requires that the mean of the wells posttreatment exceeds the mean of the wells pretreatment by at least 3 standard deviations. Rule 2 requires that the mean of the wells posttreatment is more than three times as large as the mean pretreatment. Rule 3 combines features of 1 and 2. Rule 4 is a hybrid that considers the difference between the reactions to the specific and irrelevant peptides. Table 4 evaluates the four rules described above in terms of the probability of declaring that a patient has experienced an immunological response (based on the one ELISPOT assay and according to the rule). Two variations of the rules are also evaluated (*see* footnotes in Table 4): rule 1a requires that the mean of the wells posttreatment exceeds the mean of the wells pretreatment by at least 2 standard deviations (instead of 3), and rule 2a requires that the mean of the wells posttreatment is more than two times as large as the mean pretreatment (instead of 3). The simulations in Table 4 assume that three wells were used for each experimental condition for each patient.

In Table 4, the probabilities in the rows labeled "Same as baseline" are the chances that a patient who has not had an immunological change is incorrectly labeled as an immune responder; generally, we would like this probability to be small, say less than 0.05. The other rows list the probability that a patient is correctly labeled an immune responder when the therapy has increased the mean number of spots by a factor of 2, 3, 5, or 10 over baseline; generally, we would like the probabilities in these rows to be large, say greater than 0.80 or 0.90. Inspection of the rows at baseline suggest that rules 1a, 2, and 2a may be too liberal—too likely to incorrectly declare a patient a responder when the coefficient of variation for the assay is large. Among the rules 1, 2, and 4, rule 1 has the best power to correctly identify a responder, but does not do so consistently until the therapy produces a (true) fivefold increase in the mean number of spots. In general, all rules perform well in terms of correctly identifying responders, if the therapy produces a (true) fivefold increase in the mean number of spots. Throughout the table, it is apparent that the variability (reflected by the coefficient of variation) can greatly affect the probability of correct classification. Rule 4 tends to be more conservative and is affected by the response to the specific peptide at baseline. These rules in Table 4 were reevaluated under the same conditions, but assumed that six wells were used per patient for each experiment condition. The performance of these rules did not improve appreciably with the increased number of wells.

In clinical trials, more than one assay will be used. For example, the T-cell response to several peptides will be tested using the ELISPOT assay. Because, if one performs enough tests, by chance alone, eventually one will be positive, even if there is no treatment effect, it is important to evaluate these above rules according to the likelihood that at least one response will be falsely positive when multiple peptides are tested. Table 5 summarizes the probability of at least one false-positive test when T-cell responses are tested against 5 or 10 peptides, using the ELISPOT assay in a trial. In this table, rule 3 does a better job to ensure a small probability of false-positive results. No rule is clearly

Table 4
Probability That a Patient Will Be Classified as Being an Immunological Responder, Using Six Different Rules, With Three Wells Per Assay

Mean response after treatment (relative to baseline mean)	Mean response at baseline (relative to assay threshold)	Coefficient of variation	Probability of classifying patient as being an immunological responder[a]					
			Rule 1	Rule 1a	Rule 2	Rule 2a	Rule 3	Rule 4
Same as baseline	0.50	25%	0.00	0.00	0.00	0.00	0.00	0.00
Same as baseline	0.50	50%	0.00	0.00	0.00	0.00	0.00	0.00
Same as baseline	0.50	75%	0.00	0.00	0.00	0.00	0.00	0.00
Same as baseline	1.00	25%	0.00	0.00	0.00	0.00	0.00	0.00
Same as baseline	1.00	50%	0.00	0.00	0.00	0.00	0.00	0.00
Same as baseline	1.00	75%	0.00	0.01	0.00	0.01	0.00	0.01
Same as baseline	2.00	25%	0.03	0.06	0.00	0.00	0.00	0.02
Same as baseline	2.00	50%	0.03	0.06	0.01	0.05	0.01	0.02
Same as baseline	2.00	75%	0.03	0.06	0.05	0.11	0.02	0.03
Twofold increase	0.50	25%	0.00	0.00	0.00	0.00	0.00	0.00
Twofold increase	0.50	50%	0.00	0.00	0.00	0.00	0.00	0.01
Twofold increase	0.50	75%	0.01	0.01	0.01	0.01	0.01	0.01
Twofold increase	1.00	25%	0.45	0.49	0.03	0.38	0.15	0.12
Twofold increase	1.00	50%	0.29	0.41	0.14	0.37	0.15	0.14
Twofold increase	1.00	75%	0.21	0.32	0.21	0.38	0.16	0.16
Twofold increase	2.00	25%	0.76	0.92	0.03	0.51	0.18	0.52
Twofold increase	2.00	50%	0.37	0.57	0.17	0.50	0.18	0.34
Twofold increase	2.00	75%	0.24	0.40	0.26	0.49	0.18	0.27
Threefold increase	0.50	25%	0.01	0.01	0.01	0.01	0.01	0.03
Threefold increase	0.50	50%	0.12	0.13	0.12	0.12	0.12	0.04
Threefold increase	0.50	75%	0.20	0.23	0.19	0.22	0.19	0.07
Threefold increase	1.00	25%	0.98	0.99	0.50	0.97	0.83	0.55
Threefold increase	1.00	50%	0.70	0.82	0.51	0.80	0.54	0.51
Threefold increase	1.00	75%	0.49	0.64	0.48	0.68	0.42	0.46
Threefold increase	2.00	25%	0.99	1.00	0.51	0.97	0.84	0.94
Threefold increase	2.00	50%	0.73	0.86	0.50	0.83	0.54	0.69
Threefold increase	2.00	75%	0.52	0.68	0.50	0.74	0.43	0.54
Fivefold increase	0.50	25%	0.91	0.92	0.92	0.92	0.92	0.32
Fivefold increase	0.50	50%	0.75	0.75	0.74	0.75	0.76	0.36
Fivefold increase	0.50	75%	0.65	0.68	0.65	0.68	0.64	0.37
Fivefold increase	1.00	25%	1.00	1.00	0.99	1.00	1.00	0.98
Fivefold increase	1.00	50%	0.94	0.97	0.88	0.97	0.90	0.90
Fivefold increase	1.00	75%	0.78	0.87	0.78	0.88	0.76	0.79
Fivefold increase	2.00	25%	1.00	1.00	0.99	1.00	1.00	1.00
Fivefold increase	2.00	50%	0.95	0.98	0.88	0.97	0.91	0.94
Fivefold increase	2.00	75%	0.80	0.87	0.78	0.90	0.76	0.81

[a]Rules for classifying a posttreatment change as a "response" with notations defined in Table 3:

1. $S_{post} > S_{pre} + 3 \times sd(S_{pre})$ and $S_{post} > C$;
   a. $S_{post} > S_{pre} + 2 \times sd(S_{pre})$ and $S_{post} > C$.
2. $S_{post} > 3 \times S_{pre}$ and $S_{post} > C$;
   a. $S_{post} > 2 \times S_{pre}$ and $S_{post} > C$.
3. $S_{post} > 2 \times S_{pre} + 2 \times sd(S_{pre})$ and $S_{post} > C$.
4. $(S_{post} - I_{post}) > 2(S_{pre} - I_{pre})$ and $(S_{post} - I_{post}) > I_{post} + 2 \times sd(I_{post})$ and $S_{post} > C$.

The probabilities in the table are based on 10,000 simulations with the enzyme-linked immunospot results represented by normally distributed data; the coefficient of variation was assumed the same, pre- and posttreatment. In these simulations, the value of C (for all the rules) was assumed the assay threshold. For rule 4, the mean number of spots for the irrelevant peptide was taken to be equal to the assay threshold as well, and the coefficient of variation for the distribution of the irrelevant peptide was set at 50%.

Table 5
Probability That a Patient Will Be Classified as Being an Immunological Responder
if More Than One Immune Response Assay is Used (e.g., Multiple Peptides)
and Requiring at Least One Positive Assay, When There Is No Change From Baseline,
Using Six Different Rules, With Three Wells Per Assay

Number of assays/peptides	Mean response at baseline (relative to assay threshold)	Coefficient of variation	Probability of classifying patient as being an immunological responder[a]					
			Rule 1	Rule 1a	Rule 2	Rule 2a	Rule 3	Rule 4
5	0.50	25%	0.00	0.00	0.00	0.00	0.00	0.00
5	0.50	50%	0.00	0.00	0.00	0.00	0.00	0.00
5	0.50	75%	0.00	0.00	0.00	0.00	0.00	0.00
5	1.00	25%	0.00	0.00	0.00	0.00	0.00	0.01
5	1.00	50%	0.00	0.00	0.00	0.00	0.00	0.02
5	1.00	75%	0.01	0.02	0.01	0.03	0.01	0.03
5	2.00	25%	0.14	0.27	0.00	0.01	0.00	0.05
5	2.00	50%	0.14	0.27	0.05	0.23	0.03	0.09
5	2.00	75%	0.14	0.28	0.24	0.47	0.09	0.14
10	0.50	25%	0.00	0.00	0.00	0.00	0.00	0.00
10	0.50	50%	0.00	0.00	0.00	0.00	0.00	0.00
10	0.50	75%	0.00	0.00	0.00	0.00	0.00	0.00
10	1.00	25%	0.00	0.00	0.00	0.00	0.00	0.03
10	1.00	50%	0.00	0.00	0.00	0.00	0.00	0.04
10	1.00	75%	0.02	0.04	0.03	0.06	0.02	0.05
10	2.00	25%	0.26	0.46	0.00	0.01	0.00	0.10
10	2.00	50%	0.27	0.46	0.10	0.40	0.06	0.17
10	2.00	75%	0.27	0.47	0.42	0.71	0.16	0.26

[a]Rules for classifying a posttreatment change as a "response" with notations defined in Table 3:

1. $S_{post} > S_{pre} + 3 \times sd(S_{pre})$ and $S_{post} > C$;
   a. $S_{post} > S_{pre} + 2 \times sd(S_{pre})$ and $S_{post} > C$.
2. $S_{post} > 3 \times S_{pre}$ and $S_{post} > C$;
   a. $S_{post} > 2 \times S_{pre}$ and $S_{post} > C$.
3. $S_{post} > 2 \times S_{pre} + 2 \times sd(S_{pre})$ and $S_{post} > C$.
4. $(S_{post} - I_{post}) > 2(S_{pre} - I_{pre}) + 2 \times sd(S_{pre})$ and $(S_{post} - I_{post}) > I_{post} + 2 \times sd(I_{post})$ and $S_{post} > C$.

The probabilities in the table are based on 10,000 simulations with the enzyme-linked immunospot results represented by normally distributed data; the coefficient of variation was assumed the same, pre- and posttreatment. In these simulations, the value of C (for all the rules) was assumed the assay threshold. For rule 4, the mean number of spots for the irrelevant peptide was taken to be equal to the assay threshold as well, and the coefficient of variation for the distribution of the irrelevant peptide was set at 50%.

superior; but based on Tables 4 and 5, consideration should be given to using rules 1 or 2. If it is important to include irrelevant peptides as controls, rule 4 performs well for protecting against false-positives, although it is somewhat conservative overall. If other configurations of parameters apply, then other rules may be superior.

The purpose of this example was to demonstrate that tools exist to evaluate rules for classifying immune responses that are large enough according to that prespecified rule. Other rules exist and other conditions may prevail, and simulations can be used to evaluate those. In planning the analysis of an immune response in a clinical trial or in a cohort of patients, simulations of the type in Tables 4 and 5 can be helpful for understanding the statistical properties of the rules used, in terms of correctly classifying responders.

4. CONCLUSIONS

Immune response assays play an important and growing role in the effort to develop improved immunotherapy regimens for the treatment of cancer. For these new immuno-therapies, pilot trials are needed to establish proof of principal: that the therapy can affect the patient and produce a change in the immunological status that has the potential to translate into an antitumor effect. Careful statistical analyses of these measures of immune response will increase the understanding of the biological effects of the new therapies and will expedite the evaluation of immunotherapies the clinical setting.

REFERENCES

1. Keilholz U, Weber J, Finke JH, et al. Immunologic monitoring of cancer vaccine therapy: results of a workshop sponsored by the Society of Biological Therapy. *J Immunother* 2002; 25:97–138.
2. Horig H, Lee DS, Conkright W, et al. Phase I clinical trial of a recombinant canarypoxvirus (ALVAC) vaccine expressing human carcinoembryonic antigen and the B7.1 co-stimulatory molecule. *Cancer Immunol Immunother* 2000; 49:504–514.
3. Scheibenbogen C, Schmittel A, Keilholz U, et al. Phase 2 trial of vaccination with tyrosinase peptides and granulocyte-macrophage colony-stimulating factor in patients with metastatic melanoma. *J Immunother* 2000; 23:275–281.
4. Banchereau J, Palucka AK, Dhodapkar M, et al. Immune and clinical responses in patients with meta-static melanoma to CD34$^+$ progenitor-derived dendritic cell vaccine. *Cancer Res* 2001; 61:6451–6458.
5. Pepe MS, Etzioni R, Feng Z, et al. Phases of biomarker development for early detection of cancer. *J Natl Cancer Inst* 2001; 93:1054–1061.
6. Hammond ME, Taube SE. Issues and barriers to development of clinically useful tumor markers: a devel-opment pathway proposal. *Semin Oncol* 2002; 29:213–221.
7. Prentice RL. Surrogate endpoints in clinical trials: definition and operational criteria. *Stat Med* 1989; 8: 431–440.
8. Morrison DF. *Multivariate Statistical Methods, 3rd Edition.* New York: McGraw-Hill. 1995.
9. Tooze JA, Gunward GK, Jones RH. Analysis of repeated measures data with clumping at zero. *Stat Methods Med Res* 2002; 11:341–355.
10. Rashid M. Rank-based analysis of clinical trials with unbalanced repeated measures data. *ASA Proc Joint Stat Meetings* 2002; 2838–2843.
11. Whiteside TL, Zhao Y, Tsukishiro T, Elder EM, Gooding W, Baar J. Enzyme-linked immunospot, cytokine flow cytometry, and tetramers in the detection of T-cell responses to a dendritic cell-based multi-peptide vaccine in patients with melanoma. *Clin Cancer Res* 2003; 9:641–649.
12. Simon R, Altman DG. Statistical aspects of prognostic factor studies in oncology. *Br J Cancer* 1994; 69:979–985.
13. Drew PJ, Ilstrup DM, Kerin MJ, Monson JR. Prognostic factors: guidelines for investigation design and state of the art analytical methods. *Surg Oncol* 1998; 7:71–76.
14. Schmoor C, Sauerbrei W, Schumacher M. Sample size considerations for the evaluation of prognostic factors in survival analysis. *Stat Med* 2000; 19:441–452.
15. Pajak TF, Clark GM, Sargent DJ, McShane LM, Hammond ME. Statistical issues in tumor marker studies. *Arch Pathol Lab Med* 2000; 124:1011–1015.
16. Altman DG, Royston P. What do we mean by validating a prognostic model? *Stat Med* 2000; 19:453–473.
17. Harrell FE, Lee KL, Matchar DB, Reichert TA. Regression models for prognostic prediction: advan-tages, problems, and suggested solutions. *Cancer Treat Rep* 1985; 69:1071–1077.
18. Metz CE. Basic principles of ROC analysis. *Semin Nucl Med* 1978; 8:283–298.
19. Hanley JA. (1989) Receiver operating characteristic (ROC) methodology: the state of the art. *CRC Crit Rev Diagn Imaging* 1989; 29:307–335.
20. Zhou XH, Gatsonis CA. A simple method for comparing correlated ROC curves using incomplete data. *Stat Med* 1996; 15:1687–1691.
21. Heagerty PJ, Lumley TR, Pepe MS. Time-dependent ROC curves for censored survival data and a diag-nostic marker. *Biometrics* 2000; 56:337–344.

22. Alonzo TA, Pepe MS. Distribution-free ROC analysis using binary regression techniques. *Biostatistics* 2002; 3:421–432.

23. Pepe MS. *The Statistical Evaluation of Medical Tests for Classification and Prediction, Oxford Statistical Science Series*. Oxford: Oxford University Press. 2003.

24. Halpern J. Maximally selected chi-square statistics for small samples. *Biometrics* 1982; 38:1017–1023.

25. Miller R, Siegmund D. Maximally selected chi-square statistics. *Biometrics* 1982; 38:1011–1016.

26. Altman DG, Lausen B, Sauerbrei W, Schumacher M. Dangers of using "optimal" cutpoints in the evaluation of prognostic factors. *J Natl Cancer Inst* 1994; 86:829–835.

27. Faraggi D, Simon R. A simulation study of cross-validation for selecting an optimal cutpoint in univariate survival analysis. *Stat Med* 1996; 15:2203–2213.

28. Hollander N, Schumacher M.On the problem of using "optimal" cutpoints in the assessment of quantitative prognostic factors. *Onkologie* 2001; 24:194–199.

29. Mazumdar M, Smith A, Bacik J. Methods for categorizing a prognostic variable in a multivariable setting. *Stat Med* 2003; 22:559–571.

30. Hollander N, Sauerbrei W, Schumucher M. Confidence intervals for the effect of a prognostic factor after selection of an "optimal" cutpoint. *Stat Med* 2004; 23:1701–1713.

31. Molenberghs G, Buyse M, Geys H, Renard D, Burzykowski T, Alonso A. Statistical challenges in the evaluation of surrogate endpoints in randomized trials. *Controlled Clin Trials* 2002; 23:607–625.

32. Berger VW. Does the Prentice criterion validate surrogate endpoints? *Stat Med* 2004; 23:1571–1578.

6 DNA Vaccines for Cancer Immunotherapy

Heesun Kwak and Howard L. Kaufman

SUMMARY

The introduction of selected genes by direct injection of DNA represents a general strategy for short-term gene expression in vivo. DNA vaccines may be especially useful for cancer immunotherapy because DNA allows transient expression of tumor-associated antigens and immunostimulatory proteins by a relatively nonimmunogenic vector. This chapter focuses on how DNA vaccines stimulate immune responses and how different immunization strategies may result in various types of immunity. The inclusion of chemical and genetic adjuvants as methods for enhancing DNA vaccination is also discussed. The methods currently available for constructing DNA vaccines and the implications for cancer therapy will be reviewed. Finally, some of the safety and ethical concerns generated by DNA vaccination are presented.

Key Words: Adjuvants; cancer; DNA; immunotherapy; vaccination.

1. INTRODUCTION

DNA vaccines have become a reliable and major method to elicit immune responses in the past decade. DNA vaccination has been used for gene delivery, and, combined with an increased understanding of the human genome, has provided a new technique for gene therapy. Ideal vaccines should be inexpensive, stable, and easy to manufacture and store. DNA vaccines offer many advantages over many conventional approaches: they are simple to make and deliver, and they elicit both humoral and cellular immunity. They can deliver multiple antigens that can be expressed in the same immunization.

DNA vaccines consist of a plasmid DNA backbone containing one or more genes that encode immunogenic and/or immunostimulatory proteins. DNA by itself has a much-conserved structure that may be ignored by the host's immune system. However, after delivery of DNA to an organism, the encoded message is translated into specific proteins, which can be processed and presented by professional antigen-presenting cells (APCs), providing the initiation of an antigen-specific immune response.

To date, this approach has been experimentally applied to elicit protective immunity as well as to induce therapeutically efficient immunity in several species, including humans. DNA vaccination aims at inducing the strongest possible immune response, focused precisely on a specific target, such as a specific pathogen or tumor-associated antigen, through transient expression of genes encoding antigens and/or immunostimulatory proteins.

From: *Cancer Drug Discovery and Development: Immunotherapy of Cancer*
Edited by: M. L. Disis © Humana Press Inc., Totowa, NJ

In this chapter, we focus on the therapeutic aspects of DNA vaccines with respect to tumor immunotherapy. We address some of the current problems and possible solutions. The ideal DNA vector would have certain attributes that could be predicted based on previous experience. These attributes include:

1. High transfection efficiency of specific cells.
2. Maintenance of the episomal state.
3. Levels of transgene expression corresponding to expected function.
4. Proper intra- or extracellular localization of the transgenic product.
5. Stimulation of the proper quality, antigen-specific immune response that is typically humoral for extracellular pathogens and cellular for intracellular parasites and tumor cells.

We discuss major hurdles that need to be overcome and ways to enhance the efficacy of therapeutic vaccination. Some of the issues related to safety concerns with DNA vaccines and possible future directions of DNA vaccine research will be discussed.

2. MECHANISM OF DNA VACCINE-INDUCED IMMUNITY

In general, primary protection for most viral and bacterial infections is mediated by humoral immune response. For intracellular infection, such as *Mycobacterium tuberculosis*, *Leishmania major*, or other cellular parasites, protection is mediated by cellular immunity. However, for some diseases, such as HIV, herpes, or malaria, both humoral and cellular responses are likely to be required. Cellular immune response comprises primarily CD4+ and CD8+ T-cells. These cells recognize the foreign antigens that have been processed and presented by APCs in the context of major histocompatibility complex (MHC) class II or MHC class I molecules, respectively. Exogenous antigens provided by killed pathogens or proteins derived from live vaccines are taken up by APCs by phagocytosis or endocytosis and presented by MHC class II molecules to stimulate CD4+ T-cells, which can help generate effective antibody responses. In some cases, MHC class I molecules associate with antigens synthesized within the cytoplasm of the cell that are elicited by live or DNA vaccines (crosspriming). In this regard, DNA vaccines can induce both humoral and cellular responses.

2.1. Antigen Presentation

The ability to "sneak in" to an organism without inciting a strong immune response makes plasmid DNA unique among vaccines. In fact, complete adaptive immunity specific to plasmid DNA has not been reported. Importantly, although plasmid DNA is quickly deposited in myocytes and APCs *(1)*, there is a several-hours-long time gap between injection of DNA vaccine and the appearance of encoded antigen. This might have major consequences for the ability of DNA vaccines to prime naïve T-cells. The amount of antigen produced in vivo after DNA inoculation is in the picogram-to-nanogram range *(2)*. Equivalent amount of antigen introduced in vivo in the form of protein would probably be processed by macrophages without inducing an adaptive response, resulting in the impression that the antigen was either ignored or tolerized. These observations suggest that the plasmid itself may function as a powerful immunomodulator.

The most likely explanation for such broad and sustained immune responses from a relatively small amount of protein is related to characteristics of the DNA itself (e.g., cytosine–phosphate–guanine [CpG] motifs) and/or type of APC transfected. So far, at least three different mechanisms by which DNA antigen is processed have been described:

direct priming by somatic cells, such as myocytes or keratinocytes *(3–5)*; direct transfection of dendritic cells (DCs) *(6)*; and crosspriming.

Direct priming of somatic cells was shown in studies by Wolff et al. *(2)* and Ulmer et al. *(7)*, in which the intramuscular vaccination of naked DNA led the expression of protein in transfected cells. These studies suggested muscle cells were involved in the initiation of immune response after DNA vaccination. Because these muscle cells do not express other cell surface molecules that are critical in optimizing T-cell priming, such as CD80 and CD86, they might not be as efficient as DCs. To test whether muscle cells alone are sufficient to prime immune cells, several experiments were undertaken. One study showed the muscle cells could induce cytotoxic T-lymphocyte (CTL) responses when mice were vaccinated with DNA expressing both antigen and CD86 *(8)*. Another study showed that DNA encoding antigen and CD86, interleukin (IL)-12, or granulocyte/macrophage colony-stimulating factor (GM-CSF) failed to induce CTL responses *(9)*. Yet others demonstrated that removing muscle cells immediately (within 10 min) after immunization did not alter subsequent immune responses *(10)*, suggesting that DNA likely gains access to the lymphatic or circulatory system even after intramuscular injection. For skin injection, keratinocytes and Langerhans' cells are the major cell types that are transfected by plasmid DNA *(11,12)*. In skin biopsies after DNA vaccination, it has been suggested that the cells migrate from the epidermis within 24 h of immunization and elicit primary immune responses *(13)*.

In most cases, secreted or exogenous proteins are presented through the MHC class II pathway, whereas endogenously produced proteins or peptides are presented through MHC class I pathways. However, exogenous antigens can be presented through MHC class I pathways (crosspriming), providing an additional mechanism by which DNA immunization can enhance immune responses *(14)*. During crosspriming, antigens generated by somatic cells can be taken up by professional APCs to directly prime T-cell responses. Thus, the best evidence currently suggests that somatic cells constitute the predominant cells transfected by DNA via muscle or skin injection and immune responses are induced via crosspriming by DCs.

Successful immunization requires all steps of DC maturation from monocyte through immature DCs to mature DCs to occur, with each stage playing a critical role in DNA-elicited immunity *(15,16)*. The early presence of interferon (IFN)-γ is essential in stimulating maturation of monocytes and upregulation of several co-stimulatory and antigen-presenting molecules, such as MHC class II, B7.1/CD80, B7.2/CD86, intracellular adhesion molecule 1/CD54, and CD40 *(17)*. IFN-γ can also significantly influence the intracellular processing of antigen by inducing replacement of standard proteasomes by immunoproteasomes that are much more efficient at producing antigenic peptides presented by MHC class I to CD8$^+$ T-cells *(18,19)*, thus explaining the efficient priming of naïve CD8$^+$ T-cells by DNA vaccination *(20)*. This two-phase response allowing DCs to reach a more mature phenotype characterized by the expression of several co-stimulatory molecules at the time of antigen presentation may also have beneficial effects through lowering the threshold of MHC/peptide–T-cell receptor-binding avidity. This way, more precursors, including those with relatively low-affinity T-cell receptor, have a chance to be activated, thus increasing the polyclonality of T-cell responses.

2.2. Cellular Immunity

To provide effective protection, a vaccine should be able to induce both humoral and cell-mediated immune responses. In patients with cancer and certain infectious diseases, such as HIV, the T-cell response may be more important for long-term protection. In this sense, DNA vaccines have advantages over other types of vaccine in that they can induce strong T-helper-cell (Th) and CTL responses. DNA vaccines are therefore considered a promising alternative to attenuated live viruses and other vaccines in the field of infectious diseases and cancer.

2.2.1. CD4⁺ T-CELLS

CD4⁺ T-cells play a central role in immune homeostasis. Activated CD4⁺ T-cells promote B-cell survival and antibody production, provide helper function to CD8⁺ T-cells, and secrete myriad cytokines. Based on their production of certain cytokines, activated CD4⁺ T-cells can be divided into two distinct subsets, Th1 type and Th2 type. Th1 CD4⁺ T-cells produce IFN-γ, IL-2, IL-12, and promote cell-mediated immunity. In contrast, Th2 CD4⁺ T-cells secrete IL-4, IL-5, IL-10, IL-13, and provide help for B-cell differentiation and humoral immunity. The ability of DNA vaccines to generate Th1 responses is useful in situations, such as intracellular infectious disease and cancer, requiring Th1 responses. For example, it was shown that DNA vaccination enhanced IFN-γ and decreased IL-4 production in mice infected with *L. major (21)*. The presence of unmethylated CpG motifs in bacterial DNA can trigger the immune system to induce a variety of proinflammatory cytokines including IL-12. Thus, the generation of Th1 responses may be a general property of DNA vaccines. Activation of signaling pathways in DCs leads not only to the production of IL-12, important for skewing immune responses toward Th1 *(22)*, but also tumor necrosis factor-α and type 1 IFNs that are important for the release of IFN-γ by natural-killer cells *(23)*. Type 1 IFNs appear to be particularly important for the stimulation of Th1-type priming by immunostimulatory sequence-containing DNA vaccines. It has been shown that IFN-α and IFN-β secreted by immunostimulatory sequence-stimulated APCs can upregulate not only B7, but also the peptide transporter associated with antigen-processing expression *(24)*, which is essential for efficient antigen crosspresentation *(25)*. Moreover, recently published reports indicate the importance of IL-18 and IL-23 in the Th1-polarizing capacity of DCs *(26,27)*.

Whereas many studies of DNA vaccines demonstrated induction of Th1 responses in animal models, under certain circumstances, DNA vaccines can also induce Th2 responses. This has been reported in situations where DNA is delivered by gene gun immunization A potential explanation for this is that the gene gun delivers plasmid DNA directly into cells, bypassing surface interactions which may be important for Th1 polarization. When the plasmid is internalized directly, CpG motifs in the plasmid backbone may be unable to interact with Toll-like receptors on APCs inhibiting release of proinflammatory Th1-type cytokines. In at least one report, supplying DNA vaccines with additional CpG motifs that stimulate Th1 responses could not overrule Th2-promoting signals when the vaccine was delivered by gene gun bombardment *(28)*.

2.2.2. CD8⁺ T-CELLS

One of the major advantages of DNA vaccination is generation of endogenous antigens that are presented to CD8⁺ T-cells via the MHC class I pathway. CD8⁺ T-cell responses are easily generated by live viral vaccines, but because of safety concerns and immunity to viral components limiting the ability to boost responses against targeted antigens, DNA vaccination may represent an advantage. In addition, CTL response can be optimized relatively easily by modifying DNA encoding antigen. In a lymphocytic choriomeningitis virus murine model, although lower than live viral infection, DNA vaccination induced precursor CTLs that expanded in vivo after infectious challenge *(29–31)*. DNA vaccination also elicited CTL responses similar to live viral infection after short-term in vitro culture. Studies showed that the DNA vaccines encoding an influenza or Sendai virus nucleoprotein elicited CTL responses against both dominant and subdominant epitopes *(32,33)*. These studies suggest DNA vaccines can elicit broad precursor CTL frequency and memory responses.

2.3. Humoral Immunity

Plasmid DNA immunization can induce a strong antibody response to a variety of proteins in animal and human subjects *(34)*. The humoral response generated by DNA vaccination has been shown to be protective in several animal models in vivo *(35)*. Studies demonstrated that the dose and frequency of immunization affects the kinetics and magnitude of response. Antibody production peaked and reached a plateau between 4 and 12 wk after a single DNA immunization in mice, whereas antibody production was increased in a dose-responsive manner after multiple injections of DNA by various routes of immunization *(36,37)*. The antibody subtypes induced by DNA vaccination include immunoglobulin (Ig)G, IgM, and IgA. As mentioned in Subheading 2.2.2., because DNA vaccination generally enhanced Th1 cytokine production, the subclass of antibodies generated by plasmid DNA vaccination will be biased toward IgG2a production *(38)*. The location of antigen expression may also influence the type of response as DNA encoding-secreted antigen generates higher levels of IgG1 than membrane-bound antigen *(39)*. In addition, DNA vaccination via gene gun may also preferentially bias toward IgG1 production *(40)*.

2.4. Memory Response

Current knowledge of the mechanism by which central and effector memory cells are generated is limited *(41)*. In fact, it has been suggested that only those vaccines that induce long-term protection exert this effect through neutralizing antibodies *(42)*. Apparently, antigen-specific T-cell precursors induced by vaccines aimed at HIV or antigenic tumors do not persist long enough to maintain sufficient numbers of activated effector T-cells. Although the mechanisms of terminating immune responses are incompletely understood, it is possible that eradication of antigen from the host could be a major reason for termination of the immune response *(43)*. Whereas this explanation might be plausible for certain kinds of transient infections, there is little chance for complete elimination of an antigen in chronic infections or cancer. Along this line, efficient control of chronic infections might rely on a continued immune response maintained by functional memory B- and T-cells. Long-lasting expression of proteins provided by DNA vaccination may favor persistence of T-cell memory and consequently, effective immunity. Alternatively, providing booster antigen may also promote memory responses.

3. IMMUNIZATION REGIMENS

3.1. Administration Techniques

The most commonly used methods to date are intradermal and intramuscular needle injection of "naked" plasmid DNA or ballistic means, such as gene gun delivery. Needle injection is easily performed by preparing DNA in saline and injecting the mixture into the muscle or different layers of skin. This typically requires 10–100 µg of plasmid DNA to elicit immune responses. Gene gun uses ballistic administration of plasmid DNA-coated gold beads, fired by compressed gas *(44)*. The gene gun uses a regulated burst of helium gas to propel plasmid DNA-coated gold beads (approx 1–3 µm in diameter) directly into the cytoplasm of skin cells *(45)*. This method of vaccination typically requires as little as 0.1–1 µg of plasmid DNA to evoke substantial immune responses, and is much more reproducible than the syringe injection.

Low-volume jet injection is another mechanical method of plasmid DNA delivery *(46)*. This requires a simple, hand-held injector to deliver plasmid DNA under high pressure into the desired tissue. It is more effective than syringe injection and without the requirement for precipitation of plasmid DNA onto gold particles, and is easier to perform than particle bombardment *(47)*.

Needle-free jet injection of plasmid DNA has been tested in animals and in several human clinical trials *(48,49)*, and many studies suggest enhanced immune responses over needle injection. Aguiar et al. *(50)* showed up to a 50-fold increase in antibody titers with intramuscular jet injection (Biojector® 2000; Bioject, Portland, OR), compared with intramuscular needle injection in rabbits. In pigs and dogs immunized with a human growth hormone plasmid by subcutaneous or intramuscular injection, antigen-specific antibody titers were increased up to 20-fold with jet injection (Medi-Jector VISION®; Mediject, Minneapolis, MN) compared with needle injection *(51)*. However, the method requires large amounts of DNA (usually from 50 µg in mice to 2 mg per dose in humans) for effective immunization *(52)*. In many cases, needle injection and gene gun methods produce different types of immune responses using the same plasmid. For example, a measles antigen plasmid DNA given by intramuscular needle injection elicits Th1 responses, whereas gene gun delivery elicits Th2 or balanced Th1/Th2 responses *(53)*. Although this result is surprising, the type of antigen and the route of immunization contribute to the type of immunity generated.

To reduce the dose of plasmid DNA and enhance the efficiency, nanoparticle-based jet injection has been investigated. Nanoparticles or microspheres offer many advantages as a vaccine delivery system *(54)*. Organic microparticles, preferably positively charged to increase adsorption of negatively charged DNA molecules, is one obvious choice. These particles range in size from 1 to 10 µm in diameter and are readily phagocytosed by APCs *(55)*. They are made from poly(lactide-co-glycolide), which is a biodegradable and bio-compatible polymer *(54)*. These particles coated with cationic surfactants (e.g., 1,2-dioleoyl-1,3-trimethylammoniopropane) proved to be very efficient carriers of plasmid DNA. Moreover, particle-bound DNA induced at least 100 times higher antibody titers than soluble plasmid DNA. Similarly, DNA-coated cetyltrimethylammonium bromide/poly(lactide-coglycolide) proved to be superior to naked plasmid DNA or even lipofectamine/DNA-transfected DCs in the stimulation of IL-2 production by gag55-specific T-cell hybridomas *(56)*. Microspheres enhance immune responses to DNA plasmids by generating both cellular and humoral immune responses *(57)*. In mice, jet injection of plasmid DNA-coated nanoparticles enhanced antibody titers more than 200-fold over jet injection of plasmid DNA alone *(58–61)*. Dendritic cell-targeted plasmid DNA-coated nanoparticles significantly enhanced antibody and Th1-type immune responses *(62)*. These nanoparticles further enhanced the resulting immune responses when combined with other known adjuvants *(63)*.

Other compounds used to improve transfection through compacting DNA are cationic polymers, such as poly-L-lysine. The formation of cationic polymers substituted with sugar residues as ligands, providing a method for adding a targeting component to the complex. Along this line, plasmid DNA combined with poly- L-lysine-bearing lactose residues was found to efficiently transfect hepatocytes, probably through galactose-specific lectins, which are heavily expressed by these cells (64). Similarly, DNA in complexes with β-D-GlcNAc-substituted poly- L-lysine was efficiently incorporated by cystic fibrosis epithelial cells (65).

The use of ultrasound to increase transfection efficiency (66) or magnetofection, based on delivery of DNA-coated superparamagnetic nanoparticles by application of a magnetic field, are other interesting experimental strategies awaiting validation (67). Several techniques based on mechanical, electrical, and chemical approaches have been developed to increase the efficiency of plasmid DNA delivery. For intramuscular delivery, low uptake of DNA can be a limiting factor, and transfection of skeletal muscles can be enhanced by electroporation. This enhances movement of the DNA construct across the cytoplasmic membrane. Electroporation of plasmid DNA into variety of cells in vitro (68) has been successfully adopted for the transformation of cells in vivo (69). Although this is an efficient method for site-localized transfection, severe cytotoxicity caused by high-voltage exposure limits it applicability. As shown by Rizutto et al. (69), a significant improvement can be achieved by using low-voltage, high-frequency electric pulses that can increase efficiency of muscle cells transformation 100-fold with only transient tissue damage.

Obviously, using naked plasmid DNA, although sufficient to elicit immune responses, does not always establish a sufficient level of cell targeting. There is currently an intense focus on trying to manufacture a product that would not only improve the efficiency of plasmid delivery, but also target plasmid DNA to preferred tissues. These efforts are focused largely on the development of nonviral carriers of DNA and are extensively reviewed elsewhere (70).

3.2. Administration Route

A variety of DNA injection routes have been studied: intramuscular, intradermal, subcutaneous, intravenous, intraperitoneal, oral, intranasal, intravaginal, and intrarectal (71–80). The most widely used methods are intramuscular, subcutaneous, and intradermal. Depending on the route by which DNA is administered, different types of immune responses may be elicited, as previously discussed. Intramuscular immunization elicits predominantly Th1 immune responses, whereas gene gun predominantly elicits Th2 responses by delivering DNA directly into the cells, bypassing surface interaction of immunostimulatory CpG motifs with APCs. Further research is needed to define fully the optimal route of DNA administration for specific indications.

3.3. Prime–Boost

A number of studies demonstrated the advantage of combining two or more vaccine modalities. The basic prime–boost strategy involves priming the immune system to a target antigen delivered by one vector and then selectively boosting by readministration of the antigen in the context of a second and distinct vector. This heterologous prime–boost elicited greater levels of immunity than single administration or homologous boost vaccination and increased numbers of antigen-specific T-cells (81,82). For optimal response, the development of vectors that are not affected by prior immunity and that can elicit systemic immunity is important. A large number of alternative expression vectors have been

developed for such prime–boost vaccine approaches, including, replication-defective adenoviruses, avipoxviruses, influenza viruses, and Sendai viruses, among others *(83–86)*.
Immune responses can be qualitatively and quantitatively different with various combinations. Strategies in which a DNA prime is followed by a boost with a recombinant viral
vector expressing the antigen of interest has been shown to dramatically enhance the
protective immune response generated in several murine and primate models of intracellular infection *(87,88)*. In mice, systemic (intramuscular) prime–boost with DNA encoding glycoprotein gB of herpes simplex virus and recombinant vaccinia virus encoding gB
was more effective than DNA alone in inducing serum IgG and herpes simplex virus-
specific IFN-γ-producing splenic CD4$^+$ T-cells *(87)*. However, when these mice were
mucosally (intranasally) immunized, those primed with recombinant vaccinia virus
encoding gB and boosted with gB DNA generated higher frequencies of IFN-γ-producing CD4$^+$ T-cells than those with the reverse regimen. In macaques, a combined regimen
of vaccinia virus and DNA expressing highly pathogenic simian HIV was more effective
than DNA alone in protecting CD4$^+$ T-cells from viral challenge *(88)*. In addition, priming with vaccinia virus and boosting with DNA was more effective than the reverse regimen in decreasing postacute viral load, demonstrating that the sequence of prime–boost
affects vaccine efficacy.

4. ADJUVANTS

Adjuvants are used to modify the intensity or type of immune responses generated
with vaccines. Appropriate adjuvants must be able to promote the modulation of immune
responses and are generally effective at initiating innate immunity. They can be conventional (chemical) or genetic in form. Conventional adjuvants are chemical compounds
that enhance, prolong, and modulate immune responses. Genetic adjuvants are expression vectors encoding cytokines or other molecules that modulate antigen-specific immune
responses. In addition, DNA vaccines themselves possess adjuvant activity because of
the presence of unmethylated CpG motifs *(89)*. In choosing appropriate adjuvants, it is
important to consider which type of response provides protection and then select the best
adjuvant to help vaccine-induced immunity. Careful selection of adjuvants can significantly enhance DNA-elicited immune responses.

4.1. Conventional Adjuvants

Conventional adjuvants (Table 1) include aluminum salts, bacteria-derived adjuvants,
lipid particles, emulsifier-based adjuvants, and synthetic adjuvants. Generally, conventional adjuvant–DNA complexes are relatively easy to make, because they require simple
mixing with/without incubation or emulsification. Aluminum salts include aluminum
phosphate, aluminum hydroxide, and calcium gels, which act by adsorbing antigen on
their surfaces *(90,91)*. Co-administration of aluminum adjuvants with DNA vaccines
enhanced vaccination efficacy and is approved for human use. Bacteria-derived molecules
have been used widely as adjuvants as well. Perhaps the most well-characterized adjuvants are oil–water emulsion containing fragments of killed mycobacteria, also known as
complete Freund's adjuvant. The administration of complete Freund's adjuvant is potent,
but also causes severe local reactions prohibiting its clinical use. The less toxic incomplete
Freund's adjuvant contains the oil in water emulsion without mycobacterial components
and incomplete Freund's adjuvant is commonly used as an adjuvant for vaccination.

Table 1

Chemical Adjuvants for DNA Vaccines

Classification	Adjuvant	Specific agents	Mechanism	Toxicity
Mineral salts	Alum	Aluminum phosphate, aluminum hydroxide	Forms antigen depot at the injection site	Granulomas, increased IgE production
Glycosides	Saponins	QS-21	Strong CD8$^+$ T-cell responses	Local reactions, granulomas, hemolysis
Bacterial components	Gram-negative bacteria	LPS, MDP	Activates TLR-4 In saline, enhances humoral immunity; in glycerol, results in cellular immunity	Local reactions, multiple systemic effects
Emulsions	Oil in water	IFA, Montanide, Adjuvant 65, Lipovant	Forms a depot at injection site	Inflammatory reactions, granulomas, ulcers
Synthetic lipids	Liposomes	Doxil, Caelyx, DuanoXome, Ambisome, Amphitec, Abelect, Allovectin 7	Extends half-life of antigens in circulation; may also accumulate at sites of inflammation or tumor	Limited
Microspheres	Polymeric microspheres	Poly (DL-lactide-coglycolide)	Based on components can control rate of antigen delivery	Limited
Carbohydrates	Insulin-derived	γ-Insulin	Natural carbohydrate activates RES; activates Th1 and Th2 cellular immunity	Limited; metabolizes into simple sugars
	Polysaccharides	Glucans, dextrans, glucomannans	Activates macrophages through glucan and mannan receptors	Limited

IgE, immunoglobulin E; LPS, lipopolysaccharide; TLR-4, Toll-like receptor 4; MDP, N-acetyl-muramyl-L-alanyl-D-isoglutamine; IFA, incomplete Freund's adjuvant; RES, reticuloendothelial system; Th1 and Th2, T-helper cell 1 and T-helper cell 2.

Other examples of adjuvants include monophosphoryl lipid A and muramyl peptides *(92)*. Lipid particle-based adjuvants include cationic liposomes and mannan-coated cationic lipids *(93,94)*. These act by facilitating entry of DNA into cells by entrapping DNA within and increasing the affinity of the DNA complex for the cell membrane. The optimal ratio of liposome to DNA is a key factor when synthesizing DNA–liposome complexes. Another adjuvant, QS-21, is a highly purified saponin fraction from extracts of the *Quillaja saponaria* tree *(95)*. QS-21 enhances immune responses and is currently under investigation as a potential adjuvant in humans. Other synthetic adjuvants, such as ubenimex, have shown adjuvant effects in mice and are now in clinical trials with cancer vaccines *(96)*.

4.2. Genetic Adjuvants

Genetic adjuvants (Table 2) are immunostimulatory molecules administered as recombinant proteins or encoded by defined genes that can bias immune responses to enhance DNA vaccination. These includes cytokines, chemokines, growth factors, costimulatory molecules, complement (e.g., C3d), heat shock proteins (e.g., Hsp70), apoptosis inducers (e.g., caspase 3), and transcription factors (e.g., IFN regulator factor) that are capable of potentiating immune responses. Genetic adjuvants can be used to enhance antigen presentation, T-cell priming and differentiation, maintenance of memory responses, and antibody production. Genes encoding genetic adjuvants can be given on the same DNA plasmid as the targeted antigen or on a separate plasmid in addition to administration of recombinant or synthetic proteins immediately following DNA vaccination. Dual expression vectors encoding mutant caspase 3 and influenza genes enhanced $CD4^+$ and $CD8^+$ T-cell responses and protected against lethal influenza challenge *(97)*.

4.2.1. CYTOKINES

Cytokines play a critical regulatory role in immune responses and have been used as DNA vaccine adjuvants. Numerous studies have focused on the coadministration of antigen and cytokine-encoding plasmids. For example, plasmids encoding HIV-1 gp120 antigen and GM-CSF under a single promoter gave improved $CD4^+$ T-cell responses *(98)*. Other examples of synergy include improved $CD8^+$ T-cell immunity in mice following coadministration of IL-12 or IFN-γ with a vaccine encoding hepatitis B viral DNA and protection against experimental autoimmune encephalitis in mice treated with a DNA vaccine and IL-4 *(99,100)*. Co-administration of Th1 cytokine encoding plasmids, such as IFN-γ, IL-2, IL-12, IL-15, or IL-18, with HIV-antigen-encoding DNA in mice and primate models, showed increased antigen-specific antibody responses and Th-proliferative responses *(101,102)*. The effects of different combination of cytokines have been tested as well. Coimmunization of HIV DNA with GM-CSF combined with IL-12 or IL-15 enhanced Th1-biased HIV-specific CTL responses and delayed-type hypersensitivity tests, whereas the inflammatory response induced by herpes simplex virus in mice was significantly attenuated after intranasal vaccinations with a DNA vaccine encoding IL-10 *(103–110)*. These studies suggest cytokines may have synergistic effects and may influence Th1/Th2 balance and immunological outcome after vaccination.

4.2.2. CHEMOKINES

Chemokines are a group of small, chemotactic cytokines that play important roles in the trafficking and activation of leukocytes in both normal and pathological states. More than 50 human chemokines and 18 chemokine receptors have been discovered so far. Che-

Table 2
Genetic Adjuvants for DNA Vaccines

Classification	Name	Cell-mediated response	Humoral response
Cytokines	IL-1	↑Proliferation, ↑IFN-γ, ↑CTL	↑IgG, ↑IgG2a
	IL-2	↑Proliferation, ↑IFN-γ, ↑CTL	↑IgG, ↑IgG2a
	IL-4	↑Proliferation, ↑IL-4, ↓DTH	↑IgG, ↑IgG1
	IL-5		↑IgG
	IL-7	↑IFN-γ	↑IgG2a
	IL-8	↑Neutrophils	
	IL-10	↓Proliferation, ↓DTH	↑IgG
	IL-12	↑Proliferation, ↑IFN-γ, ↑DTH, ↑CTL	↑IgG2a
	IL-15	↑Proliferation, ↑CTL	
	IL-18	↑Proliferation, ↑CTL	↑IgG
	TNF	↑Proliferation, ↑CTL	↑IgG
	GM-CSF	↑Proliferation, ↑IFN-γ, ↑IL-4	↑IgG, ↑IgG1, ↑IgG2a
	TGF-β	↓Proliferation, ↓DTH	↑IgG1
	IFN-γ	↑IFN-γ, ↑CTL	↑IgG2a
Costimulatory molecules	CD80 (B7-1)		
	CD86 (B7-2)		
	CD40L	↑IFN-γ, ↑CTL, ↑IgG	↑IgG1, ↑IgG2a
	ICAM-1	↑Proliferation, ↑IFN-γ, ↑CTL	
	LFA-3	↑Proliferation, ↑IFN-γ, ↑CTL	
Chemokines	RANTES		
	MIP1-α		
	MCP-1		
Complement	C3d		
Heat shock protein	HSP70		
	Gp96/GRP94		
Apoptosis inducer	Bcl-xL		
	Caspase 3		
Transcriptional factors	IRF-1, IRF-3, IRF-7		

IL, interleukin; IFN, interferon; Ig, immunoglobulin; DTH, delayed-type hypersensitivity test; CTL, cytotoxic T-lymphocyte; TNF, tumor necrosis factor; GM-CSF, granulocyte/macrophage colony-stimulating factor; TGF-β, transforming growth factor-β; ICAM-1, intracellular adhesion molecule 1; LFA-3, lymphocyte function associated 3; RANTES, regulated on activation, normal T-cell-expressed and -secreted; MIP1-α, mitochondrial DNA polymerase-encoding-α; MCP-1, monocyte chemotactic protein 1; IRF, interferon regulatory factor.

mokines released in damaged or infected peripheral tissues recruit phagocytic cells and APCs to sites of injury. APCs ingest pathogenic antigens or apoptotic cells and transport them to local secondary lymphoid tissue, where they process and present antigens to prime naïve T-cells under the influence of local chemokines. The magnitude of immune induction depends on frequency of encounters between naïve T-lymphocytes and APCs within lymph nodes. Following DNA vaccination, migration of directly transfected DCs to secondary lymphoid organs is critical for priming immune responses *(111,112)*. Although the ability of naked DNA to induce migration of DCs is yet to be proved, almost certainly plasmid DNA–microparticle complexes can be phagocytosed by monocytes at the site of injection, followed by migration to lymph nodes, where they become functional DCs *(113)*. Thus, DNA vaccines can be improved by including genes encoding chemokines involved in the migration of DCs. Early studies showed that coadministration of the CC chemokine secondary lymphoid-organ chemokine or Epstein-Barr virus-induced molecule 1 ligand chemokine with a plasmid-expressing antigen resulted in profound T-cell cytokine production in vitro *(114)*. Coadministration of cDNA encoding monocyte chemoattractant protein 1α with HIV DNA-enhanced antibody and CTL responses *(115)*. Other chemokines, such as regulated-on-activation, normal T-cell-expressed and-secreted, a β-chemokine, increased CTL responses when coadministered with HIV DNA in mice and primates *(116)*.

Receptors for chemokines such as CXCR4, CCR4, and especially CCR7 are upregulated in mature DCs *(117)*. The CCR7 ligands secondary lymphoid-organ chemokine and Epstein-Barr virus-induced molecule 1 ligand chemokine have been shown to be potent immunostimulators for both humoral and T-cell-mediated immunity *(118)*. Overexpression of these chemokines in plasmid-transfected cells may increase chances of direct contact between T-cells and DCs accumulating at the site of chemokine expression, thus leading to improved presentation of coexpressed antigen and enhanced immune responses against targeted antigens.

4.2.3. Co-Stimulatory Molecules

Optimal T- and B-cell activation requires secondary signals delivered through co-stimulatory molecules, such as CD80 (B7.1) and CD86 (B7.2). It is speculated that the codelivery of plasmid-expressing co-stimulatory molecules would improve humoral and cell-mediated immune responses. When the gene for CD86 was cloned and administered with HIV *env* or *gag/pol* DNA in mice, T-cell proliferation and CTL responses were increased *(119, 120)*. Co-administration of CD40L with *LacZ* DNA in mice showed a striking increase in antigen-specific production of IFN-γ, cytolytic T-cell activity, and IgG2a antibody titers *(120)*. Co-administration of intracellular adhesion molecule 1, lymphocyte function associated 3, and HIV antigens enhanced T-cell proliferative and CTL responses with a significant increase in IFN-γ secretion from activated T-cells *(121)*.

4.2.4. Heat Shock Proteins

Heat shock proteins (HSPs) are highly conserved molecules found in eukaryotes, prokaryotes, and plants. They act as molecular chaperones, helping appropriate protein folding and subunit assembly *(122,123)*. They are involved in assembly of antibody molecules and stabilization of MHC class I and class II molecules during peptide transport, playing an important role in protective immunity. Linkage of antigens to HSPs that play a role as chaperons involved in the endogenous antigen-processing pathway represents a particularly interesting approach for increasing the potency of DNA vaccines. Several members of the HSP70 and HSP90 family have been shown to facilitate CTL priming when injected in the form of protein-based vaccines *(124)*. Incorporation of the gene encoding HSP70-antigen fusion proteins into DNA vaccines was effective in enhancing CTL priming, followed by potent antitumor immunity against established tumors *(125)*. Similarly, fusion of the antigen to the N-terminal HSP-binding domain of the simian virus 40 (SV40) large T-antigen to increase chaperoning by endogenous HSPs, led to increased activity of antigen-specific CTLs *(126)*.

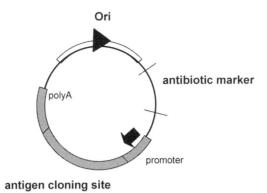

Fig. 1. Composition of a basic expression vector for DNA vaccine construction. A DNA plasmid is composed of bacterial origin of replication (Ori) for amplication in bacterial cultures, antibiotic selection marker, and antigen cloning site. In the simplest construction, the antigen-encoding gene is cloned between a promoter (arrow) and polyadenylation (polyA) signal.

Peptides are bound to HSPs and transferred to MHC class I molecules, leading to efficient crosspresentation of selected epitopes *(127)*. In several systems, immunization with HSP70-peptide complexes activated the innate immune response and led to maturation of immunized DCs, resulting in enhanced CTL responses *(128–131)*. When immunized mice with several plasmid-based vectors encoding chimeric proteins containing a chimeric prostate-specific antigen (PSA) fused to *Mycobacterium tuberculosis* HSP70, *M. bovis* HSP65, *E. coli* DnaK (HSP70), or human HSP70, human PSA-specific CD8+ CTL responses were induced, and mice were protected from a subsequent subcutaneous challenge with PSA-expressing tumors *(132)*. HSPs isolated from tumors have been under clinical investigation, and encouraging results form early phase trials have led to phase III clinical trials in renal cell carcinoma and melanoma *(133–135)*.

5. CONSTRUCTION OF DNA VACCINES

Construction of plasmid DNA vaccines requires certain minimum components (Fig. 1). These include bacterial origin of replication and selection marker for efficient large-scale production; expression cassette comprising a promoter, cloning sites and coding sequence for antigen; and a polyadenylation (poly [A]) signal to achieve adequate levels of protein expression. Other considerations in designing DNA vaccines are the choice of antigen(s), additional adjuvant genes, and the form of the gene(s).

5.1. Origins and Selection Systems

The success of DNA vaccines is largely dependent on the design and development of the gene delivery vector. Important considerations in the construction of a long-lasting gene-expression system include tissue specificity, ability for self-replication, and degree of integration possible with selected vectors. DNA vaccines also include a gene or genes of interest (antigen) cloned into the bacterial plasmid and engineered for optimal gene expression in eukaryotic cells. Hence, for growth in bacteria, an origin of replication is needed. For large-scale production of plasmid DNA vaccines, a high-copy number origin is required and origin in a *pUC* plasmid (*E.coli*:Col1E1 origin) is generally used for this purpose. To select plasmid-containing cells from bacterial cultures, antibiotic resistance markers are required. Ampicillin resistance markers are commonly used in mice and kana-mycin or neomycin resistance markers are often used in plasmids destined for humans.

5.2. Antigen-Expression Cassette

Antigen-expression cassettes are composed of promoter, multiple cloning sites for antigen(s), and a poly (A) signal. DNA encoding the antigen of interest is placed between the promoter and poly (A) signal, with a complete open reading frame for single genes, single epitopes, minigenes, or strings of open reading frames for polyproteins, ensuring Kozak consensus sequences are aligned ([136]; see Fig. 1). Sequences flanking the AUG initiator codon within mRNA influence its recognition by eukaryotic ribosomes, and it has been shown that the defined translational initiating sequence ($^{-6}$GCCA/GCCAUGG^{+}4) should be included in vertebrate mRNA located around the initiator codon. The antigen-expression system is a key element affecting the outcome of DNA immunization, and to activate the host immune system efficiently, sufficient antigen expression is important. Studies have emphasized the importance of the antigen-expression system in efforts to pursue stronger DNA-induced immunity (137).

5.2.1. PROMOTER AND POLY (A) SIGNALS

Protein levels are largely determined by the promoter, and generally, a strong pro-moter is used to give the maximum expression of antigens. The most commonly used in DNA vaccines are viral promoters, such as the human cytomegalovirus (CMV) immedi-ate–early promoter (IE-CMV), the Rous sarcoma virus, long terminal repeat Rous sarcoma virus, and the SV40 promoter. Among these, the most popular is the IE-CMV promoter, often used with an adjacent enhancer (138). In monocytes, the activity of IE-CMV pro-moter is strongly influenced by mobilization of nuclear factor (NF)-κB by tumor necrosis factor-α (139). It appears that other transcription factors, such as C/EBP-α and -β, involved in maturation of monocytes, can suppress NF-κB-mediated upregulation of the IE-CMV promoter (140). This pattern of IE-CMV promoter regulation may have major conse-quences for the expression of transgene(s) delivered by plasmid DNA to APCs. Such a mechanism may not only facilitate IE-CMV promoter-controlled transgene expression in directly transfected immature DCs, but may also ensure its transient expression in mature DC. This might help to explain the relatively high efficiency after delivery of a plasmid DNA-containing IE-CMV promoter by intramuscular or intradermal injection. Thus, the efficiency of the IE-CMV promoter in eliciting an immune response may be based on the high level of expression in transfected cells or may be because of the selec-tive expression in specific tissues.

To maintain tissue specificity the presence of many upstream regulatory elements are required, and if truncated to fit the right size of the plasmid, such promoters often lose their strength and specificity (141). Nevertheless, an inducible expression system based on the combination of hypoxia-responsive element and hypoxia inducible factor 1 has been shown to be effective for driving transgene expression in usually hypoxic, solid tumor tissue (142). This system might be particularly useful for the introduction of MHC class I/II or co-stim-ulatory molecules into tumor cells to enable efficient presentation of tumor-associated antigens (TAAs) and activation of effector T-cells.

Different sources of poly (A) signals have been used. These include viral signals (e.g., SV40), mammalian signals (e.g., rabbit globin), and most widely used, bovine growth hor-mone, or BGHpA. These poly (A) sequences provide stabilization of mRNA transcripts.

Table 3
Partial Listing of Antigens Used in DNA Vaccines

Classification	Disease	Antigen
Infectious disease	Tuberculosis	ESAT6
		pHsp65
	Malaria	
	HIV	Gag, env, pol
Autoimmunity	Allergy	
	Multiple sclerosis	
	Type I diabetes	
Cancer	Colon cancer	CEA
	Melanoma	MART-1
		MAGE
		Tyrosinase
		gp100
	Cervical cancer	HPV E6, E7
	Prostate cancer	PSA
	Breast cancer	Fra-1
	Angiogenesis	FLK-1

ESAT6, early secreted antigenic target protein; CEA, carcinoembryonic antigen; MART-1, melanoma antigen recognized by T-cells; MAGE, melanoma antigen; HPV, human papilloma virus; PSA, prostate-specific antigen; Fra-1, Fos-related antigen 1; FLK-1, fetal liver kinase 2.

5.2.2. ANTIGENS

A wide spectrum of antigens have been incorporated into DNA vaccines and tested in vivo. Table 3 displays some of the antigens that have been tested, and demonstrates the range of human diseases where DNA vaccines may be useful. The array of possible applications of such vaccines ranges from inhibition of allergic reactions and autoimmune phenomenon to boosting infectious disease vaccines and providing antitumor immunity.

5.3. Immunostimulatory Sequences

DNA vaccines possess their own adjuvant activity because of the presence of unmethylated CpG motifs. Unmethylated CpG motifs are known as immunostimulatory sequence DNA. The family of unmethylated CpG dinucleotides with a consensus sequence of 5'-pur-(pur or T)-CpG-pyr-pyr-3' are common in certain bacterial and viral genomes but suppressed in mammalian genomes *(143)*. These CpG sequences have a broad range of stimulatory effects on natural-killer cells, B-cells, and APCs, with potent effects on both innate and adaptive cellular immunity by enhancing antigen presentation, upregulating co-stimulatory molecules, and increasing local cytokine production *(144)*. These effects may be mediated largely through Toll-like receptor 9 expressed on DCs and other cells, with resultant secretion of proinflammatory cytokines. Preclinical studies in which additional CpG motifs were cloned into a plasmid vector and coadministered with a separate DNA vaccine encoding HIV protein antigen resulted in significantly enhanced HIV immunity *(145)*. Hence, proper positioning of CpG motifs in DNA vaccines might have beneficial effect on their efficacy.

5.4. Delivery of Multiple Antigens

DNA vaccines are usually in the same form, and there are no issues of incompatibility. This property allows DNA vaccines to encode multiple antigens or combinations of antigens with immunostimulatory molecules, which provides many benefits. Strategies to deliver more than one gene in a DNA vaccine can include:

1. Multiple plasmids.
2. Bicistronic expression of two antigens using a single plasmid with an internal ribosome entry site to initiate translation of the second gene.
3. A single plasmid with multiple expression cassettes.
4. Fusion proteins comprising whole antigens.
5. Subcloning sequences encoding polyepitopes (*see* Fig. 2).

Multiple plasmids (*see* Fig. 2A) can be easily administered together and provide flexibility in choosing different routes of administration, but production can be costly. In rhesus monkeys, the immunization of a trivalent construct encoding antigens from both the pre-erythrocytic and erythrocytic stages together with three immunostimulatory cytokines resulted in significant protection against *Plasmodium knowlesi* sporozoite challenge *(146)*.

Alternatively, the use of bicistronic plasmids (*see* Fig. 2B) proved to be a powerful method for vaccinating with multiple genes. Immunization of mice with a bicistronic plasmid that coexpressed HIV-1 gp120 and GM-CSF under control of a single promoter was superior to an admixture of separate plasmids expressing GM-CSF and gp120 in stimulating gp120-specific CD4$^+$ T-cell responses *(147)*. However, the selection of genes should be carefully considered. For example, the combination of HIV-1 gp120 and IL-2 in a bicistronic vector induced weaker specific immune responses than the monocistronic plasmid coding for gp120 alone *(148)*. Another method for coexpressing multiple genes is the use of additional expression cassettes (promoter-gene-poly [A]) in a single vector (*see* Fig. 2C). Although appealing, this approach needs to be developed cautiously, because it can result in crosspromoter silencing. Studies with dual-antigen-expression systems that consist of two antigen-expression cassettes induced stronger immune responses than those of an ordinary antigen-expression plasmid. Bidirectional promoters have also been used for unilateral expression of two transgenic proteins: hepatitis B surface antigen and hepatitis B core antigen *(149)*.

Another strategy is based on covalent linking of two or more proteins (*see* Fig. 2D). A number of DNA vaccines containing genes encoding fusion proteins have been generated. The access of antigens to APCs appears to be a rate-limiting step in the generation of immune responses by DNA vaccines. Fusion of genes encoding an antigen with a common ligand of receptors present on the surface of APCs may enhance the processing and presentation of the antigen. Drew et al. reported enhanced responses to DNA vaccines encoding a fusion protein composed of an antigen and the CTL antigen 4 that binds with high affinity to the B7 membrane receptor on APCs *(150)*. This novel approach serves two purposes at the same time: it facilitates uptake of antigen by APCs, and blocks interactions that provides inhibitory signals to activated T-lymphocytes through CTL antigen 4 *(151,152)*. Similarly, other co-stimulatory molecules, such as CD40L, have been fused

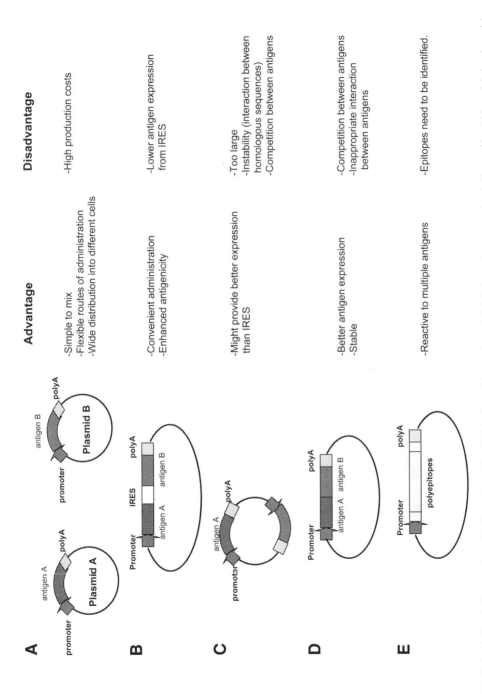

Fig. 2. Methods for delivery of multiple antigens by DNA plasmid vaccines. Multiple antigens can be delivered by (**A**) multiple plasmids encoding each antigen, (**B**) bicistronic plasmids using an IRES to separate the genes, (**C**) single plasmid with two separate cloning sites, (**D**) plasmids encoding fusion proteins, or (**E**) plasmids encoding a single polyepitope "chain" from various genes.

to selected tumor antigens in an effort to improve immunogenicity *(153)*. In this case, CD40–CD40L interaction improves antigen presentation and consequently enhances priming of T-cells because of CD40L-stimulated maturation of APCs *(154)*.

Finally, using fusions of different coding sequences to improve potency of DNA vaccines was applied to minigene-encoded T-cell epitopes (*see* Fig. 2E). Numerous immunogenic epitopes have now been identified in many potential antigenic targets ranging from important clinical pathogens, such as HIV, to antigens from a wide variety of tumors. Instead of using the entire coding region of an antigen in plasmid DNA, only a single epitope or several epitopes with known immunogenicity can be sequentially arranged into a single polypeptide, thus forming a string of epitopes. This so-called minigene, or minimal-epitope, approach takes advantage of the fact that plasmid DNA-encoded antigenic peptides can be loaded onto MHC class I molecules via the endogenous antigen-processing pathway. The safety and efficiency of this vaccine was confirmed in several preclinical studies *(155,156)*.

5.5. *Optimization of Vaccine Efficacy*

To design DNA vaccines with enhanced efficacy, a series of approaches have been suggested. These approaches emphasize:

1. The importance of optimizing the antigen-expression system.
2. Choice of optimal immunomodulators.
3. Coexpression of stimulatory sequences.
4. Selection of delivery system used for vaccination.
5. Manipulating antigen-specific host immune interactions.

One of the most important factors in optimizing DNA vaccines is the selection of a vector for gene expression. Increased antigen expression results in enhanced antigen-specific immune responses and numerous ways to enhance antigen expression have been demonstrated. These include the optimization of regulatory elements, such as promoter–enhancer complexes, transcription termination signals, and modifying the plasmid backbone itself. When using the IE-CMV, insertion of the first intron of the immediate early gene from CMV produced higher antigen expression *(157,158)*. Different sources of terminal sequences have been studied for the effects on gene expression. Native codons for encoded antigen can be substituted by more frequently used codons to optimize codon usage. In mice, the use of synthetic HIV-1 gp120 with codons from highly expressed human genes resulted in significantly increased antibody titers and CTL responses *(159)*. Plasmids may also be engineered to manipulate antigen secretion or localization depending on the desired outcome *(160–162)*.

The application of immunomodulators and the optimization of the delivery system have been emphasized for effective manipulation of host immune system for improved vaccine immunogenicity. DNA vaccines encoding an antigen and IFN-γ-inducible protein (IP)-10, that causes retention of Th1 lymphocytes in draining lymph nodes, facilitated their contact with DCs and improved presentation of weak antigens *(163)*. This kind of vaccine formulation might be particularly useful for tumor vaccines, because it combines weak TAAs with IP-10, and has already demonstrated an effective tumor-protective CD8+ T-cell response in mice.

To date, the efficacy of at least 60 different combinations of cytokines, chemokines, and co-stimulatory molecules were examined in several experimental settings, with most demonstrating improved vaccine-induced immunity *(164,165)*. One unique approach was the fusion of different immunomodulatory cytokines to the Fc portion of an Ig molecule. The major advantage of using Fc–cytokine fusion proteins is their prolonged half-life and the ability to cluster receptors because of dimerization of the Fc segment *(166, 167)*. Interestingly, not only Fc, but also Ig single-chain variable fragments (sFvs) have been used to improve vaccine immunogenicity. Lymphoma sFvs were fused respectively to two chemokines, IP-10 and monocyte chemotactic protein 3. The sFv–chemokine fusion proteins elicited chemotactic responses in vitro and induced inflammatory responses in vivo. These fusion proteins showed superior chemoattractive properties and subsequent tumor protection as compared with the chemokine alone *(168)*.

Despite the numerous approaches to improve vaccine efficacy, evaluating the optimal composition of DNA vaccines for possible use in humans is challenging because of the enormous heterogeneity of individual host molecular and clinical profiles, and may require a more targeted approach in the future.

6. DNA VACCINES FOR CANCER THERAPY

Despite myriad approaches to therapy and prevention, cancer remains one of the major causes of death worldwide. Increased knowledge of the immune system and identification of TAAs ignited interest in immunological approaches to target and eliminate cancer cells. However, cancer cells are derived from host cells with most of their macromolecules being normal self-antigens. In addition, many potential tumor antigens are not exposed on the surface of tumor cells and are inaccessible to antibodies. Similarly, unless these antigens are degraded by the immunoproteasome, they may also fail to be presented by class I MHC molecules and will be ignored by T-cells. Thus, major hurdles in developing cancer vaccines include the following:

1. Identification of tumor-specific antigens.
2. Confirming expression of antigens on tumor cells.
3. Development of methods to overcome peripheral tolerance.
4. Avoiding the mechanisms by which tumors evade the host immune response.

DNA vaccines encoding tumor antigen have been shown to generate immune responses. DNA vaccines may introduce tumor antigens directly into DCs for endogenous processing and presentation to T-cells in draining lymph nodes. Alternatively, DNA vaccines may reach DCs after injection into other cells for crosspresentation by DCs. Several different DNA vaccines have been tested in animal and human studies for various cancers including melanoma, prostate, cervical, and breast cancer. Vaccination of BALB–NeuT transgenic mice with a DNA plasmid encoding the extracellular and transmembrane domain of rat p185 elicited antirat p185 antibody and CTL responses, resulting in tumor rejection *(169)*. The combination of DNA (extracellular and transmembrane domain) vaccination with lymphocyte activation gene 3 provided longer protection and mice remained tumor-free. Injection of plasmid DNA encoding a xenogeneic differentiation antigen (human prostate-specific membrane antigen) into mice induced antibody and T-cell responses *(170)*.

Inhibition of tumor growth by attacking the tumor's vascular supply offers another antitumor strategy that can be exploited with DNA vaccines. Orally delivered DNA vaccines that target the vascular endothelial growth factor receptor 2 or transcription factor Fos-related antigen 1 induced a robust T-cell-mediated immune response, leading to

Table 4
Selected DNA Vaccine Clinical Trials for Cancer

Disease	Antigen	Trial phase
Prostate cancer	PSMA	I/II
	PSA	
Ovarian cancer	HER-2/*neu*	I
Cervical cancer	HPV E6 and E7	II
Colon cancer	CEA	

PSMA, prostate-specific membrane antigen; PSA, prostate-specific antigen; HPV, human papilloma virus; CEA, carcino-embryonic antigen.

effective suppression of tumor growth and metastases *(171)*. Cytokine–antigen fusion proteins have been shown to be especially effective in stimulating cellular immunity. Among several ovalbumin (OVA)-cytokine fusion proteins, those containing GM-CSF, IL-10, and IL-12, proved to be the most efficient in an OVA-expressing murine tumor model. Interestingly, a nanopeptide from IL-1β (amino acids 163–171) fused to OVA was as potent as IL-12 in inducing a Th1-type response *(172)*. This approach might be especially interesting for tumor therapy.

Prime–boost vaccination strategies are another innovative approach in early clinical development. Priming with DNA followed by boosting with the same antigen delivered by viral vectors, such as nonreplicating poxviruses or adenoviruses, was effective in inducing protective immune responses *(20,173)*. Table 4 documents several DNA vaccine clinical trials conducted in patients with a variety of different cancers.

7. SAFETY CONCERNS, ETHICAL ISSUES, AND LIMITATIONS

The feasibility of DNA vaccines has raised ethical and safety concerns. Genomic integration of plasmid DNA is among several concerns connected to the application of DNA vaccines. The probability of plasmid integration into genomic DNA is known to be very low *(174,175)*, and, considering the small percentage of coding and regulatory sequences in the human genome *(176)*, the probability of sustained plasmid integration into these functionally important regions is practically negligible. Still, the Food and Drug Administration recommends avoiding the incorporation of sequences homologous to human DNA and to keep the size of plasmids to a minimum to reduce the possibility of homologous recombination. Other concerns, such as the potential for induction of immunological tolerance or autoimmunity, and possible induction of anti-DNA antibodies, also have little scientific confirmation at this time *(177)*.

Owing to the rapid development of DNA microarrays and proteomics technology, it has become clear that unlike other epidemic diseases, the treatment of cancer requires an individualized approach. Because of the enormous molecular heterogeneity of cancer and individual variations in the human genome, no single drug or even combination of drugs will be able to eradicate phenotypically similar tumors in all patients *(178)*. The same may apply to other immunotherapeutic methods as well. However, DNA vaccines, unlike other therapeutics, can be customized relatively easily according to individual needs.

Other issues facing DNA vaccine development are current procedures involved in early stage research and development that often require lengthy procedures of preclinical evaluation and complex patenting requirements resulting in excessive costs. This might pose major drawbacks for obtaining new therapeutically valuable vaccines. Obviously, more studies are required to ensure the safety of plasmid DNA inoculation in humans. Along with the continued debate by ethicists and legal scholars, the scientific support for DNA vaccines and the low cost of production will be needed to push the field forward.

8. CONCLUSION

The identification and cloning of tumor-associated antigens from a variety of cancers has resulted in intense interest in developing vaccines for cancer. The simplicity, cost, and feasibility of expressing antigens in bacterial plasmids have resulted in a wide array of molecular approaches for DNA vaccine development. DNA vaccines offer many advantages over more complex vaccines, including the ease of construction, high levels of gene expression in targeted tissues, the opportunity to express multiple genes, and the ability to induce strong immune responses in vivo. Depending on the type and dose of antigen, the route of administration, and the addition of chemical or genetic adjuvants, DNA vaccines can be engineered to initiate humoral or cell-mediated immune responses against expressed antigens. This has important implications for the treatment or prevention of human diseases, including infectious diseases, autoimmunity, and cancer.

The last decade witnessed significant advances in molecular biology that have resulted in numerous advances in DNA vector design. Several strategies for coexpression of multiple antigens or immunomodulatory molecules are now possible. The addition of chemical or genetic adjuvants can improve the immunogenicity of DNA vaccines and influence the type and magnitude of immune response generated. Further research is needed to define the role of novel administration techniques, routes of administration, and the optimal prime–boost protocol in selected situations. Despite the lack of optimal conditions, several clinical trials employing a variety of DNA vaccines for cancer immunotherapy have begun. These trials will be pivotal for documenting the safety of DNA vaccination and should lead to well-designed later stage clinical investigation in patient populations more likely to benefit from early vaccination. Once safety is established, DNA vaccines will be evaluated for antitumor activity as single agent vaccines and in combination with other immunotherapeutic and conventional cancer therapeutic agents.

REFERENCES

1. Dupuis M, Denis-Mize K, Woo C, et al. McDonald DM. Distribution of DNA vaccines determines their immunogenicity after intramuscular injection in mice. *J Immunol* 2000; 165:2850–2858.
2. Wolff JA, Malone RW, Williams P, et al. Direct gene transfer into mouse muscle in vivo. *Science* 1990; 247:1465–1468.
3. Corr M, Lee DJ, Carson DA, Tighe H. Gene vaccination with naked plasmid DNA: mechanism of CTL priming. *J Exp Med* 1996; 184:1555–1560.
4. Iwasaki A, Torres CA, Ohashi PS, Robinson HL, Barber BH. The dominant role of bone marrow-derived cells in CTL induction following plasmid DNA immunization at different sites. *J Immunol* 1997; 159:11–14.
5. Doe B, Selby M, Barnett S, Baenziger J, Walker CM. Induction of cytotoxic T lymphocytes by intramuscular immunization with plasmid DNA is facilitated by bone marrow-derived cells. *Proc Natl Acad Sci USA* 1996; 93:8578–8583.
6. Tuting T, Wilson CC, Martin DM, et al. Autologous human monocyte-derived dendritic cells genetically modified to express melanoma antigens elicit primary cytotoxic T cell responses in vitro: enhancement by cotransfection of genes encoding the Th1-biasing cytokines IL-12 and IFN-alpha. *J Immunol* 1998;160:1139–1147.

7. Ulmer JB, Donnelly JJ, Parker SE, et al. Heterologous protection against influenza by injection of DNA encoding a viral protein. *Science* 1993; 259:1745–1749.

8. Agadjanyan MG, Kim JJ, Trivedi N, et al. CD86 (B7-2) can function to drive MHC-restricted antigen-specific CTL responses in vivo. *J Immunol* 1999; 162:3417–3427.

9. Iwasaki A, Stiernholm BJ, Chan AK, Berinstein NL, Barber BH. Enhanced CTL responses mediated by plasmid DNA immunogens encoding costimulatory molecules and cytokines. *J Immunol* 1997; 158: 4591–45601.

10. Torres CA, Iwasaki A, Barber BH, Robinson HL. Differential dependence on target site tissue for gene gun and intramuscular DNA immunizations. *J Immunol* 1997; 158:4529–4532.

11. Yang NS, Burkholder J, Roberts B, et al. In vivo and in vitro gene transfer to mammalian somatic cells by particle bombardment. *Proc Natl Acad Sci USA* 1990; 87:9568–9572.

12. Raz E, Carson DA, Parker SE, et al. Intradermal gene immunization: the possible role of DNA uptake in the induction of cellular immunity to viruses. *Proc Natl Acad Sci USA* 1994; 91:9519–9523.

13. Klinman DM, Sechler JM, Conover J, Gu M, Rosenberg AS. Contribution of cells at the site of DNA vaccination to the generation of antigen-specific immunity and memory. *J Immunol* 1998; 160:2388–2392.

14. Moron G, Dadaglio G, Leclerc C. New tools for antigen delivery to the MHC class I pathway. *Trends Immunol* 2004; 25:92–97.

15. Banchereau J, Steinman RM. Dendritic cells and the control of immunity. *Nature* 1998; 392:245–252.

16. Pulendran B, Palucka K, Banchereau J. Sensing pathogens and tuning immune responses. *Science* 2001; 293:253–256.

17. Lanzavecchia A, Sallusto F. Dynamics of T lymphocyte responses: intermediates, effectors, and memory cells. *Science* 2000; 290:92–97.

18. Hwang LY, Lieu PT, Peterson PA, Yang Y. Functional regulation of immunoproteasomes and transporter associated with antigen processing. *Immunol Res* 2001; 24:245–272.

19. Van den Eynde BJ, Morel S. Differential processing of class-I-restricted epitopes by the standard proteasome and the immunoproteasome. *Curr Opin Immunol* 2001; 13:147–153.

20. Ramshaw IA, Ramsay AJ. The prime-boost strategy: exciting prospects for improved vaccination. *Immunol Today* 2000; 21:163–165.

21. Zimmermann S, Egeter O, Hausmann S, Lipford GB, Rocken M, Wagner H, Heeg K. CpG oligodeoxynucleotides trigger protective and curative Th1 responses in lethal murine leishmaniasis. *J Immunol* 1998; 160:3627–3630.

22. Ma X, Trinchieri G. Regulation of interleukin-12 production in antigen-presenting cells. *Adv Immunol* 2001; 79:55–92.

23. Roman M, Martin-Orozco E, Goodman JS, et al. Immunostimulatory DNA sequences function as T helper-1-promoting adjuvants. *Nat Med* 1997; 3:849–854.

24. Cho HJ, Hayashi T, Datta SK, et al. IFN-alpha beta promote priming of antigen-specific CD8[+] and CD4[+] T lymphocytes by immunostimulatory DNA-based vaccines. *J Immunol* 2002; 168:4907–4913.

25. Heath WR, Carbone FR. Cross-presentation in viral immunity and self-tolerance. *Nat Rev Immunol* 2001; 1:126–134.

26. Stoll S, Jonuleit H, Schmitt E, et al. Production of functional IL-18 by different subtypes of murine and human dendritic cells (DC): DC-derived IL-18 enhances IL-12-dependent Th1 development. *Eur J Immunol* 1998; 28:3231–3239.

27. Oppmann B, Lesley R, Blom B, et al. Novel p19 protein engages IL-12p40 to form a cytokine, IL-23, with biological activities similar as well as distinct from IL-12. *Immunity* 2000; 13:715–725.

28. Weiss R, Scheiblhofer S. Gene gun bombardment with gold particles displays a particular Th2-promoting signal that over-rules the Th1-inducing effect of immunostimulatory CpG motifs in DNA vaccines. *Vaccine* 2002; 3277:1–7.

29. Martins LP, Lau LL, Asano MS, Ahmed R. DNA vaccination against persistent viral infection. *J Virol* 1995; 69:2574–2582.

30. Yokoyama M, Zhang J, Whitton JL. DNA immunization confers protection against lethal lymphocytic choriomeningitis virus infection. *J Virol* 1995; 69:2684–2688.

31. Zarozinski CC, Fynan EF, Selin LK, Robinson HL, Welsh RM. Protective CTL-dependent immunity and enhanced immunopathology in mice immunized by particle bombardment with DNA encoding an internal virion protein. *J Immunol* 1995; 154:4010–4017.

32. Chen Y, Webster RG, Woodland DL. Induction of CD8[+] T cell responses to dominant and subdominant epitopes and protective immunity to Sendai virus infection by DNA vaccination. *J Immunol* 1998; 160: 2425–2432.

33. Fu TM, Friedman A, Ulmer JB, Liu MA, Donnelly JJ. Protective cellular immunity: cytotoxic T-lymphocyte responses against dominant and recessive epitopes of influenza virus nucleoprotein induced by DNA immunization. *J Virol* 1997; 71:2715–2721.
34. Calarota SA, Weiner DB. Enhancement of human immunodeficiency virus type 1-DNA vaccine potency through incorporation of T-helper 1 molecular adjuvants. *Immunol Rev* 2004; 199:84–99.
35. Hermanson G, Whitlow V, Parker S, et al. A cationic lipid-formulated plasmid DNA vaccine confers sustained antibody-mediated protection against aerosolized anthrax spores. *Proc Natl Acad Sci USA* 2004; 101:13,601–13,606.
36. Deck RR, DeWitt CM, Donnelly JJ, Liu MA, Ulmer JB. Characterization of humoral immune responses induced by an influenza hemagglutinin DNA vaccine. *Vaccine* 1997; 15:71–78.
37. Robinson HL, Boyle CA, Feltquate DM, Morin MJ, Santoro JC, Webster RG. DNA immunization for influenza virus: studies using hemagglutinin- and nucleoprotein-expressing DNAs. *J Infect Dis* 1997; 176(Suppl 1):S50–S55.
38. Hovav AH, Mullerad J, Davidovitch L, et al. The Mycobacterium tuberculosis recombinant 27-kilodalton lipoprotein induces a strong Th1-type immune response deleterious to protection. *Infect Immun* 2003; 71:3146–3154.
39. Boyle JS, Koniaras C, Lew AM. Influence of cellular location of expressed antigen on the efficacy of DNA vaccination: cytotoxic T lymphocyte and antibody responses are suboptimal when antigen is cytoplasmic after intramuscular DNA immunization. *Int Immunol* 1997; 9:1897–1906.
40. Feltquate DM, Heaney S, Webster RG, Robinson HL. Different T helper cell types and antibody isotypes generated by saline and gene gun DNA immunization. *J Immunol* 1997; 158:2278–2284.
41. Lefrancois L, Masopust D. T cell immunity in lymphoid and non-lymphoid tissues. *Curr Opin Immunol* 2002; 14:503–508.
42. Zinkernagel RM. On differences between immunity and immunological memory. *Curr Opin Immunol* 2002; 14:523–536.
43. Zinkernagel RM, Hengartner H. Regulation of the immune response by antigen. *Science* 2001; 293:251–253.
44. Sasaki S, Takeshita F, Xin KQ, Ishii N, Okuda K. Adjuvant formulations and delivery systems for DNA vaccines. *Methods* 2003; 31:243–254.
45. Johnston SA, Tang DC. Gene gun transfection of animal cells and genetic immunization. *Methods Cell Biol* 1994; 43:353–365.
46. Furth PA, Kerr D, Wall R. Gene transfer by jet injection into differentiated tissues of living animals and in organ culture. *Mol Biotechnol* 1995; 4:121–127.
47. Ren S, Li M, Smith JM, DeTolla LJ, Furth PA. Low-volume jet injection for intradermal immunization in rabbits. *BMC Biotechnol* 2002; 2:10.
48. Cui Z, Baizer L, Mumper RJ. Intradermal immunization with novel plasmid DNA-coated nanoparticles via a needle-free injection device. *J Biotechnol* 2003; 102:105–115.
49. Epstein JE, Gorak EJ, Charoenvit Y, et al. Safety, tolerability, and lack of antibody responses after administration of a PfCSP DNA malaria vaccine via needle or needle-free jet injection, and comparison of intramuscular and combination intramuscular/intradermal routes. *Hum Gene Ther* 2002; 13:1551–1560.
50. Aguiar JC, Hedstrom RC, Rogers WO, et al. Enhancement of the immune response in rabbits to a malaria DNA vaccine by immunization with a needle-free jet device. *Vaccine* 2001; 20:275–280.
51. Anwer K, Earle KA, Shi M, et al. Synergistic effect of formulated plasmid and needle-free injection for genetic vaccines. *Pharm Res* 1999; 16:889–895.
52. Wang R, Epstein J, Baraccros FM, et al. Induction of CD4(+) T cell-dependent CD8(+) type 1 responses in humans by a malaria DNA vaccine. *Proc Natl Acad Sci USA* 2001; 98:10,817–10,822.
53. Tabata Y, Ikada Y. Effect of the size and surface charge of polymer microspheres on their phagocytosis by macrophage. *Biomaterials* 1988; 9:356–362.
54. Singh M, Briones M, Ott G, O'Hagan D. Cationic microparticles: a potent delivery system for DNA vaccines. *Proc Natl Acad Sci USA* 2000; 97:811–816.
55. Denis-Mize KS, Dupuis M, MacKichan ML, et al. Plasmid DNA adsorbed onto cationic microparticles mediates target gene expression and antigen presentation by dendritic cells. *Gene Ther* 2000; 7:2105–2112.
56. Falo LD Jr, Kovacsovics-Bankowski M, Thompson K, Rock KL. Targeting antigen into the phagocytic pathway in vivo induces protective tumour immunity. *Nat Med* 1995; 1:649–653.
57. O'Hagan DT. Recent advances in vaccine adjuvants for systemic and mucosal administration. *J Pharm Pharmacol* 1998; 50:1–10.

58. Cui Z, Mumper RJ. Genetic immunization using nanoparticles engineered from microemulsion precursors. *Pharm Res* 2002; 19:939–946.

59. Cui Z, Mumper RJ. Topical immunization using nanoengineered genetic vaccines. *J Control Release* 2002; 81:173–184.

60. Cui Z, Mumper RJ. Intranasal administration of plasmid DNA-coated nanoparticles results in enhanced immune responses. *J Pharm Pharmacol* 2002; 54:1195–1203.

61. Mumper RJ, Cui Z. Genetic immunization by jet injection of targeted pDNA-coated nanoparticles. *Methods* 2003; 31:255–262.

62. Cui Z, Mumper RJ. The effect of co-administration of adjuvants with a nanoparticle-based genetic vaccine delivery system on the resulting immune responses. *Eur J Pharm Biopharm* 2003; 55: 11–18.

63. Midoux P, Mendes C, Legrand A, et al. Specific gene transfer mediated by lactosylated poly- L-lysine into hepatoma cells. *Nucleic Acids Res* 1993; 21:871–878.

64. Fajac I, Briand P, Monsigny M, Midoux P. Sugar-mediated uptake of glycosylated polylysines and gene transfer into normal and cystic fibrosis airway epithelial cells. *Hum Gene Ther* 1999; 10:395–406.

65. Taniyama Y, Tachibana K, Hiraoka K, et al. Local delivery of plasmid DNA into rat carotid artery using ultrasound. *Circulation* 2002; 105:1233–1239.

66. Scherer F, Anton M, Schillinger U, et al. Magnetofection: enhancing and targeting gene delivery by magnetic force in vitro and in vivo. *Gene Ther* 2002; 9:102–109.

67. Wong TK, Neumann E. Electric field mediated gene transfer. *Biochem Biophys Res Commun* 1982; 107:584–587.

68. Titomirov AV, Sukharev S, Kistanova E. In vivo electroporation and stable transformation of skin cells of newborn mice by plasmid DNA. *Biochim Biophys Acta* 1991; 1088:131–134.

69. Rizzuto G, Cappelletti M, Maione D, et al. Efficient and regulated erythropoietin production by naked DNA injection and muscle electroporation. *Proc Natl Acad Sci USA* 1999; 96:6417–6422.

70. Brown MD, Schatzlein AG, Uchegbu IF. Gene delivery with synthetic (non viral) carriers. *Int J Pharm* 2001; 229:1–21.

71. Fynan EF, Webster RG, Fuller DH, Haynes JR, Santoro JC, Robinson HL. DNA vaccines: protective immunizations by parenteral, mucosal, and gene-gun inoculations. *Proc Natl Acad Sci USA* 1993; 90: 11478–11,482.

72. Jones DH, Corris S, McDonald S, Clegg JC, Farrar GH. Poly(dl-lactide-co-glycolide)-encapsulated plasmid DNA elicits systemic and mucosal antibody responses to encoded protein after oral administration. *Vaccine* 1997; 15:814–817.

73. Chen SC, Jones DH, Fynan EF, et al. Protective immunity induced by oral immunization with a rotavirus DNA vaccine encapsulated in microparticles. *J Virol* 1998; 72:5757–5761.

74. Herrmann JE, Chen SC, Jones DH, et al. Immune responses and protection obtained by oral immunization with rotavirus VP4 and VP7 DNA vaccines encapsulated in microparticles. *Virology* 1999; 259: 148–153.

75. Roy K, Mao HQ, Huang SK, Leong KW. Oral gene delivery with chitosan—DNA nanoparticles generates immunologic protection in a murine model of peanut allergy. *Nat Med* 1999; 5:387–391.

76. Klavinskis LS, Gao L, Barnfield C, Lehner T, Parker S. Mucosal immunization with DNA-liposome complexes. *Vaccine* 1997; 15:818–820.

77. Ban EM, van Ginkel FW, Simecka JW, Kiyono H, Robinson HL, McGhee JR. Mucosal immunization with DNA encoding influenza hemagglutinin. *Vaccine* 1997; 15:811–813.

78. Kuklin N, Daheshia M, Karem K, Manickan E, Rouse BT. Induction of mucosal immunity against herpes simplex virus by plasmid DNA immunization. *J Virol* 1997; 71:3138–3145.

79. Sasaki S, Hamajima K, Fukushima J, et al. Comparison of intranasal and intramuscular immunization against human immunodeficiency virus type 1 with a DNA-monophosphoryl lipid A adjuvant vaccine. *Infect Immun* 1998; 66:823–826.

80. McShane H. Prime-boost immunization strategies for infectious diseases. *Curr Opin Mol Ther* 2002; 4:23–27.

81. Estcourt MJ, Ramsay AJ, Brooks A, Thomson SA, Medveckzy CJ, Ramshaw IA. Prime-boost immunization generates a high-frequency, high-avidity CD8(+) cytotoxic T lymphocyte population. *Int Immunol* 2002; 14:31–37.

82. Ramshaw IA, Ramsay AJ. The prime-boost strategy: exciting prospects for improved vaccination. *Immunol Today* 2000; 21:163–165.

83. Takeda A, Igarashi H, Nakamura H, et al. Protective efficacy of an AIDS vaccine, a single DNA priming followed by a single booster with a recombinant replication-defective Sendai virus vector, in a macaque AIDS model. *J Virol* 2003; 77:9710–9715.

84. Nakaya Y, Zheng H, Garcia-Sastre A. Enhanced cellular immune responses to SIV Gag by immunization with influenza and vaccinia virus recombinants. *Vaccine* 2003; 21:2097–2106.

85. Gherardi MM, Najera JL, Perez-Jimenez E, Guerra S, Garcia-Sastre A, Esteban M. Prime-boost immunization schedules based on influenza virus and vaccinia virus vectors potentiate cellular immune responses against human immunodeficiency virus Env protein systemically and in the genitorectal draining lymph nodes. *J Virol* 2003; 77:7048–7057.

86. Eo SK, Gierynska M, Kamar AA, Rouse BT. Prime-boost immunization with DNA vaccine: mucosal route of administration changes the rules. *J Immunol* 2001; 166:5473–5479.

87. Doria-Rose NA, Ohlen C, Polacino P, et al. Multigene DNA priming-boosting vaccines protect macaques from acute CD4+-T-cell depletion after simian-human immunodeficiency virus SHIV89.6P mucosal challenge. *J Virol* 2003; 77:11,563–11,577.

88. Krieg AM. CpG motifs in bacterial DNA and their immune effects. *Annu Rev Immunol* 2002; 20:709–760.

89. Ulmer JB, DeWitt CM, Chastain M, et al. Enhancement of DNA vaccine potency using conventional aluminum adjuvants. *Vaccine* 1999; 18:18–28.

90. Lindblad EB. Aluminium compounds for use in vaccines. *Immunol Cell Biol* 2004; 82:497–505.

91. Kuklin N, Daheshia M, Karem K, Manickan E, Rouse BT. Induction of mucosal immunity against herpes simplex virus by plasmid DNA immunization. *J Virol* 1997; 71:3138–3145.

92. Sasaki S, Hamajima K, Fukushima J, et al. Comparison of intranasal and intramuscular immunization against human immunodeficiency virus type 1 with a DNA-monophosphoryl lipid A adjuvant vaccine. *Infect Immun* 1998; 66:823–826.

93. Denis-Mize KS, Dupuis M, Singh M, et al. Mechanisms of increased immunogenicity for DNA-based vaccines adsorbed onto cationic microparticles. *Cell Immunol* 2003; 225:12–20.

94. Toda S, Ishii N, Okada E, et al. HIV-1-specific cell-mediated immune responses induced by DNA vaccination were enhanced by mannan-coated liposomes and inhibited by anti-interferon-gamma antibody. *Immunology* 1997; 92:111–117.

95. Sasaki S, Sumino K, Hamajima K, et al. Induction of systemic and mucosal immune responses to human immunodeficiency virus type 1 by a DNA vaccine formulated with QS-21 saponin adjuvant via intramuscular and intranasal routes. *J Virol* 1998; 72:4931–4939.

96. Sasaki S, Fukushima J, Hamajima K, et al. Adjuvant effect of Ubenimex on a DNA vaccine for HIV-1. *Clin Exp Immunol* 1998; 111:30–35.

97. Sasaki S, Amara RR, Oran AE, Smith JM, Robinson HL. Apoptosis-mediated enhancement of DNA-raised immune responses by mutant caspases. *Nat Biotechnol* 2001; 19:543–547.

98. Barouch DH, Santra S, Tenner-Racz K, et al. Potent CD4+ T cell responses elicited by a bicistronic HIV-1 DNA vaccine expressing gp120 and GM-CSF. *J Immunol* 2002; 168:562–568.

99. Kim JJ, Yang JS, Lee DJ, et al. Macrophage colony-stimulating factor can modulate immune responses and attract dendritic cells in vivo. *Hum Gene Ther* 2000; 11:305–321.

100. Chow YH, Chiang BL, Lee YL, et al. Development of Th1 and Th2 populations and the nature of immune responses to hepatitis B virus DNA vaccines can be modulated by codelivery of various cytokine genes. *J Immunol* 1998; 160:1320–1329.

101. Garren H, Ruiz PJ, Watkins TA, et al. Combination of gene delivery and DNA vaccination to protect from and reverse Th1 autoimmune disease via deviation to the Th2 pathway. *Immunity* 2001; 15:15–22.

102. Prayaga SK, Ford MJ, Haynes JR. Manipulation of HIV-1 gp120-specific immune responses elicited via gene gun-based DNA immunization. *Vaccine* 1997; 15:1349–1352.

103. Hengge UR, Chan EF, Foster RA, Walker PS, Vogel JC. Cytokine gene expression in epidermis with biological effects following injection of naked DNA. *Nat Genet* 1995; 10:161–166.

104. Daheshia M, Kuklin N, Kanangat S, Manickan E, Rouse BT. Suppression of ongoing ocular inflammatory disease by topical administration of plasmid DNA encoding IL-10. *J Immunol* 1997; 159:1945–1952.

105. Tsuji T, Hamajima K, Fukushima J, et al. Enhancement of cell-mediated immunity against HIV-1 induced by coinoculation of plasmid-encoded HIV-1 antigen with plasmid expressing IL-12. *J Immunol* 1997; 158:4008–4013.

106. Xin KQ, Hamajima K, Sasaki S, et al. IL-15 expression plasmid enhances cell-mediated immunity induced by an HIV-1 DNA vaccine. *Vaccine* 1999; 18:858–866.

107. Billaut-Mulot O, Idziorek T, Loyens M, Capron A, Bahr GM. Modulation of cellular and humoral immune responses to a multiepitopic HIV-1 DNA vaccine by interleukin-18 DNA immunization/viral protein boost. *Vaccine* 2001; 19:2803–2811.

108. Okada E, Sasaki S, Ishii N, et al. Intranasal immunization of a DNA vaccine with IL-12- and granulocyte-macrophage colony-stimulating factor (GM-CSF)-expressing plasmids in liposomes induces strong mucosal and cell-mediated immune responses against HIV-1 antigens. *J Immunol* 1997; 159:3638–3647.

109. Kusakabe K, Xin KQ, Katoh H, et al. The timing of GM-CSF expression plasmid administration influences the Th1/Th2 response induced by an HIV-1-specific DNA vaccine. The timing of GM-CSF expression plasmid administration influences the Th1/Th2 response induced by an HIV-1-specific DNA vaccine. *J Immunol* 2000; 164:3102–3111.

110. Liu LJ, Watabe S, Yang J, et al. Topical application of HIV DNA vaccine with cytokine-expression plasmids induces strong antigen-specific immune responses. *Vaccine* 2001; 20:42–48.

111. Akbari O, Panjwani N, Garcia S, Tascon R, Lowrie D, Stockinger B. DNA vaccination: transfection and activation of dendritic cells as key events for immunity. *J Exp Med* 1999; 189:169–178.

112. Condon C, Watkins SC, Celluzzi CM, Thompson K, Falo LD Jr. DNA-based immunization by in vivo transfection of dendritic cells. *Nat Med* 1996; 2:1122–1128.

113. Randolph GJ, Inaba K, Robbiani DF, Steinman RM, Muller WA. Differentiation of phagocytic monocytes into lymph node dendritic cells in vivo. *Immunity* 1999; 11:753–761.

114. Eo SK, Kumaraguru U, Rouse BT. Plasmid DNA encoding CCR7 ligands compensate for dysfunctional CD8+ T cell responses by effects on dendritic cells. *J Immunol* 2001; 167:3592–3599.

115. Lu Y, Xin KQ, Hamajima K, et al. Macrophage inflammatory protein-1alpha (MIP-1alpha) expression plasmid enhances DNA vaccine-induced immune response against HIV-1. *Clin Exp Immunol* 1999; 115:335–341.

116. Boyer JD, Kim J, Ugen K, et al. HIV-1 DNA vaccines and chemokines. *Vaccine* 1999; 17(Suppl 2): S53–S64.

117. Lanzavecchia A, Sallusto F. From synapses to immunological memory: the role of sustained T cell stimulation. *Curr Opin Immunol* 2000; 12:92–98.

118. Eo SK, Lee S, Kumaraguru U, Rouse BT. Immunopotentiation of DNA vaccine against herpes simplex virus via co- delivery of plasmid DNA expressing CCR7 ligands. *Vaccine* 2001; 19:4685–4693.

119. Kim JJ, Bagarazzi ML, Trivedi N, et al. Engineering of in vivo immune responses to DNA immunization via codelivery of costimulatory molecule genes. *Nat Biotechnol* 1997; 15:641–646.

120. Kim JJ, Nottingham LK, Wilson DM, et al. Engineering DNA vaccines via co-delivery of co-stimulatory molecule genes. *Vaccine* 1998; 16:1828–1835.

121. Kim JJ, Tsai A, Nottingham LK, et al. Intracellular adhesion molecule-1 modulates beta-chemokines and directly costimulates T cells in vivo. *J Clin Invest* 1999; 103:869–877.

122. Smith DF, Whitesell L, Katsanis E. Molecular chaperones: biology and prospects for pharmacological intervention. *Pharmacol Rev* 1998; 50:493–514.

123. Melnick J, Argon Y. Molecular chaperones and the biosynthesis of antigen receptors. *Immunol Today* 1995; 16:243–250.

124. Srivastava PK, Menoret A, Basu S, Binder RJ, McQuade KL. Heat shock proteins come of age: primitive functions acquire new roles in an adaptive world. *Immunity* 1998; 8:657–665.

125. Chen CH, Wang TL, Hung CF, et al. Enhancement of DNA vaccine potency by linkage of antigen gene to an HSP70 gene. *Cancer Res* 2000; 60:1035–1042.

126. Kammerer R, Stober D, Riedl P, Oehninger C, Schirmbeck R, Reimann J. Noncovalent association with stress protein facilitates cross-priming of CD8+T cells to tumor cell antigens by dendritic cells. *J Immunol* 2002; 168:108–117.

127. Noessner E, Gastpar R, Milani V, et al. Tumor-derived heat shock protein 70 peptide complexes are cross-presented by human dendritic cells. *J Immunol* 2002; 169:5424–5432.

128. Singh-Jasuja H, Hilf N, Arnold-Schild D, Schild H. The role of heat shock proteins and their receptors in the activation of the immune system. *Biol Chem* 2001; 382:629–636.

129. Chu NR, Wu HB, Wu T, Boux LJ, Siegel MI, Mizzen LA. Immunotherapy of a human papillomavirus (HPV) type 16 E7-expressing tumour by administration of fusion protein comprising Mycobacterium bovis bacilli Calmette-GUA(C)rin (BCG) hsp65 and HPV16 E7. *Clin Exp Immunol* 2000; 121:216–225.

130. Somersan S, Larsson M, Fonteneau JF, Basu S, Srivastava P, Bhardwaj N. Primary tumor tissue lysates are enriched in heat shock proteins and induce the maturation of human dendritic cells. *J Immunol* 2001; 167:4844–4852.

131. Kuppner MC, Gastpar R, Gelwer S, et al. The role of heat shock protein (hsp70) in dendritic cell maturation: hsp70 induces the maturation of immature dendritic cells but reduces DC differentiation from monocyte precursors. *Eur J Immunol* 2001; 31:1602–1609.

132. Pavlenko M, Roos AK, Leder C, et al. Comparison of PSA-specific CD8(+) CTL responses and anti-tumor immunity generated by plasmid DNA vaccines encoding PSA-HSP chimeric proteins. *Cancer Immunol Immunother* 2004; 53:1085–1092.

133. Srivastava PK. Immunotherapy of human cancer: lessons from mice. *Nat Immunol* 2000; 1:363–66.

134. Srivastava PK, Amato RJ. Heat shock proteins: the "Swiss Army Knife" vaccines against cancers and infectious agents. *Vaccine* 2001; 19:2590–2597.

135. Janetzki S, Palla D, Rosenhauer V, Lochs H, Lewis JJ, Srivastava PK. Immunization of cancer patients with autologous cancer-derived heat shock protein gp96 preparations: a pilot study. *Int J Cancer* 2000; 88:232–238.

136. Kozak M. Adherence to the first-AUG rule when a second AUG codon follows closely upon the first. *Proc Natl Acad Sci USA* 1995; 92:2662–2666.

137. Sasaki S, Takeshita F, Oikawa T, et al. Improvement of DNA vaccine immunogenicity by a dual anti-gen expression system. *Biochem Biophys Res Commun* 2004; 315:38–43.

138. Nelson JA, Gnann JW Jr, Ghazal P. Regulation and tissue-specific expression of human cytomegalo-virus. *Curr Top Microbiol Immunol* 1990; 154:75–100.

139. Prosch S, Staak K, Stein J, et al. Stimulation of the human cytomegalovirus IE enhancer/promoter in HL-60 cells by TNF alpha is mediated via induction of NF-kappaB. *Virology* 1995; 208:197–206.

140. Prosch S, Heine AK, Volk HD, Kruger DH. CCAAT/enhancer-binding proteins alpha and beta nega-tively influence the capacity of tumor necrosis factor alpha to up-regulate the human cytomegalovirus IE1/2 enhancer/promoter by nuclear factor kappaB during monocyte differentiation. *J Biol Chem* 2001; 276:40,712–40,720.

141. Nettelbeck DM, Jerome V, Muller R. Gene therapy: designer promoters for tumour targeting. *Trends Genet* 2000; 16:174–181.

142. Dachs GU, Patterson AV, Firth JD, et al. Targeting gene expression to hypoxic tumor cells. *Nat Med* 1997; 3:515–520.

143. Sasaki S, Amara RR, Yeow WS, Pitha PM, Robinson HL. Regulation of DNA- raised immune responses by cotransfected interferon regulatory factors. *J Virol* 2002; 76:6652–6659.

144. Klinman DM, Yamshchikov G, Ishigatsubo Y. Contribution of CpG motifs to the immunogenicity of DNA vaccines. *J Immunol* 1997; 158:3635–3639.

145. Yamada H. Gursel I, Takeshita F, et al. Effect of suppressive SNA on CpG-induced immune activation. *J Immunol* 2002; 169:5590–5594.

146. Kumar S, Epstein JE, Richie TL, et al. A multilateral effort to develop DNA vaccines against falciparum malaria. *Trends Parasitol* 2002; 18:129–135.

147. Barouch DH, Santra S, Tenner-Racz K, et al. Potent CD4+ T cell responses elicited by a bicistronic HIV-1 DNA vaccine expressing gp 120 and GM-CSF. *J Immunol* 2002; 168:562–568.

148. Barouch DH, Santra S, Steenbeke TD, et al. Augmentation and suppression of immune responses to an HIV-1 DNA vaccine by plasmid cytokine/Ig administration. *J Immunol* 1998; 161:1875–1882.

149. Kwissa M, Unsinger J, Schirmbeck R, Hauser H, Reimann J. Polyvalent DNA vaccines with bidirec-tional promoters. *J Mol Med* 2000; 78:495–506.

150. Drew DR, Boyle JS, Lew AM, Lightowlers MW, Chaplin PJ, Strugnell RA. The comparative efficacy of CTLA-4 and L-selectin targeted DNA vaccines in mice and sheep. *Vaccine* 2001; 19:4417–4428.

151. Chambers CA, Kuhns MS, Egen JG, Allison JP. CTLA-4 mediated inhibition in regulation of T cell re-sponses: mechanisms and manipulation in tumor immunotherapy. *Annu Rev Immunol* 2001; 19:565–594.

152. Egen JG, Kuhns MS, Allison JP. CTLA-4: new insights into its biological function and use in tumor immunotherapy. *Nat Immunol* 2002; 3:611–618.

153. Xiang R, Primus FJ, Ruehlmann JM, et al. A dual-function DNA vaccine encoding carcinoembryonic antigen and CD40 ligand trimer induces T cell-mediated protective immunity against colon cancer in carcinoembronic antigen-transgenic mice. *J Immunol* 2001; 167:4560–4565.

154. van Kooten C, Banchereau J. CD40-CD40 ligand. *J Leukoc Biol* 2000; 67:2–17.

155. Hanke T, Neumann VC, Blanchard TJ, et al. Effective induction of HIV-specific CTL by multi-epitope using gene gun in a combined vaccination regime. *Vaccine* 1999; 17:589–596.

156. Wee EG, Patel S, McMichael AJ, Hanke T. A DNA/MVA-based candidate human immunodeficiency virus vaccine for Kenya induces multi-specific T cell responses in rhesus macaques. *J Gen Virol* 2002; 83:75–80.

157. Manthorpe M, Cornefert-Jensen F, Hartikka J, et al. Gene therapy by intramuscular injection of plasmid DNA: studies on firefly luciferase gene expression in mice. *Hum Gene Ther* 1993; 4:419–431.

158. Cheng L, Ziegelhoffer PR, Yang NS. In vivo promoter activity and transgene expression in mammalian somatic tissues evaluated by using particle bombardment. *Proc Natl Acad Sci USA* 1993; 90:4455–4559.

159. Andre S, Seed B, Eberle J, Schraut W, Bultmann A, Haas J. Increased immune responses elicited by DNA vaccination with a synthetic gp120 sequence with optimized codon usage. *J Virol* 1998; 72:1497–1503.

160. Boyle JS, Koniaras C, Lew AM. Influence of cellular location of expressed antigen on the efficacy of DNA vaccination: cytotoxic T lymphocyte and antibody responses are suboptimal when antigen is cytoplasmic after intramuscular DNA immunization. *Int Immunol* 1997; 9:1897–1906.

161. Lewis PJ, Cox GJ, van Drunen Little-van den Hurk S, Babiuk LA. Polynucleotide vaccines in animals: enhancing and modulating responses. *Vaccine* 1997; 15:861–864.

162. Rice J, King CA, Spellerberg MB, Fairweather N, Stevenson FK. Manipulation of pathogen-derived genes to influence antigen presentation via DNA vaccines. *Vaccine* 1999; 17:3030–3038.

163. Yoneyama H, Narumi S, Zhang Y, et al. Pivotal role of dendritic cell-derived CXCL10 in the retention of T helper cell 1 lymphocytes in secondary lymph nodes. *J Exp Med* 2002; 195:1257–1266.

164. Gurunathan S, Klinman DM, Seder RA. DNA vaccines: immunology, application, and optimization. *Annu Rev Immunol* 2000; 18:927–974.

165. Scheerlinck JY. Genetic adjuvants for DNA vaccines. *Vaccine* 2001; 19:2647–2656.

166. Strom TB, Steele AW, Nichols J. Genetically engineered proteins for immunoregulation. *Transplant Proc* 1995; 27:18–20.

167. You Z, Huang X, Hester J, Toh HC, Chen SY. Targeting dendritic cells to enhance DNA vaccine potency. *Cancer Res* 2001; 61:3704–3711.

168. Biragyn A, Tani K, Grimm MC, Weeks S, Kwak LW. Genetic fusion of chemokines to a self-tumor antigen induces protective, T-cell dependent antitumor immunity. *Nat Biotechnol* 1999; 17:253–258.

169. Cappello P, Triebel F, Iezzi M, et al. LAG-3 enables DNA vaccination to persistently prevent mammary carcinogens in HER-2/*neu* transgenic BALB/c mice. *Cancer Res* 2003; 63:2518–2525.

170. Wolchok JD, Gregor PD, Nordquist LT, Slovin SF, Scher HI. DNA vaccines: an active immunization strategy for prostate cancer. *Semin Oncol* 2003; 30:659–666.

171. Reisfeld RA, Niethammer AG, Luo Y, Xiang R. DNA vaccines designed to inhibit tumor growth by suppression of angiogenesis. *Int Arch Allergy Immunol* 2004; 133:295–304.

172. Maecker HT, Umetsu DT, DeKruyff RH, Levy S. DNA vaccination with cytokine fusion constructs biases the immune response to ovalbumin. *Vaccine* 1997; 15:1687–1696.

173. McConkey SJ, Reece WH, Moorthy VS, et al. Enhanced T-cell immunogenicity of plasmid DNA vaccines boosted by recombinant modified vaccinia virus Ankara in humans. *Nat Med* 2003; 9:729–735.

174. Nichols WW, Ledwith BJ, Manam SV, Troilo PJ. Potential DNA vaccine integration into host cell genome. *Ann NY Acad Sci* 1995; 772:30–39.

175. Ledwith BJ, Manam S, Troilo PJ, et al. Plasmid DNA vaccines: assay for integration into host genomic DNA. *Dev Biol* 2000; 104:33–43.

176. Subramanian G, Adams MD, Venter JC, Broder S. Implications of the human genome for understanding human biology and medicine. *JAMA* 2001; 286:2296–2307.

177. Donnelly JJ, Ulmer JB, Shiver JW, Liu MA. DNA vaccines. *Annu Rev Immunol* 1997; 15:617–648.

178. Roses AD. Genome-based pharmacogenetics and the pharmaceutical industry. *Nat Rev Drug Discov* 2002; 1:541–549.

7 Dendritic Cells

Weiping Zou and Tyler J. Curiel

SUMMARY

Dendritic cells (DCs) have been called "nature's adjuvant" because of their remarkable ability to elicit adaptive, antigen-specific immunity. Immature DCs are highly specialized to capture antigens, but are poor at priming or activating T-cells. Following antigen capture or in a proinflammatory environment, DCs undergo a process of maturation in which antigen-carrying capacity is greatly reduced as T-cell priming and activating capacity are increased.

DCs are tightly regulated by expression of chemokine receptors whose expression varies according to the maturation state, microenvironmental milieu, and type of DC. Three principal subsets of human DCs are recognized: Langerhans' DCs, myeloid DCs, and plasmacytoid DCs. Much is now known regarding the lineage origins and specialized functions of these subsets, although much remains to be learned, and controversies abound.

Key Words: Human; dendritic cell; adaptive immunity; T cell; immunotherapy; chemokines; Langerhans' cells; clinical trial; cancer.

1. INTRODUCTION

Dendritic cells (DCs) have been called "nature's adjuvant" because of their remarkable capacity to elicit adaptive, antigen-specific immunity. They originate in the bone marrow as proliferating hematopoietic bone marrow cells, enter blood as nonproliferating precursor cells and seed most tissue as quiescent, nonproliferating immature DCs poised to sample the environment for evidence of immunopathology. Immature DCs are highly specialized to capture antigens, but are poor at priming or activating T-cells. Following antigen capture or in a proinflammatory environment, DCs undergo a process of maturation in which antigen-carrying capacity is greatly reduced as T-cell priming and activating capacity are increased.

DC trafficking is tightly regulated by expression of chemokine receptors whose expression varies according to the maturation state, microenvironmental milieu, and type of DC. Three principal subsets of human DCs are recognized: Langerhans' DCs, myeloid DCs, and plasmacytoid DCs. Much is now known regarding the lineage origins and specialized functions of these subsets, although much remains to be learned, and controversies abound. Dysfunctional DCs in tumors contribute to immunopathology. DCs grown ex vivo are now in clinical trials to treat cancers and other diseases.

From: *Cancer Drug Discovery and Development: Immunotherapy of Cancer*
Edited by: M. L. Disis © Humana Press Inc., Totowa, NJ

While examining skin in 1868, Paul Langerhans originally described the cells that we now recognize as Langerhans' DCs. He identified them as neural cells and failed to link between them to immune responses. DC studies languished for 90 yr, until Ralph Steinman and colleagues rediscovered them in 1972 at the Rockefeller University (NY). The role of DCs in immunity was thereafter quickly established, but progress in understanding DC function was hampered by their rarity in vivo, and because adequate means for in vitro propagation were not available. Research discoveries quickened with the finding that bone marrow cells and blood monocytes differentiated into DCs in vitro when cultured with recombinant cytokines including granulocyte-macrophage colony-stimulating factor (GM-CSF), interleukin (IL)-4, or tumor necrosis factor (TNF)-α.

2. DC DIFFERENTIATION

The terms *differentiation*, *activation*, and *maturation* are often incorrectly used interchangeably when describing DCs. The following will help to clarify these distinct events and the use of these terms. Bone marrow contains a population of proliferating CD34+ hematopoietic progenitor cells that give rise to the cellular elements of blood, including DCs. *Differentiation* refers to the process by which distinct cell lineages arise from these precursor cells to become lymphocytes, monocytes, DCs, and other cellular elements. As these progenitor cells differentiate, recently differentiated cells in the DC lineage exit marrow and enter blood as nonproliferating DC precursor cells *(1,2)*. Two principal types DC precursor cells circulate in human blood, giving rise to apparently distinct DC lineages. Myeloid DCs (MDCs) arise from lineage-negative precursor cells expressing the major histocompatibility complex (MHC) class II molecule human leukocyte antigen (HLA)-DR (as well as other class I and II molecules) and CD11c, whereas plasmacytoid DC (PDCs) arise from lineage-negative precursor cells expressing HLA-DR (as well as other class I and II molecules), but lacking CD11c *(3)*. (*See* Fig. 1 for a graphic illustration.) A hallmark of PDC precursor cells is their striking production of type I interferons (IFNs) following viral infection *(4,5)*, which is used to confirm their functional identity in vitro.

PDCs and MDCs differ with respect to expression of Toll-like receptors, which in part, accounts for their functional differences *(4)*. Although there are clear functional differences between MDCs and PDCs *(5)*, these lineage distinctions are still controversial *(6)* and are likely to be modified as new data emerge. For example, MDCs may become the principal type I IFN-producing cell in some viral infections *(7)*.

3. DC MATURATION AND ACTIVATION

Nonproliferating DC precursor cells exit blood to reside in essentially all lymphoid and nonlymphoid tissues. There they remain as nonmigratory, immature DCs, poised to sample the environment for foreign antigens or signs of danger. Proinflammatory stimuli including IL-1β and TNF-α, viral and bacterial products, such as cytosine-phosphate-guanine (CpG), and bacterial cell wall components, such as lipopolysaccharide ([LPS] endotoxin), elicit DC maturation. DC maturation is a complex, coordinated process in which cells specifically lose antigen-capture capacity in favor of T-cell stimulating activity, accompanied by morphologic and phenotypic changes to be detailed below. For full DC activation (such as to elicit CD8+ cytotoxic T-lymphocyte activity, a CD40 signal (usually delivered through T-cell CD40L) is also required. This activation signal has

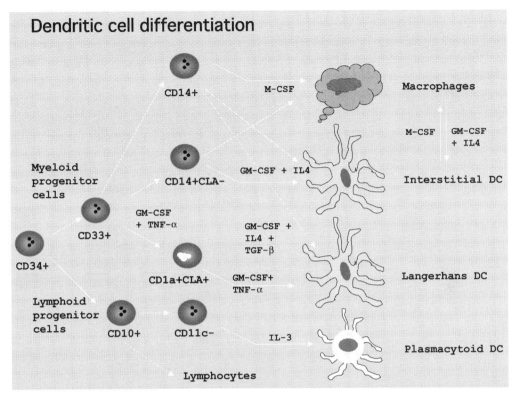

Fig. 1. Dendritic cells (DCs) arise from proliferating CD34[+] hematopoietic progenitor cells in bone marrow. They enter blood as nonproliferating precursor cells expressing either expressing CD11c (giving rise to myeloid DCs and Langerhans' DCs) or lacking CD11c expression (giving rise to plasmacytoid DCs). Various cytokines as shown can be added to DCs to induce their terminal differentiation in various DC subsets in vitro.

been termed "the license to kill." Following activation through CD40, DCs acquire a significant capacity to activate cytotoxic T-lymphocytes *(8,9)*.

Immature DCs are highly specialized to capture antigens, but are poor at priming naïve T-cells. As DCs mature, they lose their capacity to capture antigen and simultaneously acquire an extraordinary capacity to prime naïve T-cells. Mechanisms to capture antigen include pinocytosis, phagocytosis, and receptor-mediated mechanisms *(1,2)*. Immature DCs are highly migratory cells, although factors controlling their mobilization are poorly understood. Migration is dictated by expression of chemokine receptors, integrins, and selectins *(1,2,10,11)*. Migration signals in human cancers may differ compared to homeostatic signals *(12)*. DC migration likely also depends on the tissue origin of the DC, local factors, and specific characteristics of the mobilizing/migratory signals. Figure 2 depicts critical events in DC migration.

4. DC MOBILIZATION

The growth factors granulocyte colony-stimulating factor (G-CSF), GM-CSF and Fms-like tyrosine kinase 3 ligand (Flt3L) were originally developed to help mobilize granulo-

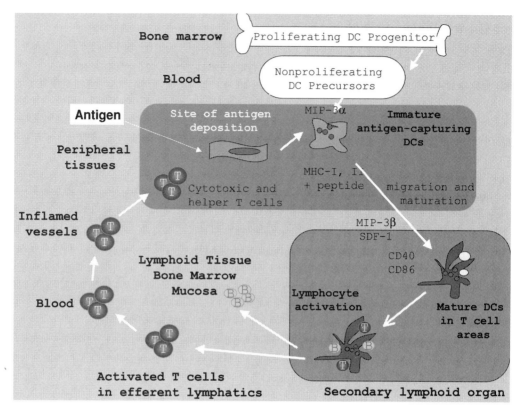

Fig. 2. Immature dendritic cells (DCs) are present in peripheral tissue, attracted by local monocyte chemoattractant protein 1α production. They wait, poised to capture antigen and continuously sample for antigens in the environment. Following exposure to proinflammatory danger signals or foreign antigens, DCs undergo maturation as they exit into draining lymph channels to migrate to local draining lymph nodes. Following maturation, high antigen-capture capacity is replaced by strong T- or B-cell-activating capacity. Matured and activated DCs in lymph nodes instruct antigen-specific cells to exit, and then migrate to sites of danger or foreign antigen expression to affect their specific functions. Mature DCs are then removed from lymph nodes by apoptosis.

cytes and myeloid cells to prevent or treat infection in leukopenic patients, as when, for example, following cytotoxic chemotherapy.

We now know that these growth factors also mobilize circulating DCs into peripheral blood. G-CSF preferentially mobilizes CD11c⁻ PDC precursor cells (although it also mobilizes CD11c⁺ DC precursor cells). GM-CSF preferentially mobilizes CD11c⁺ MDCs and their precursor cells. Flt3L mobilizes large numbers of both MDCs and PDCs in human administration *(1,13,14)*.

5. MYELOID DCs

MDCs occur either as interstitial DCs in the dermis of skin or in most organs or as Langerhans' DCs, which populate and survey skin epidermis. Interstitial DCs are the same as the well-known in vitro monocyte-derived DCs *(1,2)*. Humoral responses might preferentially be regulated by interstitial DC. Langerhans' DCs are poor at apoptotic body capture and pinocytosis, but excellent in inducing cytotoxic T-lymphocytes or CD4+ and CD8+ T-cell proliferation. Experimental evidence also suggests that Langerhans' DCs are better than interstitial DCs in elicitation of cytotoxic T-lymphocytes (1,2).

6. PLASMACYTOID DCs

Human PDCs derive from circulating precursor cells lacking lineage marker and CD11c expression but expressing HLA-DR. They are further identified by expression of CD123, the IL-3R-α-chain (12). Blood PDC lineage cells appear primarily to circulate as precursor cells. These precursor cells were identified as high-type I IFN-producing cells following virus infection (15). This type I IFN induces significant T-helper cell (Th)1 polarization (16,17). When activated through CD40 or CpG motifs, murine PDCs (CD40 or CpG can not stimulate human PDC IL-12) may also induce T-cell IFN-α through IL-12 secretion (18). PDCs may also mediate antigen-specific tolerance (19) and can induce CD4+ (20) as well as CD8+ (21) regulatory T-cells in vitro. The murine equivalent of human PDCs has been described (22–24), which may help allow more detailed in vivo studies of this rare and little-known DC subset.

7. LANGERHANS' DCs

Langerhans' DCs populate epidermal layers of skin, where they form a first line of defense against infection and inflammation (1,2). Langerhans' DCs are easily cultivated from murine ear explants (25) and from CD34+ bone marrow progenitor cells (26), making their study relatively easy. Transforming growth factor (TGF)-β is an important factor in in vivo Langerhans' cell differentiation (27). IL-15 contributes to Langerhans' DC differentiation in vitro and contributes to the cells' migration (28). Langerhans' DCs may be especially suited to activate cytotoxic T-lymphocytes (1,2).

8. T-CELL ACTIVATION

Immature MDCs express low levels of T-cell co-stimulatory molecules, such as CD40, CD54, CD80, CD86, and MHC classes I and II. Following maturation, through a variety of mechanisms, MDCs greatly increase expression of all of these T-cell co-stimulatory molecules and also express CD83, a molecule with a function that is incompletely understood, but which is a hallmark of mature MDCs (1,2). PDCs express these molecules, as well and upregulate them following maturation, and they are less potent than MDCs in priming naïve T-cells (1,2). The capacity of MDCs or PDCs to prime naïve T-lymphocytes forms the basis of the standard mixed lymphocyte reaction (MLR). Immature MDCs are relatively poor at inducing naïve CD4+ T-cell proliferation compared with matured/activated MDCs and induce T-cell IL-4 and IFN-γ, but no significant T-cell IL-10. Following maturation, their capacity to induce T-cell IFN-γ increases substantially. Immature MDCs secrete little IL-12 and IL-10. Following maturation, they greatly increase IL-12 secretion, which is critical to their capacity to induce Th1 polarization and T-cell IFN-γ secretion, and increase IL-10 secretion, but to a much lesser degree. Mature MDCs also secrete a variety of other soluble factors, such as IL-6, IL-18, TNF-α, and chemokines. The immunobiological roles of all of these factors remain to be fully defined. The murine counterparts of human MDCs are similar in most of these important aspects (29,30).

Immature (precursor) PDCs secrete little type I IFN, but secrete enormous quantities following virus infection when exposed to CpG motifs *(4,31)*. These type I IFNs can induce Th1 polarization of T-cells *(17)*. Mature PDCs also secrete the chemokines IP-10 and IL-8 and the cytokines TNF-α and IL-6, which may have effects on T-cell activation or polarization *(18)*. Murine PDCs are similar to human PDCs in many regards, but do express CD11c and, more importantly, do secrete significant IL-12 *(22,23)*.

9. ANTIGEN PROCESSING AND PRESENTATION

DCs prime or activate a variety of antigen-specific immune cells through presentation of antigen in the context of both MHC class I and class II. Thus, DCs possess a variety of mechanisms by which antigen is introduced into the MHC class I or II pathways for eventual presentation to antigen-specific cells. DCs use classic antigen-processing pathways for processing endogenous antigen into MHC class II and endogenous antigen into class I *(1,2)*. Further, they may capture apoptotic bodies through the surface receptors CD36 or αvβ5 integrins for processing and presentation in the MHC class I pathway *(32,33)*. Several DC-specific antigen-capture receptors or processing mechanisms have been identified, including DC-lysosome-associated membrane glycoprotein *(34)* and DC-specific intracellular adhesion molecule 1-grabbing nonintegrin *(35)*. Thus, DCs can present antigen in a class I- or class II-restricted fashion to activate CD4+ or CD8+ T-cells, respectively.

10. MICROENVIRONMENTAL INFLUENCES

The ultimate differentiation potential and effector function of MDCs or PDCs is dictated by microenvironmental conditions and signals. For example, MDCs differentiating and maturing under homeostatic conditions generally induce potent Th1 polarization *(5)*. However, when matured in the presence of prostaglandins, they may induce Th2 polarization *(36,37)*. MDCs exposed to IL-10 may induce T-cell anergy or tolerance, which can impede tumor-specific immunity *(38)*. T-cells repeatedly stimulated with immature, rather than mature, MDCs may induce IL-10-secreting regulatory T-cells with a type 1 regulatory T-cell phenotype *(38,39)*. Immature PDCs in blood may induce a Th0 phenotype characterized by T-cell secretion of both IFN-γ and IL-4. However, following activation by virus infection, they induce potent Th1 polarization through IFN-α secretion *(17)*. In tumors, PDCs may induce T-cell IL-10, contributing to tumor-mediated immune suppression *(12)*.

11. IN VITRO GENERATION OF DCs

11.1. Introduction

Study of DCs was hampered for decades by lack of sufficient numbers owing to their scarcity in vivo. It is now possible to generate large numbers of DCs in vitro using techniques that have revolutionized their study. Generally, the easiest way to generate DCs in vitro is to culture precursor cells in recombinant GM-CSF plus IL-4. Different cytokine manufacturers may use different units to measure potency, so care should be taken to ensure that correct concentrations of cytokines are used if products are purchased from vendors with methods that differ from published methods. DC phenotype and function can be affected by the precursor cells from which they are derived by any growth factors used to mobilize precursor cells, differentiation, or maturation factors, or the anatomic location from which the DC or its precursor cell was recovered (1,2). All these factors must be considered when choosing a DC system for a specific application.

Monocytes reverse transmigrating across endothelial surfaces will differentiate into MDCs in the absence of exogenous cytokines (40,41), which may be a mechanism by which DC precursor cells differentiate into DCs in vivo.

11.2. Cultivation of Human DCs

11.2.1. CLASSICAL MONOCYTE-DERIVED DCS

The best-studied human DCs are those derived from monocytes, which may be obtained by plastic adherence. Various methods to deplete contaminating lymphocytes, platelets, and other cells include plastic adherence, sorting, paramagnetic beads, neuraminidase-treated sheep red blood cells, and other techniques. However, significant differences in DCs differentiated from these monocytes collected and purified in these distinct ways have not generally been noted. Fetal calf serum may contain trace amounts of endotoxin, TGF-β, or other factors (42). Some investigators thus use serum-free medium or autologous plasma instead of fetal calf serum.

To produce immature DCs, monocytes are cultured with GM-CSF plus IL-4 for 5–7 d. Maturation can be effected with LPS or a variety of other agents, well described elsewhere. It is not clear that specific culture systems are advantageous over others, aside from cost considerations.

11.2.2. MONOCYTES TO DIFFERENTIATE LANGERHANS' DCS

Circulating monocytes will differentiate into cells with many features of immature Langerhans' DCs on culture with GM-CSF, IL-4 and TGF-β (43). These monocyte-derived Langerhans' DC effect a significant allogeneic MLR comparable to classical monocyte-derived DC described in Subheading 11.2.1.

11.2.3. CD34+ CELL-DERIVED DCS

DC progenitor cells differ from precursor cells in that they proliferate. Thus, DC yields can be increased if the progenitor pool is first expanded before differentiation into DCs. In this regard, CD34+ cells from leukapheresis, bone marrow, or umbilical cord blood serve as an excellent source of proliferating DC progenitor cells for DC generation. The yield of CD34+ cells in blood can be increased greatly by treating donors with factors, such as Flt3L or G-CSF, before leukapheresis. Umbilical cord blood contains many more CD34+ cells than normal adult blood.

11.2.4. CONSIDERATIONS FOR THERAPEUTIC USE OF HUMAN DCS

If human DCs grown ex vivo are to be transfused adoptively back into human subjects, special attention must be paid to the nature of the cell collection, culture conditions, differentiation agents, maturation agents, and antigens used. In the United States, the Food and Drug Administration closely scrutinizes human trials involving transfused, manipulated cells, particularly when gene therapy is involved, and must approve such trials before they can be effected. Cells and viruses must be cultivated and prepared in specialized, good-laboratory-practice facilities, which are loosely defined and not as stringently controlled as good-manufacturing-process facilities used in manufacture of drugs and biologics by pharmaceutical and biotechnology companies.

11.3. Murine DC Cultivation

11.3.1. CULTURED DCs

Inaba and associates described an in vitro technique *(44)* that is still used, with minor modifications. Bone marrow cells are cultured with recombinant murine GM-CSF to induce DC differentiation. These DCs can be matured by LPS or TNF-α treatment or other means. CD34+ cells obtained from murine bone marrow will differentiate into DCs when cultured with GM-CSF plus Flt3L *(45)*. CD34+ cells may be obtained from murine marrow by depletion of lineage+, nonadherent cells, followed by sorting. These cells will differentiate into CD11b+CD11c+ and CD11b−/dullCD11c+ subsets on culture with GM-CSF, TNF-α, and CSF *(46)*. Addition of TGF-β to these three cytokines preferentially drives precursors down a Langerhans' DC differentiation pathway *(47)*. Contaminating macrophages and granulocytes are greatly reduced by sorting CD34+ cells.

11.3.2. DIRECTLY ISOLATED DCs

Spleen cells contain variable amounts of CD4−CD8α−DEC-205loCD11bhi and CD4−CD8α+DEC-205hiCD11blo DCs that can be sorted to high purity for immediate use or cultured in GM-CSF overnight before use *(48)*. Flt3L or GM-CSF treatment of animals significantly increases the number of both types of DCs, which may then be sorted from spleen for immediate use *(30,49)*. A third major spleen DC subset, which is CD4+CD8α−DEC-205loCD11bhi, was recently reported *(50)*.

The skin is a significant source of both Langerhans' DCs (isolated from epidermis) and interstitial DCs (isolated from dermis).

12. TUMOR EFFECTS ON DCs

It is well-known that microenvironmental factors influence DC differentiation and function. Thus, it is reasonable to expect that DCs from tumors may behave differently compared with DCs isolated from normal subjects. In fact, the tumor microenvironment produces a number of factors that inhibit DC differentiation or maturation including vascular endothelial growth factor *(51,52)*, and M-CSF and IL-6 *(53)*. Tumor stromal derived factor 1 alters the function of PDCs to make them dysfunctional *(12)*. Tumor IL-10 and vascular endothelial growth factor contribute to induce B7-H1 expression on tumor-associated MDCs, which helps suppress host antitumor immunity *(54)*. Blocking DC B7-H1 augments antitumor immunity *(54)*, demonstrating that inhibition of DC dysfunction may be a novel therapeutic strategy. Breast carcinomas appear preferentially to attract immature DCs while excluding trafficking of mature DCs, which may prevent ignition of effective antitumor immunity *(55)*. Immature myeloid cells in tumors with features of DCs inhibit host antitumor immunity *(56)*.

13. DCs IN CONTROL OF TOLERANCE

Although DCs are primarily considered to be immune-activating cells, they also play a significant role in inducing and maintaining tolerance in normal and pathological conditions *(1,2)*. Immature DCs injected into humans induce antigen-specific tolerance *(57)*. Specialized DCs in gut may mediate oral tolerance *(58)*. Additional roles for DCs in tolerizing in other anatomic compartments are being defined *(1,2)*. Roles for PDCs and MDCs normally and in tumor to mediate tolerance or induce regulatory T-cells have been discussed.

14. ADDITIONAL CONSIDERATIONS

HLA-DR$^+$lin$^-$CD11c$^-$ cells with features of PDCs have been demonstrated in cord blood cells, where they compose about 0.3% of the total cell population *(59)*. CD2$^+$ monocytes may represent circulating MDCs, and effect an efficient allogeneic MLR, without culture in cytokines *(60)*. Macrophages also serve as DC precursor cells, which have novel T-cell-activating properties *(61)*. Some leukemia and lymphoma cells may be induced to differentiate in vitro into cells with DC features, which may have therapeutic potential. Thus, peripherally circulating CD34$^+$ leukemic blasts from both myeloid and lymphoid leukemias will differentiate into DCs in vitro under appropriate conditions *(62,63)*.

Adherent peripheral blood mononuclear cells or CD34$^+$ cells from patients with chronic myelogenous leukemia will differentiate into DCs that express the Philadelphia chromosome *(64)* and stimulate tumor-specific immunity *(65,66)*. Myeloid precursor cells in acute myelogenous leukemias also differentiate into DCs, some of which express tumor-specific genetic defects *(67)*. Progenitor cells in chronic myelogenous leukemia differentiate into DC-like cells with calcium ionophores *(68)*.

ACKNOWLEDGMENTS

We acknowledge the tremendous efforts of our colleagues, from whose work we have extracted summaries. We regret not mentioning the work of others owing to space limitations. This work was supported by National Institutes of Health, the Department of Defense, and the Tulane Endowment.

REFERENCES

1. Banchereau J, Briere F, Caux C, et al. Immunobiology of dendritic cells. *Annu Rev Immunol* 2000; 18: 767–811.
2. Banchereau J, Steinman RM. Dendritic cells and the control of immunity. *Nature* 1998; 392:245–252.
3. Kohrgruber N, Halanek N, Groger M, et al. Survival, maturation, and function of CD11c$^-$ and CD11c$^+$ peripheral blood dendritic cells are differentially regulated by cytokines. *J Immunol* 1999; 163:3250–3259.
4. Liu YJ. IPC: professional type 1 interferon-producing cells and plasmacytoid dendritic cell precursors. *Annu Rev Immunol* 2004; 23:275–306.
5. Rissoan MC, Soumelis V, Kadowaki N, et al. Reciprocal control of T helper cell and dendritic cell differentiation. *Science* 1999; 283:1183–1186.
6. Shigematsu H, Reizis B, Iwasaki H, et al. Plasmacytoid dendritic cells activate lymphoid-specific genetic programs irrespective of their cellular origin. *Immunity* 2004; 21:43–53.
7. Diebold SS, Montoya M, Unger H, et al. Viral infection switches non-plasmacytoid dendritic cells into high interferon producers. *Nature* 2003; 424:324–328.
8. Bennett SR, Carbone FR, Karamalis F, Flavell RA, Miller JF, Heath WR. Help for cytotoxic-T-cell responses is mediated by CD40 signalling. *Nature* 1998; 393:478–480.
9. Ridge JP, Di Rosa F, Matzinger P. A conditioned dendritic cell can be a temporal bridge between a CD4$^+$ T- helper and a T-killer cell. *Nature* 1998; 393:474–478.
10. Sallusto F, Palermo B, Lenig D, et al. Distinct patterns and kinetics of chemokine production regulate den-dritic cell function. *Eur J Immunol* 1999; 29:1617–1625.
11. Sallusto F, Schaerli P, Loetscher P, et al. Rapid and coordinated switch in chemokine receptor expression during dendritic cell maturation. *Eur J Immunol* 1998; 28:2760–2769.
12. Zou W, Machelon V, Coulomb-L'Hermin A, et al. Stromal-derived factor-1 in human tumors recruits and alters the function of plasmacytoid precursor dendritic cells. *Nat Med* 2001; 7:1339–1346.
13. Pulendran B, Banchereau J, Burkeholder S, et al. Flt3-ligand and granulocyte colony-stimulating factor mobilize distinct human dendritic cell subsets in vivo. *J Immunol* 2000; 165:566–572.

14. Arpinati M, Green CL, Heimfeld S, Heuser JE, Anasetti C. Granulocyte-colony stimulating factor mobilizes T helper 2-inducing dendritic cells. *Blood* 2000; 95:2484–2490.
15. Siegal FP, Kadowaki N, Shodell M, et al. The nature of the principal type 1 interferon-producing cells in human blood. *Science* 1999; 284:1835–1837.
16. Cella M, Jarrossay D, Facchetti F, et al. Plasmacytoid monocytes migrate to inflamed lymph nodes and produce large amounts of type I interferon. *Nat Med* 1999; 5:919–923.
17. Cella M, Facchetti F, Lanzavecchia A, Colonna M. Plasmacytoid dendritic cells activated by influenza virus and CD40L drive a potent TH1 polarization. *Nat Immunol* 2000; 1:305–310.
18. Krug A, Towarowski A, Britsch S, et al. Toll-like receptor expression reveals CpG DNA as a unique microbial stimulus for plasmacytoid dendritic cells which synergizes with CD40 ligand to induce high amounts of IL-12. *Eur J Immunol* 2001; 31:3026–3037.
19. Kuwana M, Kaburaki J, Wright TM, Kawakami Y, Ikeda Y. Induction of antigen-specific human CD4(+) T cell anergy by peripheral blood DC2 precursors. *Eur J Immunol* 2001; 31:2547–2557.
20. Moseman EA, Liang X, Dawson AJ, et al. Human plasmacytoid dendritic cells activated by CpG oligodeoxynucleotides induce the generation of CD4+CD25+ regulatory T cells. *J Immunol* 2004; 173:4433–4442.
21. Gilliet M, Liu YJ. Generation of human CD8 T regulatory cells by CD40 ligand-activated plasmacytoid dendritic cells. *J Exp Med* 2002; 195:695–704.
22. Nakano H, Yanagita M, Gunn MD. CD11c+B220+Gr-1+ cells in mouse lymph nodes and spleen display characteristics of plasmacytoid dendritic cells. *J Exp Med* 2001; 194:1171–1178.
23. Asselin-Paturel C, Boonstra A, Dalod M, et al. Mouse type I IFN-producing cells are immature APCs with plasmacytoid morphology. *Nat Immunol* 2001; 2:1144–1150.
24. Asselin-Paturel C, Brizard G, Pin JJ, Briere F, Trinchieri G. Mouse strain differences in plasmacytoid dendritic cell frequency and function revealed by a novel monoclonal antibody. *J Immunol* 2003; 171: 646–6477.
25. Schuler G, Steinman RM. Murine epidermal Langerhans cells mature into potent immunostimulatory dendritic cells in vitro. *J Exp Med* 1985; 161:526–546.
26. Caux C, Dezutter-Dambuyant C, Schmitt D, Banchereau J. GM-CSF and TNF-alpha cooperate in the generation of dendritic Langerhans cells. *Nature* 1992; 360:258–261.
27. Borkowski TA, Letterio JJ, Farr AG, Udey MC. A role for endogenous transforming growth factor beta 1 in Langerhans cell biology: the skin of transforming growth factor beta 1 null mice is devoid of epidermal Langerhans cells. *J Exp Med* 1996; 184:2417–2422.
28. Mohamadzadeh M, Berard F, Essert G, et al. Interleukin 15 Skews monocyte differentiation into dendritic cells with features of Langerhans cells. *J Exp Med* 2001; 194:1013–1020.
29. Pulendran B, Lingappa J, Kennedy MK, et al. Developmental pathways of dendritic cells in vivo: distinct function, phenotype, and localization of dendritic cell subsets in FLT3 ligand- treated mice. *J Immunol* 1997; 159:2222–2231.
30. Pulendran B, Smith JL, Caspary G, et al. Distinct dendritic cell subsets differentially regulate the class of immune response in vivo. *Proc Natl Acad Sci USA* 1999; 96:1036–1041.
31. Liu Y-J. Directing T-cell responses by human dendritic cell subsets. American Association of Immunologists 2000 Meeting. 2000; S165.
32. Albert ML, Pearce SF, Francisco LM, et al. Immature dendritic cells phagocytose apoptotic cells via alphavbeta5 and CD36, and cross-present antigens to cytotoxic T lymphocytes. *J Exp Med* 1998; 188: 1359–1368.
33. Albert ML, Sauter B, Bhardwaj N. Dendritic cells acquire antigen from apoptotic cells and induce class I-restricted CTLs. *Nature* 1998; 392:86–89.
34. de Saint-Vis B, Vincent J, Vandenabeele S, et al. A novel lysosome-associated membrane glycoprotein, DC-LAMP, induced upon DC maturation, is transiently expressed in MHC class II compartment. *Immunity* 1998; 9:325–336.
35. Geijtenbeek BHT. DC-SIGN-ICAM-2 interaction mediates dendritic cell trafficking. *Nature* 2000; 1: 353–357.
36. Kalinski P, Schuitemaker JH, Hilkens CM, Kapsenberg ML. Prostaglandin E2 induces the final maturation of IL-12-deficient CD1a+CD83+ dendritic cells: the levels of IL-12 are determined during the final dendritic cell maturation and are resistant to further modulation. *J Immunol* 1998; 161:2804–2809.
37. Kalinski P, Hilkens CM, Snijders A, Snijdewint FG, Kapsenberg ML. IL-12-deficient dendritic cells, generated in the presence of prostaglandin E2, promote type 2 cytokine production in maturing human naive T helper cells. *J Immunol* 1997; 159:28–35.

38. Steinbrink K, Wolfl M, Jonuleit H, Knop J, Enk AH. Induction of tolerance by IL-10-treated dendritic cells. *J Immunol* 1997; 159:4772–4780.

39. Levings MK, Gregori S, Tresoldi E, Cazzaniga S, Bonini C, Roncarolo MG. Differentiation of Tr1 cells by immature dendritic cells requires IL-10 but not CD25$^+$CD4$^+$ Tr cells. *Blood* 2005; 105:1162–1169.

40. Randolph GJ, Beaulieu S, Lebecque S, Steinman RM, Muller WA. Differentiation of monocytes into dendritic cells in a model of transendothelial trafficking. *Science* 1998; 282:480–483.

41. Randolph GJ, Inaba K, Robbiani DF, Steinman RM, Muller WA. Differentiation of phagocytic monocytes into lymph node dendritic cells in vivo. *Immunity* 1999; 11:753–761.

42. Strobl H, Bello-Fernandez C, Riedl E, et al. flt3 ligand in cooperation with transforming growth factor-beta1 potentiates in vitro development of Langerhans-type dendritic cells and allows single-cell dendritic cell cluster formation under serum-free conditions. *Blood* 1997; 90:1425–1434.

43. Geissmann F, Prost C, Monnet JP, Dy M, Brousse N, Hermine O. Transforming growth factor beta1, in the presence of granulocyte/macrophage colony-stimulating factor and interleukin 4, induces differentiation of human peripheral blood monocytes into dendritic Langerhans cells. *J Exp Med* 1998; 187: 961–966.

44. Inaba K, Inaba M, Romani N, et al. Generation of large numbers of dendritic cells from mouse bone marrow cultures supplemented with granulocyte/macrophage colony-stimulating factor. *J Exp Med* 1992; 176:1693–1702.

45. Vecchi A, Massimiliano L, Ramponi S, et al. Differential responsiveness to constitutive vs. inducible chemokines of immature and mature mouse dendritic cells. *J Leukoc Biol* 1999; 66:489–494.

46. Zhang Y, Harada A, Wang JB, et al. Bifurcated dendritic cell differentiation in vitro from murine lineage phenotype-negative c-kit$^+$ bone marrow hematopoietic progenitor cells. *Blood* 1998; 92:118–128.

47. Zhang Y, Zhang YY, Ogata M, et al. Transforming growth factor-beta1 polarizes murine hematopoietic progenitor cells to generate Langerhans cell-like dendritic cells through a monocyte/macrophage differentiation pathway. *Blood* 1999; 93:1208–1220.

48. Maldonado-Lopez R, De Smedt T, Michel P, et al. CD8alpha$^+$ and CD8alpha$^-$ subclasses of dendritic cells direct the development of distinct T helper cells In vivo. *J Exp Med* 1999; 189:587–592.

49. Maraskovsky E, Brasel K, Teepe M, et al. Dramatic increase in the numbers of functionally mature dendritic cells in Flt3 ligand-treated mice: multiple dendritic cell subpopulations identified. *J Exp Med* 1996; 184:1953–1962.

50. Vremec D, Pooley J, Hochrein H, Wu L, Shortman K. CD4 and CD8 expression by dendritic cell subtypes in mouse thymus and spleen. *J Immunol* 2000; 164:2978–2986.

51. Gabrilovich D, Ishida T, Oyama T, et al. Vascular endothelial growth factor inhibits the development of dendritic cells and dramatically affects the differentiation of multiple hematopoietic lineages in vivo. *Blood* 1998; 92:4150–4166.

52. Gabrilovich DI, Chen HL, Girgis KR, et al. Production of vascular endothelial growth factor by human tumors inhibits the functional maturation of dendritic cells (published erratum appears in *Nat Med* 1996 Nov;2[11]:1267). *Nat Med* 1996; 2:1096–1103.

53. Menetrier-Caux C, Montmain G, Dieu MC, et al. Inhibition of the differentiation of dendritic cells from CD34(+) progenitors by tumor cells: role of interleukin-6 and macrophage colony-stimulating factor. *Blood* 1998; 92:4778–4791.

54. Curiel TJ, Wei S, Dong H, et al. Blockade of B7-H1 improves myeloid dendritic cell-mediated antitumor immunity. *Nat Med* 2003; 9:562–567.

55. Bell D, Chomarat P, Broyles D, et al. In breast carcinoma tissue, immature dendritic cells reside within the tumor, whereas mature dendritic cells are located in peritumoral areas. *J Exp Med* 1999; 190:1417–1426.

56. Almand B, Clark JI, Nikitina E, et al. Increased production of immature myeloid cells in cancer patients: a mechanism of immunosuppression in cancer. *J Immunol* 2001; 166:678–689.

57. Dhodapkar MV, Steinman RM, Krasovsky J, Munz C, Bhardwaj N. Antigen-specific inhibition of effector T cell function in humans after injection of immature dendritic cells. *J Exp Med* 2001; 193:233–238.

58. Bilsborough J, Viney JL. Gastrointestinal dendritic cells play a role in immunity, tolerance, and disease. *Gastroenterology* 2004; 127:300–309.

59. Sorg RV, Kogler G, Wernet P. Identification of cord blood dendritic cells as an immature CD11c$^-$ population. *Blood* 1999; 93:2302–2307.

60. Crawford K, Gabuzda D, Pantazopoulos V, et al. Circulating CD2$^+$ monocytes are dendritic cells. *J Immunol* 1999; 163:5920–5928.

61. Zou W, Borvak J, Marches F, et al. Macrophage-derived dendritic cells have strong Th1-polarizing potential mediated by beta-chemokines rather than IL-12. *J Immunol* 2000; 165:4388–4396.

62. Cignetti A, Bryant E, Allione B, Vitale A, Foa R, Cheever MA. CD34(+) acute myeloid and lymphoid leukemic blasts can be induced to differentiate into dendritic cells. *Blood* 1999; 94:2048–2055.

63. Mutis T, Schrama E, Melief CJ, Goulmy E. CD80-transfected acute myeloid leukemia cells induce primary allogeneic T-cell responses directed at patient specific minor histocompatibility antigens and leukemia-associated antigens. *Blood* 1998; 92:1677–1684.

64. Heinzinger M, Waller CF, von den Berg A, Rosenstiel A, Lange W. Generation of dendritic cells from patients with chronic myelogenous leukemia. *Ann Hematol* 1999; 78:181–186.

65. Eibl B, Ebner S, Duba C, et al. Dendritic cells generated from blood precursors of chronic myelogenous leukemia patients carry the Philadelphia translocation and can induce a CML-specific primary cytotoxic T-cell response. *Genes Chromosomes Cancer* 1997; 20:215–223.

66. Choudhury A, Gajewski JL, Liang JC, et al. Use of leukemic dendritic cells for the generation of anti-leukemic cellular cytotoxicity against Philadelphia chromosome-positive chronic myelogenous leukemia. *Blood* 1997; 89:1133–1142.

67. Choudhury BA, Liang JC, Thomas EK, et al. Dendritic cells derived in vitro from acute myelogenous leu-kemia cells stimulate autologous, antileukemic T-cell responses. *Blood* 1999; 93:780–786.

68. Engels FH, Koski GK, Bedrosian I, et al. Calcium signaling induces acquisition of dendritic cell charac-teristics in chronic myelogenous leukemia myeloid progenitor cells. *Proc Natl Acad Sci USA* 1999; 96: 10,332–10,337.

8

Different Approaches to Dendritic Cell-Based Cancer Immunotherapy

Noweeda Mirza and Dmitry Gabrilovich

SUMMARY

In this chapter, we discuss the development of cancer vaccines, using as an example a vaccine based on dendritic cells transduced with wild-type p53. We discuss requirements for tumor-associated antigens, antigen carriers, and selection of patients. Theoretical considerations are supported by specific experiments testing p53 vaccine in preclinical settings in vitro and in vivo.

Key Words: Cancer vaccines; tumor immunology; dendritic cells; p53; adenovirus; small cell lung cancer.

1. INTRODUCTION

Immunotherapy can be a very powerful tool in controlling tumor progression. It has now become increasingly clear that the success of immunotherapy of cancer depends on several major factors:

1. Discovery of suitable tumor-associated antigens (TAAs). An ideal TAA should have several important features:
   a. Immune response against this TAA should recognize the tumor, but not normal cells.
   b. It is important that this TAA should not be relatively rare, and it should be expressed in a significant proportion of cancer patients.
   c. If the chosen TAA is part of a self-protein, then the immune response against this TAA should not lead to severe autoimmune abnormalities.
   d. It is important that the survival of tumor cells depend on the presence of molecules containing chosen TAA, and in this way tumor cells will not be able to escape immune recognition by losing this molecule.
2. An adequate carrier for TAA. This vehicle should help to activate the primary immune response and if necessary, to overcome tolerance to self-proteins. This carrier should be relatively easy to manufacture and standardize, and it should not be toxic to patients.
3. Selection of the patients. In the past, most of the clinical trials were performed in patients with bulky disease or metastatic cancer. It is clear now that even these effectively activated cytotoxic T-cells (CTLs) had very little opportunity to penetrate large, solid tumors. In addition, patients at terminal stages of cancer had profound abnormalities in their metabolism, hence limiting their ability to develop and maintain effective antitumor immune responses. It is clear that immunotherapy of cancer can be the most effective in neoadjuvant settings or in combination with other treatment options like chemotherapy or radiation.

From: *Cancer Drug Discovery and Development: Immunotherapy of Cancer*
Edited by: M. L. Disis © Humana Press Inc., Totowa, NJ

4. Host immune system of cancer patients does not function normally. A large number of different defects in T-cells, natural-killer cells, and antigen-presenting cells (APCs) have been described *(1)*. These defects impair the ability of the immune system to amass anti-tumor immunity. It appears that successful immunotherapy of cancer will require correction of these defects.

This chapter discusses one experimental strategy to develop a cancer vaccine, and traces the development of the vaccine from the conception of scientific hypothesis through preclinical experiments to the design of the clinical trial.

1.1. The Development of the Hypothesis: p53 as a Target for Cancer Immunotherapy

The *p53* gene plays a central role in the control of cell growth and differentiation. The biological functions of wild-type p53 are related to cell cycle arrest/growth arrest, the induction of apoptosis, and maintenance of genetic stability by modulation of DNA repair, replication, and recombination pathways. Normally, p53 is a short-lived protein localized in the nuclei of cells. In response to DNA damage, p53 becomes stabilized and can induce either cell cycle arrest or apoptosis. Cell cycle arrest is mediated by the ability of p53 to form homodimers that bind to specific DNA sequences and activate transcription of cycle-control genes, such as *p21* and cdk-interacting protein 1. These proteins, in turn, induce a block at a G_1/S or G_2/M phases of the cell cycle and lead to growth arrest. Although the mechanisms for the induction of apoptosis remain unclear, it is evident that p53 upregulates the expression of p21, B-cell lymphoma 2-associated X protein, and fatty acid synthase and downregulates expression of B-cell lymphoma 2, all of which are implicated in the modulation of apoptosis. Overall, p53 plays a key regulatory role in many of the biochemical processes, including DNA repair, cell cycle control, apoptosis, and genomic stability, which are integral to the development of human carcinogenesis.

Approximately 50% of all human cancers have altered p53 function resulting from stable sense mutations. These mutations in the *p53* gene result in the accumulation of mutant p53 protein in the nuclei and cytoplasm of tumor cells. Alterations in the *p53* gene usually result in the accumulation of both mutated and/or wild-type p53 molecules in tumor cells. Therefore, potentially both mutant and wild-type p53 peptide sequences can be processed and presented by major histocompatibility complex (MHC) class I molecules of tumor cells *(2)*. Normal tissues have low to undetectable levels of p53 protein expression compared with tumor cells. The high frequency of mutations in the *p53* gene in cancer, as well as underlying differences in the level of p53 expression between neoplastic and normal cells, raises the potential for p53-based cancer immunotherapy. Importantly, the abnormalities in the *p53* gene are critically important for the survival of tumor cells, because restoration of wild-type p53 in tumor cells results in their apoptosis. It is highly unlikely that tumor cells will be able to escape effective anti-p53 CTL by restoring wild-type p53 status.

2. SELECTION OF THE ANTIGENS FOR VACCINATION

2.1. Limitations of Targeting Mutant p53-Derived Peptides in Immunotherapy

It has been known for some time now that p53 can be utilized as target for immune recognition and over the last several years, different approaches to p53-based immunotherapy have been explored. In 1979, DeLeo and colleagues first described p53 as a tumor antigen *(3)*, and circulating antibodies to p53 are found in a variety of malignancies, including lung, breast, colorectal, hepatoma, and head and neck cancers *(4,5)*. However, whereas the ability of lung cancer patients to develop anti-p53 antibodies correlated with the type of *p53* mutation, many patients have tumors with missense *p53* mutations and did not develop anti-p53 antibodies. The presence of p53 antibodies does not correlate to stage, prior treatment, sex, or survival *(6)*. One of the first experimental approaches to capitalize on this information was to use mutant p53 epitopes. These epitopes would span the site of point mutation and would be highly specific for each patient. Mutant p53 peptide pulsed dendritic cells (DCs) were used in a number of animal studies, and good antitumor responses were obtained *(7–10)*. However, there were serious limitations in translating this approach to human studies. This approach would require the identification of the mutational site for each patient before matching the mutant p53 peptide to the respective patient's MHC class I motif. Custom-made p53 mutant epitopes would have to be designed for each individual patient. In addition, mutant p53 epitope may not necessarily match any of MHC class I molecules in individual patients, and that would make the entire approach ineffective. Furthermore, a single peptide epitope may not generate an effective immune response as a multiepitope.

2.2. Wild-Type p53-Derived Peptides in Immunotherapy of Cancer

Several groups investigated the use of wild-type p53 peptide sequences in the induction of antitumor CTL responses in humans and animals in the in vitro setting. The rationale behind this approach is that because most of the mutations in the *p53* gene are single-nucleotide substitutions, most of the epitopes expressed in tumor cells will be derived from wild-type sequences. Therefore, CTLs generated after immunization with wild-type p53-derived epitopes could recognize and eliminate tumor cells. This approach has been tested in number of studies. Both murine and human studies in vitro demonstrated that this approach could be effective. Immunization of mice with wild-type p53 peptides resulted in the development of CTLs recognizing these epitopes and eradication of p53-expressing tumors *(9,11–13)*. Human leukocyte antigen (HLA)-A2- and HLA-A24-restricted CTLs recognizing the wild-type sequence p53 can be generated using autologous DCs from precursors present in peripheral blood lymphocytes obtained from normal donors *(2,14)*. In a phase I study, the toxicity and efficacy of autologous DCs loaded with a cocktail of three wild-type and three modified p53 peptides was analyzed in six HLA-A2+ patients with progressive advanced breast cancer. Vaccinations were well tolerated, and no toxicity was observed. Disease stabilization was seen in two of six patients, one patient had a transient regression of a single lymph node, and one had a mixed response. Enzyme-linked immunospot analyses showed that the p53-peptide-loaded DCs were able to induce specific T-cell responses against modified and unmodified p53 peptides in three patients, including two of the patients with a possible clinical benefit from the treatment *(15)*.

However, despite obvious advantages, this approach has significant limitations. First, the necessity for patient selection based on the correct MHC class I motif remains a prerequisite. Second, the accumulation of specific, predefined p53-derived epitopes in tumor cells is a prerequisite for this immunization to work *(16)*. However, these defined peptides may not be presented by tumor cells and thus serve as a target for CTLs. This can be illustrated in the case of wild-type p53 sequence (264–272). Missense mutation at the p53 codon 273 blocks processing of the $p53_{264-272}$ epitope, and consequently, cells accumulating p53 molecules expressing this mutation are not recognized by anti-$p53_{264-272}$ CTLs *(17)*. In addition, posttranslational modifications may affect the recognition of tumor-associated peptides. Furthermore, MHC class I-restricted peptides do not engage CD4[+] lymphocytes, which are critical in the induction of an effective immune response.

2.3. Use of Full-Length p53 in Cancer Immunotherapy

Another approach to cancer immunotherapy utilizes the full-length *p53* gene. The rationale for this approach is based on the assumption that multiple MHC class I- and class II-matching p53-derived epitopes will be presented on the surface of DCs, which will eliminate the necessity of selecting MHC class I-matching patients as well as provide conditions for activation of CD4[+] T-cells. Previous studies have demonstrated that each of the different minimal epitopes combined to a single fusion protein can be presented separately on the cell surface and be recognized by specific CTLs *(18)*. In a recent clinical trial a recombinant canary poxvirus (ALVAC) vaccine encoding wild-type human p53 was used in 15 patients with advanced colorectal cancer. A phase I/II dose-escalation study was performed that evaluated the effect of this ALVAC vaccine. Each group of five patients received three intravenous doses at one-tenth of a dose, one-third of a dose, or a single dose of the vaccine. Potent T-cell and immunoglobulin G antibody responses against the vector component of the ALVAC vaccine were induced in the majority of the patients. Enzyme-linked immunospot analysis of vaccine-induced immunity revealed the presence of interferon (IFN)-γ-secreting T-cells against both ALVAC and p53. Vaccine-mediated enhancement of p53-specific T-cell immunity was found in two patients in the highest-vaccine-dose group *(19)*.

Another approach utilizes adenovirus. Adenovirus provides a high-level transduction efficacy of many cell types, regardless of the mitotic status of the cell *(20)*. Replication defective adenoviruses with deletions in the E1 region have been directly injected into people in several human clinical trials (reviewed in ref. *21*). Successful transduction of APCs—DCs in particular—with green fluorescent protein and model antigens has been reported *(22–24)*. Transduced DCs were able to present effectively the recombinant protein antigens. In our preclinical studies, we have demonstrated that DCs transduced with wild-type p53 using adenoviral vector were able to induce potent antitumor responses *(25)*. This response recognized epitopes associated with different mutant p53 and led to tumor protection from p53-associated tumors, as well as to a significant decrease in the growth of already established tumors *(25,26)*.

Thus, each form of p53-derived antigens has their positive and negative characteristics (summarized in Fig. 1). However, it appears that full-length p53 may provide the most effective usage of antigens for vaccination.

3. SEARCH FOR THE MOST EFFECTIVE VEHICLE FOR ANTIGEN DELIVERY: DCs IN IMMUNOTHERAPY

DCs are scattered throughout many tissues of the body, as well as bone marrow and peripheral blood. The cytokine granulocyte-macrophage colony-stimulating factor has been found to induce the maturation and enhance the viability of dendritic cells isolated from peripheral blood. DCs are the most potent antigen-processing cells capable of sensitizing T-cells to new and recall antigens. DCs express high levels of MHC class I and

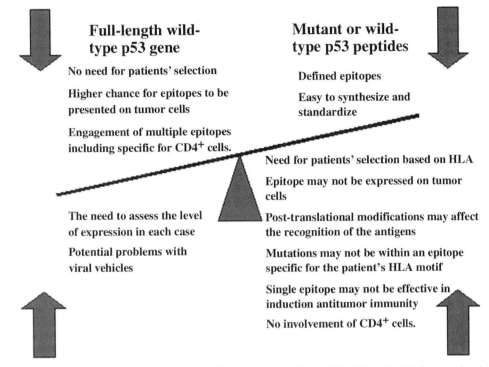

Fig. 1. Comparison between the use of p53-derived peptides and full-length p53 for vaccination.

II antigens, which are crucial to cancer immunotherapy, as well as a variety of important co-stimulatory and adhesion molecules. They also produce a number of cytokines, for instance, interleukin (IL)-12—critically important for the development and maintenance of the effective immune response (reviewed in ref. *27*).

3.1. Short Overview of DC Biology

DCs are bone marrow-derived APCs that play a critical role in the induction and regulation of immune responses. DCs are a heterogeneous population of cells produced in the bone marrow in response to growth and differentiation factors Fms-like tyrosine kinase 3 ligand and granulocyte-macrophage colony-stimulating factor. There are three generally accepted stages of differentiation for all DCs: DC precursors, immature DCs, and mature DCs. DCs capture bacteria, viruses, dead or dying cells, proteins, and immune complexes through phagocytosis, endocytosis, and pinocytosis. They have an array of surface receptors for antigen uptake, many of which are involved in signaling or cell–cell interactions. DCs process captured proteins into peptides that are loaded onto MHC class I and II molecules, and these peptide–MHC complexes (pMHC I and II) are transported to the cell surface for recognition by antigen-specific T-cells (pMHC I and pMHC II are recognized by $CD8^+$ and $CD4^+$ T-cells, respectively). Antigens acquired endogenously within the DC cytosol are processed and loaded onto MHC I molecules, whereas exogenous antigens obtained from the extracellular environment are processed and loaded onto MHC II molecules. Exogenous antigens can also be processed by DCs and loaded onto MHC I. This pathway is called crosspresentation, and permits DCs to engage both

CD8[+] and CD4[+] T-cell responses to exogenous antigens like apoptotic or necrotic tumor cells, virus-infected cells, and immune complexes. DCs can also present lipid and glyco-lipid antigens to T-cells on CD1d molecules, which are structurally similar to MHC I but specialized in binding of lipids instead of peptides. CD1d molecules present lipid anti-gens to a variety of lymphocytes including T-cells and natural-killer T-cells (27–29).

Maturation is a terminal differentiation process that transforms DCs from cells spe-cialized in antigen capture into cells specialized in T-cell stimulation. On maturation DCs, develop an enhanced ability to form pMHC II and pMHC I, migrate to lymphoid tissues, and prime naïve and memory T-cells. The strength of the T-cell response is dependent on the concentration of pMHC, the state of DC maturation, and the affinity of the T-cell receptor for the corresponding pMHC. For example, T-cell stimulation by immature DCs results in T-cell proliferation but only short-term survival, whereas stimu-lation by mature DCs results in long-term T-cell survival and differentiation into memory and effector T-cells. Maturation of DCs also results in the increased expression of surface adhesion and co-stimulatory molecules and induces DCs to secrete cytokines and che-mokines important in the recruitment of monocytes and specific T-cells subsets into the local environment.

3.2. Use of DCs in Immunotherapy Trials and the Role of DC Activation

Despite great progress made in the field of tumor immunology, objective response to cancer vaccine remains relatively low (30). It is imperative to use the most effective way to deliver TAAs. Therefore, DC-based cancer vaccines attract special attention. By this time, a number of clinical trials utilized DC-based vaccines in various types of cancers. These studies show that antigen-loaded DC vaccinations are safe and promising in the treatment of cancer. They include trials in non-Hodgkin's lymphoma, B-cell lymphoma, multiple myeloma, prostate cancer, malignant melanoma, colorectal cancer, and so on. Currently, it appears that one of the critical factors in DC-based vaccination is the activa-tion status of DCs. Immature DCs are not able to stimulate potent immune responses. Moreover, they may induce inhibition of antigen-specific T-cells (31). Adenovirus pro-vides a unique opportunity to combine antigen delivery and DC activation. DCs trans-duced with adenovirus clearly become more mature by the phenotypic criterion of upreg-ulation of CD83 and downregulation of CD14. Transduced DCs also decrease production of IL-10, and a subset of transduced DCs produce increased levels of IL-12 p70. This level of maturation is superior to that achieved by treatment of these cells with tumor necro-sis factor (TNF)-α or IFN-α but less pronounced than with CD40L trimer or a combina-tion of CD40L plus IFN-γ (32). Maturation by adenovirus transduction alone leads to efficient stimulation of antigen-specific T-cells from both healthy donors and patients with advanced cancer, using two defined human tumor-associated antigens, melanoma antigen recognized by T-cells 1 and α-fetoprotein (32). Recent studies demonstrated that infection of DCs with adenovirus induced high levels of TNF-α expression by DCs, comparable to levels observed with lipopolysaccharide exposure. Unlike TNF-α production associated with exposure to lipopolysaccharide, adenovirus induction of TNF-α was not dependent on the MyD88 signaling pathway. In contrast, adenovirus-induced TNF-α production and DC maturation were dependent on signaling by phosphoinositide-3-OH kinase. The ade-novirus capsid protein penton contains a well-characterized arginine–glycine–aspartic acid integrin-binding domain that stimulates phosphoinositide-3-OH kinase in fibroblast cell lines (33). The ability of adenovirus to induce DC maturation/activation was established by several other groups *(25,34–36)*. These data indicate that adenoviral construct can provide additional benefits for DC based cancer immunotherapy.

The above-presented data suggest that DCs may serve as an effective vehicle for antigen delivery. It appears that use of adenoviral constructs may provide additional benefits in form of maturation/activation of DCs.

4. TESTING THE HYPOTHESIS: THE NECESSITY TO OVERCOME TOLERANCE TO SELF-PROTEIN

Wild-type p53 is expressed by bone marrow-derived cells in the thymus. This causes negative selection of immature thymic T-cells with high avidity for p53, which results in deletion of T-cells able to recognize natural wild-type p53 epitopes presented by MHC class I molecules on tumor cells and thus prevents immune response. Only low-avidity CTLs survive the induction of self-tolerance (*[37]; see* Fig. 2). CD4+ T-cells reactive to p53 exist in cancer patients *(38)*, and the epitopes are probably ignored by the immune system under normal physiological conditions. Zwaveiling and colleagues have investigated the involvement of CD4+ T-helper in the antitumor response *(12)*. They have demonstrated that CD4+ T-helper cells having a high affinity for the naturally processed epitopes $p53_{108-122}$ were elicited in both p53-bearing and p53-deficient mice, and that the CD4+ T-helper response was unaffected by self-tolerance. These $p53_{108-122}$-specific CD4+ T-helper cells were effective in enabling p53-specific CTLs to control the growth of p53-overexpressing tumors in vivo *(12)*. Thus, the tolerance against wild-type p53 is not complete and may be overcome under certain conditions. From this study, it seems that exploiting the p53-specific CD4+ T-helper response will be a useful aspect of immunotherapeutic strategies against cancers. Initially, we tested the concept of using the wild-type *p53* gene for immunotherapy of cancer. DCs were transduced with a human wild-type p53 containing recombinant adenovirus (Ad-p53). About a half of DCs transduced with this virus expressed p53 protein by fluorescence-activated cell sorting analysis 48 h after infection. Mice immunized twice with Ad-p53 DC developed substantial CTL responses against tumor cells expressing wild-type and different mutant human and murine *p53* genes *(26)*. Very low CTL responses were observed against target cells infected with control adenovirus. Immunization with Ad-p53 provided complete tumor protection in 85% of mice challenged with tumor cells expressing human mutant p53 and in 72.7% of mice challenged with tumor cells with murine mutant p53 *(26)*. Treatment with Ad-p53-transduced DCs significantly slowed the growth of established tumors. In a recent study, murine DCs transduced with full-length murine wild-type p53 were used for vaccination *(25)*. Murine DCs were transduced with adenoviral construct containing murine full-length wild-type Ad-p53. Repeated immunizations with these cells protected 60% of mice against challenge with MethA sarcoma cells bearing point mutations in the *p53* gene. Activation of DCs via ligation of CD40 significantly improved the results of immunization: all mice were protected against MethA sarcoma *(25)*. The treatment of MethA tumor-bearing mice with activated Ad-p53-transduced DCs showed complete tumor rejection in four out of six mice. The specificity of antitumor immune response was confirmed by CTL assay. The analysis of phenotype and function of DCs demonstrated that the effect of CD40 ligation on these cells was enhanced by their infection with Ad-p53 *(25)*. The level of neutralizing antiadenovirus antibody was moderately elevated in these mice. No signs of autoimmune reaction were evident during detailed pathological evaluation of treated

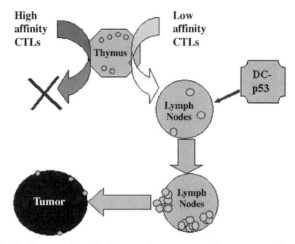

Fig. 2. Generation of p53-specific response in cancer patients.

mice *(25)*. These data demonstrate that activated Ad-p53-infected DCs are able to break tolerance to this protein and can be used in immunotherapy of cancer.

The ability of DCs transduced with full-length p53 to stimulate specific immune response was investigated in an ex vivo study of cancer patients. T-cells obtained from nine HLA-A2-positive cancer patients and three HLA-A2-positive healthy individuals were stimulated twice with DCs transduced with a wild-type Ad-p53 construct. Significant cytotoxicity was detected against HLA-A2-positive tumor cells with accumulation of mutant or wild-type p53, but not against HLA-A2-positive tumor cells with normal (undetectable) levels of p53 or against HLA-A2-negative tumor cells *(39)*. This response was specific and mediated by CD8+ CTLs. These CTLs recognized HLA-A2-positive tumor cells expressing normal levels of p53 protein after their transduction with Ad-p53, but not with control adenovirus. Stimulation of T-cells with Ad-p53-transduced DCs resulted in generation of CTLs specific for p53-derived peptide *(39)*.

Thus, these studies provided proof of concept for using DC transduced with wild-type full-length p53 in cancer immunotherapy. The mechanism of the generation of antitumor response is illustrated in Fig. 2. The next question is the selection of patients for clinical trial.

5. SELECTION OF THE PATIENTS FOR VACCINATION: SMALL-CELL LUNG CANCER AS TARGET FOR CANCER IMMUNOTHERAPY

5.1. Historical Prospective

Small-cell lung carcinoma (SCLC) was considered to be a potentially curable cancer in the 1970s, because it was responsive to chemotherapy and radiation, and dramatic tumor shrinkage was achieved. Depending on its severity, SCLC is clinically presented as either early disease (limited stage) or late disease (or extensive-stage disease). Early disease is confined to one side of the thorax and includes the regional lymph nodes. Late- or extensive-stage disease extends beyond the thorax, and involves drainage from both the lymphatics and circulation. From 1973 to 1993, an analysis of patients with SCLC treated at the

National Cancer Institute indicated no significant improvement in the survival in patients with either limited or extensive disease. However, despite the impressiveness of the initial response rates, patients are rarely cured, and the median survival is less than 1 yr for most patients who present with late disease and 18 mo for patients with early disease. There has been some recent progress in the area of long-term survival for early disease. A regimen of combination chemotherapy usually using etoposide and a platinum-based agent (cisplatin or carboplatin), and concurrent thoracic radiation have improved 2- and 5-yr survival rates to 44% and 22%, respectively, for some patients experiencing remission in early disease.

Even so, it is imperative to realize that long-term outcomes for late disease remain quite poor. The median survival of untreated extensive stage SCLC patients is 6–12 wk; for patients receiving treatment median survival is still less than 1 yr, and with recurrent disease survival is only about 4 mo. Clearly, alternative forms of treatments must be addressed to improve long-term patient survival. It has been proposed that manipulation of DCs as a natural vaccine adjuvant may prove to be a particularly attractive way to stimulate antitumor immunity.

5.2. Pathology of SCLC

SCLC is characterized by the presence of atypical small cells twice the size of lymphocytes in which the cytoplasm is sparse and the nuclei display dispersed chromatin, giving a salt-and-pepper appearance on histological examination. The chromatin is condensed, and therefore, these small cells are in a rapid state of mitoses (40). These small cells exhibit properties similar to neuroendocrine cells, and it is hypothesized that they have originated from a neuroendocrine precursor cell, the Kulchitsky cell, which resides in the airway epithelium (41). However, data gathered from the careful examination of various cell types within small cell tumors indicate that either a pluripotent cell or multiple cell types are involved and dispute that these atypical cells arise from a single cell type alone.

Given the poor long-term survival and the propensity for the development of drug resistance in SCLC, there have been major efforts toward understanding some of the known genetic alterations of SCLC. SCLC is associated with frequent abnormalities in p53. Takahashi and colleagues examined 17 SCLC tumor samples taken directly from 15 patients, as well as the corresponding nine tumor cell lines. Mutations changing the *p53* coding sequence were found in 11 of 15 patients (73.3%) (42). In another study, the *p53* open reading frame was studied in 16 SCLC cell lines and 20 SCLC tumors. Abnormalities of p53 were found in 16/16 cell lines (100%) and in 16/20 tumors (80%) (43). No p53 mutations were found in the corresponding normal tissue from 19 patients whose tumors had p53 lesions, indicating that the mutations were all somatically acquired (43). Similar (more than 80%) prevalence of mutations was found in SCLC by Fujita and colleagues (44).

5.3. Immunotherapy of SCLC

Several biological agents targeting cell cycle regulation, angiogenesis, and signal transduction pathways have reached clinical testing in lung cancer and have been introduced into clinical trials in SCLC. To date, no DC-based therapy has been employed in the treatment of patients with SCLC. One novel approach to the treatment of lethal residual disease in patients with SCLC relies on the induction of a host immune response to attack chemoresistant tumor cells. Because of its neuroectodermal origin, SCLC has a number of specific antigens that could be capitalized on as immune targets. Two vaccine strategies are currently in clinical study. The anti-idiotype vaccine to the GD3 ganglioside BEC-2 has recently been tested in a phase III trial. In this trial, patients with SCLC who had completed initial chemotherapy were vaccinated with BEC-2 plus bacillus of Calmette–Guerin adjuvant. A series of other trials have established the immunogenicity of several vaccines relevant to SCLC, including GM2, Globo H, fucosyl GM1, and polysialic acid. To optimize an immune response against a broad range of tumor phenotypes, these components will be combined into a polyvalent vaccine *(45)*.

6. DESIGN OF THE CLINICAL TRIAL

We selected patients with extensive-stage SCLC based on several characteristics described above: more than 80% of patients with SCLC have abnormalities in p53; SCLC patients are highly responsive to first-line chemotherapy that decreases tumor burden. Time to disease progression and survival is short in these patients, which would allow for clinical evaluation of the response within a relatively short period of time. We have designed a phase I–II trial. In this trial, patients with extensive stage SCLC who responded to chemotherapy were vaccinated with autologous DCs transduced with an adenoviral vector carrying the intact normal human *p53* gene. These modified DCs have the ability to endogenously process and present p53 epitopes in the correct context to each patient's individual HLA type. Nontransduced DCs expressed no detectable level of p53. After infection with Ad-p53, 20–30% of the cells were p53-positive as was evaluated by intracellular staining. DCs (5×10^6 p53-positive DCs) are injected intradermally. Three doses of this vaccine are administered to the patients on days 1, 14, and 28. The first vaccination dose is administered 9 wk after the last dose of chemotherapy. We are currently monitoring a p53-specific immune response, antiadenoviral antibody response, and clinical response to the treatment. Preliminary data from this trial are encouraging, but obviously more data need to be obtained before any conclusions can be made.

REFERENCES

1. Gabrilovich D, Pisarev V. Tumor escape from immune response: mechanisms and targets of activity. *Curr Drug Targets* 2003; 4:525–536.
2. Chikamatsu K, Nakano K, Storkus W, et al. Generation of anti-p53 cytotoxic T lymphocytes from human peripheral blood using autologous dendritic cells. *Clin Cancer Res* 1999; 5:1281–1288.
3. DeLeo AB, Jay G, Appella E, Dubois GC, Law LW, Old LJ. Detection of a transformation-related antigen in chemically induced sarcomas and other transformed cells of the mouse. *Proc Natl Acad Sci USA* 1979; 76:2420–2424.
4. Crawford LV, Pim DC, Bulbrook RD. Detection of antibodies against the cellular protein p53 in sera from patients with breast cancer. *Int J Cancer* 1982; 30:403–408.
5. Soussi T. The humoral response to the tumor-suppressor gene product p53 in human cancer: implications for diagnosis and therapy. *Immunol Today* 1996; 17:354–356.
6. Winter SF, Minna JD, Johnson BE, Takahashi T, Gazdar AF, Carbone DP. Development of antibodies against p53 in lung cancer patients appears to be dependent on the type of p53 mutation. *Cancer Res* 1992; 52:4168–4174.
7. Noguchi Y, Chen Y, Old L. A mouse mutant p53 product recognized by CD4+ and CD8+ T cells. *Proc Natl Acad Sci USA* 1994; 91:171–175.
8. Yanuck M, Carbone DP, Pendleton D, et al. Mutant p53 tumor suppressor protein is a target for peptide-induced CD8+ cytotoxic T-cells. *Cancer Res* 1993; 53:3257–3261.
9. Mayordomo JI, Loftus DJ, Sakamoto H, et al. Therapy of murine tumors with p53 wild-type and mutant sequence peptide-based vaccines. *J Exp Med* 1996; 183:1357–1365.

10. Gabrilovich DI, Cunningham HT, Carbone DP. IL-12 and mutant p53 peptide-pulsed dendritic cells for the specific immunotherapy of cancer. *J Immunother* 1997; 19:414–418.

11. Vierboom MPM, Nijman HW, Offringa R, et al. Tumor eradication by wild-type p53-specific cytotoxic T lymphocytes. *J Exp Med* 1997; 186:695–704.

12. Zwaveling S, Vierboom MP, Ferreira Mota SC, et al. Antitumor efficacy of wild-type p53-specific CD4(+) T-helper cells. *Cancer Res* 2002; 62:6187–6193.

13. Parajuli P, Pisarev V, Sublet J, et al. Immunization with wild-type p53 gene sequences coadministered with Flt3 ligand induces an antigen-specific type 1 T-cell response. *Cancer Res* 2001; 61:8227–8234.

14. Eura M, Chikamatsu K, Katsura F, et al. A wild-type sequence p53 peptide presented by HLA-A24 induces cytotoxic T lymphocytes that recognize squamous cell carcinomas of the head and neck. *Clin Cancer Res* 2000; 6:979–986.

15. Svane IM, Pedersen AE, Johnsen HE, et al. Vaccination with p53-peptide-pulsed dendritic cells, of patients with advanced breast cancer: report from a phase I study. *Cancer Immunol Immunother* 2004; 53:633–641.

16. Vierboom MPM, Gabrilovich DI, Offringa R, Kast WM, Melief CJM. p53: a target for T-cell mediated immunotherapy. In: Kast WM, ed. *Peptide-Based Cancer Vaccines*. Georgetown: Landes Bioscience. 2000: pp. 40–55.

17. Theobald M, Ruppert T, Kuckelkorn U, et al. The sequence alteration associated with a mutational hot-spot in p53 protects cells from lysis by cytotoxic T lymphocytes specific for a flanking peptide epitope. *J Exp Med* 1998; 188:1017–1728.

18. Thomson SA, Khanna R, Gardner J, et al. Minimal epitopes expressed in a recombinant polyepitope protein are processed and presented to CD8[+] cytotoxic T cells: implications for vaccine design. *Proc Natl Acad Sci USA* 1995; 92:5845–5849.

19. van der Burg SH, Menon AG, Redeker A, et al. Induction of p53-specific immune responses in colorectal cancer patients receiving a recombinant ALVAC-p53 candidate vaccine. *Clin Cancer Res* 2002; 8:1019–1027.

20. Becker TC, Noel RJ, Coats WS, et al. Use of recombinant adenovirus for metabolic engineering of mammalian cells. *Methods Cell Biol* 1994; 43:161–176.

21. Roth JA, Cristiano RJ. Gene therapy for cancer: what have we done and where are we going? *J Natl Cancer Inst* 1997; 89:21–39.

22. Brossart P, Goldrath AW, Butz EA, Martin S, Bevan MJ. Virus-mediated delivery of antigenic epitopes into dendritic cells as a means to induce CTL. *J Immunol* 1997; 158:3270–3276.

23. Dietz AB, Vuk-Pavlovic S. High efficiency adenovirus-mediated gene transfer to human dendritic cells. *Blood* 1998; 91:392–398.

24. Wan Y, Bramson J, Carter R, Graham F, Gauldie J. Dendritic cells transduced with an adenoviral vector encoding a model tumor-associated antigen for tumor vaccination. *Hum Gene Ther* 1997; 8:1355–1363.

25. Nikitina EY, Chada S, Muro-Cacho C, et al. An effective immunization and cancer treatment with activated dendritic cells transduced with full-length wild-type p53. *Gene Ther* 2002; 9:345–352.

26. Ishida T, Chada S, Stipanov M, et al. Dendritic cells transduced with wild type p53 gene elicit potent anti-tumor immune responses. *Clin Exp Immunol* 1999; 117:244–251.

27. Banchereau J, Briere F, Caux C, et al. Immunobiology of dendritic cells. *Ann Rev Immunol* 2000; 18: 767–812.

28. Steinman RM, Inaba K, Turley S, Pierre P, Mellman I. Antigen capture, processing, and presentation by dendritic cells: recent cell biological studies. *Hum Immunol* 1999; 60:562–567.

29. Steinman RM. Some interfaces of dendritic cell biology. *APMIS* 2003; 111:675–697.

30. Rosenberg SA, Yang JC, Restifo NP. Cancer immunotherapy: moving beyond current vaccines. *Nat Med* 2004; 10:909–915.

31. Dhodapkar MV, Steinman RM, Krasovsky J, Munz C, Bhardwaj N. Antigen-specific inhibition of effector T cell function in humans after injection of immature dendritic cells. *J Exp Med* 2001; 193:233–238.

32. Schumacher L, Ribas A, Dissette VB, et al. Human dendritic cell maturation by adenovirus transduction enhances tumor antigen-specific T-cell responses. *J Immunother* 2004; 27:191–200.

33. Philpott NJ, Nociari M, Elkon KB, Falck-Pedersen E. Adenovirus-induced maturation of dendritic cells through a PI3 kinase-mediated TNF-alpha induction pathway. *Proc Natl Acad Sci USA* 2004; 101:6200–6255.

34. Miller G, Lahrs S, Shah AB, DeMatteo RP. Optimization of dendritic cell maturation and gene transfer by recombinant adenovirus. *Cancer Immunol Immunother* 2003; 52:347–358.

35. Miller G, Lahrs S, Pillarisetty VG, Shah AB, DeMatteo RP. Adenovirus infection enhances dendritic cell immunostimulatory properties and induces natural killer and T-cell-mediated tumor protection. *Cancer Res* 2002; 62:5260–5266.
36. Korst RJ, Mahtabifard A, Yamada R, Crystal RG. Effect of adenovirus gene transfer vectors on the immunologic functions of mouse dendritic cells. *Mol Ther* 2002; 5:307–315.
37. Theobald M, Biggs J, Hernandez J, Lustgarten J, Labadie C, Sherman LA. Tolerance to p53 by A2.1-restricted cytotoxic T lymphocytes. *J Exp Med* 1997; 185:833–841.
38. van der Burg SH, de Cock K, Menon AG, et al. Long-lasting p53-specific T cell memory responses in the absence of anti-p53 antibodies in patients with resected primary colorectal cancer. *Eur J Immunol* 2001; 31:146–155.
39. Nikitina EY, Clark JI, van Beynen J, et al. Dendritic cells transduced with full-length wild-type p53 generate antitumor cytotoxic T lymphocytes from peripheral blood of cancer patients. *Clin Cancer Res* 2001; 7:127–135.
40. Campbell AM, Campling BG, Algazy KM, el-Deiry WS. Clinical and molecular features of small cell lung cancer. *Cancer Biol Ther* 2002; 1:105–112.
41. Lee JS, Mao L, Hong WK. Biology of preneoplastic lesions. In: Roth A, Cox JD, Hong WK, eds. *Lung Cancer, 2nd Edition*. Malden: Blackwell Science. 1998: 45–46.
42. Takahashi T, Takahashi T, Suzuki H, et al. The *p53* gene is very frequently mutated in small-cell lung cancer with a distinct nucleotide substitution pattern. *Oncogene* 1991; 6:1775–1778.
43. D'Amico D, Carbone DP, Mitsudomi T, et al. High frequency of somatically acquired *p53* mutations in small cell lung cancer cell lines and tumors. *Oncogene* 1992; 7:339–346.
44. Fujita T, Kiyama M, Tomizawa Y, Kohno T, Yokota J. Comprehensive analysis of p53 gene mutation characteristics in lung carcinoma with special reference to histological subtypes. *Int J Oncol* 1999; 15: 927–934.
45. Krug LM. Vaccine therapy for small cell lung cancer. *Semin Oncol* 2004; 31:112–116.

9 Anti-Idiotype Antibody Vaccines for the Immunotherapy of Cancer

Malaya Bhattacharya-Chatterjee,
Nitin Rohatgi, Sunil K. Chatterjee,
Asim Saha, Rakesh Shukla,
and Kenneth A. Foon

SUMMARY

Certain anti-idiotypic (Id) antibodies that bind to the antigen-combining sites of antibodies can effectively mimic the three-dimensional structures and functions of the external antigens and can be used as surrogate antigens for active specific immunotherapy. Several monoclonal anti-Id antibodies that mimic distinct human tumor-associated antigens have been developed and characterized by others and us. CeaVac (anti-Id 3H1) is an internal image anti-Id antibody that mimics a distinct and specific epitope of carcinoembryonic antigen (CEA) and can be used as a surrogate for CEA. Extensive preclinical studies, as well as results obtained from clinical trials, suggest that vaccination with 3H1 has the potential to augment survival benefits. Anti-Id 3H1 easily breaks immune tolerance to CEA and induces anti-CEA antibody, as well as CD4+ T-helper, responses in colorectal cancer patients and also in mice transgenic for CEA. This chapter summarizes the science behind the development of anti-Id 3H1 and updates our clinical experience that includes all the patients entered on the study thus far.

Key Words: Anti-idiotype antibody; cancer; immunotherapy; CEA; vaccine.

1. INTRODUCTION

The idiotype (Id) network offers an elegant approach to transforming epitope structures into idiotypic determinants expressed on the surface of antibodies. According to the network concept, as proposed by Lindemann *(1)* and Jerne *(2)*, immunization with a given tumor-associated antigen (TAA) will generate production of antibodies against these TAAs, which are termed Ab1; the Ab1 is then used to generate a series of anti-Id antibodies against the idiotypic determinants of the Ab1, termed Ab2. Some of these Ab2 molecules can effectively mimic the three-dimensional structure of the TAA identified by the Ab1. These particular anti-Ids, called Ab2β, which fit into the paratopes of Ab1, can induce specific immune responses similar to the responses induced by nominal antigens. Other

From: *Cancer Drug Discovery and Development: Immunotherapy of Cancer*
Edited by: M. L. Disis © Humana Press Inc., Totowa, NJ

anti-Ids generated, designated as Ab2α and Ab2γ, may not mimic the TAAs. Anti-idiotypic antibodies of the β-type express the internal image of the antigen recognized by the Ab1 antibody and can be used as surrogate antigens. Immunization with Ab2β can lead to the generation of anti-anti-Id antibodies (Ab3) that recognize the corresponding original antigen identified by Ab1. Because of this Ab1-like reactivity, Ab3 is also called Ab1' to indicate that it might differ in its other idiotopes from Ab1. Several such Ab2βs have been used in animal models to trigger the immune system to induce specific and protective immunity against bacterial, viral, and parasitic infections, as well as cancer (reviewed in ref. *3*).

Anti-Id antibodies that mimic distinct TAAs expressed by malignant cells of different histology or distinct determinants of a TAA have been used to implement active specific immunotherapy in patients with malignant diseases. A number of anti-Ids to a variety of solid tumors (predominantly colon cancer and melanoma) have demonstrated active immune responses in patients *(4–25)*. The putative immune pathways triggered by an anti-Id antibody may be summarized as follows: Anti-Id antibodies that are exogenous proteins are endocytosed by antigen-presenting cells and degraded to 14- to 25-mer peptides that are presented by major histocompatibility complex class II antigens to activate CD4 T-helper (Th) cells. Activated Th2 CD4 Th cells secrete cytokines, such as interleukin (IL)-4 and IL-10, that stimulate B-cells that have been directly activated by the anti-Id (Ab2β) to produce Ab1'. The Ab1' binds to the original antigen on tumor cells identified by the Ab1 (original immunizing murine antibody). In addition, activated Th1 CD4 Th cells secrete cytokines that activate T-cells, macrophages, and natural-killer cells. The latter may lyse target cells directly and/or serve as effector cells for antibody-dependent, cell-mediated cytotoxicity. Th1 cytokines, such as IL-2 also contribute to the activation of a CD8 cytotoxic T-cell (CTL) response. A second pathway is feasible by the induction by anti-idiotypic antibodies of human leukocyte antigen class I antigen-restricted TAA-specific CTLs because of amino acid sequence homology with TAAs. Furthermore, investigators *(26)* have shown that a conformational and a linear peptide derived from an antigenic moiety may express the same determinant, despite the lack of amino acid sequence homology. Therefore, peptides derived from the heavy and/or light chain of the anti-Id antibody may mimic the corresponding antigen, despite the lack of amino acid sequence homology with the Id mimicking the antigen and with the antigen itself. Peptides that are 9/10-mer and contain human leukocyte antigen class I antigen-binding motifs may be presented in the context of major histocompatibility complex class I antigens to activate CD8 CTLs that are also stimulated by IL-2 secreted by CD4 Th cells. Activated CD8 CTLs secrete perforin, granzymes, interferon-γ, and tumor necrosis factor-β and make direct contact with tumor cells leading to direct cell lysis. This mechanism may account for the generation of TAA-specific CTLs after immunizations with anti-Id antibodies that has been described both in animal model systems *(27,28)* and in patients with malignant diseases *(8,20,25)*.

2. DEVELOPMENT AND CHARACTERIZATION OF CEAVAC

The murine anti-Id monoclonal antibody (MAb) designated 3H1, or CeaVac, was generated against an anticarcinoembryonic antigen (anti-CEA) antibody, designated 8019, which identifies a specific epitope on CEA that is highly restricted to tumor cells and not found on normal tissues *(9)*. 3H1 anti-Id antibody functioned as an internal image of CEA by generating Ab3 responses that recognized the CEA in mice, rabbits, and monkeys, and had a major antitumor effect in a murine tumor model *(10)*.

3. CEA AS A TARGET FOR IMMUNOTHERAPY

CEA is a 180-kDa glycoprotein tumor-associated antigen present on endodermally derived neoplasms of the gastrointestinal tract, as well as other adenocarcinomas *(29)*. CEA is considered a self-antigen by the immune system, and patients with CEA-positive tumors are typically immunologically "tolerant" to CEA. CEA is an excellent tumor-associated antigen for active immunotherapy because it is typically present in high levels on the tumor cell surface. CEA is also very well characterized with a known gene sequence, and its three-dimensional structure has been reported *(30)*. CEA is a member of the immunoglobulin gene superfamily located on chromosome 19, which is thought to be involved in cell–cell interactions *(31,32)*. It is also an adhesion molecule and may play a role in the metastatic process by mediating attachment of tumor cells to normal cells *(32,33)*. Active immunotherapy targeting CEA might be particularly beneficial in the prevention of metastases. For all of these reasons, we have chosen CEA as the target antigen for generating an anti-Id antibody.

4. CLINICAL STUDIES IN PATIENTS WITH ADVANCED COLORECTAL CANCER CEAVAC

In a phase I clinical trial, among 23 patients with advanced colorectal cancer, 17 generated Ab3 responses, and 13 of these responses were proven to be true anti-CEA responses (Ab1' *[11,12]*). The antibody response was polyclonal, and sera from 11 patients mediated antibody-dependent cellular cytotoxicity. Ten patients had idiotypic T-cell responses, and five had specific T-cell responses to CEA. None of the patients had objective clinical responses, but, overall, the median survival for the 23 evaluable patients was 11.3 mo, with 44% having a 1-yr survival (95% confidence interval, 23–64%). Toxicity was limited to local swelling and minimal pain. The overall survival of 11.3 mo was comparable with other phase II clinical data in which patients with advanced colorectal cancer were treated with a variety of chemotherapy agents, including irinotecan, and had considerably less toxicity.

5. CLINICAL STUDIES WITH CEAVAC IN PATIENTS WITH RESECTED COLORECTAL CANCER

We previously reported the clinical and immune data on patients with metastatic disease *(11,12)* and 32 patients with resected Dukes' B, C, and D colorectal cancer treated with CeaVac, with or without 5-fluorouracil (5-FU)-based chemotherapy regimens *(13)*. We now present long-term follow up of these patients plus an additional 22 patients treated on this trial.

5.1. Selection of Patients

All patients had CEA-positive resected colorectal cancer, including resected Dukes' stage D with minimal residual disease, completely resected Dukes' D, Dukes' C, and Dukes' B disease. Baseline studies included a complete physical examination; computed tomography (CT) scans of the chest, abdomen, and pelvis; serum CEA level; and routine blood counts and chemistries. Staging was repeated 1 mo after the fourth immunization and every 3 mo thereafter for patients with Dukes' D disease, and every 6 mo for those with Dukes' B and C disease. All patients signed informed consent forms approved by the University of Kentucky and University of Cincinnati Institutional Review Boards.

5.2. Treatment Schedule

The majority of patients were treated intracutaneously with 2 mg of aluminum hydroxide (Alu-Gel)-precipitated CeaVac (Titan Pharmaceuticals, South San Francisco, CA) every other week for four injections. Some patients were treated subcutaneously with 2 mg of CeaVac mixed with 100 μg QS-21 (Aquila Biopharaceuticals, Worcester, MA) on the same dosing schedule. A third group of patients enrolled later in the trial were treated with 2 mg of CeaVac mixed with 100 μg of granulocyte-macrophage colony-stimulating factor ([GM-CSF] Leukine; Immunex, Seattle, WA). Patients continued to receive a monthly booster injection and were clinically reevaluated every 3 (Dukes' D) or 6 mo (Dukes' B and C) with physical examination, blood chemistries, and CT scans until the time of tumor recurrence or disease progression. Patients were allowed to be treated concurrently or previously with chemotherapy. Patients were monitored for clinical and immunological responses as described previously (13).

5.3. Statistical Analysis

For the purpose of statistical analysis, patients with Dukes' B and C were considered together so that there would be adequate numbers to generate survival curves. For patients in this group, days to progression and death were calculated from the time of initial diagnosis, whereas for patients with Dukes' D these end points were calculated from the time of diagnosis of metastatic disease. Kaplan–Meier curves were generated for each of these end points, using a statistical software package.

6. RESULTS

6.1. Clinical Outcome

There were 24 Dukes' B and C patients, 10 patients with completely resected Dukes' D disease (D_{cr}), and 20 with incompletely resected Dukes' D disease (D_{ir}). None of these patients had measurable disease by CT scan before entry, although three patients with D_{ir} had elevated CEA levels. Among the patients with Dukes' B and C disease, six of them had Dukes' B disease, six had Dukes' C1 disease, and 12 had Dukes' C2 disease. Patients with D_{cr} had either liver or extrahepatic (five patients, including those with lung, bladder, and ovary) metastases that were completely resected. All of the patients with D_{ir} had either evidence of residual tumor after resection (positive margins, elevated CEA) or soft tissue metastases. Seventeen of the 24 patients with Dukes' B and C received 5-FU-based chemotherapy regimens, as did 16 of the 30 patients with Dukes' D. Median follow-up for the entire cohort was 37 mo. Relapse-free (RFS) and overall (OS) survival data is presented in Table 1.

For Dukes' B and C disease, there were four deaths among the 24 patients, all of them in the Dukes' C2 group, and seven patients relapsed. Of the patients with D_{cr}, there were two deaths, and six patients relapsed. In the D_{ir} group, there were 10 deaths, and 16 patients relapsed. Interestingly, four of the patients with D_{ir} did not have CEA or CT scan evidence of disease progression at 35, 45, 57, and 72 mo. A Kaplan–Meier overall survival curve is presented in Fig. 1. For the patients with Dukes' B and C, the median RFS

Table 1
Clinical Outcome for Resected Colorectal Cancer Patients Treated With CeaVac

Stage	Number	Chemotherapy	Mo of RFS (median)	Relapses	Mo of OS (median)	Deaths
B and C	24	17	16–65	7	19–65 (58)	4
D_{cr}	10	4	11–42 (34)	6	16–64 (47)	2
D_{ir}	20	12	7–72 (18)	16	24–72 (40)	10

RFS, Relapse-free survival; OS, overall survival; B & C, Dukes' B and C colorectal cancer; D_{cr}, completely resected Dukes' D colorectal cancer; D_{ir}, incompletely resected Dukes' D colorectal cancer.

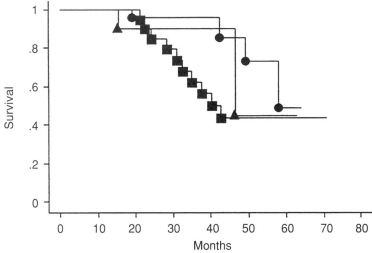

Fig. 1. Kaplan–Meier curves for overall survival. (●–●, Dukes' B and C colorectal cancer; ▲–▲, completely resected Dukes' D colorectal cancer; ■–■, incompletely resected Dukes' D colorectal cancer).

has not been reached. For the patients with D_{cr}, the median RFS was 34 mo, whereas it was 18 mo for the D_{ir} cohort. Median OS for the patients with Dukes' B and C was 58 mo; for the patients with D_{cr}, 47 mo; and for the patients with D_{ir}, 40 mo.

6.2. Immune Responses

All 54 patients generated active immune responses with robust anti-CEA immunoglobulin G responses and CD4 T-cell responses. These immune responses persisted as long as patients continued on vaccine therapy. Thirty-three patients received 5-FU-based chemotherapy regimens, and the majority of these were in combination with leucovorin. We found no differences in the anti-CEA humoral or cellular responses in any of these patients compared with patients not treated with chemotherapy. These data have been previously presented *(13)*.

We compared immune responses in patients treated with three different adjuvants including Alu-Gel, QS-21, and GM-CSF. Forty patients were treated with 2 mg of CeaVac-AluGel, five patients were treated with 2 mg of CeaVac plus QS-21, and nine patients were treated with CeaVac plus GM-CSF. We found no major difference in the humoral (Fig. 2) or cellular (Fig. 3) immune response among these patients. Most of the patients reached a peak anti-CEA humoral immune response after nine vaccinations, and the titer remained constant with monthly booster injections of CeaVac. The T-cell assays were performed on fresh cells and showed some variation, but responses persisted in individual patients throughout the course of therapy. Some patients, such as patient 5 in Fig. 3A, did not generate a T-cell response to the idiopeptide. This peptide could be substituted for the CEA protein in these T-cell assays and has previously been described (14). All patients' T-cells responded to the idiotype protein (data not shown), suggesting a genetically restricted response to the peptide.

6.3. Toxicity

Toxicity was typically mild erythema and induration at the injection site. Some patients developed larger local reactions with swelling that resolved within a few days. The most severe local reactions were seen with the combination of CeaVac and GM-CSF, whereas CeaVac combined with AluGel and QS-21 had less local toxicity. Mild fever and chills relieved by acetaminophen occurred in a minority of patients. There were no deleterious side effects on hematopoietic, renal, or hepatic function. There was no clinical or laboratory evidence of serum sickness in any of these patients.

7. DISCUSSION

We have shown that it is possible to break immune tolerance to a variety of self-tumor antigens using the anti-idiotypic approach (11–13,23,34). Both T- and B-cell responses can be generated against tumor antigens, and these responses are strong and well maintained. It has previously been demonstrated that GM-CSF can enhance the immune response to a murine MAb (35). In the current study, however, we saw no difference in efficacy among the three adjuvants including Alu-Gel, QS-21, or GM-CSF, although local reactions were most severe with GM-CSF.

It would be optimal to initiate vaccine therapy immediately after tumor resection as it would, theoretically, be most effective against minimal residual disease. We allowed patient entry onto our trial for up to 12 mo postsurgery. For patients with Dukes' B and C, the median duration from resection to vaccine was 4.7 mo, and 7.6 mo for patients with Dukes' D. Whereas it may be argued that such a delay in enrolling patients may result in a selection bias favoring those with less aggressive disease, we allowed this in order to provide patients with access to a novel therapy. We also considered it unlikely that completely resected patients with minimal residual disease would recur within the first few months. Patients with Dukes' B and C were analyzed as a single group in order to have sufficient patients to generate meaningful survival curves for these groups. Theoretically, all patients with resected Dukes' D disease who have no evidence of tumor postsurgery can be considered to have minimal residual disease. However, we separated those with a more favorable prognosis from those at higher risk of a poor outcome. Thus, the D_{cr} group included patients with three or fewer resected liver lesions, solitary metastases at other sites (except soft tissue), negative margins at surgery, and a normal postoperative CEA. All other resected patients with Dukes' D were considered incompletely resected.

Two patients in the Dukes' B and C group and two in the D_{ir} group had local recurrences (three of these were rectal, and one T4 colon). These patients were considered to have progressed and were taken off protocol. However, adjuvant immunotherapy may afford little protection against such recurrences, as was seen in the phase III study of the murine

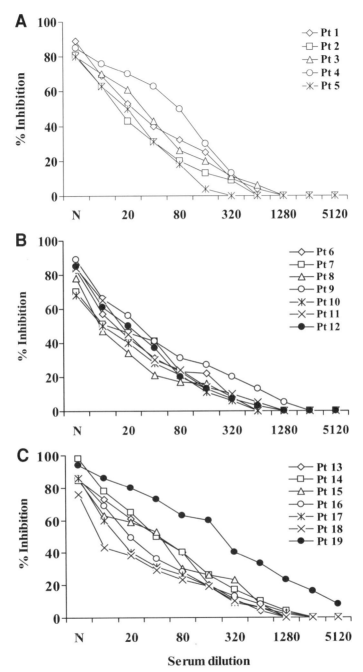

Fig. 2. Inhibition of anti-tumor-associated antigen antibodies binding to carcinoembryonic antigen by the immune sera of patients treated with (**A**) 3H1-QS21, (**B**) 3H1-aluminum hydroxide, and (**C**) 3H1-granulocyte/macrophage colony-stimulating factor. Data from representative patients are shown.

MAb 17-1A *(36,37).* Even adjuvant chemotherapy has little impact on the local recurrence rate *(38).* Such recurrences are more common in rectal cancer, and their frequency probably depends on the adequacy of surgical resection and the use of adjuvant radiotherapy.

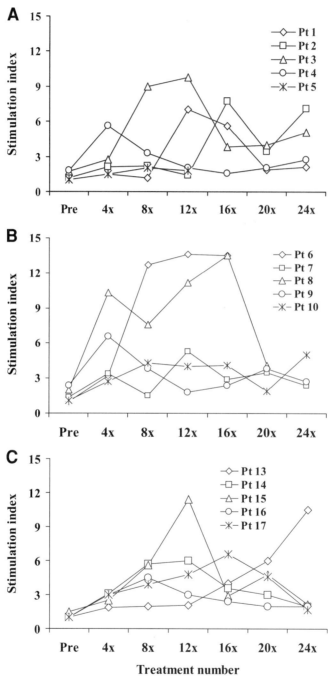

Fig. 3. Peptide-specific proliferation of peripheral blood mononuclear cells in patients treated with (**A**) 3H1-QS21, (**B**) 3H1-aluminum hydroxide, and (**C**) 3H1-granulocyte-macrophage colony-stimulating factor. Data from representative patients are shown.

In patients with Dukes' B and C, at a median follow-up of 38 mo, the median RFS had not been reached, although the median OS was 58 mo. At a median follow-up of 36 mo, 40% of the patients with D_{cr} were free from progression, as were 20% of the patients with

D_{ir}, at a median of 37 mo. At these time points, 80% of the D_{cr} and 50% of the D_{ir} patients were still alive. Our results for RFS appear to be similar to those reported in patients with completely or incompletely resected liver metastases in the literature *(39,40)*.

However, it is noteworthy that half of our patients with D_{cr} and a similar proportion of those with D_{ir} had resection of extrahepatic disease. Such patients have a poorer prognosis. Furthermore, with regard to OS, our results with adjuvant CeaVac appear to be superior to those previously obtained with surgical resection alone *(39,40)*. This conclusion is limited by the fact that this is a phase II study with relatively small numbers of patients in each group. Nevertheless, all of these patients generated active humoral and cellular immunity against CEA, and many patients had an excellent clinical result. A phase III study would be required to confirm the observed benefit in these groups of patients.

8. CONCLUSION

The anti-Id vaccine approach may have an important role in the treatment of human cancer. Anti-Id vaccines are effective at stimulating both humoral and cellular antitumor immune responses, which are long lasting. Future studies should be directed at improving the antitumor activities of anti-Id antibodies and should be tested in combination with other conventional and experimental therapies to overcome the multiple mechanisms by which tumor cells escape immune recognition and destruction. The problem of heterogeneity of TAA expression may be addressed by utilizing cocktails of anti-Id vaccine preparations directed against multiple target antigens collectively expressed by the vast majority of tumor cells. The characteristics of the TAA are also important for the preparation of an anti-Id antibody for active specific immunotherapy. Anti-Id antibodies directed against growth factor receptors such as Her-2/*neu* and epidermal growth factor receptor, may be more efficient than some other TAAs. We are characterizing several anti-Id antibodies directed against Her-2/*neu* for exploring this possibility *(41,42)*.

ACKNOWLEDGMENTS

This work was supported in party by the following grants from the National Institutes of Health (NIH): R01 CA 85025, R01 CA 91878, and R01 CA 104804. We would like to thank Audrey Morrison for typing the manuscript.

REFERENCES

1. Lindemann J. Speculations on idiotypes of homebodies. *Ann Immunol (Paris)* 1973; 124:171–184.
2. Jerne NK. Towards a network theory of the immune system. *Ann Immunol (Paris)* 1974; 125C:373–389.
3. Bhattacharya-Chatterjee M, Chatterjee SK, Foon KA. Anti-idiotype antibody therapy for cancer. *Expert Opin Biol Ther* 2002; 2:869–881.
4. Fagerberg J, Steinmetz M, Wigzell H, Askelof P, Mellstedt H. Human anti-idiotypic antibodies induced a humoral and cellular immune response against a colorectal carcinoma-associated antigen in patients. *Proc Natl Acad Sci USA* 1995; 92:4773–4777.
5. Herlyn D, Harris D, Zaloudik J, et al. Immunomodulatory activity of monoclonal anti-idiotypic antibody to anti-colorectal carcinoma antibody CO17-1A in animals and patients. *J Immunother* 1994; 15: 303–311.
6. Durrant LG, Doran M, Austin EB, Robins RA. Induction of cellular immune responses by a murine monoclonal anti-idiotypic antibody recognizing the 791Tgp72 antigen expressed on colorectal, gastric and ovarian human tumors. *Int J Cancer* 1995; 61:62–66.
7. Durrant LG, Maxwell-Armstrong C, Buckley D, et al. A neoadjuvant clinical trial in colorectal cancer patients of the human anti-idiotypic antibody 105AD7, which mimics CD55. *Clin Cancer Res* 2000; 6: 422–430.

8. Durrant LG, Buckley DJ, Robins RA, Spendlove I. 105AD7 cancer vaccine stimulates anti-tumor helper and cytotoxic T-cell responses in colorectal cancer patients but repeated immunizations are required to maintain these responses. *Int J Cancer* 2000; 85:87–92.

9. Bhattacharya-Chatterjee M, Mukherjee S, Biddle W, Foon KA, Kohler H. Murine monoclonal anti-idiotype antibody as a potential network antigen for human carcinoembryonic antigen. *J Immunol*1990; 145: 2758–2765.

10. Pervin S, Chakraborty M, Bhattacharya-Chatterjee M, Zeytin H, Foon KA, Chatterjee S. Induction of antitumor immunity by an anti-idiotype antibody mimicking carcinoembryonic antigen. *Cancer Res* 1997; 57:728–734.

11. Foon KA, Chakraborty M, John WJ, Sherratt A, Kohler H, Bhattacharya-Chatterjee M. Immune response to the carcinoembryonic antigen in patients treated with an anti-idiotype antibody vaccine. *J Clin Invest* 1995; 96:334–342.

12. Foon KA, John WJ, Chakraborty M, et al. Clinical and immune responses in advanced colorectal cancer patients treated with anti-idiotype monoclonal antibody vaccine that mimics the carcinoembryonic antigen. *Clin Cancer Res* 1997; 3:1267–1276.

13. Foon KA, John WJ, Chakraborty M, et al. Clinical and immune responses in resected colon cancer patients treated with anti-idiotype monoclonal antibody vaccine that mimics the carcinoembryonic antigen. *J Clin Oncol* 1999; 17:2889–2895.

14. Chatterjee SK, Tripathi PK, Chakraborty M, et al. Molecular mimicry of carcinoembryonic antigen by peptides derived from the structure of an anti-idiotype antibody. *Cancer Res* 1998; 58:1217–1224.

15. Reece DE, Foon KA, Bhattacharya-Chatterjee M, et al. Use of the anti-idiotype antibody vaccine TriAb after autologous stem cell transplantation in patients with metastatic breast cancer. *Bone Marrow Transplant* 2000; 26:729–735.

16. Grant SC, Kris MG, Houghton AN, Chapman PB. Long survival of patients with small cell lung cancer after adjuvant treatment with the anti-idiotype antibody BEC2 plus Bacillus Calmette-Guerin. *Clin Cancer Res* 1999; 5:1319–1323.

17. Mittleman A, Chen ZJ, Yang H, Wong GY, Ferrone S. Human high molecular weight melanoma-associated antigen (HMW-MAA) mimicry by mouse anti-idiotypic monoclonal antibody MK2-23: induction of humoral anti-HMW-MAA immunity and prolongation of survival in patients with stage IV melanoma. *Proc Natl Acad Sci USA* 1992; 89:455–470.

18. Mittleman A, Chen ZJ, Liu CC, Hirai S, Ferrone S. Kinetics of the immune response and regression of metastatic lesions following development of humoral anti-high molecular weight melanoma-associated antigen immunity in three patients with advanced malignant melanoma immunized with mouse anti-idiotypic monoclonal antibody MK2-23. *Cancer Res* 1994; 54:415–421.

19. Auan WD Jr, Dean GE, Spears L, Mitchell M. Active specific immunotherapy of metastatic melanoma with an anti-idiotype vaccine: a Phase I/II trial of I-Mel-2 plus SAF-m. *J Clin Oncol* 1997; 15:2103–2110.

20. Pride MW, Shuey S, Grillo-Lopez A, et al. Enhancement of cell-mediated immunity in melanoma patients immunized with murine anti-idiotypic monoclonal antibodies (MELIMMUNE) that mimic the high molecular weight proteoglycan antigen. *Clin Cancer Res* 1998; 4:2363–2370.

21. Saleh MN, Lalisan DY Jr, et al. Immunologic response to the dual murine anti-Id vaccine Melimmune-1 and Melimmune-2 in patients with high-risk melanoma without evidence of systemic disease. *J Immunother* 1998; 21:379–388.

22. Yao TJ, Meyers M, Livingston PO, Houghton AN, Chapman PB. Immunization of melanoma patients with BEC2-key-hole limpet hemocyanin plus BCG intradermally followed by intravenous booster immunizations with BEC2 to induce anti-GD3 ganglioside antibodies. *Clin Cancer Res* 1999; 5:77–81.

23. Foon KA, Lutzky J, Baral RN, et al. Clinical and immune responses in advanced melanoma patients immunized with an anti-idiotype antibody mimicking disialoganglioside GD2. *J Clin Oncol* 2000; 18: 376–384.

24. Cheung NV, Guo H, Heller G, Cheung IY. Induction of Ab3 and Ab1' antibody was associated with long-term survival after anti-GD2 antibody therapy of stage 4 neuroblastoma. *Clin Cancer Res* 2000; 6:2653–2660.

25. Wagner U, Kohler S, Reinartz S, et al. Immunological consolidation of ovarian carcinoma recurrences with monoclonal anti-idiotype antibody ACA125: immune responses and survival in palliative treatment. *Clin Cancer Res* 2001; 7:1154–1162.

26. Desai SA, Wang X, Noronha EJ, Ferrone S. Structural relatedness of distinct determinants recognized by mAb TP25.99 on β2-μ associated and β2-μ free HLA class I heavy chains. *J Immunol* 2000; 165:3275–3283.

27. Ruiz PJ, Wolkowicz R, Waisman A, et al. Idiotypic immunization induces immunity to mutated p53 and tumor rejection. *Nat Med* 1998; 4:710–712.

28. Saha A, Chatterjee SK, Foon KA, et al. Dendritic cells pulsed with an anti-idiotype antibody mimicking carcinoembryonic antigen (CEA) can reverse immunological tolerance to CEA and induce antitumor immunity in CEA transgenic mice. *Cancer Res* 2004; 64:4995–5003.

29. Gold P, Freedman SO. Demonstration of tumor-specific antigens in human colonic carcinomata by immunological tolerance and absorption techniques. *J Exp Med* 1965; 121:439–462.

30. Paxton RJ, Mooser G, Pande H, et al. Sequence analysis of carcinoembryonic antigen: Identification of glycosylation sites and homology with the immunoglobulin super-gene family. *Proc Natl Acad Sci USA* 1987; 84:920–924.

31. Thompson J, Zimmerman W. The carcinoembryonic antigen gene family: structure, expression and evolution. *Tumor Biol* 1988; 9:63–83.

32. Benchimol S, Fuks A, Jothy S, et al. Carcinoembryonic antigen, a human tumor marker, functions as an intercellular adhesion molecule. *Cell* 1989; 57:327–334.

33. Oikawa S, Inuzuka C, Kuroki M, et al. Cell adhesion activity of non-specific cross-reacting antigen (NCA) and carcinoembryonic antigen (CEA) expressed on CHO cell surface. Homophilic and heterophilic adhesion. *Biochem Biophys Res Commun* 1989; 164:39–45.

34. Foon, KA, Oseroff AR, Vaickus L, et al. Immune responses in patients with T-cell lymphoma treated with an anti-idiotype antibody mimicking a highly restricted T-cell antigen. *Clin Cancer Res* 1995; 1: 1285–1294.

35. Faberberg J, Ragnhammar P, Liljefors M, et al. Humoral anti-idiotypic and anti-anti-idiotypic immune response in cancer patients treated with monoclonal antibody 17-1A. *Cancer Immunol Immunother* 1996; 42:81–87.

36. Reithmuller G, Schneider-Gadicke E, Schlimok G, et al. Randomized trial of monoclonal antibody for adjuvant therapy of resected Dukes' C colorectal carcinoma. German Cancer Aid 17-1A Study Group. *Lancet* 1994; 343:1177–1183.

37. Reithmuller G, Holz E, Schlimok G, et al. Monoclonal antibody therapy for resected Dukes' C colorectal cancer: seven-year outcome of a multicenter randomized trial. *J Clin Oncol* 1998; 16:1788–1794.

38. Moertel CG, Fleming TR, MacDonald JS, et al. Levamisole and fluorouracil for adjuvant therapy of resected colon carcinoma. *N Engl J Med* 1990; 322:352–358.

39. Steele G, Bleday R, Mayer RJ, et al. A prospective evaluation of hepatic resection for colorectal carcinoma metastases to the liver: Gastrointestinal Tumor Study Group protocol 6584. *J Clin Oncol* 1991; 9: 1105–1112.

40. Fong Y, Cohen AM, Fortner JG, et al. Liver resection for colorectal metastases. *J Clin Oncol* 1997; 15: 938–946.

41. Baral R, Sherrat A, Das R, Foon KA, Bhattacharya-Chatterjee M. Murine monoclonal anti-idiotype antibody as a surrogate antigen for human Her-2/*neu*. *Int J Cancer* 2001; 92:88–95.

42. Pal S, Mohanty K, Chatterjee SK, Saha A, Foon KA, Bhattacharya-Chatterjee M. Generation of anti-idiotypic antibody vaccine mimicking human HER2/*neu*. *Proc Am Assoc Cancer Res* 2003; 44:196.

10

Autologous Tumor-Derived Heat Shock Protein Vaccine as a New Paradigm for Individualized Cancer Therapeutics

Jie Dai and Zihai Li

SUMMARY

Heat shock proteins (HSPs) are a group of highly conserved and abundant molecules across all organisms. HSPs are molecular chaperones that are further induced in response to the accumulation of misfolded proteins in the cell. They are essential in chaperoning proteins and maintaining the correct conformation of protein substrates. Recently, these molecules have been implicated in bridging innate and adaptive immunity, owing to their ability to chaperone antigenic peptides and their surprising property of being able to modulate the functional status of professional antigen-presenting cells. This chapter will summarize the immunological properties and mechanisms of HSPs and highlight the interests of autologous tumor-derived HSP–peptide complexes in the treatment of a variety of human cancers.

Key Words: Heat shock proteins; gp96; HSP70; cancer vaccine; dendritic cell; HSP–peptide complex; MHC; immunotherapy.

1. INTRODUCTION TO THE CONCEPT OF HEAT SHOCK PROTEIN-BASED TUMOR VACCINE

During the past decades, our knowledge about tumor biology has greatly expanded. However, the treatment modalities for cancers are still limited to traditional therapeutic approaches including surgery, radiation therapy, chemotherapy, or the combinations thereof. Lack of safe and effective cures for a majority of cancers is calling for more and rapid translation of the knowledge of cancer biology into novel therapeutic strategies of cancer, which can be used either as alternative approaches independent of traditional methods or in combination with them.

The concept of immunotherapy of cancers was established from observations more than half a century ago. It was demonstrated that mice immunized with irradiated syngenic tumor cells were resistant to rechallenge with tumor cells of the same origin (1–4). These experiments revealed that the immune system could recognize tumors and mount effective

From: *Cancer Drug Discovery and Development: Immunotherapy of Cancer*
Edited by: M. L. Disis © Humana Press Inc., Totowa, NJ

immune responses to eradiate tumor cells in the experimental settings. It is now known that there is an active interaction between tumors and the host immune system during oncogenesis. The list of discovered tumor antigens is growing (5). The cellular components of immune system, for instance, cytotoxic T-lymphocytes and natural-killer (NK) cells, are crucial not only for the effective killing of tumors (6,7), but also for tumor surveillance—the very first step to prevent the emergence of cancer cells (7–10). Soluble factors, such as antibody and cytokines, are also contributing to antitumor immunity (6).

A majority of heat shock proteins (HSPs) are constitutively expressed, although some of them are induced strongly by raising the temperature above the normal range for growth in both prokaryotic and eukaryotic cells. They are highly conserved across all species (11). HSPs are localized intracellularly in various subcellular compartments, including the cytosol (such as HSP70, HSP90) and the endoplasmic reticulum (such as gp96 and GRP170). The primary function of HSPs is to promote protein folding and unfolding (12), which are essential for thermotolerance (11), buffering of mutations (13) and protecting cells from apoptosis (14).

The roles of HSPs as immune modulators were not recognized until two decades ago, when Srivastava and his colleagues described that mice immunized with gp96 of the tumor origin could effectively reject subsequent tumor challenge from which gp96 was purified (15–17). Tumor-derived HSPs as cancer vaccines were quickly expanded into HSP70 (17,18), HSP90 (17,19), calreticulin (CRT) (20, 21), HSP110, and GRP170 (22, 23). It was demonstrated subsequently that HSPs could be a link between innate and adaptive immunity (summarized in Fig. 1A and discussed further under the following heading), based on two major observations. First, HSPs carry antigenic peptides by virtue of their ability to form HSP–peptide complexes (HSPPCs) intracellularly. Extracellular HSP-associated peptides can be further presented onto the class I and II molecules of the major histocompatibility complex (MHC) of the professional antigen-presenting cells (APCs), such as dendritic cells (DCs). Second, HSPs can stimulate APC maturation, resulting in the production of cytokines, upregulation of surface co-stimulatory molecules, and migration of APCs from tissues to the draining lymphoid organs. This maturation process of APCs is essential for optimal T-cell priming (24).

2. MECHANISM OF HSP-BASED TUMOR VACCINE

2.1. HSPs Are Intracellular Carriers for an Antigenic Peptide Pool

In search for tumor antigens that can immunize mice for tumor rejections, several potential target proteins of nonviral origin were identified. A significant number of them were HSPs, including gp96, HSP90 and HSP70 (15,16,18,19). Vaccination of mice with HSPs isolated from tumor cells induced strong tumor protective immunity to the original tumor from which HSPs were isolated, but not to antigenetically distinct tumors (16,18, 19,22). HSPs derived from normal tissues were unable to elicit tumor protection (17,18, 20,22). Moreover, no tumor-specific mutations of HSP genes were reported (25,26). Thus, it was proposed that HSPs were not antigenic per se; rather, HSPs were chaperones for antigenic peptides (25,27). Such a hypothesis, although purely speculative at its inception, later gained experimental support. Antigenic peptides were naturally associated with, and could be eluted from, HSPs chromatographically (18,28–30). Furthermore, HSPPCs could be reconstituted in vitro to immunize for antigen-specific CD8$^+$ T-cell responses and productive immunity in vivo (20,23,31). Importantly, tumor-derived HSP70

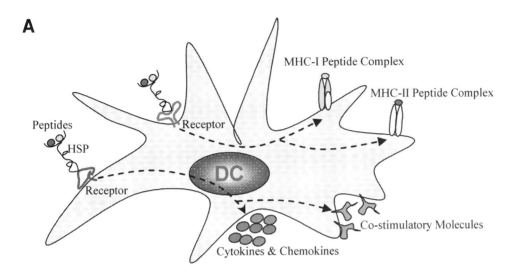

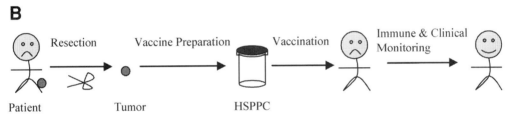

Fig 1. Schematic depiction of basic mechanism and strategy of heat shock protein (HSP)-based cancer vaccination. **(A)** HSPs play roles in both innate and adaptive immunity. HSP–peptide complex (HSPPC) interacts with receptors on dendritic cells, resulting in the endocytosis of HSPPC and cross-presentation of HSP-chaperoned peptides to major histocompatibility complex class I and class II molecules for recognition by and activation of CD8$^+$ and CD4$^+$ T-cells. Interaction of HSPPC with the same or different sets of receptors induces dendritic cell activation, manifested by upregulation of surface co-stimulatory molecules and production of cytokines and chemokines for optimal T-cell priming. (*See* Heading 2. for detailed discussion.) **(B)** A simplified schema demonstrating the basic strategy of autologous HSPPC vaccine against cancer.

stripped off peptides by adenosine triphosphate lost its immunogenicity in tumor challenge experiments *(18)*. It was noted that HSPs bind peptides promiscuously, without obvious preference for a particular sequence/size of peptides *(31–33)*. Although many of these original studies were in murine models, it was found later that HSPs from human cancers also chaperone antigenic peptides. For example, virus-specific peptides could be biochemically isolated from gp96 preparation of patients with hepatitis B virus-induced hepatocellular carcinoma *(34)*. HSP70 or gp96 purified from human lung cancer, breast cancer, and melanoma were able to stimulate T-cell responses to respective tumors *(35–38)*. Such an immunological activity of HSP70 was also abrogated by treatment with adenosine triphosphate *(35,38)*.

The peptide-binding property of HSPs forms the basis of HSPPC vaccines. In theory, HSPs derived from tumor cells contain all cellular peptides, including peptides of normal proteins, as well as of mutated proteins. Antigenicity of any given cancer cell therefore could be represented by the HSPPC purified from it. In this regard, HSPPCs obviously offer an advantage over epitope-defined vaccines because of the potential of HSPPCs to stimulate immune responses against multiple epitopes.

Tumors are known for a long time to be antigenetically distinct *(39)*. The molecular heterogeneity of histologically indistinguishable tumors is now confirmed by DNA array analysis of gene expression profiles of cancers *(40)*. In addition, the collection of mutations is expected to be different from tumor to tumor because of randomness of mutations resulting from the genetic instability of cancer genome. Therefore, the best tumor vaccines have to be derived from the original tumors. Most of HSPPC vaccines in current clinical trials are therefore purified from autologous tumors of patients. This customized strategy of autologous tumor vaccine represents a significant paradigm shift from the traditional cancer therapeutics, such as chemotherapy, when a large number of patients were treated with the same regimen.

2.2. Antigenic Peptides Chaperoned by HSPs Can Be Presented to Both MHC Class I and II Molecules to Prime CD8+ and CD4+ T-Cells

Early experiments using minor histocompatibility antigens (mHAgs) showed that mHAgs could be transferred from antigen-carrying cells to host APCs with a MHC haplotype different from antigen-carrying cells. This process was coined crosspresentation to differentiate it from direct presentation by the MHC compatible cells naturally expressing these mHAgs *(41)*. In vivo depletion of various cellular subsets of the immune system demonstrated that CD8+ T-cells were essential for rejection of tumors after immunization with gp96, HSP70, or HSP110 of tumor origin *(23,42–44)*. HSP70–, gp96–, HSP110–, or CRT–peptide complexes reconstituted in vitro could immunize for peptide-specific cytotoxic T-lymphocytes in vivo *(20,23,31)*. Subsequent in vitro and in vivo experiments demonstrated that exogenous peptide chaperoned by HSPs were taken up by APCs and crosspresented onto MHC I molecules *(45,46)*. These observations led to the proposal that HSPs are able to chaperone peptides for crosspriming of antigen-specific CD8+ T-cell responses, which is an area of intense investigation.

In contrast to CD8+ T-cell responses, limited attention was paid to presentation of HSP-associated peptides to MHC class II pathways to activate CD4+ T-cell responses. Mice depleted of CD4+ T-cells were functionally impaired in rejecting tumor challenge from which HSP110, gp96, or HSP70 were isolated and used for vaccinations *(23,42–44)*. Recently, it was found that gp96 and HPS70 could chaperone peptides to MHC II pathways. In one case, gp96 was purified from Meth A fibrosarcoma, which harbors a mutated cytosolic ribosomal protein L11. It was found that Meth A-derived gp96 was able to pulse APCs to stimulate the proliferation of a CD4+ T-cell clone specific for the mutated L11 epitope. The proliferation was mediated by MHC class II molecules and was dependent on an acidic microenvironment *(47)*. In another case, gp96 was complexed with a peptide derived from the hemagglutinin of the influenza virus. Such a complex was able to vaccinate and stimulate the proliferation of adoptively transferred hemagglutinin-specific transgenic CD4+ T-cells *(48)*. In addition, when HSP70 was loaded with glycoprotein D peptides of herpes simplex virus (HSV)-1 and used to immunize mice, epitope-specific CD4+ T-cell proliferation and antibody production were observed. Furthermore, coimmunization of HSP70 loaded with both CD4 (HSV-glycoprotein D) and CD8 (HSV-ICP27) peptide epitopes greatly increased precursor frequency and cytolytic activity of

ICP27-spcific memory CD8[+] T-cells in vivo. Taken together, these data argued that in addition to stimulating CD8[+] T-cell responses, HSPPC could also prime CD4[+] T-cells, which, in turn, deliver helper signals to optimize CD8[+] T-cell functions *(49)*. All of these experiments were performed without the use of exogenous adjuvant, suggesting that HSPs may activate APCs to provide the signal that was supplied by adjuvant. In addition to the peptide-binding property, it was reasoned that HSP might indeed serve as an endogenous adjuvant.

2.3. HSPs Modulate Innate Immunity

The innate immune cells of the immune system consist of MΦs, DCs, polymorphonuclear neutrophils and NK cells. Innate immunity does not need to be primed and does not have secondary memory response, both of which are characteristics of the adaptive immunity. However, activation of innate cells is crucial for initiation and optimal priming/memory of adaptive immune responses. For example, without DCs, T-cells are poorly primed. It was suspected very early on that HSPs might have important roles in modulate innate immunity, because the early form of the HSPPC vaccine was given without the exogenous adjuvant. It was reasoned perhaps that HSP can bind to receptors on APCs and activate them to provide proinflammatory molecules *(50)*. It is now demonstrated that on exposure to HSPs, DCs undergo maturation process, as indexed by upregulation of their surface molecules (such as CD40, CD80, CD86, and MHC class II) and production of cytokines and chemokines *(51,52)*. It was also shown that gp96 induced the migration of DCs from the peripheral tissues to secondary lymphoid organs *(53)*. Additionally, HSPs can activate other cellular components of the innate immunity, such as MΦs and polymorphonuclear neutrophils, leading to the release of nitric oxide *(54)*, cytokines *(51)*, and chemokines *(55)*. Activation of DCs by gp96 was demonstrated by the use of soluble gp96, as well as cells that were engineered to secret gp96 or express gp96 on cell surfaces *(56–59)*. Recently, there have been attempts to separate the innate functions of HSPs from the peptide-dependent functions. For example, the N-terminal domain of gp96 (gp96-NTD) has been shown to be able to mature DCs in vitro *(56)* and stimulate APCs to produce cytokines in vivo *(57)*. The gp96-NTD also transiently increased lytic activity of NK cells to a moderate extent *(57)*. It is unclear however whether gp96-NTD can bind to peptides, given the recent finding that the N-terminal fragment (N34–355) does contain peptide-binding pocket *(60,61)*. Interestingly, full-length human HSP70 protein, as well as its 14-mer peptide TKD (amino acids 450–463), have been shown to specifically bind CD94 on human NK cells in a dose-dependent fashion *(62,63)*, and to stimulate the proliferation, chemotaxis and cytolytic activity of human NK cells *(64–66)*.

2.4. The Immunomodulating Properties of HSPs Depend on Their Interaction With Receptor-Like Molecules on Immune Cells

The very effectiveness of the induction of antigen-specific T-cell responses by HSPPCs suggested the presence of receptor(s) on APCs for HSPs *(50)*. Binding of HSPs to APCs was specific, saturable, and competitive *(67,68)*. HSPPCs were rapidly endocytosed via a receptor-mediate mechanism *(69,70)*. In particular, gp96 has been shown to be colocalized with MHC class I and MHC class II molecules in endosomal compartments after internalization *(70)*, whereas peptides associated with HSP70 were presented onto MHC class I molecules in a manner that is both dependent and independent of transporters associated with antigen processing, indicating that HSP70–peptide complexes could enter endosomes or endoplasmic reticulum *(69)*. By gp96-affinity column, it was revealed that CD91 in a murine macrophage cell lysate was able to bind gp96 *(71)*. CD91 is previously known as the receptor for α_2-macroglobulin (α_2M). It is also a receptor for gp96, because both the binding of gp96 to and crosspresentation of gp96–peptide complexes by MΦs were inhibited by α_2M as well as a monoclonal antibody against CD91 *(71)*. Furthermore, both representation of gp96- and α_2M-chaperoned peptides were drastically diminished when CD91 expression was suppressed by small RNA interference technique *(72)*. In the murine system, CD91 has been shown to be a common receptor for gp96, HSP90, HSP70, and CRT *(73)*.

However, CD91 does not seem to be the only receptor for HSPs. Other groups also described CD91-independent binding and endocytosis of HSPs by APCs, suggesting that receptors for HSPs are more diverse than expected. Four groups of receptors have been implicated to interact with HSPs in a CD91-independent manner. The first group comprises the scavenger receptor lectin-like oxidized LDL (LOX)-1 *(74)* and scavenger receptor class A (SR-A) *(75)*. LOX-1 was specific for human HSP70. Both HSP70 binding to DCs and HSP70-mediated cross-presentation of antigens can be inhibited by a monoclonal antibody to LOX-1 *(74)*. SR-A was also identified as a receptor for murine HSP. Gp96 or CRT binding and uptake, as well as crosspresentation of peptides chaperoned by gp96, were substantially impaired in macrophages that are either genetically deficient of SR-A or when the scavenger receptor was blocked by its ligand, fucoidin *(75)*. The second class of receptors was represented by CD40 of the tumor necrosis receptor family. The N-terminal nucleotide-binding domain of human HSP70 was found to bind CD40, which was significantly increased in the presence of adenosine diphosphate and peptides *(76)*. Interestingly, in a model of T-cell-mediated diabetes mellitus, diseases can be induced by coinjection of HSP70 and the cognate peptide in CD40-dependent manner *(77)*. Toll-like receptors (TLRs)-2 and -4 have also been implicated as receptors for HSP60, HSP70, and gp96 *(78–81)*. Transfection of HEK293T human embryonic kidney cells with TLR2 or TLR4 expression vector conferred responsiveness to HSP60, HSP70, and gp96, as evidenced by the activation of reporter genes *(78–81)*. Incubation of MΦ cell line with HSP60 and gp96 triggered phosphorylation of c-Jun N-terminal kinases 1 and 2, extracellular signal-regulated kinases 1 and 2, and p38 *(78,80)*. In concord with these findings, TLR2- or TLR4-deficient APCs had decreased cytokine productions in response to HSP60, HSP70, or gp96 stimulation *(78–80)*. MyD88, adaptive molecules utilized by all TLRs for signaling, was essential for HSP60- and HSP70-mediated responses *(78,79,81)*. Furthermore, it was found that constitutive expression of cell surface gp96 in a transgenic murine model induced a MyD88-dependent lupus-like disease *(82)*. Noticeably, MD2 and CD14 were reported to be necessary for the signaling pathway initiated by HSP60, HSP70, and gp96 *(78–80)*, or HSP60 and HSP70 *(81,83,84)*, respectively. Whether HSPs can signal through TLRs directly remains a question, because HSPs have been found to chaperone TLR ligands, such as lipopolysaccharide *(85–88)*. Finally, CD94 of the C-type lectin receptor family on human NK cells has been shown to bind human HSP70 and its C-terminal 14-mer peptide, TKD *(62)*. The increased density of surface CD94 on NK cells was associated with various stimulatory functions of human HSP70 and TKD *(63)*. Physiologically, it is unclear how much contribution this interaction might have in the HSP70-mediated immune response.

Table 1
Heat Shock Protein–Peptide Complex-Based Vaccination
Against a Variety of Experimental Tumors in Prophylactic or Therapeutic Setting

Animal	Tumor type	Model	Vaccine	References
Rat	Hepatoma	Zajdela	gp96	15
	Prostate cancer	Dunning G	gp96	96[a]
Mouse	Fibrosacoma	Meth A	gp96	16,17,43[a],90[a]
			HSP70	17,18
			HSP90	17,19
			Calreticulin	20
			HSP110	22
			Grp170	22
		CSM5	gp96	16
		CSM13	gp96	91
	Squamous cell	UV6138	gp96	92
	carcinoma	UV6139	gp96	43[a]
	Colon cancer	CT26	gp96	43[a]
			HSP110	22[a]
			Grp170	22[a]
	Thymoma	N1	gp96	31
			HSP70	31
	Melanoma	B16	gp96	43[a]
			HSP110	23[a]
	Lung carcinoma	D122	gp96	43[a],90[a]
			HSP70	43[a]
	Leukemia	A20	gp96	44[a],93
			HSP70	44[a],93
			HSP90	93
			Calreticulin	93
	Spontaneous mammary		HSP110	94
	adenocarcinoma			
	Prostate cancer	TRAMP-C2	HSP70	89
Frog	Lymphoma	15/0	gp96	95
			HSP70	95

HSP, heat shock protein.
[a]Immunotherapy of established tumors.

3. IMMUNOTHERAPY
OF PRE-EXISTING TUMORS IN MURINE MODELS

Tumor-derived HSPPC vaccines were effective in rejecting tumor challenge in a variety of preclinical models. Furthermore, HSPPCs were also effective in the treatment of established tumors, leading to either complete tumor regression, or significantly delayed tumor progression *(43)*. These studies are summarized in Table 1 *(89–96)*, without detailed discussion because of space constraints. Because the biochemical and immunological properties of HSPs are conserved across species, it was asked if HSP vaccines are also effective in the treatment of human cancers. Numerous clinical trials have been launched to address this question.

4. HSPPC TUMOR VACCINES
AS A NEW PARADIGM FOR CANCER THERAPEUTICS

4.1. General Strategies for Autologous HSPPC Vaccination

Methods to purify different species of peptide-bound HSPs, such as HSP70, HSP90, and gp96, were well established and standardized *(97)*. Care was taken to ensure that purified HSPPCs retain immunological activities. For example, no detergent was used during any steps of purifications to avoid potential dissociation between HSP and peptides. The general schema, stepwise, for autologous HSPPC vaccination is outlined as follows (*see* Fig. 1B):

1. Surgical resection of solid tumors or leukapheresis of leukemic cells.
2. Vaccine preparation from tumor cells by established methods.
3. Sterility testing and quality assurance of the vaccine product.
4. Vaccination of patients.
5. Clinical and immunological evaluation of responses to the vaccine.

4.2. Feasibility, Safety, and Tolerability

The first pilot trial of HSPPC-96 was conducted in 16 patients with different advanced cancers that were refractory to the standard therapy *(98)*. All resected tumor samples were sufficient for HSPPC-96 preparation, with the yield of HSPPC-96 ranging from 13 to 150 μg/g sample. Weekly subcutaneous injection of 25 μg of autologous tumor-derived HSPPC-96 was performed for 4 wk. No serious side effect was observed except minor and transient flu-like symptoms *(98)*. No evidence of autoimmunity was found. In other phase I clinical trials in patients with gastric cancer *(99)* or renal cell carcinoma *(100)*, doses for vaccination were escalated from weekly 2.5, 15, 25, or 100 μg/ dose for at least 4 wk. No obvious side effect was reported, even at the highest dose. Overall, preparations of autologous HSPPC-96 from resected solid tumor tissues or HSPPC-70 *(101)* from leukapheresed peripheral blood samples were feasible. Administration of autologous HSPPC had no significant clinical toxicities. No autoimmunity has been observed.

4.3. Clinical Evaluation of HSPPC Vaccination

Most ongoing trials are in phase I/II stages, except melanoma and renal cell carcinoma, which have entered into phase III. These uncontrolled single-arm studies were undertaken principally to evaluate the feasibility and toxicity of autologous HSPPC vaccine. It is therefore too early to comment on the clinical efficacy of this strategy. Furthermore, most of the studies were published in abstract form only. Caution must be exercised in evaluating the data from these trials, which are summarized in Table 2.

4.3.1. MELANOMA

The phase I trial recruited a total of 36 patients with stage III/IV diseases. HSPPC-96 was purified from resected tumors and given 2.5, 25 or 100 μg/dose intradermally and weekly for four doses (Q1W × 4). One patient at each dose level had stabilization or mixed response after initial progression in nodal or lung metastases. Twenty-nine (80%) patients were alive for a median of 9 mo, whereas 11 out of 12 stage IV patients remained free of disease at a median of more than 11 mo *(102)*.

In a phase II study, 64 patients were enrolled after surgical resection of metastatic cancers. Among them, 42 patients were able to receive the vaccine, and 39 were assessable

Table 2
Summary of Clinical Trials Using Autologous Heat Shock Protein-Based Tumor Vaccines[a]

Cancer type	State	Phase	Dose schedule	Patient number[b]	Clinical responses[c] +	Clinical responses[c] −	Immunological responses[d] +	Immunological responses[d] −	References
Melanoma[e]	III/IV	Phase I	2.5/25/100 µg QW × 4	36	NA	NA	NA		102
	IV	Phase II	5/50 µg QW × 4, then Q2W × 4	39	5 (18%)	23 (82%)	11 (48%)	12 (52%)	103
RCC[e]	IV	Phase I	2.5/25/100 µg QW × 4	39	22 (76%)	7 (24%)	NA	NA	100
	IV	Phase II	25 µg QW × 4, then Q2W	61	21 (34%)	40 (66%)	NA		104
	IV	Phase II	25 µg QW × 4, then Q2W	59	8 (32%)	17 (68%)	NA		105
Gastric	Advanced	Phase I	2.5/15/25/100 µg QW × 4–9	18	3 (20%)	12 (80%)	8 (73%)	3 (27%)	99
Colorectal[f]	IV	Phase I/II	2.5/25/100 µg QW × 4, then Q2W	29	11 (38%)	18 (62%)	17 (59%)	12 (41%)	106
Pancreatic	I–III	Phase I	5 µg QW × 4	10	3 (30%)	7 (70%)	NA		107
Lymphoma	Low grade	Phase II	25 µg QW × 4, then Q2W	10	6 (60%)	4 (40%)	NA		108
CML	Chronic	Phase I	50 µg QW × 8	21	13 (65%)	7 (35%)	11 (55%)	9 (45%)	101

QW, weekly; NA, not available; RCC, renal cell carcinoma; CML, chronic myeloid leukemia.

[a]In all trials vaccines are HSPPC-96, except in CML, where HSPPC-70 was used.

[b]Number of patients indicted in this column were of successful vaccine preparations.

[c,d]Number of patients indicated in these columns were those who completed vaccination as scheduled and were evaluable; positive response means either complete/partial response or stabilization unless specified.

[e]Currently in phase III trials. NA, not available.

[f]Here, positive clinical response is defined as lack of tumor recurrence.

159

after one cycle of vaccination (5 or 50 µg, Q1W × 4), and 21 patients were able to receive a second cycle (biweekly × 4) of injection. Of 28 patients with measurable diseases, two had a complete response, and three had stabilization of diseases for more than 5 mo. Therefore, the total response rate was 18%. In parallel to clinical response, 11 out of 23 patients (47.8%) showed increased number of melanoma-specific T-cells in the peripheral blood post-vaccination, as was assessed by interferon (IFN)-γ enzyme-linked immunospot (ELISPOT) assay. The clinical responses were correlated with the increased frequency of T-cell activity *(103)*.

4.3.2. Renal Cell Carcinoma

The vaccination schedule for the phase I trial in patients with renal cell carcinoma consisted of intradermal and weekly injection of 2.5, 25, or 100 µg of HSPPC-96 per dose for four doses. Among 42 enrolled patients, 29 patients completed the treatment. One patient had a complete response, 3 had a partial response, and 18 showed stable diseases or slight disease progressions *(100)*.

In the two subsequent phase II studies, vaccination schedules consisted of 25 µg of HSPPC-96 given Q1W × 4, followed by Q2W injection until disease progression or exhaustion of the vaccine. In the case of metastatic renal cell carcinoma, 61 patients received at least one dose of vaccine. One of them had a complete remission, 2 had a partial remission, and 18 were stable. Thirty percent of patients were still alive 2 yr after the vaccination *(104)*. In the other trial, 70 patients were enrolled, and 25 patients completed the therapy. Eight patients (32%) showed clinical responses: one had a complete response, 1 had a partial response, and 6 patients remained stable *(105)*.

4.3.3. Gastric Cancer

A phase I clinical trial in gastric cancer patients was conducted *(99)*. Four to 8 wk after curative surgery, 2.5, 15, 25, or 100 µg of HSPPC-96 was given intradermally to patients Q1W four to nine times. Fifteen patients received vaccinations. After a median follow-up 32 mo from surgery, 3 patients were disease-free, and 12 patients had tumor recurrence. The median disease-free and overall survival of the 15 vaccinated patients was 7 mo and more than 16 mo, respectively, with 9 out of 15 patients still alive at the time of report of this study. Immunological tests showed an expansion of CD8+CD45RO+ memory T-cells in 8 out of 11 patients and an expansion of CD8+ T-cells with specific T-cell receptor-Vβ subtypes in two out of nine patients evaluated.

4.3.4. Colorectal Cancer

HSPPC-96 vaccine was used in a phase I/II study on patients with liver metastatic colorectal cancer. Twenty-nine patients were recruited after liver resection of metastatic tumor. All patients completed vaccination Q1W × 4 with 2.5, 25, or 100 µg of HSPPC-96 by the intradermal route, and then with Q2W × 4 injections 8 wk after the first cycle. Two-year overall survival and disease-free survival were evaluated. Human leukocyte antigen class I-restricted and colon cancer-specific T-cell responses in peripheral blood mononuclear cells (PBMCs), before and after vaccination, were assayed by IFN-γ ELISPOT. A significant increase of T-cell responses was observed in 17 out of 29 (59%) patients. Tumor recurrence occurred in 18 patients (62%), whereas 11 patients (38%) were tumor-free. The overall survival of all patients was 79%, and disease-free survival was 33%. These data were encouraging, in that patients who had immunological responses had significant survival advantage over nonresponders. At the time of the report of this study, the overall survival is 100% for responders vs 50% for nonresponders; the disease-free survival is 51% for responders vs 8% for nonresponders *(106)*.

4.3.5. Pancreatic Cancer

Pancreatic cancer is often associated with an advanced stage and very poor prognosis. HSPPC-96 vaccine was used in a phase I trial. Owing to the small size and presence of proteolytic enzymes in tumor samples, preparation of vaccines was more difficult when compared with other types of tumors. In 10 patients receiving 5 µg of autologous HSPPC-96 Q1W × 4, three were alive and free of disease at 5.0, 1.7, and 1.6 yr. Median overall survival was 2.0 yr, and mean overall survival was 2.0 yr *(107)*.

4.3.6. Lymphoma

The phase II study of HSPPC-96 was conducted on patients with either newly diagnosed or relapsed low-grade non-Hodgkin's lymphoma. Vaccines were prepared from 10 patients and given 25 µg Q1W × 4, followed by a Q2W schedule. Patients were then evaluated at week 14 after the start of treatment. Treatment continued if patients were improving or stable, but not longer than 1 yr. Of the 10 patients, 1 patient had a partial response, 2 had minor responses, and 3 additional patients had stable diseases *(108)*.

4.3.7 Chronic Myeloid Leukemia in Chronic Phase

Currently, completed or ongoing HSP-based vaccines were/are using HSPPC-96, with the exception of the chronic myeloid leukemia trial, in which HSPPC-70 was used. A phase I trial was initiated to test the roles of combination therapy of autologous HSPPC-70 vaccine and imatinib mesylate, a B-cell receptor/Abelson leukemia virus tyrosine kinase inhibitor. Autologous HSPPC-70 was purified from PBMCs obtained by leukapheresis. Patients were vaccinated by intradermal injection of 50 µg of HSPPC-70 Q1W × 8. Of the 21 eligible patients, 20 patients completed the study. Vaccines were successfully prepared from all patients and were well tolerated. At the end of vaccinations, all patients remained in chronic phase. Thirteen out of 20 patients had either a reduced number of Philadelphia chromosome-positive cells or a decreased level of B-cell receptor/Abelson leukemia virus transcripts by a polymerase chain reaction-based assay. Immunological measurements (IFN-γ ELISPOT assay) were performed on PBMCs in response to prevaccination autologous leukocytes at baseline, before the fifth vaccination and 2 wk after the eighth vaccination. Nine out of 16 patients had an increased number of IFN-γ-producing cells. For the other four patients with available data at only two time points, two of them showed significant postvaccination responses. These increased immune activities were associated with both NK cells and CD8+ T-cells against chronic myeloid leukemia. In addition, a significant correlation between clinical responses and immunological responses was observed *(101)*. A phase II study is ongoing to determine the efficacy of HSPPC-70 vaccine against imatinib-resistant chronic myeloid leukemia.

5. CONCLUDING REMARKS

HSPPC is a personalized vaccine derived from autologous tumor tissues. The antigenicity of the vaccine is toward HSP-chaperoned peptides from tumor cells. HSPPC vaccines require no epitope identification and have a potential to generate immunity against multiple epitopes, such as shared tumor antigens or unique tumor antigens. The immunogenicity of HSPPC vaccine depends on the proinflammatory properties of HSPs to activate professional APCs. The mechanisms of HSP-mediated immunomodulations are complex and are a fruitful field for further investigations. It is clear now that HSPPC-based vaccination is feasible and effective against many types of cancers in preclinical models. Phase I/II human studies have not generated any surprises, which shows that autologous HSPPC vaccine is feasible and in many cases, induces immune responses that were predicable from preclinical experience. The results of phase III data in melanoma and renal cell carcinoma are eagerly anticipated, and which will undoubtedly stimulate more interests in understanding the physiological roles of HSPs in immune responses.

REFERENCES

1. Gross L. Intradermal immunization of C3H mice against a sarcoma that originated in an animal of the same line. *Cancer Res* 1943; 3:323–326.
2. Baldwin RW. Immunity to methylcholanthrene-induced tumours in inbred rats following atrophy and regression of the implanted tumours. *Br J Cancer* 1955; 9:652–657.
3. Prehn RT, Main JM. Immunity to methylcholanthrene-induced sarcomas. *J Natl Cancer Inst* 1957; 18: 769–778.
4. Klein G, Sjogren HO, Klein E, Hellstrom KE. Demonstration of resistance against methylcholanthrene-induced sarcomas in the primary autochthonous host. *Cancer Res* 1960; 20:1561–1572.
5. van Der Bruggen P, Zhang Y, Chaux P, et al. Tumor-specific shared antigenic peptides recognized by human T cells. *Immunol Rev* 2002; 188:51–64.
6. Blattman JN, Greenberg PD. Cancer immunotherapy: a treatment for the masses. *Science* 2004; 305: 200–205.
7. Smyth MJ, Hayakawa Y, Takeda K, Yagita H. New aspects of natural-killer-cell surveillance and therapy of cancer. *Nat Rev Cancer* 2002; 2:850–861.
8. Street SE, Hayakawa Y, Zhan Y, et al. Innate immune surveillance of spontaneous B cell lymphomas by natural killer cells and gammadelta T cells. *J Exp Med* 2004; 199:879–884.
9. Shankaran V, Ikeda H, Bruce AT, et al. IFNgamma and lymphocytes prevent primary tumour development and shape tumour immunogenicity. *Nature* 2001; 410:1107–1111.
10. Dunn GP, Old LJ, Schreiber RD. The immunobiology of cancer immunosurveillance and immuno-editing. *Immunity* 2004; 21:137–148.
11. Lindquist S, Craig EA. The heat-shock proteins. *Annu Rev Genet* 1988; 22:631–677.
12. Gething MJ, Sambrook J. Protein folding in the cell. *Nature* 1992; 355:33–45.
13. Rutherford SL, Lindquist S. Hsp90 as a capacitor for morphological evolution. *Nature* 1998; 396:336–342.
14. Jaattela M, Wissing D, Kokholm K, Kallunki T, Egeblad M. Hsp70 exerts its anti-apoptotic function downstream of caspase-3-like proteases. *EMBO J* 1998; 17:6124–6134.
15. Srivastava PK, Das MR. The serologically unique cell surface antigen of Zajdela ascitic hepatoma is also its tumor-associated transplantation antigen. *Int J Cancer* 1984; 33:417–422.
16. Srivastava PK, DeLeo AB, Old LJ. Tumor rejection antigens of chemically induced sarcomas of inbred mice. *Proc Natl Acad Sci USA* 1986; 83:3407–3411.
17. Udono H, Srivastava PK. Comparison of tumor-specific immunogenicities of stress-induced proteins gp96, hsp90, and hsp70. *J Immunol* 1994; 152:5398–5403.
18. Udono H, Srivastava PK. Heat shock protein 70-associated peptides elicit specific cancer immunity. *J Exp Med* 1993; 178:1391–1396.
19. Ullrich SJ, Robinson EA, Law LW, Willingham M, Appella E. A mouse tumor-specific transplantation antigen is a heat shock-related protein. *Proc Natl Acad Sci USA* 1986; 83:3121–3125.
20. Basu S, Srivastava PK. Calreticulin, a peptide-binding chaperone of the endoplasmic reticulum, elicits tumor- and peptide-specific immunity. *J Exp Med* 1999; 189:797–802.
21. Nair S, Wearsch PA, Mitchell DA, Wassenberg JJ, Gilboa E, Nicchitta CV. Calreticulin displays in vivo peptide-binding activity and can elicit CTL responses against bound peptides. *J Immunol* 1999; 162: 6426–6432.

22. Wang XY, Kazim L, Repasky EA, Subjeck JR. Characterization of heat shock protein 110 and glucose-regulated protein 170 as cancer vaccines and the effect of fever-range hyperthermia on vaccine activity. *J Immunol* 2001; 166:490–497.

23. Wang XY, Chen X, Manjili MH, Repasky E, Henderson R, Subjeck JR. Targeted immunotherapy using reconstituted chaperone complexes of heat shock protein 110 and melanoma-associated antigen gp100. *Cancer Res* 2003; 63:2553–2560.

24. Srivastava P. Roles of heat-shock proteins in innate and adaptive immunity. *Nat Rev Immunol* 2002; 2:185–194.

25. Srivastava PK, Maki RG. Stress-induced proteins in immune response to cancer. *Curr Top Microbiol Immunol* 1991; 167:109–123.

26. Srivastava PK. Peptide-binding heat shock proteins in the endoplasmic reticulum: role in immune response to cancer and in antigen presentation. *Adv Cancer Res* 1993; 62:153–177.

27. Srivastava PK, Heike M. Tumor-specific immunogenicity of stress-induced proteins: convergence of two evolutionary pathways of antigen presentation? *Semin Immunol* 1991; 3:57–64.

28. Li Z, Srivastava PK. Tumor rejection antigen gp96/grp94 is an ATPase: implications for protein folding and antigen presentation. *EMBO J* 1993; 12:3143–3151.

29. Nieland TJ, Tan MC, Monne-van Muijen M, Koning F, Kruisbeek AM, van Bleek GM. Isolation of an immunodominant viral peptide that is endogenously bound to the stress protein GP96/GRP94. *Proc Natl Acad Sci USA* 1996; 93:6135–6139.

30. Ishii T, Udono H, Yamano T, et al. Isolation of MHC class I-restricted tumor antigen peptide and its precursors associated with heat shock proteins hsp70, hsp90, and gp96. *J Immunol* 1999; 162:1303–1309.

31. Blachere NE, Li Z, Chandawarkar RY, et al. Heat shock protein-peptide complexes, reconstituted in vitro, elicit peptide-specific cytotoxic T lymphocyte response and tumor immunity. *J Exp Med* 1997; 186:1315–1322.

32. Li Z, Dai J, Zheng H, Liu B, Caudill M. An integrated view of the roles and mechanisms of heat shock protein gp96-peptide complex in eliciting immune response. *Front Biosci* 2002; 7:d731–d751.

33. Grossmann ME, Madden BJ, Gao F, et al. Proteomics shows Hsp70 does not bind peptide sequences indiscriminately in vivo. *Exp Cell Res* 2004; 297:108–117.

34. Meng SD, Gao T, Gao GF, Tien P. HBV-specific peptide associated with heat-shock protein gp96. *Lancet* 2001; 357:528–529.

35. Castelli C, Ciupitu AM, Rini F, et al. Human heat shock protein 70 peptide complexes specifically activate antimelanoma T cells. *Cancer Res* 2001; 61:222–227.

36. Noessner E, Gastpar R, Milani V, et al. Tumor-derived heat shock protein 70 peptide complexes are cross-presented by human dendritic cells. *J Immunol* 2002; 169:5424–5432.

37. Triozzi PL, Khurram R, Aldrich WA, Walker MJ, Kim JA, Jaynes S. Intratumoral injection of dendritic cells derived in vitro in patients with metastatic cancer. *Cancer* 2000; 89:2646–2654.

38. Michils A, Dutry D, de Beyl VZ, Remmelink M, de Maertelaer V, Rocmans P. Peripheral blood mononuclear cell proliferation to heat shock protein-70 derived from autologous lung carcinoma. *Am J Respir Crit Care Med* 2002; 166:749–753.

39. Srivastava PK, Menoret A, Basu S, Binder RJ, McQuade KL. Heat shock proteins come of age: primitive functions acquire new roles in an adaptive world. *Immunity* 1998; 8:657–665.

40. Alizadeh AA, Eisen MB, Davis RE, et al. Distinct types of diffuse large B-cell lymphoma identified by gene expression profiling. *Nature* 2000; 403:503–511.

41. Bevan MJ. Cross-priming for a secondary cytotoxic response to minor H antigens with H-2 congenic cells which do not cross-react in the cytotoxic assay. *J Exp Med* 1976; 143:1283–1288.

42. Udono H, Levey DL, Srivastava PK. Cellular requirements for tumor-specific immunity elicited by heat shock proteins: tumor rejection antigen gp96 primes CD8+ T cells in vivo. *Proc Natl Acad Sci USA* 1994; 91:3077–3081.

43. Tamura Y, Peng P, Liu K, Daou M, Srivastava PK. Immunotherapy of tumors with autologous tumor-derived heat shock protein preparations. *Science* 1997; 278:117–120.

44. Sato K, Torimoto Y, Tamura Y, et al. Immunotherapy using heat-shock protein preparations of leukemia cells after syngeneic bone marrow transplantation in mice. *Blood* 2001; 98:1852–1857.

45. Suto R, Srivastava PK. A mechanism for the specific immunogenicity of heat shock protein-chaperoned peptides. *Science* 1995; 269:1585–1588.

46. Arnold D, Faath S, Rammensee H, Schild H. Cross-priming of minor histocompatibility antigen-specific cytotoxic T cells upon immunization with the heat shock protein gp96. *J Exp Med* 1995; 182:885–889.

47. Matsutake TS, P. K. CD91 is involved in MHC class II presentation of gp96-chaperoned peptides. *Cell Stress Chaperones* 2000; 5:378.
48. Doody AD, Kovalchin JT, Mihalyo MA, Hagymasi AT, Drake CG, Adler AJ. Glycoprotein 96 can chaperone both MHC class I- and class II-restricted epitopes for in vivo presentation, but selectively primes CD8$^+$ T cell effector function. *J Immunol* 2004; 172:6087–6092.
49. Kumaraguru U, Suvas S, Biswas PS, Azkur AK, Rouse BT. Concomitant helper response rescues otherwise low avidity CD8$^+$ memory CTLs to become efficient effectors in vivo. *J Immunol* 2004; 172:3719–3724.
50. Srivastava PK, Udono H, Blachere NE, Li Z. Heat shock proteins transfer peptides during antigen processing and CTL priming. *Immunogenetics* 1994; 39:93–98.
51. Basu S, Binder RJ, Suto R, Anderson KM, Srivastava PK. Necrotic but not apoptotic cell death releases heat shock proteins, which deliver a partial maturation signal to dendritic cells and activate the NF-kappa B pathway. *Int Immunol* 2000; 12:1539–1546.
52. Somersan S, Larsson M, Fonteneau JF, Basu S, Srivastava P, Bhardwaj N. Primary tumor tissue lysates are enriched in heat shock proteins and induce the maturation of human dendritic cells. *J Immunol* 2001; 167:4844–4852.
53. Binder RJ, Anderson KM, Basu S, Srivastava PK. Cutting edge: heat shock protein gp96 induces maturation and migration of CD11c$^+$ cells in vivo. *J Immunol* 2000; 165:6029–6035.
54. Panjwani NN, Popova L, Srivastava PK. Heat shock proteins gp96 and hsp70 activate the release of nitric oxide by APCs. *J Immunol* 2002; 168:2997–3003.
55. Radsak MP, Hilf N, Singh-Jasuja H, et al. The heat shock protein Gp96 binds to human neutrophils and monocytes and stimulates effector functions. *Blood* 2003; 101:2810–2815.
56. Baker-LePain JC, Sarzotti M, Fields TA, Li CY, Nicchitta CV. GRP94 (gp96) and GRP94 N-terminal geldanamycin binding domain elicit tissue nonrestricted tumor suppression. *J Exp Med* 2002; 196:1447–1459.
57. Baker-LePain JC, Sarzotti M, Nicchitta CV. Glucose-regulated protein 94/glycoprotein 96 elicits by-stander activation of CD4$^+$ T cell Th1 cytokine production in vivo. *J Immunol* 2004; 172:4195–4203.
58. Zheng H, Dai J, Stoilova D, Li Z. Cell surface targeting of heat shock protein gp96 induces dendritic cell maturation and antitumor immunity. *J Immunol* 2001; 167:6731–6735.
59. Strbo N, Oizumi S, Sotosek-Tokmadzic V, Podack ER. Perforin is required for innate and adaptive immunity induced by heat shock protein gp96. *Immunity* 2003; 18:381–390.
60. Vogen S, Gidalevitz T, Biswas C, et al. Radicicol-sensitive peptide binding to the N-terminal portion of GRP94. *J Biol Chem* 2002; 277:40,742–40,750.
61. Gidalevitz T, Biswas C, Ding H, et al. Identification of the N-terminal peptide binding site of glucose-regulated protein 94. *J Biol Chem* 2004; 279:16,543–16,552.
62. Gross C, Hansch D, Gastpar R, Multhoff G. Interaction of heat shock protein 70 peptide with NK cells involves the NK receptor CD94. *Biol Chem* 2003; 384:267–279.
63. Gross C, Schmidt-Wolf IG, Nagaraj S, et al. Heat shock protein 70-reactivity is associated with increased cell surface density of CD94/CD56 on primary natural killer cells. *Cell Stress Chaperones* 2003; 8:348–360.
64. Multhoff G, Mizzen L, Winchester CC, et al. Heat shock protein 70 (Hsp70) stimulates proliferation and cytolytic activity of natural killer cells. *Exp Hematol* 1999; 27:1627–1636.
65. Multhoff G, Pfister K, Gehrmann M, et al. A 14-mer Hsp70 peptide stimulates natural killer (NK) cell activity. *Cell Stress Chaperones* 2001; 6:337–344.
66. Gastpar R, Gross C, Rossbacher L, Ellwart J, Riegger J, Multhoff G. The cell surface-localized heat shock protein 70 epitope TKD induces migration and cytolytic activity selectively in human NK cells. *J Immunol* 2004; 172:972–980.
67. Arnold-Schild D, Hanau D, Spehner D, et al. Cutting edge: receptor-mediated endocytosis of heat shock proteins by professional antigen-presenting cells. *J Immunol* 1999; 162:3757–3760.
68. Binder RJ, Harris ML, Menoret A, Srivastava PK. Saturation, competition, and specificity in interaction of heat shock proteins (hsp) gp96, hsp90, and hsp70 with CD11b$^+$ cells. *J Immunol* 2000; 165:2582–2587.
69. Castellino F, Boucher PE, Eichelberg K, et al. Receptor-mediated uptake of antigen/heat shock protein complexes results in major histocompatibility complex class I antigen presentation via two distinct processing pathways. *J Exp Med* 2000; 191:1957–1964.

70. Singh-Jasuja H, Toes RE, Spee P, et al. Cross-presentation of glycoprotein 96-associated antigens on major histocompatibility complex class I molecules requires receptor-mediated endocytosis. *J Exp Med* 2000;191:1965–1974.

71. Binder RJ, Han DK, Srivastava PK. CD91: a receptor for heat shock protein gp96. *Nat Immunol* 2000; 1:151–155.

72. Binder RJ, Srivastava PK. Essential role of CD91 in re-presentation of gp96-chaperoned peptides. *Proc Natl Acad Sci USA* 2004; 101:6128–6133.

73. Basu S, Binder RJ, Ramalingam T, Srivastava PK. CD91 is a common receptor for heat shock proteins gp96, hsp90, hsp70, and calreticulin. *Immunity* 2001; 14:303–313.

74. Delneste Y, Magistrelli G, Gauchat J, et al. Involvement of LOX-1 in dendritic cell-mediated antigen cross-presentation. *Immunity* 2002; 17:353–362.

75. Berwin B, Hart JP, Rice S, et al. Scavenger receptor-A mediates gp96/GRP94 and calreticulin internalization by antigen-presenting cells. *EMBO J* 2003; 22:6127–6136.

76. Becker T, Hartl FU, Wieland F. CD40, an extracellular receptor for binding and uptake of Hsp70-peptide complexes. *J Cell Biol* 2002; 158:1277–1285.

77. Millar DG, Garza KM, Odermatt B, et al. Hsp70 promotes antigen-presenting cell function and converts T-cell tolerance to autoimmunity in vivo. *Nat Med* 2003; 9:1469–1476.

78. Vabulas RM, Ahmad-Nejad P, da Costa C, et al. Endocytosed HSP60s use toll-like receptor 2 (TLR2) and TLR4 to activate the toll/interleukin-1 receptor signaling pathway in innate immune cells. *J Biol Chem* 2001; 276:31,332–31,339.

79. Vabulas RM, Ahmad-Nejad P, Ghose S, Kirschning CJ, Issels RD, Wagner H. HSP70 as endogenous stimulus of the Toll/interleukin-1 receptor signal pathway. *J Biol Chem* 2002; 277:15,107–15,112.

80. Vabulas RM, Braedel S, Hilf N, et al. The endoplasmic reticulum-resident heat shock protein Gp96 activates dendritic cells via the Toll-like receptor 2/4 pathway. *J Biol Chem* 2002; 277:20,847–20,853.

81. Asea A, Rehli M, Kabingu E, et al. Novel signal transduction pathway utilized by extracellular HSP70: role of toll-like receptor (TLR) 2 and TLR4. *J Biol Chem* 2002; 277:15,028–15,034.

82. Liu B, Dai J, Zheng H, Stoilova D, Sun S, Li Z. Cell surface expression of an endoplasmic reticulum resident heat shock protein gp96 triggers MyD88-dependent systemic autoimmune diseases. *Proc Natl Acad Sci USA* 2003; 100:15,824–15,829.

83. Kol A, Lichtman AH, Finberg RW, Libby P, Kurt-Jones EA. Cutting edge: heat shock protein (HSP) 60 activates the innate immune response: CD14 is an essential receptor for HSP60 activation of mononuclear cells. *J Immunol* 2000; 164:13–17.

84. Asea A, Kraeft SK, Kurt-Jones EA, et al. HSP70 stimulates cytokine production through a CD14-dependant pathway, demonstrating its dual role as a chaperone and cytokine. *Nat Med* 2000; 6:435–442.

85. Bausinger H, Lipsker D, Ziylan U, et al. Endotoxin-free heat-shock protein 70 fails to induce APC activation. *Eur J Immunol* 2002; 32:3708–3713.

86. Gao B, Tsan MF. Recombinant human heat shock protein 60 does not induce the release of tumor necrosis factor alpha from murine macrophages. *J Biol Chem* 2003; 278:22,523–22,529.

87. Gao B, Tsan MF. Endotoxin contamination in recombinant human heat shock protein 70 (Hsp70) preparation is responsible for the induction of tumor necrosis factor alpha release by murine macrophages. *J Biol Chem* 2003; 278:174–179.

88. Gao B, Tsan MF. Induction of cytokines by heat shock proteins and endotoxin in murine macrophages. *Biochem Biophys Res Commun* 2004; 317:1149–1154.

89. Huang XF, Ren W, Rollins L, et al. A broadly applicable, personalized heat shock protein mediated oncolytic tumor vaccine. *Cancer Res* 2003; 63:7321–7329.

90. Kovalchin JT, Murthy AS, Horattas MC, Guyton DP, Chandawarkar RY. Determinants of efficacy of immunotherapy with tumor-derived heat shock protein gp96. *Cancer Immun* 2001; 1:7.

91. Palladino MA Jr, Srivastava PK, Oettgen HF, DeLeo AB. Expression of a shared tumor-specific antigen by two chemically induced BALB/c sarcomas. *Cancer Res* 1987; 47:5074–5079.

92. Janetzki S, Blachere NE, Srivastava PK. Generation of tumor-specific cytotoxic T lymphocytes and memory T cells by immunization with tumor-derived heat shock protein gp96. *J Immunother* 1998; 21: 269–276.

93. Graner M, Raymond A, Romney D, He L, Whitesell L, Katsanis E. Immunoprotective activities of multiple chaperone proteins isolated from murine B-cell leukemia/lymphoma. *Clin Cancer Res* 2000; 6: 909–915.

94. Manjili MH, Wang XY, Chen X, et al. HSP110-HER2/*neu* chaperone complex vaccine induces protective immunity against spontaneous mammary tumors in HER-2/*neu* transgenic mice. *J Immunol* 2003; 171:4054–4061.

95. Robert J, Menoret A, Basu S, Cohen N, Srivastava PR. Phylogenetic conservation of the molecular and immunological properties of the chaperones gp96 and hsp70. *Eur J Immunol* 2001; 31:186–195.

96. Yedavelli SP, Guo L, Daou ME, Srivastava PK, Mittelman A, Tiwari RK. Preventive and therapeutic effect of tumor derived heat shock protein, gp96, in an experimental prostate cancer model. *Int J Mol Med* 1999; 4:243–248.

97. Srivastava PK. Purification of heat shock protein-peptide complexes for use in vaccination against cancers and intracellular pathogens. *Methods* 1997; 12:165–171.

98. Janetzki S, Palla D, Rosenhauer V, Lochs H, Lewis JJ, Srivastava PK. Immunization of cancer patients with autologous cancer-derived heat shock protein gp96 preparations: a pilot study. *Int J Cancer* 2000; 88:232–238.

99. Hertkorn C, Lehr A, Woelfel T, et al. Phase I trial of vaccination with autologous tumor-derived gp96 (oncophage) in patients after surgery for gastric cancer. *Proc Am Soc Clin Oncol* 2002; 21:30a (abstract no. 117).

100. Amato R, Murray L, Wood L, Savary C, Tomasovic S, Reitsma D. Active specific immunotherapy in patients with renal cell carcinoma (RCC), using autologous tumor derived heat shock protein–peptide complex–96 (HSPP-96) vaccine. *Proc Am Soc Clin Oncol* 1999; 18:332a (abstract no. 1278).

101. Li Z, Qiau Y, Liu B, et al. Combination of imatinib mesylate with autologous leukocyte-derived heat shock proteins and chronic myelogenous leukemia. *Clin Cancer Res* 2005; 11:4460–4468.

102. Eton O, East M, Ross MI, et al. Autologous tumor-derived heat-shock protein peptide complex-96 (HSPPC-96) in patients with metastatic melanoma. *Proc Ann Meet Am Assoc Cancer Res* 2000; 41:543 (abstract no. 3463).

103. Belli F, Testori A, Rivoltini L, et al. Vaccination of metastatic melanoma patients with autologous tumor-derived heat shock protein gp96-peptide complexes: clinical and immunologic findings. *J Clin Oncol* 2002; 20:4169–4180.

104. Assikis VJ, Daliani D, Pagliaro L, et al. Phase II study of an autologous tumor derived heat shock protein-peptide complex vaccine (HSPPC-96) for patients with metastatic renal cell carcinoma (mRCC). *Proc Am Soc Clin Oncol* 2003; 22:386(abstract no. 1552).

105. Amato RL, Wood C, Savary C, et al. (2000) Patients with renal cell carcinoma (RCC) using auto-logous tumor-derived heat shock protein-peptide complex (HSPPC-96) with or without interleukin-2 (IL-2). *Proc Am Soc Clin Oncol* 2000; 19:454a (abstract no. 1782).

106. Mazzaferro V, Coppa J, Carrabba MG, et al. Vaccination with autologous tumor-derived heat-shock protein gp96 after liver resection for metastatic colorectal cancer. *Clin Cancer Res* 2003; 9:3235–3245.

107. Maki RG, Lewis JJ, Janetzki S, et al. Phase I study of HSPPC-96 (Oncophage® vaccine in patients with completely resected pancreatic adenocarcinoma. *Eur J Cancer Suppl* 2003; 1:S19.

108. Younes A, Fayad LE, Pro B, et al. Safety and efficacy of heat shock protein-peptide 96 complex (HSPPC-96) in low-grade lymphoma. *Proc Am Soc Clin Oncol* 2003; 22:570(abstract no. 2294).

11 Tumor-Reactive T-Cells for Adoptive Immunotherapy

Helga Bernhard, Julia Neudorfer,
Kerstin Gebhard, Heinke Conrad,
Dirk H. Busch, and Christian Peschel

SUMMARY

Adoptive T-cell therapy is based on specificity and efficacy, two essentials known to be necessary for successful cancer therapy. Tumor-reactive T-cells potentially display both characteristics in terms of antigen recognition and antitumor activity. In recent years, novel technologies have been established for the identification, isolation, activation, and expansion of human T-cells, which have greatly facilitated the further development of adoptive T-cell transfer regimens. Lessons learned from the first clinical trials revealed that the complexity of the in vivo environment interferes with the efficacy of transferred T-cells, such as tolerance induction and outgrowth of tumor escape variants. The results from these studies can be concluded by the following critical, but nevertheless encouraging, statement: "Tumor regressions observed after adoptive T-cell transfer are too frequent to be spontaneous." As these trials are not solely conducted for treating cancer patients, but also for research on human beings, the resulting scientific observations have increased our understanding of T-cell activation, homing, and survival, as well as of the possibility of disrupting regulatory mechanisms. The knowledge drawn from the first generation of transfer studies can be implemented in the next generation of clinical trials. T-cell-based immunotherapy regimens are currently being combined with other immunological strategies in order to coordinate an effective attack against tumors. Further development of combinatorial therapies involving immunological and molecular technologies will offer the means to tailor adoptive transfer of T-cell immunity for each cancer patient.

Key Words: Cancer; immunotherapy; T-lymphocytes; cytokines; immunity.

1. RATIONALE FOR ADOPTIVE T-CELL TRANSFER

The immune system is capable of recognizing and eliminating malignant cells. Favorable courses of metastatic disease or even spontaneous regressions of malignant tumors indicate that an effective tumor-specific immune response may be elicited in some patients *(1)*. This hypothesis has been supported by the detection of tumor-directed T-lymphocytes

From: *Cancer Drug Discovery and Development: Immunotherapy of Cancer*
Edited by: M. L. Disis © Humana Press Inc., Totowa, NJ

and antibodies in cancer patients *(2,3)*. However, physiological and pathological mechanisms both can inhibit an adequate antitumor response. In particular, the tumor itself interferes with the development and function of immunological responses. New technologies have provided evidence that antigen-specific T-cells present at high levels in the blood or in tumor-draining lymph nodes of tumor patients have functional defects *(4,5)*.

The rationale for adoptive T-cell therapy is based on the attempt to circumvent the tolerizing environment by taking out the ignorant/anergic, but potentially tumor-lytic, T-cells from the cancer-bearing patient and by subsequently activating these T-cells ex vivo. Following the expansion of the tumor-reactive T-cells in vitro, great numbers of T-cells can be adoptively transferred to the immunosuppressed patient. In this way, a high frequency level of ex vivo-activated tumor-directed T-cells can be achieved in vivo.

Adoptive transfer of T-lymphocytes is not only a passive transfer of immunity, but is also a potential activation of the host immune system. The transferred T-cells may induce a cascade of cellular interactions, leading to the initiation of an endogenous immune response. It is known that the dynamic interaction of CD8$^+$ cytotoxic T-cells (CTLs), CD4$^+$ T helper (Th) cells and antigen-presenting dendritic cells (DCs) is required for the initiation of an immune response. DCs take up tumor-derived antigens and subsequently process and present antigenic peptides in context with human leukocyte antigen (HLA) and costimulatory molecules to CD8$^+$ and CD4$^+$ T-cells. Antigen-specific CD4$^+$ T-cells then provide direct and indirect help to CD8$^+$ effector T-cells *(6)*. During this three-cell interaction, CD8$^+$ CTLs are not a passive partner, but are able to activate naive CD4$^+$ Th cells *(7)*. Therefore, adoptively transferred CD4$^+$ Th cells may help pre-existing CD8$^+$ CTLs and vice versa. The overall goal of T-cell therapy for cancer is the establishment of a long-term antigen-specific cellular immune response against tumor cells.

2. IDENTIFYING TUMOR-REJECTION ANTIGENS FOR TARGETED T-CELL THERAPY

During the last decade, a great number of tumor-associated antigens have been identified that are recognized by human T-lymphocytes. An actual overview of the defined T-cell epitopes is in the database established by Benoit Van den Enden and Pierre van der Bruggen (www.cancerimmunity.org/peptidedatabase/Tcellepitopes.htm). Antigenic peptides presented with HLA class I and II can serve as targets for antigen-specific T-killer and Th cells, respectively. Meanwhile, various families of tumor-associated antigens have been classified, e.g., differentiation antigens, overexpressed antigens, cancer–testis antigens, mutated antigens, and viral antigens *(8,9)*. The identification of these cancer antigens has been the first step for the development of adoptive immunotherapy regimens using T-cells with defined antigen specificity. However, it is still an open question as to which kind of tumor antigen can function as a tumor-rejection antigen in the context of adoptive T-cell transfer. As the immune system evolved to fight against pathogens, viral antigens associated with tumors, such as Epstein-Barr virus (EBV), have been attractive candidates for antigen-specific T-cell therapy. Indeed, the clinical research group of Rooney and Heslop has recently shown that the transfer of autologous EBV-reactive T-cells to patients with EBV$^+$ Hodgkin's disease can promote tumor regression *(10)*. However, viral-derived antigens represent only a small fraction of tumor-associated antigens. The majority of defined tumor antigens belongs to the group of self-antigens, which are shared antigens either expressed in a tissue-restricted matter, such as Melan-A *(11)*, overexpressed in tumor compared to normal tissues, such as HER-2 *(12)*, or aberrantly expressed in malignant cells, such as cancer–testis antigens *(13)*. An even larger number of yet undefined antigens might belong to the class of mutated antigens that are difficult to identify, because mutations often occur individually and are less frequently shared by tumors *(14)*. These private antigens are potentially very immunogenic, because the host's tolerance to a self-antigen is broken as soon as it is mutated. Therefore, it has been a matter of debate whether mutated antigens are superior to nonmutated self-antigens regarding T-cell-mediated tumor rejection *(15,16)*. A recent clinical trial conducted by Rosenberg and coworkers has demonstrated that the adoptive transfer of tumor-infiltrating lymphocytes leads to clonal repopulation, with T-lymphocytes directed against both shared and private, nonmutated and mutated, self-antigens and that the persistence of clonotypes further correlated with tumor regression *(17,18)*. Moreover, a clinical study performed by Greenberg and colleagues documented that clonal T-cell populations directed against the melanocyte differentiation antigen Melan-A can promote remissions of metastatic melanoma lesions after adoptive transfer *(19)*. The studies with melanoma patients also documented that the physiological expression pattern of the targeted self-antigen contributes to the balance/imbalance of tumor immunity and autoimmunity induced by T-cell transfer *(17,20)*.

An exceptional clinical and immunological situation for T-cell therapy is the relapse of leukemia after allogeneic stem cell transplantation, where donor lymphocyte infusions can reinduce complete remissions *(21)*. It has been proposed that one of the underlying mechanisms for this graft-vs-leukemia effect might be because of donor T-cells recognizing antigens derived from polymorphic genes in context with self or non-self HLA molecules. It has been speculated that these so-called minor histocompatibility antigens (mHAgs) may be able to induce the graft-vs-leukemia effect without graft-vs-host disease (GVHD), if T-cells recognize mHAgs restricted to hematopoietic cell lineages *(22)*. This hypothesis has been strengthened by the fact that following donor lymphocyte infusions, the rise of T-cells specific for hematopoiesis-restricted mHAgs correlates with complete remissions of relapsed leukemia without inducing GVHD *(23)*.

Regardless of the type of antigen being recognized by the adoptively transferred T-cells, it cannot be ruled out that secondary events might be responsible for the final hit during the process of tumor rejection. Following adoptive T-cell transfer, endogenous T-cells may be stimulated, and antitumor clonotypes may arise, displaying antigen specificities distinct from the transferred T-cells. This theory has been supported by observations made in the course of peptide-based vaccines, where antigen spreading is associated with T-cell-mediated tumor regression *(24,25)*. In conclusion, multiple characteristics of the antigen will influence its making as a tumor-rejection antigen, including its contribution to the malignant phenotype of the tumor cell and subsequently, the likelihood of selecting antigen loss variants following T-cell transfer *(26,27)*. Future in vivo studies in humans have to explore further which tumor antigens are suitable targets for T-cell therapy.

3. SELECTING T-CELL POPULATIONS FOR IMMUNOTHERAPY

Attempts to treat patients with antigen-specific T-lymphocytes have been limited because of the difficulty of detecting and isolating functionally active T-cells, which are present at extremely low frequencies in the peripheral blood. Recently, a novel method of identifying antigen-specific T-lymphocytes has been described using tetrameric major histocompatibility complex (MHC)–peptide complexes, so-called tetramers or multimers, that bind stably and specifically to appropriate MHC-peptide-specific T-cells *(28)*. This technique permits both the detection and isolation of antigen-specific T-cells present at low frequencies *(29)*. However, the functional activity of MHC multimer-labeled cells is hampered by the persistence of T-cell receptor (TCR)–MHC interactions and subsequently induced signaling events *(30,31)*. This intrinsic problem can be circumvented by reversible MHC–peptide multimers, so-called streptamers, that can be dissociated from the T-cells and, therefore, preserve T-cell function *(32)*.

As the natural frequency of tumor-reactive T-cells in the blood is often too low to be directly detectable by multimers, the number of antigen-specific peripheral blood T-lymphocytes can be enhanced by repetitive in vitro stimulations with antigen-loaded antigen-presenting cells (APCs) before isolation. Currently, one of the most widely used methods for stimulating T-lymphocytes in vitro is the use of peptide-pulsed DCs as APCs. One advantage of using peptide-pulsed DCs is the ability to isolate T-cells recognizing subdominant epitopes to which T-cells are not naturally activated in vivo. This peptide-based stimulation method, however, often promotes the growth of peptide-specific T-cells with low-affinity TCRs that are unable to lyse tumor cells. This major disadvantage can be partly circumvented by cloning the peptide-stimulated T-cells and further expanding only those T-cell clones with high functional avidity *(33)*. A promising attempt to exclusively stimulate tumor-lytic T-cells might be the usage of protein-pulsed DCs known to be able to present and crosspresent antigenic peptides to MHC class II- and class I-restricted T-cells, respectively *(34,35)*. An additional mode of antigen loading is the transfection of DCs with genes coding for tumor antigens. Genetically modified DCs take advantage of the endogenous antigen-processing machinery for presenting T-cell epitopes in the context of HLA molecules and, therefore, should preferentially stimulate T-cells capable of recognizing peptides also being processed and presented by tumor cells *(36)*. In addition, gene-modified DCs have the capacity to present multiple epitopes and to subsequently induce cytotoxic and Th cells both recognizing the same antigen in context with different HLA molecules *(37,38)*.

An alternative method to repetitive in vitro antigen stimulations might be in vivo immunizations of the patients in order to enhance the starting numbers of antigen-specific T-cells before the T-cell isolation procedure. Clearly, the vaccination of cancer patients can increase the number of immune T-cells capable of recognizing and responding to the tumor antigens that has been used as a vaccine *(25,39,40)*. Moreover, it has been shown in a murine model that vaccine-stimulated, adoptively transferred CD8+ T-cells can mediate antigen-specific tumor destruction *(41)*.

Tumor tissue or tumor-infiltrated lymph nodes are an alternative source to peripheral blood for isolating potentially tumor-reactive T-cells, because tumor-directed T-cells can migrate to, and accumulate at, the tumor site *(42)*. However, tumor progression is often observed even in the presence of these so-called tumor-infiltrating T-cells (TILs) and, therefore, TILs have been nicknamed tumor-observing lymphocytes, pointing out their poor functionality in terms of tumor defense. Based on these observations, the use of TILs for adoptive transfer requires the isolation and ex vivo activation in order to stimulate them in the absence of the tolerizing tumor environment. First attempts to treat patients with TILs showed a confined efficacy *(43)*, which might be explained by the deficient effector functions *(44,45)* that were not fully overcome by ex vivo stimulation when given back to the patients' tolerizing environment. More recently, a clinical trial regarding adoptive transfer of ex vivo-activated TILs into melanoma patients elicited very encouraging results that tolerizing factors can be overcome by conditioning the recipients before TIL transfer (17).

Studies in mice and humans are currently investigating whether culturing and transferring T-lymphocytes as monoclonal or polyclonal lines leads to superior tumor cell elimination. Both attempts may have advantages and disadvantages. Cloning CTLs and/or Th cells before transfer is a sophisticated method to investigate the efficacy of a homogeneous T-cell population with defined specificity, avidity, and effector function. Moreover, certain medical indications may even require cloning before T-cell transfer, such as adoptive T-cell transfer for allogeneic stem cell recipients, where specificity of donor-derived T-cells should be ensured in order to avoid GVHD. One advantage of using antigen-specific T-cell lines might be the transfer of CD8$^+$ and CD4$^+$ T-cells both being present in a polyclonal T-cell line, which may support the efficacy of T-cell transfer. In addition, a cocktail of T-cells with different antigen specificities will help to avoid antigen selection and tumor-escape phenotypes (26,27).

Once antigen-specific T-cells are selected, these T-cells can be expanded in an antigen-independent way. Several culture protocols have been established, based mainly on the usage of cytokines, such as interleukin (IL)-2, and stimulating antibodies to CD3 (46). Additional, yet unknown, T-cell growth factors and co-stimulatory factors can be provided by co-culturing T-cells with so-called feeder cells, including irradiated EBV-transformed B-cells and peripheral blood mononuclear cells. Using this method, antigen-specific T-cells derived from the blood, as well as from tumor lesions, can be expanded as clonal and polyclonal T-cell lines to numbers up to 10^{10} T-cells. In this manner, a high frequency level of ex vivo-activated antigen-specific T-cells can be achieved in vivo, following the adoptive transfer to cancer patients (17,19).

Recent strategies focus on changing the recipient's environment in order to improve the proliferation and survival of transferred T-cells in vivo (17,47). Using this approach, even a relatively small number of transferred T-cells might be sufficient to proliferate in vivo. Therefore, T-cell expansion before the adoptive transfer might not be obligatory for a conditioned recipient. T-cells that have been heavily expanded in vitro might become dependent on particular culture conditions, and perhaps be unable to adapt to the physiological milieu following the transfer. This further emphasizes the need to continue studies on how the recipient's environment can best be prepared for adoptive transfer.

There is no doubt that the continuous development of novel technologies for isolating and propagating tumor-reactive T-lymphocytes will facilitate the transfer of T-cells as a therapeutic option for cancer patients (48). Nevertheless, transfer of naturally occurring antigen-specific T-cells may not become a treatment for the masses, because it may remain difficult to generate antigen-specific, tumor-reactive T-cells from every single patient being eligible for adoptive T-cell therapy. An alternative approach is to provide T-cells with the desired antigen specificity and avidity by TCR gene transfer, thereby redirecting T-cell populations to tumor cells (49). Recently developed retroviral vectors provide high-level gene expression in primary human T-lymphocytes, being a prerequisite for TCR transfer, because T-cell efficacy depends on the amount of the TCR transgene product (50). In preclinical studies, HLA-restricted, antigen-specific TCR genes isolated from human TILs could endow peripheral blood lymphocytes with the ability to recognize antigen-expressing tumor cells following retroviral gene transfer (51,52). This genetic approach also bears the possibility to select high-avidity TCRs from MHC-allorestricted T-cells, as these T-cells may display enhanced avidity to certain antigens, in particular to tumor/self-antigens, because the allorestricted T-cells are not tolerant *(53,54)*. The selection of the allorestricted tumor-reactive TCRs will be dominated by the flexibility of TCR allorecognition and by the molecular mimicry of MHC–peptide complexes *(55)*. In addition, the genetic engineering has been used to express so-called chimeric TCRs redirecting primary T-cells to cancer cells *(56)*, e.g., by tumor-antigen-specific, chimeric single-chain receptors capable of delivering TCR ζ-chain-activation signals *(57)*.

The knowledge of recently defined molecules physiologically expressed by T-cells allows for searching and selecting for T-cells, which may have the potential to survive long term in vivo. Therefore, culture conditions are currently being optimized in order to manipulate the up- and downregulation of the molecules involved in T-cell survival and death. Candidate T-cells for adoptive transfer may be those that transiently express molecules upon antigen stimulation, which are known to promote the survival and differentiation of activated lymphocytes into memory CD8[+] T-cells *(58)*. Attractive molecules for positively selecting T-cells include cytokine receptors, such as CD127 (IL-7 receptor) and CD27 *(59,60)*. An alternative method to selecting naturally occurring T-cells is genetically engineering T-cells by introducing molecules into T-cells that promote function and/or prolong survival of T-cells. T-cells can be modified by gene insertion to express molecules that mediate signaling, homing, and maintenance following transfer *(61)*. Adoptive transfer of T-cells naturally or artificially equipped with survival molecules may contribute to a population of effector and/or memory T-cells and subsequently mediate a long-lasting tumor remission in patients.

4. MANIPULATING SURVIVAL AND EFFICACY OF T-CELLS FOLLOWING ADOPTIVE TRANSFER

From adoptive T-cell transfer studies, it appears that identification of tumor antigens and generation of tumor-reactive lymphocytes are necessary, but not sufficient, for treatment efficiency. The induction of tolerance by the host in general and the tumor in particular are important mechanisms limiting the efficacy of adoptive T-cell therapy *(15,62)*. Therefore, a number of strategies are currently being developed in order to retain the function of adoptively transferred T-cells. The efficacy of transferred T-cells—regardless of the antigen specificity or the source of population—depends strongly on their ability to retain function and survive long-term in the host. As CD4[+] Th cells play an important role for improving the persistence of adoptively transferred antigen-specific CTL clones *(63)*, it has been proposed that the administration of T-cell growth factor IL-2 may be able to mimic the naturally existing help by IL-2-producing CD4[+] T-lymphocytes. Indeed, systemic application of IL-2 improved survival of transferred melanoma-reactive CD8[+] CTL clones *(19)*. Other T-cell growth factors involved in T-cell homeostasis, including IL-7, IL-15, and IL-21, have been shown to enhance the efficacy of transferred antigen-specific T-cells in tumor-bearing mice *(64,65)*. Based on these preclinical data, combinatory immunotherapy regimens with tumor-reactive T-cells and cytokines are currently being investigated for cancer patients.

However, the systemic administration of cytokines may not be able to mimic fully the physiological situation, as the dynamic interaction of immune cells and soluble factors is required for effective tumor rejection. A logical consequence for substituting antigen-specific T-cell help might be the simultaneous transfer of CD4+ and CD8+ T-cell populations both recognizing antigens presented by the tumor cells *(38)*. This assumption has already been supported by studies both in animals and humans, demonstrating that the immunization with Th and CTL epitopes derived from the same tumor antigen resulted in a synergistic antitumor activity *(37,66)*. Moreover, it has been shown in murine models that the transfer of solely antigen-specific CD4+ T-cells can mediate the regression of antigen-positive, but MHC class II-negative, tumors, presumably via targeting tumor stroma *(67,68)*.

Another method of improving antigen-specific T-cell function might be the concurrent therapy with T-lymphocytes and antibodies directed against the same antigen. The presence of simultaneous humoral and cellular immune responses against identical antigens in cancer patients suggests that the antitumor activity of antibodies and T-lymphocytes might be intertwined *(69,70)*. Indeed, it has been demonstrated for multiple myeloma that antitumor monoclonal antibodies (MAbs) can enhance crosspresentation of cellular antigens and subsequently, the stimulation of antigen-specific killer T-cells *(71)*. Moreover, we have shown for the HER-2 antigen that the cytolytic activity of human, HER-2-specific CD8+ CTLs is augmented by anti-HER-2 MAb trastuzumab *(72)*. The underlying mechanism remains unclear. We propose that tumor cells become more susceptible to CTL-mediated lysis, because antibody-induced internalization and degradation of HER-2 is likely to be accompanied with increased numbers of HER-2 peptides presented with HLA molecules. The potentially synergistic activity of antigen-specific antibodies and CTLs encourages the development of targeted immunotherapy regimens based on the combination of MAbs and T-lymphocytes both directed against the same antigen.

Despite the fact that the in vivo persistence of transferred T-cells is crucial for efficiently targeting tumor cells, the mere presence of tumor-reactive T-cells might not be sufficient to induce tumor regression. This concern seems to be a major hurdle, because T-cell transfer experiments in mice have recently shown that CTLs, which recognize a tumor/self-antigen and do lyse tumor cells in vitro, were rendered unresponsive in vivo *(15)*. One strategy to reverse the functionally tolerant state of transferred antigen-specific T-cells may be the active immunization with the T-cell-recognized antigen. It has recently been shown in a murine model that vaccination after T-cell transfer can greatly improve the efficacy of adoptive T-cell therapy in terms of tumor destruction *(73)*. Repetitive and continuous antigen vaccines might boost the transferred T-cell immunity, thereby helping to keep a high-frequency level of functionally active tumor-reactive T-cells in vivo *(74)*.

In recent years, it has become evident that a variety of factors regulates the size and composition of the entire T-cell pool resulting in a physiologically steady T-cell homoeostasis including proliferation, diversity, and functionality *(75)*. A balanced T-cell pool has a vital influence on the capacity of the host to respond to tumor-associated antigens. Subsequently, the pre-existing equilibrium also has an essential impact on promoting the survival and function of adoptively transferred T-cells. Strategies are being developed in order to manipulate host factors known to limit the in vivo persistence of transferred T-cells. Indeed, conditioning primates with an immunosuppressive regimen promotes the long-term survival of autologous T-cells following transfer *(47)*. Moreover, it has been shown in humans that a nonmyeloablative conditioning regimen leads to a milieu that enables the in vivo expansion of individual T-cell clones following transfer *(17,76,77)*. The underlying mechanism is not fully understood, but it has been hypothesized that the lympho-depleting conditioning therapy may have altered homoeostatic mechanisms that are responsible for limiting lymphocyte numbers. There is accumulating evidence that certain T-cell populations suppress the activation and proliferation of antigen-specific T-cells in vivo and consecutively, may also inhibit tumor immunity mediated by adoptively transferred T-cells *(78)*. Recent studies in animals have shown that in vivo depletion of T-regulatory (Treg) cells before T-cell transfer can facilitate the persistence and amplification of the transmitted T-cells, subsequently leading to the regression of established tumors *(79)*. As in vivo depletion of all lymphocytes or even of CD25[+] T-cells is a rather crude method to purge suppressive T-lymphocytes, more sophisticated methods are currently being evaluated to selectively deplete Treg cells by targeting markers restricted to Treg cells.

5. OVERCOMING THE TUMOR-INTRINSIC BARRIER TO T-CELL INFILTRATION

As we have outlined, persistently high levels of activated tumor-specific T-lymphocytes are an essential requirement for successful T-cell therapy. However, this may not be sufficient to eliminate solid tumors. Established tumors surrounded by pathological stromal and endothelial cells are intrinsically resistant to infiltration and destruction by tumor-specific T-lymphocytes. Targeting the tumor barrier is supposed to be an effective strategy for promoting the extravasation of T-cells from tumor vessels to the tumor cells, and thereby enhances the efficacy of adoptive T-cell transfer in cancer patients *(62,80)*. In mice, such resistance can be overcome and evident barriers erected by solid tumors can be disrupted by tumor irradiation. The combination of T-cell transfer and tumor irradiation leads to lymphocyte infiltration into solid tumors and subsequently to tumor rejection. The underlying mechanism may be that irradiation triggers remodeling of the vasculature and leads to a proinflammatory micro-environment that permits T-cells to extravasate and to destroy the tumor cells *(81)*. Adjuvants, such as unmethylated cytosine–phosphate–guanine-containing oligodeoxynucleotides and antiangiogenic molecules, also normalize the vascular structure of the tumor stroma, and thereby augment the susceptibility of the tumor endothelium for lymphocyte extravasation *(82)*. Moreover, it has recently been shown that the induction of certain molecules in the tumor stroma leads to a massive infiltration of adoptively transferred T-cells into the tumor, which correlates with the tumor rejection in these mice *(83)*.

These observations made in murine models have been supported by preliminary data derived from a patient with metastatic HER-2-overexpressing breast cancer, who received ex vivo-activated autologous HER-2-specific CTL clones *(84)*. The clinical response evaluation correlated with the migration behavior of adoptively transferred T-cells. The trafficking of HER-2-specific T-cells evaluated by [111]indium labeling demonstrated that HER-2-specific T-cells migrated from the blood into the lung, and then to other organs including liver, spleen, and bone marrow. However, the transferred T-cells were not able to penetrate into the solid metastases in the liver. The assessment of the clinical responses revealed progressive disease of liver metastases despite T-cell therapy. Of note, disseminated tumor cells present in the patient's bone marrow before T-cell transfer were no longer detectable after T-cell transfer. This observation supports the hypothesis that adoptively transferred T-cells might be able to eradicate disseminated tumor cells, but not tumor cells forming a solid tumor mass.

The concept of targeting the tumor barrier for improved T-cell infiltration merits further investigation in clinical trials. The usage of combinational therapies, such as "angioimmunotherapies," will provide new knowledge on migration and efficacy of adoptively transferred tumor-reactive T-cells. It also strengthens the point that the monitoring of transferred T-cells is mandatory during combinatorial immunotherapies in order to observe the capacity of T-cells to infiltrate into the tumor. A panel of technologies have been developed that allow to monitor migration, survival, and function of ex vivo-stimulated T-cells following transfer, such as radiolabeling methods *(85)*, staining with fluorochrome-labeled MHC–peptide multimers *(19,32)*, immunohistochemistry of tumor biopsies *(17)*, gene marker studies *(10)*, and enzyme-linked immunospot *(86,87)*.

6. CONCLUDING REMARKS

More than 20 yr ago, it was shown in mice that cancer can be cured by adoptive T-cell transfer *(88)*. The first human studies regarding T-cell therapy were disappointing. Based on negative results derived from a series of clinical studies, the therapeutic potential of adoptive T-cell transfer for cancer patients has been questioned. However, during the last years, it has become clear that the knowledge drawn from murine experiments cannot easily be translated to the human situation. Human-oriented research is hindered by obstacles of both intrinsic and extrinsic nature, as outlined by Steinman and Mellman *(89)*. The intrinsic problems are related to the unique features of the individual human beings, such as the heterogeneity of the study population, the difficulty to biopsy critical tissues, and the time required for each "experiment." The extrinsic obstacles to human research are less scientific, but often dominate the planning and outcome of the human experiment. Examples for extrinsic hurdles include the requirement for good manufacturing practice, the diminishing species of professionals doing both clinical practice and scientific work, and the lack of talk between clinical departments and scientific institutes. These problems need to be solved in order to continue clinical research on cellular immunotherapy. The often cited "bench-to-bedside concept" must be replaced by turning the "translational research standard" into a "reciprocal research paradigm" as suggested by Drake and Pardoll *(90)*. The implication of this reciprocal model is the cooperative understanding for the complexity of T-cell-based immunotherapy. This will help to overcome intrinsic and extrinsic hurdles and will subsequently lead to exciting progress in the field of cancer treatment based on adoptive T-cell therapy.

ACKNOWLEDGMENTS

This work has been supported by grants from the Research Council of Germany SFB 456 (HB), the Wilhelm Sander Foundation (HB) and the GSF National Research Center for Environment and Health–Clinical Cooperation Group Vaccinology (HB, JN, KG, and DHB). We thank Wendy Batten and Matthias Wolfe for helpful discussion and critical reading of the manuscript.

REFERENCES

1. Gromet MA, Epstein WL, Blois MS. The regressing thin malignant melanoma: a distinctive lesion with metastatic potential. *Cancer* 1978; 42:2282–2292.
2. Old LJ. Cancer immunology: the search for specificity. *Cancer Res* 1981; 41:361–375.
3. Knuth A, Danowski B, Oettgen HF, Old LJ. T-cell mediated cytotoxicity against autologous malignant melanoma: analysis with interleukin-2-dependent T-cell cultures. *Proc Natl Acad Sci USA* 1984; 81: 3511–3515.

4. Lee PP, Yee C, Savage PA, et al. Characterization of circulating T cells specific for tumor-associated antigens in melanoma patients. *Nat Med* 1999; 5:677–685.
5. Pittet MJ, Zippelius A, Speiser DE, et al. Ex vivo IFN-γ secretion by circulating CD8 lymphocytes: implications of a novel approach for T cell monitoring in infectious and malignant diseases. *J Immunol* 2001; 166:7634–7640.
6. Ridge JP, DiRosa F, Matzinger P. A conditioned dendritic cell can be a temporal bridge between a CD4+ T-helper and a T-killer cell. *Nature* 1998; 303:474–478.
7. Stuhler G, Zobywalski A, Grünebach F, et al. Immune regulatory loops determine productive interactions within human T lymphocyte-dendritic cell clusters. *Proc Natl Acad Sci USA* 1999; 96:1532–1535.
8. Gilboa E. The makings of a tumor rejection antigen. *Immunity* 1999; 11:263–270.
9. Renkvist N, Castelli C, Robbins PF, Parmiani G. A listing of human tumor antigens recognized by T cells. *Cancer Immunol Immunother* 2001; 50:3–15.
10. Bollard CM, Aguilar L, Straathof KC, et al. Cytotoxic T lymphocyte therapy for Epstein-Barr virus Hodgkin's disease. *J Exp Med* 2004; 200:1623–1633.
11. Coulie PG, Brichard V, VanPel A, et al. A new gene coding for a differentiation antigen recognized by autologous cytolytic T lymphocytes on HLA-A2 melanomas. *J Exp Med* 1994; 180:35–42.
12. Slamon DJ, Clark GM. Amplification of c-erbB-2 and aggressive human breast tumors. *Science* 1988; 240:1795–1798.
13. Gotter J, Brors B, Hergenhahn M, Kyewski B. Medullary epithelial cells of the human thymus express a highly diverse selection of tissue-specific genes colocalized in chromosomal clusters. *J Exp Med* 2004; 199:155–166.
14. Wölfel T, Hauer M, Schneider J, et al. A p16INK-4a-insensitive CDK4 mutant targeted by cytolytic T lymphocytes in a human melanoma. *Science* 1995; 269:1281–1284.
15. Bendle GM, Holler A, Pang L-K, et al. Induction of unresponsiveness limits tumor protection by adoptively transferred MDM2-specific cytotoxic T lymphocytes. *Cancer Res* 2004; 64:8052–8056.
16. Nanda NK, Sercarz EE. Induction of anti-self-immunity to cure cancer. *Cell* 1995; 82:13–17.
17. Dudley ME, Wunderlich JR, Robbins PF, et al. Cancer regression and autoimmunity in patients after clonal repopulation with antitumor lymphocytes. *Science* 2002; 298:850–854.
18. Huang J, El-Gamil M, Dudley ME, Li YF, Rosenberg SA, Robbins PF. T cells associated with tumor regression recognize frameshift products of the CDKN2A tumor suppressor gene locus and a mutated HLA class I gene product. *J Immunol* 2004; 172:6057–6064.
19. Yee C, Thompson JA, Byrd D, et al. Adoptive T cell therapy using antigen-specific CD8+ T cell clones for the treatment of patients with metastatic melanoma: In vivo persistence, migration, and antitumor effect of transferred T cells. *PNAS* 2002; 99:16,168–16,173.
20. Yee C, Thompson JA, Roche P, et al. Melanocyte destruction after antigen-specific immunotherapy of melanoma: direct evidence of T cell-mediated vitiligo. *J Exp Med* 2000; 192:1637–1643.
21. Kolb HJ, Mittermüller J, Clemm C, et al. Donor leukocyte transfusions for treatment of recurrent chronic myelogenous leukemia in marrow transplant patients. *Blood* 1990; 76:2462–2465.
22. Goulmy E. Human histocompatibility antigens: new concepts for marrow transplantation and adoptive immunotherapy. *Immunol Rev* 1997; 157:125–140.
23. Marijt WA, Heemskerk MHM, Kloosterboer FM, et al. Hematopoiesis-restricted minor histocompatibility antigens HA-1- or HA-2-specific T cells can induce complete remissions of relapsed leukemia. *PNAS* 2003; 100:2742–2747.
24. Disis ML, Grabstein KH, Sleath PR, Cheever MA. Generation of immunity to the HER-2/*neu* oncogenic protein in patients with breast and ovarian cancer using a peptide-based vaccine. *Clin Cancer Res* 1999; 5:1289–1297.
25. Germeau C, Ma W, Schiavetti F, et al. High frequency of antitumor T cells in the blood of melanoma patients before and after vaccination with tumor antigens. *J Exp Med* 2005; 201:241–248.
26. Khong HT, Restifo NP. Natural selection of tumor variants in the generation of "tumor escape" phenotypes. *Nat Immunol* 2002; 3:999–1005.
27. Dunn GP, Bruce AT, Ikeda H, Old LJ, Schreiber RD. Cancer immunoediting: from immuno-surveillance to tumor escape. *Nat Immunol* 2002; 3:991–998.
28. Altman JD, Moss PA, Goulder PJ, et al. Phenotypic analysis of antigen-specific T lymphocytes. *Science* 1996; 274:94–96.
29. Busch DH, Philip IM, Vijh S, Pamer EG. Coordinate regulation of complex T cell populations responding to bacterial infection. *Immunity* 1998; 8:353–362.

30. Whelan JA, Dunbar PR, Price DA, et al. Specificity of CTL interactions with peptide-MHC class I tetrameric complexes is temperature dependent. *J Immunol* 1999; 163:4342–4348.
31. Daniels MA, Jameson SC. Critical role for CD8 in T cell receptor binding and activation by peptide/major histocompatibility complex multimers. *J Exp Med* 2000; 191:335–345.
32. Knabel M, Franz TJ, Schiemann M, et al. Reversible MHC multimer staining for functional isolation of T-cell populations and effective adoptive transfer. *Nat Med* 2002; 8:631–637.
33. Bernhard H, Schmidt B, Busch DH, Peschel C. Isolation and expansion of tumor-reactive cytotoxic T cell clones for adoptive immunotherapy. In: Ludewig B, Hoffmann MW, eds. *Adoptive Immunotherapies: Methods and Protocols, Methods Molecular Medicine, Volume 109*. Totowa, NJ: Humana Press. 2005: pp. 175–184.
34. Inaba K, Metlay JP, Crowley MT, Steinman RM. Dendritic cells pulsed with protein antigens in vitro can prime antigen-specific, MHC-restricted T cells *in situ*. *J Exp Med* 1990; 172:631–640.
35. Belz GT, Carbone FR, Heath WR. Cross-presentation of antigens by dendritic cells. *Crit Rev Immunol* 2002; 22:439–448.
36. Meyer zum Büschenfelde C, Nicklisch N, Rose-John S, Peschel C, Bernhard H. Generation of tumor-reactive cytotoxic T lymphocytes against the tumor-associated antigen HER2 using retrovirally transduced dendritic cells derived from CD34+ hemopoietic progenitor cells. *J Immunol* 2000; 165:4133–4140.
37. Ossendorp F, Mengedé E, Camps M, Filius R, Melief CJM. Specific T helper cell requirement for optimal induction of cytotoxic T lymphocytes against major histocompatibility complex class II negative tumors. *J Exp Med* 1998; 187:693–702.
38. Meyer zum Büschenfelde C, Metzger J, Hermann C, Nicklisch N, Peschel C, Bernhard H. The generation of both T killer and T helper cell clones specific for the tumor-associated antigen HER2 using retrovirally transduced dendritic cells. *J Immunol* 2001; 167:1712–1719.
39. Schuler-Thurner B, Dieckmann D, Keikavoussi P, et al. Mage-3 and influenza-matrix peptide-specific cytotoxic T cells are inducible in terminal stage HLA-A2.1+ melanoma patients by mature monocyte-derived dendritic cells. *J Immunol* 2000; 165:3492–3496.
40. Bernhard H, Knutson KL, Salazarm L, Schiffman K, Disis ML. Vaccination against the HER-2/*neu* oncogenic protein. *Endocr Relat Cancer* 2002; 9:33–44.
41. Palmer DC, Balasubramaniam S, Hanada K, et al. Vaccine-stimulated, adoptively transferred CD8+ T cells traffic indiscriminately and ubiquitously while mediating specific tumor destruction. *J Immunol* 2004; 173:7209–7216.
42. Lurquin C, Lethé B, DePlaen E, et al. Contrasting frequencies of antitumor and anti-vaccine T cells in metastases of a melanoma patient vaccinated with MAGE tumor antigen. *J Exp Med* 2005; 201:249–257.
43. Rosenberg SA, Lotze MT, Muul LM, et al. A progress report on the treatment of 157 patients with advanced cancer using lymphokine-activated killer cells and interleukin 2 or high-dose interleukin 2 alone. *N Engl J Med* 1987; 316:889–897.
44. Radoja S, Saio M, Schaer D, Koneru M, Vukmanovic S, Frey AB. CD8+ tumor-infiltrating T cells are deficient in perforin-mediated cytolytic activity due to defective microtubule-organizing center mobilization and lytic granule exocytosis. *J Immunol* 2001; 167:5042–5051.
45. Kolenko V, Wang Q, Riedy MC, et al. Tumor-induced suppression of T lymphocyte proliferation coincides with inhibition of Jak3 expression and IL-2 receptor signaling: role of soluble products from human renal cell carcinomas. *J Immunol* 1997; 159:3057–3067.
46. Riddell SR, Watanabe KS, Goodrich JM, Li CR, Agha ME, Greenberg PD. Restoration of viral immunity in immunodeficient humans by the adoptive transfer of T cell clones. *Science* 1992; 257:238–241.
47. Berger C, Huang M-L, Gough M, Greenberg PD, Riddell SR, Kiem H-P. Nonmyeloablative immunosuppressive regimen prolongs in vivo persistence of gene-modified autologous T cells in a nonhuman primate model. *J Virol* 2000; 75:799–808.
48. Riddell SR. Finding a place for tumor-specific T cells in targeted cancer therapy. *J Exp Med* 2004; 200:1533–1537.
49. Schumacher TNM. T-cell-receptor gene therapy. *Nat Rev Immunol* 2002; 2:512–519.
50. Engels B, Cam H, Schuler T, et al. Retroviral vectors for high-level transgene expression in T lymphocytes. *Hum Gene Ther* 2003; 14:1155–1168.
51. Morgan RA, Dudley ME, Yu YYL, et al. High efficiency TCR gene transfer into primary human lymphocytes affords avid recognition of melanoma tumor antigen glycoprotein 100 and does not alter the recognition of autologous melanoma antigens. *J Immunol* 2003; 171:3287–3295.

52. Clay TM, Custer MC, Sachs J, Hwu P, Rosenberg SA, Nishimura MI. Efficient transfer of a tumor antigen-reactive TCR to human peripheral blood lymphocytes confers anti-tumor reactivity. *J Immunol* 1999; 163:507.
53. Sadovnikova E, Jopling LA, Soo KS, Stauss HJ. Generation of human tumor-reactive cytotoxic T cells against peptides presented by non-self HLA class I molecules. *Eur J Immunol* 1998; 28:193–200.
54. Stanislawski T, Voss R-H, Lotz C, et al. Circumventing tolerance to a human MDM2-derived tumor antigen by TCR gene transfer. *Nat Immunol* 2001; 2:962–970.
55. Whitelegg A, Barber LD. The structural basis of T-cell allorecognition. *Tissue Antigens* 2004; 63:101–108.
56. Rossig C, Brenner MK. Chimeric T-cell receptors for the targeting of cancer cells. *Acta Haematol* 2003; 110:154–159.
57. Teng MW, Kershaw MH, Moeller M, Smyth MJ, Darcy PK. Immunotherapy of cancer using systemically delivered gene-modified human T lymphocytes. *Hum Gene Ther* 2004; 15:699–708.
58. Madakamutil LT, Christen U, Lena CJ, et al. CD8α-mediated survival and differentiation of CD8 memory T cell precursors. *Science* 2004; 304:590–593.
59. Powell DJ, Dudley ME, Robbins PF, Rosenberg SA. Transition of late-stage effector T cells to CD27+ CD28+ tumor-reactive effector memory T cells in humans after adoptive cell transfer therapy. *Blood* 2005; 105:241–250.
60. Huster KM, Busch V, Schiemann M, et al. Selective expression of IL-7 receptor on memory T cells identifies early CD40L-dependent generation of distinct CD8+ memory T cell subsets. *PNAS* 2004; 101:5610–5615.
61. Blattman JN, Greenberg PD. Cancer immunotherapy: a treatment for the masses. *Science* 2004; 305:200–205.
62. Ganss R, Arnold B, Hämmerling GJ. Overcoming tumor-intrinsic resistance to immune effector function. *Eur J Immunol* 2004; 34:2635–2641.
63. Walter EA, Greenberg PD, Gilbert MJ, et al. Reconstitution of cellular immunity against cytomegalovirus in recipients of allogeneic bone marrow by transfer of T-cell clones from the donor. *N Engl J Med* 1995; 333:1038–1044.
64. Zeng R, Spolski R, Finkelstein SE, et al. Synergy of IL-21 and IL-15 in regulating CD8+ T cell expansion and function. *J Exp Med* 2005; 201:139–148.
65. Roychowdhury S, May KF, Tzou KS, et al. Failed adoptive immunotherapy with tumor-specific T cells: reversal with low-dose interleukin 15 but not low-dose interleukin 2. *Cancer Res* 2004; 64:8062–8067.
66. DeVeerman M, Heirman C, VanMeirvenne S, et al. Retrovirally transduced bone marrow-derived dendritic cells require CD4+ T cell help to elicit protective and therapeutic antitumor immunity. *J Immunol* 1999; 162:144–151.
67. Greenberg PD, Kern DE, Cheever MA. Therapy of disseminated murine leukemia with cyclophosphamide and immune Lyt-1+,2– T cells. Tumor eradication does not require participation of cytotoxic T cells. *J Exp Med* 1985; 161:1122–1134.
68. Toes RE, Ossendorp F, Offringa R, Melief CJ. CD4 T cells and their role in antitumor immune responses. *J Exp Med* 1999; 189:693–702.
69. Disis ML, Calenoff E, McLaughlin G, et al. Existent T cell and antibody immunity to HER-2/*neu* protein in patients with breast cancer. *Cancer Res* 1994; 54:16–20.
70. Montgomery RB, Makary E, Schiffman K, Goodell V, Disis ML. Endogenous anti-HER2 antibodies block HER2 phosphorylation and signaling through extracellular signal-regulated kinase. *Cancer Res* 2005; 65:650–656.
71. Dhodapkar KM, Krasovsky J, Williamson B, Dhodapkar MV. Antitumor monoclonal antibodies enhance cross-presentation of cellular antigens and the generation of myeloma-specific killer T cells by dendritic cells. *J Exp Med* 2002; 195:125–133.
72. Meyer zum Büschenfelde C, Hermann C, Schmidt B, Peschel C, Bernhard H. Antihuman epidermal growth factor receptor 2 (HER2) monoclonal antibody trastuzumab enhances cytolytic activity of class I-restricted HER2-specific T lymphocytes against HER2-overexpressing tumor cells. *Cancer Res* 2002; 62:2244–2247.
73. Overwijk WW, Theoret MR, Finkelstein SE, et al. Tumor regression and autoimmunity after reversal of a functionally tolerant state of self-reactive CD8+ T cells. *J Exp Med* 2003; 198:569–580.
74. Matzinger P. An innate sense of danger. *Semin Immunol* 1998; 10:399–415.
75. Jameson SC. Maintaining the norm: T-cell homeostasis. *Nat Rev Immunol* 2002; 2:547–556.
76. Robbins PF, Dudley ME, Wunderlich J, et al. Persistence of transferred lymphocyte clonotypes correlates with cancer regression in patients receiving cell transfer therapy. *J Immunol* 2004; 173:7125–7130.

77. Zhou J, Dudley ME, Rosenberg SA, Robbins PF. Selective growth, in vitro and in vivo, of individual T cell clones from tumor-infiltrating lymphocytes obtained from patients with melanoma. *J Immunol* 2004; 173:7622–7629.
78. Sakaguchi S, Sakaguchi N, Shimizu J, et al. Immunologic tolerance maintained by CD25+ CD4+ regulatory T cells: their common role in controlling autoimmunity, tumor immunity, and transplantation tolerance. *Immunol Rev* 2001; 182:18–32.
79. Antony PA, Piccirillo CA, Akpinarli A, et al. CD8+ T cell immunity against a tumor/self-antigen is augmented by CD4+ T helper cells and hindered by naturally occurring T regulatory cells. *J Immunol* 2005; 174:2591–2601.
80. Ganss R, Limmer A, Sacher T, Arnold B, Hämmerling GJ. Autoaggression and tumor rejection: it takes more than self-specific T-cell activation. *Immunol Rev* 1999; 169:263–272.
81. Ganss R, Ryschich E, Klar E, Arnold B, Hämmerling GJ. Combination of T-cell therapy and trigger of inflammation induces remodeling of the vasculature and tumor eradication. *Cancer Res* 2002; 62: 1462–1470.
82. Kawarada Y, Ganss R, Garbi N, Sacher T, Arnold B, Hämmerling GJ. NK- and CD8+ T cell-mediated eradication of established tumors by peritumoral injection of CpG-containing oligodeoxynucleotides. *J Immunol* 2001; 167:5247–5253.
83. Yu P, Lee Y, Liu W, et al. Priming of naive T cells inside tumors leads to eradication of established tumors. *Nat Immunol* 2004; 5:141–149.
84. Bernhard H, Schmidt B, Busch DH, Harbeck N, Peschel C. Isolation and expansion of HER2-specific, tumor-reactive T cell clones from patients with HER2-overexpressing breast cancer: prospects for adoptive T cell therapy. *Breast Cancer Res Treat* 2002; 76(Suppl 1):S79.
85. Meidenbauer N, Marienhagen J, Laumer M, et al. Survival and tumor localization of adoptively transferred melan-A-specific T cells in melanoma patients. *J Immunol* 2003; 170:2161–2169.
86. Zhang Y, Sun Z, Nicolay H, et al. Monitoring of anti-vaccine CD4 T cell frequencies in melanoma patients vaccinated with a MAGE-3 protein. *J Immunol* 2005; 174:2404–2411.
87. Meyer RG, Britten CM, Siepmann U, et al. A phase I vaccination study with tyrosinase in patients with stage II melanoma using recombinant modified vaccinia virus Ankara (MVA-hTyr). *Cancer Immunol Immunother* 2005; 54:453–467.
88. Cheever M, Greenberg P, Fefer A. Specific adoptive therapy of established leukemia with syngeneic lymphocytes sequentially immunized in vivo and in vitro and nonspecifically expanded by culture with interleukin-2. *J Immunol* 1981; 126:1318–1322.
89. Steinman RM, Mellman I. Immunotherapy: bewitched, bothered, and bewildered no more. *Science* 2004; 305:197–200.
90. Drake CG, Pardoll DM. Tumor immunology towards a paradigm of reciprocal research. *Semin Cancer Biol* 2002; 12:73–80.

12

T-Cell Adoptive Immunotherapy of Cancer

From Translational Models to Clinical Significance

Peter A. Cohen, Mohamed Awad, and Suyu Shu

SUMMARY

The T-cells of many cancer patients are naturally sensitized to tumor-associated antigens or can readily be sensitized with even simple vaccination maneuvers. Adoptive immunotherapy (AIT) constitutes a coordinated effort to harvest and activate such T-cells, propagate them in culture, and adoptively transfer them back into patients as therapy. Recent modifications in culture techniques, coupled with the administration of nonmyeloablative chemotherapy, have markedly improved the clinical impact of AIT in melanoma patients. Whereas such results clearly validate the capacity of AIT to cause regression of macroscopic tumors, not just micrometastases, it remains difficult to predict which patients receiving autologous T-cells will respond to AIT, and it remains poorly understood why tumor regressions tend to be partial and impermanent at best in the clinical setting. Continuing insights from preclinical mouse studies illuminate the complexities of AIT treatment failure and point to many underlying correctable elements, such as the inadvertent coadoptive transfer of passenger suppressor cells and both positive and negative impacts of culture on effector T-cell trafficking and apoptotic susceptibility. In addition, current investigations demonstrate distinctive and often synergistic roles for CD4$^+$ and CD8$^+$ subsets in AIT, which have so far not been superseded merely by giving higher doses of either subset alone. Despite the currently nonoverlapping contributions of CD4$^+$ and CD8$^+$ subsets to therapeutic outcome, it is anticipated that continuing strides in culture techniques may ultimately produce CD4$^+$ and CD8$^+$ subsets that each possess true stand-alone potency as adoptive monotherapy.

Key Words: Adoptive immunotherapy; dendritic cells; tumor-infiltrating lymphocytes; suppressor T-cells.

1. INTRODUCTION

Adoptive immunotherapy (AIT) is a treatment strategy for cancer in which T-cells derived from tumor-bearing hosts are activated and numerically expanded, and then reinfused into the host with a goal of obtaining tumor regressions *(1,2)*. Pioneering investigations in the late 1970s demonstrated that noncultured or briefly cultured T-cells from animals vaccinated to a syngeneic transplantable tumor could be adoptively transferred to cure syngeneic animals of the same tumor *(3)*. Such transferable therapeutic

From: *Cancer Drug Discovery and Development: Immunotherapy of Cancer*
Edited by: M. L. Disis © Humana Press Inc., Totowa, NJ

potency proved to reside in the T-cell component of therapy and was variably attributable to the transfer of CD4$^+$ and/or CD8$^+$ T-cells (3–10). After it became apparent that the therapeutic impacts of AIT were dose-dependent, a multi-investigator effort emerged to identify culture techniques that would link T-cell numeric expansion to preserved therapeutic potency (11–15). This effort remains ongoing and is the subject of this chapter.

The translational value of preclinical animal tumor models for AIT clinical trials has long been recognized. Mouse models such as the weakly immunogenic National Cancer Institute (NCI) methylcholanthrene sarcoma series have proved particularly predictive during the past 20 yr for clinical trials in melanoma (13,16,17). With the opportunity for scrutiny in retrospect, it is apparent that the outcomes of failed trials could largely have been anticipated from the mouse work on which they were based (1,2). Conversely, recent therapeutic breakthroughs in the same animal tumor models serve to validate scientifically the exciting results now being observed in an ongoing melanoma trial at the NCI Surgery Branch (18,19). In composite, the progress observed in both animal models and clinical trials has led to a striking surge of optimism for the clinical future of AIT.

Our main goal in this chapter is to provide a historical perspective on animal tumor models and clinical trials in AIT that portrays the challenges confronted, the puzzles solved, and the therapeutic advances that fuel the current optimism. This chapter will particularly focus on the ways in which CD4$^+$ and CD8$^+$ T-cell subsets demonstrate either independence or interdependence when they are employed as AIT to treat macroscopic established tumors. Historically, it has proved easier to culture expand antitumor CD8$^+$ effector T-cells (T$_E$s) than CD4$^+$ T$_E$s, but recent advances in both mouse and human cultures indicate that tumor-specific CD4$^+$ T$_E$s can, in fact, be numerically expanded, maintained in culture, and impact the therapeutic outcome of AIT (1,18–24). Of necessity, comparative analyses of CD4$^+$ and CD8$^+$ T$_E$ function are observational, and are highly contingent to not only the tumor models or patients being studied, but also to the experimental conditions under which the T-cells are prepared for therapy. Several trends will nonetheless be apparent among these observations:

1. Improving culture conditions have given rise to more frequent observations of CD4$^+$ and CD8$^+$ subset independence.
2. Currently achievable CD4$^+$ and CD8$^+$ subsets still demonstrate functional differences and complementarity, even though future culture advances may ultimately eradicate such differences.
3. The role of nonmyeloablative chemotherapy or radiotherapy in maximizing responses to AIT will be highlighted, because this phenomenon long observed in animal models is finally proving to play a pivotal role in several clinical trials.

The historical challenges to successful AIT in animal models and patients have been elaborated in several recent reviews (1,2), but must be briefly recounted here to underscore several major challenges that persist to present day.

2. PRECLINICAL MODELS OF AIT: THE HISTORICAL PERSPECTIVE

2.1. Formative AIT Challenges:
Generating Therapeutically Potent T-Cells From Tumor-Bearing Mice

In pioneering experiments, it proved easiest to generate tumor-specific T$_E$s when mice were challenged with readily rejectable tumor cells. Such facilitated rejection was observed when the challenging tumors expressed highly immunogenic viral antigens (Ags), and/or when tumor growth was preattenuated by irradiation *(3–10)*. To extend T_{ES} sensitization to less-antigenic tumor models more representative of human cancer, mice were vaccinated with a mix of viable tumor cells and killed *Corynebacterium parvum* bacteria *(25)*, the latter added to facilitate complete host rejection of the growing tumor challenge. T-cells freshly obtained from successfully vaccinated mice proved capable of mediating rejection of both established pulmonary and established extrapulmonary tumors when transferred into syngeneic mice bearing the relevant tumor *(1,2,25)*. Such fresh, uncultured T-cells constituted therapeutically effective AIT even without coadministration of adjunct cytokines, such as recombinant interleukin (rIL)-2. Nonetheless, with the exception of early pulmonary tumors, efficacy required that recipients receive adjunct nonmyeloablative irradiation (500 cGy) or chemotherapy, such as cyclophosphamide (100 mg/kg) *(1,2,25–27)*. The mechanisms by which such adjuncts facilitated AIT were not understood, but their predominant impact was clearly on normal host cells, because irradiation was often fully potentiating even when administered before the tumor challenge *(28)*.

Considerable excitement was engendered by the therapeutic potency of such T_{ES}, but enthusiasm was tempered by several additional observations. It was observed that when fresh T_{ES} were carried in culture for a period as brief as 5 d before adoptive transfer, their efficacy against extrapulmonary tumors became dependent not only on adjunct nonmyeloablative radiation/chemotherapy, but also on adjunct systemic administration of rIL-2 *(13)*. Moreover, extending culture beyond 5 d led to a marked loss of therapeutic efficacy against extrapulmonary tumors, whether or not rIL-2 was administered *(29)*. Such extended culture also caused T_{ES} to become relatively or completely ineffective against even pulmonary tumors unless adjuvant rIL-2 was coadministered to the recipient host *(27,30)*.

It was not immediately clear why the act of culturing T-cells *per se* led to a progressive diminution in therapeutic potency. It was nonetheless also apparent from the translational perspective that culture expansion would remain an unavoidable component of AIT. Even in the case of fresh T-cells from vaccinated mice, therapeutic efficacy proved highly dose-dependent, defining a role for in vitro numeric expansion if therapeutic potency could also be maintained. Second, in contrast to fresh T-cells from vaccinated mice, T-cells from tumor-bearing mice displayed no therapeutic potency unless they were first culture-activated in rIL-2 before adoptive transfer *(29)*. Unsurprisingly, the therapeutic efficacy of T_{ES} cultured from tumor-bearing mice was as limited as that observed when T_{ES} were cultured from vaccinated mice, i.e., markedly reduced efficacy against extrapulmonary tumors and highly dependent on the coadministration of adjunct IL-2 *(29)*. It was therefore apparent that new techniques would need to be developed before cultured T-cells could constitute truly effective AIT.

2.2. Potentially Reversible Effector T-Cell Abnormalities Are Identified in the Tumor-Bearing Host

In the 1990s, investigators began to report the occurrence of T-cell receptor (TCR) signal transduction abnormalities when T-cells were harvested from tumor-bearing animals and cancer patients, rendering more comprehensible the difficulties encountered in isolating therapeutically active fresh T-cells from such hosts *(31–34)*. Further studies demonstrated that impaired effector function was more frequent in tumor-bearing hosts than a failure to sensitize to tumor Ags *(35–39)*. Such observations raised the hope that even in the absence of clinically detectable T_E responses, there could be steady-state sources of T_E precursors available for remedial in vitro activation *(40,41)*.

It is now understood that most natural T-cell sensitization to tumor Ags occurs at a site removed from the tumor bed itself, namely tumor-draining lymph nodes (TDLNs). Extirpation experiments have demonstrated that the tumor bed itself need only be present for 3 d to enable such T-cell sensitization, whereas TDLNs must remain undisturbed for almost 2 wk to propagate complete resistance to subsequent tumor challenges *(42)*. Such data support the importance of a transient event at the tumor site, followed by a sustained event at the TDLNs, after which sensitized T-cells distribute much more widely in the host.

That transient event within the tumor bed often appears to be processing of tumor-associated Ags by transiting host Ag-presenting cells (APCs), which subsequently transport the Ags to TDLNs. T-cell sensitization within TDLNs occurs regardless of whether tumor cells themselves actually metastasize to the lymph nodes. Experiments from several groups confirm the capacity of host APCs to "crosspresent" tumor Ags both to CD4+ and to CD8+ T-cells *(1,2,18,43)*. Dendritic cells (DCs) are the host APCs best equipped physiologically to accomplish the multiple stepwise migrations necessary for this sequence of events *(1,2,18,44,45)*.

Within TDLNs, proliferative expansion of antitumor T-cells proceeds despite the looming presence of growing upstream tumor. Somewhat surprisingly, faster-growing upstream tumor burdens appear to hasten and even enhance the phase of T_E sensitization and proliferative expansion within TDLNs, possibly because of a more robust delivery of tumor Ags to the TDLNs by DCs *(40,41)*. In fact, challenges with growing tumors are more effective for sensitization than challenges with irradiated (nongrowing) tumor cells. Current evidence suggests that proliferation of the CD8+ component in TDLNs is often strongly facilitated by activation of the CD4+ subset *(40,41)*. This is consistent with several studies that have demonstrated that CD4+ T-cells can "condition" DCs through CD40–CD40 ligand or other interactions to promote CD8+ T-cell sensitization *(46–49)*. Nonetheless, at least a subset of CD8+ T-cells is helper-independent, and is effectively sensitized to tumor Ags even in CD4 knockout animals *(18,40)*.

Although a persistent tumor burden is permissive and even stimulatory for T-cell sensitization, it also typically inhibits subsequent mounting of the effector response. In many instances, such effector inhibition is not systemic, but rather confined to the end target, e.g., the tumor bed. As demonstrated by Wick et al., concomitant challenges of normal skin allografts that are antigenically crossreactive with tumor can still be rejected, confirming the tumor host's enduring capacity for an undiminished effector response *(50)*. Therefore, it is not surprising that upstream tumor progression does not prevent sensitized T-cells from redistributing to extranodal locations, including even to the tumor bed itself. In weakly immunogenic mouse tumor models, sensitized T-cells can be cultured out both from TDLNs and from the growing tumor bed, despite the absence of a therapeutically evident antitumor response *(26,51,52)*. Similarly, the ability to culture activate tumor-specific T-cells from the long-standing nodules of melanoma patients (called tumor-infiltrating lymphocytes [TILs]) demonstrates that even tumor progression does not preclude T-cell sensitization, redistribution in the patient, and continuing accumulation within diverse tumor beds *(19)*.

A growing tumor's capacity to evade immune rejection through effector fatigue was elegantly demonstrated by Speiser et al. in a rat model of spontaneous insulinoma development *(35)*. Mice were rendered transgenic for the tumor-promoting simian virus 40 virus

Tag, expressed under control of the rat insulin promoter. Resultant "spontaneous" insulinomas were rendered more antigenic by crossing these rats with rats transgenic for a strongly antigenic viral glycoprotein (lymphocytic choriomeningitis virus glycoprotein [LCMV-GP]) also under rat insulin promoter control. Finally, these rats were crossed with rats transgenic for a TCR enabling major histocompatibility complex (MHC) class I-restricted recognition of an LCMV-GP-derived peptide. The latter rats spontaneously developed insulinomas expressing LCMV-GP, but also possessed CD8+ T-cells capable of recognizing the tumor so long as tumor cells continued to express LCMV-GP. These rats displayed no spontaneous tumor rejection, but did display transient partial tumor regressions when they were vaccine challenged with intact LCMV virus. Such vaccination acutely increased the anti-LCMV cytolytic activity of CD8+ T-cells, but this activity spontaneously subsided in the host after several weeks, with concomitant reinitiation of tumor progression. Remarkably, however, repetitive vaccinations resulted in additional episodes of transient tumor regressions and cytolytic reactivation of anti-LCMV CD8+ T-cells, indicating that tumor escape was not caused by apoptotic deletion of the anti-LCMV CD8+ T-cell repertoire. Furthermore, the insulinomas continued to express LCMV-GP at each subsequent recurrence, demonstrating that tumor escape was not accomplished through deleted expression of LCMV-GP. Anti-LCMV CD8+ T-cells remained in evidence during each subsequent tumor progression, but no longer in a fully activated effector state *(35)*.

These studies clearly demonstrated that even continuous expression of strong viral Ags by established tumors was insufficient to stimulate a sustained and strongly activated T_E response. Whereas the mechanism of effector fatigue remained unclear, transiently successful activations or reactivations of the effector response could readily be accomplished by presenting the Ags more potently and repetitively in the form of virus infection *(35)*. Similar observations have recently been extended to the activation and reactivations of *Pmel 1* transgenic T-cells in the B16 tumor model *(53,54)*.

Additional studies from Shrikant et al. and Deeths et al. have elegantly monitored the sequence of events that occur when naïve CD8+ T-cells are first exposed to an antigenically relevant tumor challenge *(37–39)*. CD8+ T-cells from OT1 transgenic mice express TCRs that recognize an MHC class I-restricted ovalbumin (OVA) peptide, and enable recognition of syngeneic EL-4 lymphoma transfected to express OVA (EL-4-OVA). Such T-cells are Thy 1.2^{pos}, enabling precise monitoring of their fate when they are adoptively transferred into otherwise syngeneic Thy 1.1^{pos} hosts. One day after adoptive transfer of naïve OT1 CD8+ T-cells, recipient mice were challenged intraperitoneally with EL-4-OVA or parent EL-4.

The adoptively transferred naïve OT1 CD8+ T-cells transiently accumulated at the intraperitoneal site of tumor, increased in numbers, and controlled tumor growth when the challenge was the antigenically relevant EL4-OVA, but not the unrecognized parent line. Such T-cell activation included conversion from a naïve to a memory (CD44^{pos}) phenotype. However, this activation did not result in a sustained antitumor response. Rather, the OT1 CD8+ T-cells activated within the peritoneum spontaneously migrated away from the tumor challenge to remote lymphoid locations, resulting in unfettered tumor progression. When tumor-vacating OT1 CD8+ T-cells were later recovered from host spleen, they retained their capacity to lyse specifically EL-4-OVA targets, but had lost their capacity to proliferate spontaneously when exposed to OVA peptide. This was deemed split anergy, or antigen-induced nonresponsiveness (AINR) *(38)*.

Subsequent studies demonstrated that elements of such AINR reflected a normal T-cell response to Ag encounter, rather than a pathological aberration of the tumor environment *(37)*. Naïve CD8+ T-cells subjected in vitro to primary TCR stimulation and co-stimulation responded with transient IL-2 production, proliferation, interferon (IFN)-γ production, and acquisition of lytic activity against the appropriate targets. After several additional days of culture, however, proliferation ceased, yielding CD8+ T-cells that could be restimulated to produce IFN-γ or lyse targets, but not to produce IL-2 or proliferate. Addition of exogenous rIL-2 reversed such split anergy and transiently enabled CD8+ T-cells not only to produce IL-2 and proliferate on TCR restimulation, but also transiently to forego co-stimulatory requirements *(37)*. Parallel in vivo data suggested that after primary activation of naive CD8+ T-cells, CD4+ T-cells might normally be required to provide a burst of exogenous IL-2 and reverse split anergy, thereby freeing memory CD8+ to undergo a period of reduced signaling requirements and autocrine IL-2-driven proliferation *(39)*. Nonetheless, similar episodes of "split anergy" have also been described for CD4+ T-cells themselves, suggesting a more complicated phenomenon than mere CD4+ "helper dependence" *(37)*.

In summary, preclinical tumor models have graphically illustrated the challenge of sustaining an effective antitumor response, even when initial sensitization and effector activation are brisk and effective due to physiological fatigue and/or pathological blunting of the effector response.

2.3. In Vitro Anti-Cd3 Activation Renders Cultured T-Cells From Tumor-Bearing Mice Therapeutically Equivalent to Fresh T-Cells From Vaccinated Mice

In an attempt both to reverse T-cell abnormalities, such as AINR, and to numerically expand competent T_Es, Shu and coworkers incorporated novel culture-activation stimuli, such as immobilized anti-CD3 monoclonal antibody (MAb) or bacterial superantigens *(16,32,55–74)*. The addition of such novel polyclonal stimuli to conventional rIL-2 treatment demonstrably reversed tumor-induced T-cell signaling abnormalities *(32)*. Furthermore, for the first time in AIT experiments, T-cells culture-activated from tumor-bearing mice displayed a therapeutic potency equivalent or superior to fresh T-cells from tumor-vaccinated mice *(16,20,75)*. Anti-CD3 or superantigen-activated TDLN T_Es could be adoptively transferred to cure tumors established not only at the pulmonary location, but even at extrapulmonary locations, such as the brain, a location notorious as an immunotherapy-resistant relapse site in cancer patients *(20,76)*. Furthermore, T_Es activated by these novel culture methods did not require co-administration of rIL-2 or other cytokines for their therapeutic effect *(16,20,75)*. As previously observed for fresh T-cells from vaccinated mice, however, the global efficacy of anti-CD3 activated T_Es depended on, or was highly facilitated by, nonmyeloablative irradiation or chemotherapy *(16,18,20,75)*.

Important consequences of this culture breakthrough included the first successful in vitro propagations of both CD4+ and helper-independent CD8+ T_Es from tumor-bearing mice *(18,20)*. Similarly potent CD4+ T-cells had previously been detected in vaccinated but not in tumor-bearing mice *(1,17,77)*. Anti-tumor CD8+ T-cells with helper-independent features had previously been detected only when vaccinations included strong viral Ags *(1,2,12,78)*. Now, for the first time, it was apparent that potent antitumor CD4+ T-cells and helper-independent CD8+ T-cells were also naturally sensitized and present as pre-effector

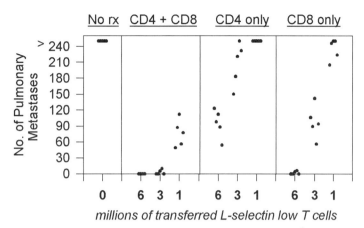

Fig. 1. Treatment of 10-d pulmonary metastases with activated L-selectin^low tumor-draining lymph node (TDLN) effector T-cell subsets. Syngeneic C57BL/6 (B6) mice were injected with viable methylcholanthrene (MCA)-205 cells and TDLNs were harvested 12 d later. L-selectin^low TDLN T-cells containing both CD4+ and CD8+ cells ("CD4+CD8"), as well as individual L-selectin^low CD4+ and CD8+ subsets ("CD4","CD8") were isolated for 5-d culture-activation with anti-CD3/recombinant interleukin-2. Each cultured T-cell group was harvested and adoptively transferred into syngeneic mice with 10-d established (advanced) MCA-205 pulmonary metastases. Recipient mice received 500 cGy nonmyeloablative radiation therapy before adoptive transfer. Mice received 1 million (1E6), 3E6, or 6E6 T-cells. Ordinate shows number of pulmonary metastases observed in mice sacrificed 11 d after adoptive therapy. Each point represents a single mouse (five mice per treatment group). Mice received no recombinant interleukin-2 treatment during adoptive therapy.

T-cells even in mice bearing progressive, weakly immunogenic tumors *(18,20)*. These potent pre-effectors required removal from the tumor host and in vitro activation with anti-CD3 and rIL-2 to unmask their full effector potency, but after such culture activation, either T-cell subset could often be administered as adoptive monotherapy without rIL-2 to achieve anatomically unrestricted tumor rejection (Figs. 1–6, 8 and 9 *[18,79]*).

3. PRECLINICAL MODELS OF AIT: THE CURRENT PERSPECTIVE

3.1. Antitumor L-Selectin^low Memory T_ES

Characterization of the highly potent antitumor CD4+ T-cells and helper-independent CD8+ T-cells naturally sensitized in TDLNs was facilitated by their distinctly low expression of the cell surface glycoprotein L-selectin (CD62L), which affords convenient isolation of these populations *(1,18,20)*. The per-cell therapeutic potency of purified L-selectin^low T-cells is logarithmically greater than that of unfractionated TDLN T-cells, and removal of L-selectin^high TDLN T-cells before culture activation has either no impact or a derepressive impact on subsequent adoptive therapy (*see* Subheading 5.3. *[1,18,20,29, 43,80,81]*). Because of their enhanced capacity to peripheralize, redistribute into tumors at any anatomic location, and proliferate intratumorally *(79,82–84)*, such L-selectin^low T_ES appear to be analogous to the L-selectin^low, CCR7^low memory T_ES recently described in nontumor studies *(85–87)*.

A cell surface glycoprotein critically involved in the extravasation of cells from the bloodstream, L-selectin manifests a strong, lectin-like affinity for the postcapillary venules

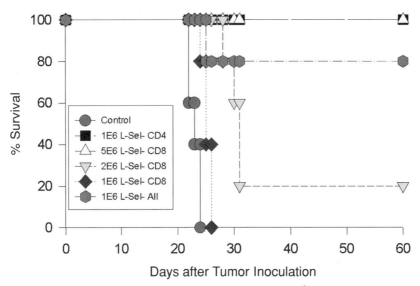

Fig. 2. Treatment of d 3 intracranial tumors with activated L-selectin^{low} tumor-draining lymph node (TDLN) effector T-cell subsets. L-Selectin^{low} T-cells unfractionated for CD4 and CD8, L-selectin^{low} CD4$^+$ T-cells, and L-selectin^{low} CD8$^+$ T-cells were each prepared from freshly harvested TDLN cells of B6 mice bearing syngeneic 12-d methylcholanthrene-205 tumors. Following 5-d culture activation with anti-CD3/interleukin-2, each T-cell group was harvested and administered to sublethally irradiated (500 cGy) B6 mice bearing d 3 intracranial tumors. The graph shows long-term survival of mice with intracranial methylcholanthrene-205 treated with 1 million (1E6) L-selectin^{low} T-cells unfractionated for CD4 and CD8 ("L-Sel-All"), 1E6 L-selectin^{low} CD4$^+$ T-cells ("L-Sel-CD4"), or 1E6, 2E6, or 5E6 L-selectin^{low} CD8$^+$ T-cells ("L-Sel-CD8)". Historically, mice surviving symptom-free at d 60 are cured in this model. Mice received no recombinant interleukin-2 treatment during adoptive therapy.

of peripheral lymph nodes *(82)*. Because L-selectin expression thus confers a homing proclivity for peripheral lymph nodes, it is not surprising that T-cells found in peripheral lymph nodes are predominantly L-selectin^{high}. However, because antigenic activation of T-cells commonly leads to downregulated L-selectin expression *(88,89)*, it is also unsurprising that the subset of T-cells with low L-selectin expression at TDLN harvest are the identified source of sensitized, tumor-specific T_E precursors *(1)*. Because L-selectin^{low} T-cells have a reduced affinity for peripheral lymph node postcapillary venules, they may conversely possess a greater freedom to traffic to extranodal locations, hence, an increased probability of random entry into tumor beds at any anatomic location *(1)*. This as yet unproven hypothesis is strongly supported by the observation that both tumor-specific and antigenically irrelevant L-selectin^{low} T-cells traffic into tumors at a much higher frequency than L-selectin^{high} T-cells following adoptive transfer *(43,82)*. However, only sensitized, tumor-specific L-selectin^{low} T-cells are subsequently observed to proliferate at a higher frequency within the tumor bed and mediate tumor rejection *(82,83)*.

As observed for L-selectin^{high} T-cells, accessory cells such as lymphokine-activated killer cells and tumoricidal, activated macrophages also appear to have a limited capacity to traffic into tumors, at least in the absence of supervisory signals from T-cells *(90,91)*. Such observations underscore the possibility that many or most components of cell-mediated immunity depend on the superior initial capacity of L-selectin^{low}, memory effec-

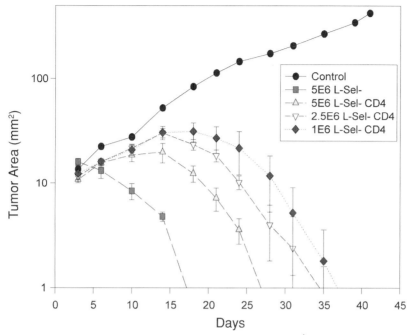

Fig. 3. Treatment of 3-d subcutaneous tumors with activated L-selectin^low tumor-draining lymph node effector T-cells: CD4+ subset vs combined CD4+ plus CD8+ T-cells. Syngeneic B6 mice were injected with viable methylcholanthrene-205 cells and tumor-draining lymph nodes harvested on d 9 to prepare purified L-selectin^low T-cells, either unfractionated for CD4 and CD8 or purified L-selectin^low CD4+ T-cells. On d 5 after anti-CD3/interleukin-2 culture activation, T-cell groups were harvested and adoptively transferred to treat syngeneic mice with 3-d established subcutaneous tumors. Recipient mice received 500 cGy before adoptive transfer. Mice received no recombinant inter-leukin-2 treatment during adoptive therapy. Subsequent growth of the subcutaneous tumors was serially evaluated. Ordinate displays tumor area determined by two perpendicular caliper measurements; abscissa displays the d following tumor inoculation. Symbols on each line display average tumor measurement of each treatment group at particular time points, five mice per treatment group, with standard deviation displayed. Data are shown in log scale to facilitate visualization of differences between groups at early time points.

tor-type T-cells to randomly enter tumor beds, react with tumor Ags, and launch a cytokine/chemokine cascade to recruit and activate the other cellular elements. An additional remarkable property of L-selectin^low T-cells is their ability to sustain and augment an antitumor response even when their initial presence in a tumor is scant. In fact, a tumor may continue to grow progressively for several weeks before L-selectin^low T-cell-initiated tumor rejection becomes detectable (*see* Fig. 3 *[18]*). The surprising capacity of L-selectin^low T-cells, especially the CD4+ subset, to proliferate within the tumor bed like memory effector T-cells *(85–87)* suggests that they are able to augment their own presence as an initial effector tactic *(18,83)*. Although L-selectin^low CD8+ T_ES are likely often to implement cytolytic T-lymphocyte (CTL) activity *(92)*, tumor-specific L-selectin^low T-cells can also remain therapeutically effective even when direct MHC-restricted interactions with tumor cells are rendered impossible either by downregulated tumor MHC expression or by experimentally generated MHC mismatches *(93)*.

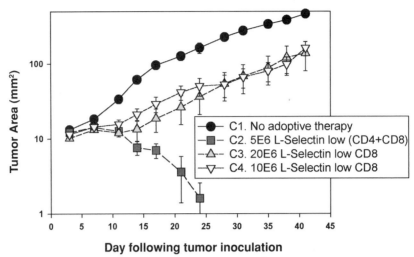

Fig. 4. Treatment of 3-d subcutaneous tumors with L-selectin^low tumor-draining lymph node effector T-cells: CD8^+ subset vs combined CD4^+ plus CD8^+ T-cells. Methods are the same as in Fig. 3, except adoptive immunotherapy with purified L-selectin^low CD8^+ subset shown. Note that for the highest CD8^+ T-cell dose (20E6), two of five mice were cured, no cures at lower doses.

3.2. Overlapping and Divergent Properties of L-Selectin^low CD4^+ and CD8^+ T_E Subsets

L-Selectin^low CD4^+ and CD8^+ T_E subsets possess several striking similarities. Knockout mouse studies have confirmed that CD8^+ L-selectin^low antitumor T-cells can be generated in the absence of CD4^+ T-cells, and vice versa, although therapeutic synergy is evident when both subsets are copresent during sensitization and/or adoptive therapy (*see* Figs. 1 and 5 *[18]*). Although some anatomic disparities are evident (discussed in following paragraphs), each anti-CD3 activated subset has proved therapeutically effective as stand-alone "adoptive monotherapy," without a need for IL-2 co-administration (e.g., *see* Figs. 1–4 *[1,8,20,94]*). Following anti-CD3 activation, each subset produces IFN-γ and granulocyte-macrophage colony-stimulating factor when cocultured with a cellular digest of relevant (sensitizing) tumor, but there is a typical absence or much lower production of IL-2, tumor necrosis factor-α, IL-4, and IL-10, as well as an absence of direct tumor target lysis (*[18] see* Fig. 7). Despite this highly circumscribed in vitro response to tumor contact at the end of culture activation, both CD4^+ and CD8^+ L-selectin^low T-cells retain the capacity for more diverse cytokine production, including IL-2, when restimulated with anti-CD3 rather than tumor digest at the end of culture *(20)*.

Despite these similarities, it is also apparent that L-selectin^low CD4^+ and CD8^+ T-cells possess significant functional differences, beginning with different practical requirements for recognizing tumor Ags. L-Selectin^low antitumor CD8^+ helper-independent T_ES produce IFN-γ when exposed either to relevant MHC class I-expressing tumor targets or to tumor-associated macrophages (TAMs); in contrast, L-selectin^low CD4^+ T-cells fail to react with relevant, MHC class II nonexpressing tumor, but produce IFN-γ when exposed to relevant MHC class II^pos TAMs (*see* Fig. 7 *[18]*). The ability to interact directly with MHC class I^pos/II^neg tumor cells may sometimes confer a therapeutic advantage to L-selectin^low CD8^+ T-cells by rendering perforin-mediated tumor cell lysis feasible. Nonetheless, AIT

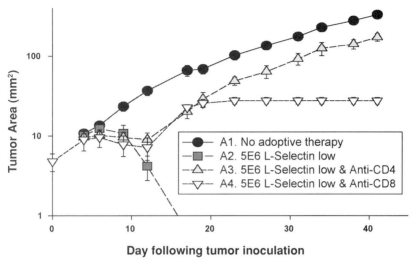

Day following tumor inoculation

Fig. 5. Effects of in vivo CD4 or CD8 depletion on treatment of 3-d subcutaneous tumor with combined CD4$^+$ plus CD8$^+$ L-selectin^{low} tumor-draining lymph node effector T-cells. Methods are the same as in Fig. 3. Mice received no adoptive therapy or 5×106 (5E6) L-selectin^{low} T-cells unfractionated for CD4 and CD8; in addition, some groups receiving T-cells received concomitant in vivo monoclonal antibody depletion ("L-Selectin low"), either anti-CD4 ("L-Selectin low & Anti-CD4"), or anti-CD8 ("L-Selectin low & Anti-CD8") monoclonal antibody depletion.

studies employing TDLN T-cells from perforin-knockout mice have demonstrated that such perforin-dependent "CTL" activity is not always essential to tumor rejection *(92,95)*.

Despite the capacities of either CD4$^+$ or CD8$^+$ L-selectin^{low} T_E subsets to provide effective adoptive monotherapy, it is evident that these subsets are not simply interchangeable as therapy. For example, adoptively transferred L-selectin^{low} CD4$^+$ T-cells have proved relatively more potent on a cell-number basis for eradicating 3-d established intracranial tumors (*see* Fig. 2), whereas L-selectin^{low} CD8$^+$ T-cells have proved more effective against 10-d pulmonary metastases (*see* Fig. 1). The most extreme differences in therapeutic performance have so far been observed for established subcutaneous tumors, probably reflecting the lower trafficking efficiency of even standardly prepared L-selectin^{low} T-cells into tumors at this anatomic site *(82)*. Although purified CD4$^+$ and CD8$^+$ L-selectin^{low} subsets are each therapeutically active against subcutaneous tumors, only the L-selectin^{low} CD4$^+$ T-cell subset has been observed to provide consistently curative adoptive therapy as single-agent therapy (*see* Figs. 3 and 4 *[18]*). The physiological basis for these observed therapeutic disparities is incompletely understood, but some mechanistic insights have already proved possible.

3.3. Mechanisms of Tumor Rejection by L-Selectin^{low} CD4$^+$ T-cells

The "helper" role of CD4$^+$ T-cells in the initial generation of CD8$^+$ CTL-type responses has long been recognized. Many animal studies have now confirmed the capacity of CD4$^+$ T-cells to facilitate initial CD8$^+$ T-cell sensitization and numeric expansion, even in the tumor-bearing setting, typically through conditioning of host APCs, such as DCs, to better prime CD8$^+$ responses *(40,48,49,96)*. Furthermore, CD4$^+$ T-cells can perform a late "helper" function even during the effector stage of tumor and/or allograft rejection by facilitating the accumulation and activation of CD8+ T-cells in the target tissue *(40,97– 99)*. However, additional roles for CD4+ T-cells apart from their helper function for CD8+ T-cells have been better appreciated in recent years. Following T-cell sensitization by vaccination maneuvers, it has been demonstrated in knockout models that sensitized CD4+ T-cells themselves play an effector role in rejecting specific tumor challenges whether or not CD8+ T-cells are present *(100)*. CD4+ effector function includes cytokine-mediated activation of accessory cells, such as host macrophages and eosinophils, and it is apparent that either T1- or T2-type cytokines can contribute to such tumor rejection *(99,100)*.

Even when CD4+ T-cells play such an effector role, it is typically not accomplished through direct MHC-restricted contact with tumor cells, at least not in the majority of animal tumor models. This is because, in contrast to human tumor cells, most studied mouse and rat tumor cells resolutely fail to express MHC class II molecules even following IFN-γ exposure *(93)*. Despite the fact that direct interactions with MHC class II^{neg} tumor cells are anomalous for CD4+ T_Es *(101,102)*, adoptively transferred L-selectin^{low} CD4+ T_Es still display therapeutic efficacy that can even exceed that observed for CD8+ T_Es *(see* Figs. 2 and 3). It is likely in such models that CD4+ T_E recognition of tumor Ags is limited to crosspresentation via host APCs *(see* Fig. 4). This limitation is likely to occur not only during initial sensitization at TDLNs, but also during the intratumoral "effector" stage of recognition, when crosspresenting host cells, such as TAMs, DCs, or other stromal components, may be the essential presenters of tumor Ags *(see* Fig. 7 *[18])*.

Recent investigations have demonstrated that L-selectin^{low} CD4+ T_Es have an enhanced capacity to proliferate intratumorally relative to CD8+ T_Es, particularly following the administration of nonmyeloablative irradiation *(83)*. Such an enhanced proliferative capacity may explain the ability of L-selectin^{low} CD4+ T_Es to persist and achieve delayed subcutaneous tumor rejection, even when T_E dosing is initially insufficient to prevent several weeks of continued tumor growth. Even at much higher doses of CD4+ T_Es, however, complete tumor rejection is not observed when the host is depleted of CD8+ T-cells *(see* Fig. 5), or when the recipient host is a CD4 and/or a CD8 knockout (Fig. 6). Therefore, curative CD4+ T_E adoptive monotherapy depends on an intact opportunity for the transferred CD4+ cells to recruit additional host CD4+ and CD8+ T-cells *(18,53)*. Even when host CD4+ and CD8+ T-cells are unavailable for recruitment, CD4+ T_E adoptive monotherapy can achieve a remarkable degree of long-term tumor regression or tumor stasis, if not actual cure *(see* Figs. 5 and 6). How can completely indirect tumor recognition lead to such effective control over tumor growth?

Profuse secretion of cytokines and chemokines within a tumor is likely to have a similar impact, whether the secretion is triggered by direct T-cell contact with tumor cells or by T-cell contact with neighboring TAMs or DCs (Fig. 7). Therefore, it is not surprising that studies employing cytokine knockout mice have confirmed that indirect tumor rejection by CD4+ T_E arises largely as a consequence of such cytokine secretion *(100)*. These mechanisms may include directly antiangiogenic and apoptotic effects of cytokines, such as tumor necrosis factor-α *(103–106)*. In addition, T_E-derived cytokines can induce activation of non-T-accessory cells, such as lymphokine-activated killer cells and tumoricidal macrophages, both of which manifest the extraordinary capacity to recognize and kill tumor cells through still obscure, MHC- and Ag-independent mechanisms (extensively reviewed in ref. *1*). In addition, activated T-cells, including CD4+ T-cells, can themselves acquire the capacity to mediate Fas ligand (APO-1 ligand)-dependent apoptosis of tumor

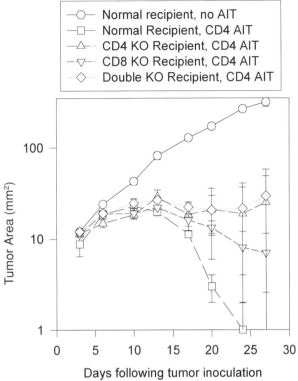

Fig. 6. Treatment of CD4 and/or CD8 syngeneic knockout mice with purified L-selectin^low CD4+ effector T-cells (T_Es). Purified, anti-CD3 activated L-selectin^low CD4+ T_Es were prepared from methylcholanthrene-205-draining tumor-draining lymph nodes, as in Fig. 3, and administered variously to normal syngeneic B6 mice, or syngeneic mice that were knockouts for CD4, CD8, or dually for CD4 and CD8. Recipient mice received 500 cGy before adoptive transfer. The dose of L-selectin^low CD4+ T_Es was 2 million per mouse, a dose that achieves delayed tumor regression in normal mice (*see* also Fig. 3). None of the knockout group mice was consistently cured of tumor, but tumor cytostasis was achieved even in the absence of recipient host T-cells.

cells. This requires reciprocal tumor cell expression of Fas but neither of specific Ag nor MHC molecules *(107–111)*.

Whereas direct recognition and perforin-mediated lysis of MHC class I-expressing tumors by CD8+ CTLs may often play a major role in tumor rejection, even following CD4+ T_E adoptive transfer *(92)*, the previously described, indirect mechanisms of tumor recognition and rejection have the theoretical advantage of remaining operative whether or not tumor cells themselves uniformly express MHC molecules. L-Selectin^low CD8+ T_Es themselves also have the option of recognizing crosspresented tumor Ag to activate indirect mechanisms of rejection *(see* Fig. 7). Furthermore, IFN-γ production arising from CD4+ or CD8+ T_E crossrecognition of tumor Ag typically results in upregulated tumor cell expression of MHC class I molecules, thereby facilitating subsequent CTL direct recognition of tumor cells *(97,112,113)*.

3.4. Mechanisms of Tumor Rejection by L-Selectin^low CD8+ T-Cells

Before the advent of anti-CD3 culture stimulation, observations of helper-independent CD8+ T_Es had been limited to mouse models employing tumor cells blatantly transformed

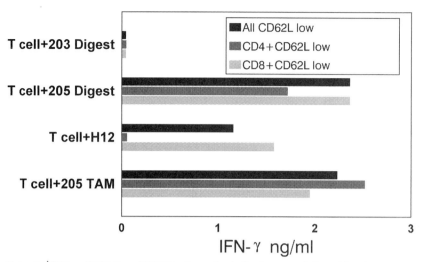

Fig. 7. L-Selectin[low] T-cell CD4[+] and CD8[+] subsets both display reactivity with relevant tumor-associated macrophages (TAMs), but only L-selectin[low] CD8[+] T-cells react directly with tumor cells. L-Selectin[low] T-cells unfractionated for CD4[+] and CD8[+] ("All CD62L low"), purified L-selectin[low] CD4[+] T-cells ("CD4[+]CD62L low"), and purified L-selectin[low] CD8[+] T-cells ("CD8[+]CD62L low") were each prepared from methylcholanthrene (MCA)-205-sensitized tumor-draining lymph nodes. At the end of 5-d culture activation with anti-CD3/interleukin 2 treatment, T-cell groups were harvested and were co-cultured with irradiated stimulator cells: either irrelevant MCA-203 whole cell digest ("T-cell[+]203 Digest"), relevant MCA-205 whole cell digest ("T-cell[+]205 Digest"), H-12 cell line (stroma-free MCA-205-derived, "T-cell[+]H12"), or MCA-205 TAMs from MCA-205 whole-cell digest ("T-cell[+]205 TAM"). Twenty-four-hour supernatants assayed by enzyme-linked immunosorbent assay; displayed is interferon-γ production in ng/106 T-cells/24 h. In this assay, production by T-cells or tumor cells alone was below the limits of assay detection (<25 pg).

by viral infection (1,12,35,78,114). The most extensively studied helper-independent CD8[+] T_Es were those generated by vaccination to the Friend leukemia virus-transformed cell line FBL-3 (1,12,78). Either CD8[+] or CD4[+] T_Es generated from FBL-3-vaccinated mice exhibited a remarkable capacity to cure widely disseminated extrapulmonary tumors when administered as adoptive monotherapy. Extensively cultured anti-FBL-3 CD8[+] T_E clones depended on co-administration of adjunct rIL-2 for their therapeutic efficacy, but still could reject widespread extrapulmonary tumors without co-administration of CD4[+] T_Es (1,12,78).

Although there was little expectation that such helper-independent CD8[+] T_Es would ever be detected in more clinically apt tumor models, the advent of anti-CD3 culture activation revealed that helper-independent CD8[+] T-cell pre-effectors were, in fact, also naturally sensitized in weakly immunogenic models, even in the face of progressively growing tumor challenges (18). It was therefore apparent that the demonstration of helper-independent CD8[+] T-cells was less dependent on tumor immunogenicity than on the capacity of culture techniques to reveal their presence.

As discussed in Subheading 3.1., helper-independent CD8[+] pre-effector T-cells reside within the L-selectin[low] fraction of TDLNs (18). Short-term (5 d) culture expansion following initial anti-CD3 stimulation generates CD8[+] T_Es that are highly effective adoptive therapy against established tumors at several anatomical locations, including lung and brain, without co-administration of either CD4[+] T_Es or adjunct cytokines, thereby fulfilling the definition of helper independence (*see* Figs. 1 and 2). Even when cultured on a protracted basis with anti-CD3 restimulations, CD8$^+$ T$_E$s can retain elements of helper-independence, although optimizing culture to prevent diminutions in per-cell therapeutic potency remains a challenge *(22)*.

Particularly illuminating are direct comparisons between L-selectin^{low} CD4$^+$ and CD8$^+$ subsets when they are respectively administered as AIT against a variety of tumor models. On a per-cell basis, L-selectin^{low} CD8$^+$ T$_E$ monotherapy is consistently more effective than CD4$^+$ T$_E$ for the treatment of 10-d established (advanced) pulmonary metastases (*see* Fig. 1). In contrast, CD8$^+$ T$_E$s are slightly less effective than CD4$^+$ T$_E$s for the treatment of 3-d intracranial tumors (*see* Fig. 2). Such distinctions are of minimal consequence because similarly curative outcomes can easily be achieved with either subset through minor dose adjustments, and in both cases, without a need to administer adjunct IL-2. In contrast, greater subset disparity is observed for subcutaneous tumors (*see* Figs. 3 and 4). Very small doses of adoptively transferred L-selectin^{low} CD4$^+$ T$_E$s (1 million) can eventually cure established subcutaneous tumors (*see* Fig. 3), whereas even 20 million L-selectin^{low} CD8$^+$ T$_E$s are often noncurative (*see* Fig. 4). In contrast to L-selectin^{low} CD4$^+$ T$_E$s monotherapy, where delayed rejection kinetics are common (*see* Fig. 3), a failure to observe rapid tumor regression following L-selectin^{low} CD8$^+$ T$_E$ adoptive transfer is predictive of treatment failure. Furthermore, carboxy-fluorescein diacetate, succinimidyl ester (CFSE)-labeled CD8$^+$ T$_E$s display a somewhat reduced capacity, compared with CD4$^+$ T$_E$s, for Ag-specific proliferation within the tumor bed *(83)*. Finally, depletion of recipient host T-cells has less negative impact on adoptively transferred CD8$^+$ T$_E$s than on CD4$^+$ T$_E$s (*see* Figs. 5 and 6), suggesting that CD8$^+$ T$_E$s have a lesser capacity to recruit host T-cells. In composite, these findings indicate that adoptively transferred CD8$^+$ T$_E$s will be at their least "helper-independent" when initial T$_E$ entry is scant, hence, most prone to require T$_E$ proliferation and host T-cell recruitment.

Given the relative insensitivity of L-selectin^{low} CD4$^+$ T-cells to trafficking variances and the observed effector impact of L-selectin^{low} CD8$^+$ T-cells even against large tumors (*see* Figs. 1 and 3), it is not surprising that these subsets are often therapeutically superior and even synergistic when administered together (*see* Figs. 1, 3, and 5). Nonetheless, because Ag availability often causes vaccination strategies to favor CD8$^+$ T-cell sensitization *(115–118)*, it is desirable to identify adjunct treatments that will ensure the sustained helper independence of L-selectin^{low} CD8$^+$ T-cells when they must be adoptively transferred without CD4$^+$ T-cells. The adjunct administration of exogenous rIL-2 to sustain helper-independent CD8$^+$ effector T-cell function is well precedented *(14,39,119, 120)*, and other CD8$^+$-facilitating agents, such as rIL-12, CD40 ligand, and anti-CTLA4, may also prove useful for this purpose *(39,117,121–125)*. However, future improvements in cell culture techniques may unmask a fuller degree of helper independence, or even elements of helper-type proficiency in L-selectin^{low} CD8$^+$ T$_E$s, ultimately obviating the need for such adjunct agents (*see* Subheading 5.4.).

In summary, these results indicate that CD8$^+$ and CD4$^+$ L-selectin^{low} T-cell subsets can play distinctive and complementary roles during adoptive therapy. Whereas the therapeutic efficacy of purified L-selectin^{low} CD8$^+$ T-cells varies strongly in proportion to the observed accumulation efficiencies of T-cells at individual anatomic sites (pulmonary tumors > intracranial tumors >> subcutaneous tumors) *(18,82)*, the therapeutic efficacy of purified L-selectin^{low} CD4$^+$ T-cells appears to be largely independent of such trafficking variances. This may reflect superior abilities of L-selectin^{low} CD4$^+$ T-cells to proliferate intratumorally, provide APC conditioning, and/or gradually recruit additional host effector elements, including CD8+ T-cells and additional CD4+ T-cells *(96,97,113,126–128)*. Nonetheless, purified L-selectin^{low} CD8+ T-cells display greater efficacy than purified L-selectin^{low} CD4+ T-cells in eradicating advanced (d 10) pulmonary tumors, even without co-administration of exogenous rIL-2 (*see* Fig. 1), and can markedly accelerate the rejection of tumors (*see* Fig. 5). Such data suggest that L-selectin^{low} CD8+ T$_E$s play an increasingly critical role when large and/or rapidly progressive tumors outstrip the CD4+ T$_E$s inability to interact directly with MHC class I^{pos}/class II^{neg} tumor cells (*see* Fig. 3). Further enhancements in L-selectin^{low} CD8+ T$_E$ stand-alone performance will likely be the result of culture modifications that enhance their capacity to accumulate more rapidly in extrapulmonary tumors (*see* Subheading 5.4.).

3.5. Adjunct Irradiation or Chemotherapy
Is Currently Essential or Highly Potentiating to Successful AIT

With the exception of early pulmonary metastases, for which T$_E$ trafficking is exceptionally robust, effective AIT has consistently benefited from or required the adjunct administration of either nonmyeloablative radiation therapy (RT) or nonmyeloablative chemotherapy before T-cell adoptive transfer *(75,129)*. This is as true for high-performance L-selectin^{low} T$_E$s as it is for less-potent T-cell preparations *(1,2,130)*.

Experiments in the mid 1980s demonstrated that adjunct nonmyeloablative total body irradiation ([TBI] 500 cGy) could potentiate AIT of methylcholanthrene-105, even when TBI was applied before tumor inoculation 5 d before adoptive transfer *(28)*. This indicated that a host alteration rather than a direct antitumor effect was vital to the observed potentiation. Although it was initially theorized that the major host alteration was elimination of suppressor T-cells (T$_S$s), reconstitution of nonirradiated lymphocytes into the irradiated host does not block the therapeutic effect of TBI *(75)*, and similar results have now been reported for high-dose cyclophosphamide *(131)*. It has also recently been observed that partial body irradiation (PBI) can be as effective an adjunct as TBI, even when such PBI excludes the tumor, thymus, spleen, and the majority of host lymph nodes and causes no detectable systemic lymphodepletion *(132)*.

Recent AIT clinical trials have begun to incorporate high-dose nonmyeloablative chemotherapy as part of their regimens (*[19,133]*; *see* Heading 4), and the remarkable objective responses observed in several trials will undoubtedly inspire the continued use of such adjunct chemotherapy, even in the absence of a sure mechanistic rationale. Clarifying the therapeutically beneficial mechanisms of nonmyeloablative RT/chemotherapy remains essential to develop less-toxic, but equally effective alternatives. Although chemotherapy is clinically more acceptable than TBI, mechanistic studies in mice are more readily accomplished with RT, because regional RT (i.e., PBI) and TBI can be comparatively administered. We recently defined several unique impacts of adjunct RT on individual elements of T-cell function:

1. Although adjunct RT itself has no discernible impact on the trafficking of adoptively transferred L-selectin^{low} T$_E$s into tumor deposits, it potentiates proliferation of adoptively transferred, fluorescently tagged (CFSE-labeled) T$_E$s. Tumor-specific proliferation within the tumor bed is especially potentiated, suggesting that adjunct RT enhances intratumoral Ag presentation or co-stimulation by an unidentified mechanism *(83)*.

2. Adjunct RT reduces the performance demands on T_Es to achieve tumor rejection. In non-irradiated hosts, others and we have demonstrated that rejection of early pulmonary tumors requires adoptively transferred T_Es to produce IFN-γ. In contrast, in irradiated hosts, T_Es or host-cell production of IFN-γ has proved completely unnecessary to tumor rejection, regardless of the site of tumor implantation (e.g., pulmonary, subcutaneous or intracranial) *(130)*. This observation was subsequently corroborated by other investigators *(106,134)*.

Administration of high-dose (100 mg/kg) cyclophosphamide several hours before adoptive therapy has proved as effective as TBI in enabling L-selectin^{low} T_Es to cure a variety of tumor models *(75)*. Furthermore, despite blood–brain barrier concerns, intra-peritoneally administered cyclophosphamide proved as effective as TBI in facilitating cure of intracranial tumors *(132)*. These studies suggest that "same-day" adjunct RT or chemotherapy may have broad therapeutic applicability, with single agent "high-dose" cyclophosphamide being clinically preferable to TBI.

Because evidence strongly suggests that the immunosensitizing effect of these adjuncts reflects host modulation rather than a direct antitumor effect, better elucidation of their mechanism(s) of action is very likely to reveal less toxic treatment alternatives. For example, nonmyeloablative RT or chemotherapy may activate stem cell DC precursors, arming the latter better to resist immunosuppression after they enter the tumor bed, thereby leading to more effective crosspresentation of tumor Ags *(132)*.

4. CLINICAL CORRELATIONS

Beginning in the 1980s, AIT trials employed rIL-2-driven culture techniques that were originally developed in mouse tumor models *(26,27,135)*. Tumor nodules were resected from melanoma patients and cultured in rIL-2 to expand autologous TILs for reinfusion into patients. Patients often received in excess of 10^{11} cultured autologous T-cells in combination with adjunct recombinant human interleukin (rhIL)-2. Not surprisingly, given the limited effect of similar treatment on extrapulmonary tumors in the mouse models, the corresponding human trials yielded disappointing results *(135)*. An underlying complete response rate of 7% was observed in melanoma patients receiving autologous TILs plus rhIL-2, a response rate identical to treatment with rhIL-2 alone. Whereas an additional 28% of patients experienced partial objective responses of tumors, such responses were typically limited in duration and often followed by tumor relapse in the central nervous system *(135)*.

Because the administered T-cells already had characteristics of mature T_Es at the time of adoptive transfer, the observed partial responses and relapses were reminiscent of the regional T_E fatigue observed by Speiser et al. and Shrikant et al. in animal models (*see* Subheading 2.2.). Additional findings consonant with intratumoral T_E fatigue were subsequently reported by Kammula et al. for vaccinated melanoma patients *(36)*. Human leukocyte antigen-tetramer and real-time polymerase chain reaction analyses revealed that melanoma patients challenged with relevant antigenic peptides transiently developed an enrichment of Ag-specific CD8$^+$ T-cells within tumor nodules, and such T-cells produced IFN-γ within the tumor bed as a transient response to the vaccination. Despite the temporal linkage of intratumoral T_E activation to treatment, no objective nodule regressions were observed in this study, indicating a failure in the scale or duration of the effector response closely paralleling that repeatedly observed in rats by Speiser et al. *(35)*.

Common to the observations of Speiser et al., Shrikant et al., and Kammula et al. is a persistence of tumor-specific host T_Es even when sustained tumor regressions do not occur. Furthermore, as shown by Speiser et al., repetitive reactivations of such T_Es resulted in indistinguishable therapeutic effects *(35)*, suggesting that no therapeutic potential was permanently lost during any of the occurrences of effector exhaustion or tolerance. Whereas the inevitable relapses in such studies might seem to suggest that definitive immunotherapy is impossible, the AIT studies of Shu et al. have demonstrated, to the contrary, that with in vitro anti-CD3 activation, adequate dosing, and nonmyeloablative chemotherapy or RT, adoptively transferred L-selectin T_Es can achieve permanent complete regressions of well-established, poorly immunogenic tumors, and subsequent tumor challenges are rejected *(18,79)*. Therefore, effector exhaustion or split anergy may not constitute inevitable sequelae of immunotherapy.

Despite the encouraging studies of Shu et al., the reality may be considerably more complex in cancer patients, where tumors can exist for many years before they are clinically evident, and immunotherapy is actually contemplated. Even if there are persistent, hypoactivated antitumor T-cells in cancer patients, are they truly representative of a T-cell repertoire that may have initially been sensitized many years previously? Because T-cell apoptosis is a well-observed and chronic event within tumors *(136–138)*, a selection process may theoretically occur in which there is clonal deletion of higher affinity or otherwise functionally superior antitumor T_Es, leaving only T_Es with a considerably reduced therapeutic potential. Fortunately, recent clinical results suggest that tumor-induced regional T_E fatigue can occur on a chronic basis without ever depleting the cancer host of essential antitumor T_Es for later ex vivo activation.

A major advance for the AIT field was triggered when Childs et al. administered nonmyeloablative chemotherapy consisting of cyclophosphamide and fludaribine to patients with advanced kidney cancer, followed by allogeneic bone marrow transplant and supplemental adoptive transfer of allogeneic T-cells *(133)*. Such therapy resulted in sustained partial regressions in approximately half of patients receiving treatment. The sustained nature and the survival prolongation implicit in these responses represented an unequivocal breakthrough for human AIT trials, regardless of its allogeneic context. Modulations in the circulating T-cell repertoires of these patients suggested that the expected graft–antihost response transiently modulated into a relatively tumor-directed response during the height of clinically observed tumor regression, then reverted to the generic graft–antihost response *(139)*. Whereas the mechanisms by which such therapy leads to tumor regression are still under analysis, the clinical impact of this approach inspired similar efforts in other cancers, variously employing either allogeneic or autologous T-cells.

Initial attempts at the NCI Surgery Branch to combine nonmyeloablative fludaribine and cyclophosphamide with conventionally prepared TILs and rhIL-2 were therapeutically unsuccessful, as was the combined administration of nonmyeloablative chemotherapy, hyperexpanded high-affinity antimelanoma T-cell clones, and rhIL-2 *(140,141)*. However, a third approach showed dramatically improved clinical results. TILs were first expanded in conventional rIL-2-driven cultures, screened for in vitro antitumor specificity, and then the most reactive cultures were activated to hyperexpansion with anti-CD3 plus IL-2. *(19)*. When such anti-CD3 activated T-cells were co-administered with nonmyeloablative fludaribine/cyclophosphamide and systemic adjunct rIL-2, dramatic and sometimes sustained body-wide objective tumor regressions were observed in approximately half of treated melanoma patients *(19)*. Although such responses have generally been confined to partial objective responses, similar to the Childs et al. kidney cancer trial *(139)*, ongoing objective responses (15–24+ mo) have occurred in melanoma patients who previously failed other immunotherapy and chemotherapy, and in several instances transferred TILs could be demonstrated in patient peripheral blood for many months following transfer *(19)*.

This improved clinical outcome appears to be linked to two specific differences from the NCI Surgery Branch's previous strategies. Patients received chemotherapy consisting of high-dose cyclophosphamide (120 mg/kg) and fludarabine instead of lower doses of cyclophosphamide alone (25 mg/kg). Nonetheless, as noted in the last paragraph, this newer chemotherapy regimen had recently proved ineffective when melanoma patients received traditionally cultured TILs or hyperexpanded autologous T-cell clones with high avidity to melanoma cells *(19,140,141)*. Therefore, the current trial's success also hinged on the distinctive culture modification in which TILs underwent anti-CD3/IL-2 activation before adoptive transfer *(19)*. This highlights the pivotal role of T-cell culture conditions on therapeutic outcome, because the ancillary procedures for TIL derivation, adoptive transfer, and IL-2 administration were identical to previous NCI TIL trials. The basis by which this culture modification gave rise to therapeutically superior T_Es in the clinical trial is under intense study, but it is hypothesized that better preservation of tumor-specific CD4$^+$ T_Es is an important consequence of the added anti-CD3 stimulation *(19)*. Certainly, in animal tumor models, the two most conspicuous benefits of in vitro anti-CD3 stimulation are the improved preservation of antitumor CD4$^+$ T_Es and emergence of antitumor CD8$^+$ T_Es with helper-independent properties *(2,18)*. Furthermore, the intrinsic polyclonality of anti-CD3 stimulation favors the in vitro preservation of antitumor TCR diversity that may already have arisen in vivo as a consequence of either tumor-bearing or superimposed vaccine maneuvers *(18,22,24)*.

This recent Surgery Branch report is probably the first compelling clinical demonstration that AIT can play a significant role in the treatment of human cancer. Furthermore, it validates the continuing importance of the weakly and poorly immunogenic mouse tumor models that have proved predictive in the development, understanding, and troubleshooting of AIT. It is essential to appreciate that the major therapeutic advance to date in mouse AIT models was the advent of anti-CD3 stimulation to activate L-selectin^{low} pre-effector T-cells from tumor-bearing mice. Secondly, maximal efficacy of AIT employing such anti-CD3 stimulated L-selectin^{low} T_Es has not depended on administration of adjunct systemic rIL-2, but remains strongly dependent on, or at least logarithmically facilitated by, the host modulations resulting from either 100 mg/kg cyclophosphamide or sublethal irradiation. Therefore, it is noteworthy that the current Surgery Branch trial is the first clinical trial to combine the preclinically identified components of in vitro anti-CD3 activation with nonmyeloablative high-dose cyclophosphamide.

5. PRECLINICAL MODELS: ONGOING AND FUTURE EFFORTS

Ongoing preclinical studies in these same animal tumor models not only corroborate the current clinical success at the Surgery Branch, but also point to the likelihood of continued clinical advances as the mechanism of successful AIT is better understood, and culture improvements further optimize T_Es function, especially intratumoral trafficking, after adoptive transfer.

As discussed under Heading 4, the adoptive transfer of T-cells following nonmyeloablative chemotherapy can exert a pronounced therapeutic effect in advanced renal cell carcinoma *(133)* or melanoma *(19)*, but for either cancer type, responses have been limited to partial responses that occur in only half the patients receiving AIT. Several inevitable questions arise, including why only partial responses, why only half of patients, and why delayed recurrences? In the case of melanoma, all patients, both responders and nonresponders, received autologous T_Es that displayed tumor-specific, T1-type cytokine secretion (e.g., IFN-γ) before adoptive transfer *(19)*. Preclinical animal studies and retrospective patient analyses have established that an absence of such in vitro reactivity portends clinical unresponsiveness to AIT *(2,92,142–144)*. Nonetheless, it is also apparent that in vitro T1-type reactivity is insufficient to ensure meaningful clinical responses, as evidenced by the large number of limited, nonenduring, or absent responses, even in patients receiving doses in excess of 10^{11} T_Es *(2,19,135,143,144)*. Current and ongoing studies in mouse tumor studies illustrate several ways in which intrinsically adequate, anti-CD3 activated T1-type T_E repertoires may fail to achieve complete and permanent tumor regressions.

5.1. AIT With L-Selectin^{low} T_Es is Highly Dose-Dependent

One striking and consistent observation in animal AIT experiments is that threshold doses of L-selectin^{low} T_Es must be adoptively transferred to achieve curative rejection of established tumors *(1,2,16,18,20)*. These doses differ for individual tumor models, and even a halving of the T_E dose can result in abject therapeutic failure (e.g., Figs. 8 and 9). The particular "impact" that the threshold T_E dose must achieve is unknown. Knockout studies have demonstrated that this impact is neither IFN-γ secretion *(130)*, nor is it linked to very high initial accumulation of T_Es within the tumor bed, because established mouse subcutaneous tumors have a notoriously low initial T_E accumulation (logs-fold less than pulmonary or intracranial tumors), yet rejection is ultimately still observed (*see* Fig. 3 *[43,82]*).

Although the mechanistic basis of this "threshold" effect is unknown, it is evident that exceeding this threshold by adoptively transferring curative doses of culture-activated T_Es is much more desirable than administering noncurative T_E doses with repetitive and indefinite vaccine maneuvers *(35,54)*. Although efforts to hyperexpand mouse L-selectin^{low} T_Es to exceed threshold are still plagued by losses in therapeutic efficacy during extended culture *(22)*, it is apparent that this is an artifact of culture that does not involve disruptions in the frequency or variable β-chain distribution of the antitumor TCR repertoire *(24)*. Such deteriorations in T_E performance during extended culture are ultimately likely to be remedied by systematic troubleshooting in preclinical models (*see* Subheading 5.4.).

5.2. Variable Efficacy of Conjunctional Treatments

Because the capacity of adoptively transferred L-selectin^{low} T_Es to mediate curative tumor rejection is highly dose-dependent, it is important to consider the capacity of conjunctional treatments to compensate for subtherapeutic T_E doses. Although rIL-2 is often administered as an AIT adjunct, its therapeutic significance in this context has not been established in randomized clinical trials. Its original testing was predicated on observations that classically derived mouse TILs lacked any therapeutic effect in the absence of rIL-2 co-administration *(26,52)*.

Because therapeutically superior L-selectin^{low} T_Es display no such absolute dependence on conjunctional rIL-2 in mouse models, we recently compared the effects of conjunctional treatments on AIT employing "therapeutic" or "subtherapeutic" doses of L-selectin^{low} T_Es.

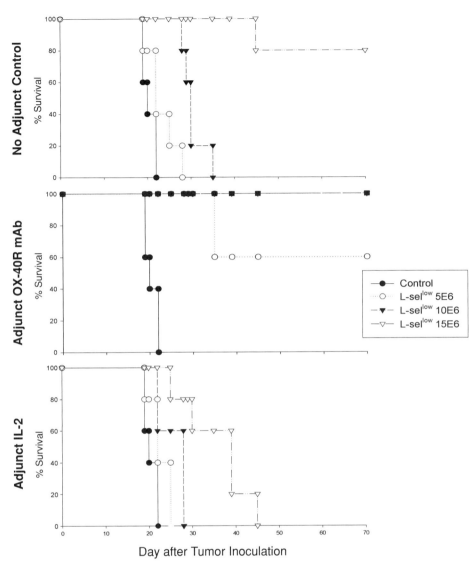

Fig. 8. Effects of conjunctional OX-40R monoclonal antibody (MAb) or recombinant interleukin-2 (rIL-2) treatment on adoptive immunotherapy of advanced (10 d) intracranial methylcholanthrene-205 tumors with L-selectin effector T-cells (T_Es). The latter were prepared as in Figs. 1–3. All mice were treated with sublethal total body irradiation (500 cGy) before intravenous infusion of T_Es. OX-40R MAbs (150 µg) was given intraperitoneally twice on d 0 and 3 after cell transfer. rIL-2 (10,000 U) was given intraperitoneally twice daily for four consecutive days commencing on the day of cell transfer. Each group consisted of five mice. A dose-dependent therapeutic effect of L-selectin^{low} T_Es is apparent. Sufficient dosing can cure without adjunct treatments. Adjunct OX-40R MAb enabled lower doses of L-selectin^{low} T_Es to be therapeutically effective, whereas adjunct rIL-2 impaired the therapeutic impact of otherwise curative doses of L-selectin^{low} T_Es.

For the treatment of advanced (10-d-established) pulmonary metastases, co-administration of either rIL-2 or the co-stimulatory ligand OX-40R MAb enhanced the therapeutic effect of suboptimal doses of L-selectin^{low} T_Es. For advanced (10 d) intracranial tumors, OX-40R MAb was similarly enhancing, but conjunctional IL-2 was nonenhancing, and

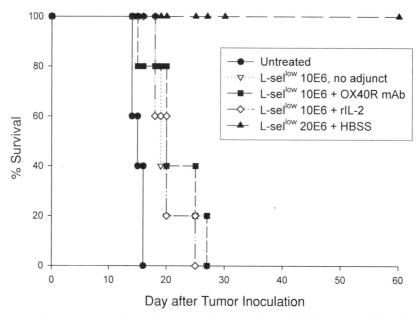

Fig. 9. Effects of conjunctional OX-40R monoclonal antibody (MAb) or recombinant interleukin (rIL)-2 treatment on adoptive immunotherapy of advanced (10 d) intrahepatic methylcholanthrene-105 tumors with L-selectin effector T-cells (T_{ES}). The latter were prepared as in Figs. 1–3. All mice were treated with sublethal total body irradiation (500 cGy) before intravenous infusion of effector cells, either a 20 million or 10 million dose. OX-40R MAb or rIL-2 was given as adjunct as in Fig. 8, commencing on the day of T_{ES} transfer. Each group consisted of five mice. A dose-dependent therapeutic effect of L-selectin^{low} T_{ES} is apparent: 20E6 T_{ES} can cure without adjunct treatments. Neither adjunct OX-40R MAb nor rIL-2 could render the 10E6 T_{ES} dose effective against this highly aggressive tumor model.

furthermore, impeded AIT by otherwise curative doses of L-selectin^{low} T_{ES} (*[79]*; *see* Fig. 8). rIL-2's therapeutic blockade was associated with inhibition of T_{ES} accumulation in intracranial tumors *(79)*. Similarly, Shrikant et al. have described undesirable proapoptotic effects of adjunct rIL-2 during AIT of malignant ascites *(145)*.

Importantly, neither adjunct IL-2 nor OX-40R MAb had any significant impact (enhancement or inhibition) on the treatment of established 10-d hepatic metastases by L-selectin^{low} T_{ES} (*see* Fig. 9). In this virtually preterminal treatment model, untreated mice survive a maximum of 2 wk past the day of therapy. Despite this disquietingly brief therapeutic window of opportunity and the inutility of conjunctional treatments, adoptive transfer of "stand-alone," adequately dosed L-selectin^{low} T_{ES} still proved curative (*see* Fig. 9). It needs to be emphasized that administration of nonmyeloablative irradiation was an essential component of this successful treatment (not shown).

Such data clearly demonstrate that the impact of adjunct treatments on AIT is vulnerable to major anatomic variances. Although modifying schedules of adjunct biological factors may address certain undesirable or paradoxical effects, the use of such adjuncts is simply unnecessary when adequate doses of L-selectin^{low} T_{ES} are administered.

5.3. Passenger T_{S}s Can Cause Effector T-Cell Blockade

As a purely pragmatic consideration, elimination of the nontherapeutic L-selectin^{high} subset at the beginning of culture markedly reduces the numbers of T-cells that must be propagated and adoptively transferred, and reduces consumption of culture medium and growth-stimulatory factors. These practical incentives become a near mandate, however, now that it has been determined that the L-selectin^{high} subset can also be a source of therapeutically ruinous passenger T_Ss (43). In contrast to previously characterized T_Ss that primarily inhibit the afferent limb of the immune response (e.g., CD4$^+$CD25$^+$ T_Ss) (146), L-selectin^{high} passenger T_Ss exert effector blockade. This poses an ultimate liability to successful AIT, because culture-activated L-selectin^{low} T_Es have remained fully vulnerable to L-selectin^{high} T_Ss, even when afferent blockade is no longer of consequence (43).

Tumor-induced L-selectin^{high} T_Ss appear in the TDLNs between d 9 and 12 following tumor challenge. They can be isolated from d 12 TDLNs, anti-CD3 activated, and co-transferred with either d 9 or d 12 L-selectin^{low} T_Es to prevent tumor rejection. These T_Ss are predominantly CD8$^+$, but CD4$^+$ participation has not been ruled out (43).

By purging L-selectin^{high} cells before culture, freshly harvested d 12 TDLNs can readily be divested of passenger T_Ss. This is only transiently available as a purging technique, however, because T_Ss downregulate L-selectin expression during culture activation. L-Selectin downregulated T_Ss are currently indistinguishable from L-selectin^{low} T_Es, showing equivalent expression patterns for CD25, CD28, CTLA4, and CD44 (43). L-Selectin downregulated T_Ss also resemble L-selectin^{low} T_Es in their superior trafficking into tumor beds, providing favorable intratumoral stoichiometrics for effector blockade (43).

Separately anti-CD3-activated L-selectin^{high} T-cells from d 12 TDLNs can already inhibit tumor-specific IFN-γ production by L-selectin^{low} T_Es before adoptive transfer. In contrast, when such T_Ss are anti-CD3-activated as a component of unfractionated d 12 TDLN T-cells, they remain functionally silent in vitro until adoptive transfer, at which time they prevent tumor rejection. A significant element of T_Ss activation therefore normally occurs following reinfusion.

In mouse models, AIT of established subcutaneous tumors is particularly vulnerable to L-selectin^{high} T_Ss, corresponding to the relatively low initial accumulation of even L-selectin^{low} T_Es at this experimental challenge site. Remarkably, mice triply challenged with subcutaneous, pulmonary, and intracranial tumors can be cured by adoptive transfer of purified L-selectin^{low} T_Es or unfractionated T-cells from d 9 TDLNs, but develop mixed responses and ultimately treatment failure when treated with unfractionated T-cells from d 12 TDLNs because of the latter's T_S content (43).

Many features augur the clinical significance of this T_S phenomenon. Historically, adoptive transfer of culture-activated T_Es to melanoma patients has typically resulted, at best, in nonsustained and/or mixed responses, with no demonstrable survival advantage (135). Even in the recent, much more promising NCI Surgery Branch trial, this has remained a problem for the majority of treated patients (19). Such disappointing or tentative clinical outcomes have occurred despite in vitro evidence that many, and sometimes all, patients received tumor-specific T-cells capable of T1-type cytokine production and direct tumor lysis (143). The therapeutic discrepancy between in vitro and in vivo performance has traditionally been attributed to a trafficking failure of cultured T-cells, even though such a trafficking defect has never been validated by clinical studies (147–149).

Mouse studies resonate disturbingly with this clinical performance discrepancy: when unfractionated T-cells from d 12 TDLNs are employed as AIT, mixed tumor responses and ultimately treatment failure are observed, despite the T-cells' strong in vitro capacity for tumor-specific IFN-γ production before infusion, and their excellent subsequent trafficking proficiency in vivo (43). Such parallels raise the hope that T_E repertoires derivable from patients are already sufficiently diverse and tumor-reactive for therapeutic purposes *(19,150–152)*, but may still be in need of T_S purging either before or following anti-CD3 activation. Because such T_Ss are functionally silent, successful purging will likely depend on the identification of distinguishing phenotypic elements. Alternatively, it may be possible to liberate T_Es from bulk cultures based on their distinguishing functional characteristics (e.g., tumor-specific IFN-γ production).

5.4. Therapeutic Potency of T_Es Is Dictated Ultimately by Culture Conditions

Culture itself is the strongest determinant of what T_E properties are in evidence for experimental characterization. Until an anti-CD3 activation step was added to conventional IL-2-driven cultures, it was unsuspected that both CD4$^+$ and helper-independent CD8$^+$ pre-T_Es were naturally sensitized even in mice with progressive, weakly immunogenic tumors. Given the major advances in T_E performance that have already been elicited solely as a consequence of culture improvements, it is inconceivable that we have yet observed the maximum therapeutic performance that can be elicited from T_Es.

Historically, extended culture of T-cells is associated with a progressive decline in per cell therapeutic performance when such cells are employed as AIT *(22)*. Despite this decline in in vivo performance, there is frequently good preservation or even enhancement of T1-type activity when long-term cultured T-cells are assayed for tumor-specific IFN-γ production or target lysis in vitro. Although it has long been recognized that an absence of in vitro T1-type activity is a negative predictor for therapeutic outcome *(2,92,142–144)*, the preservation of T1-type activity is not conversely a reliable positive indicator *(2,19,135, 143,144)*. The cultural events that diminish therapeutic potency while preserving in vitro T1-type activity remain speculative, but may include deleterious skewing of the antitumor TCR repertoire or alterations in secondary properties, such as T-cell trafficking or functional avidity.

Recent investigations have confirmed that early culture events profoundly impact T_E therapeutic potency apart from any TCR repertoire modulations. When conventional anti-CD3 activation was modified by substituting mouse serum (MS) for fetal calf serum (FCS), enhanced therapeutic potency was evident in L-selectin^{low} T_Es by d 5 of culture in MS, and was even more enhanced after an additional 7 d in MS *(24)*. In contrast to the therapeutic deterioration observed when T_Es are repetitively anti-CD3 restimulated in FCS, T_Es maintained and restimulated in MS displayed fully preserved or even enhanced therapeutic potency many weeks later in culture. Despite these therapeutic disparities, intracellular cytokine production assays coupled with variable β-chain–TCR analyses revealed that antitumor repertoires remained highly polyclonal and were indistinguishable, whether T_Es were cultured in FCS or MS *(24)*. Although repertoires were indistinguishable, several functional differences were apparent. T_E cultures propagated in conditioned media-MS displayed a consistently reduced susceptibility to apoptosis at restimulation, despite maintained or heightened T_E expression of death receptors/receptor ligands, such as PD-1, B7H1, Fas, and Fas ligand. Furthermore, CFSE-labeled, MS-propagated T_Es displayed at least a fivefold enhanced intratumoral accumulation within 2–5 d following adoptive transfer, depending on the dose administered *(24)*. The mechanisms of such enhanced resistance to apoptosis and enhanced intratumoral trafficking are under study.

Such data indicate that even when a stable antitumor T_E repertoire is verifiable, secondary culture characteristics can rapidly determine therapeutic outcome, most likely through major impacts on T_E trafficking and/or apoptotic susceptibility at antigenic restimulation. This raises the exciting hope that T_E cultures already achievable for cancer patients may often possess antitumor TCR repertoires with excellent therapeutic potential, even if the in vivo performance of such T_Es is currently disappointing because of culture-induced secondary characteristics. If this is true, eliminating detrimental culture conditions from the time of culture initiation is essential, because negative culture impacts appear to be difficult to reverse at later time points. For example, when L-selectin[low] T_Es were switched on d 9, following anti-CD3 activation from FCS to MS, then adoptively transferred on d 12, they failed to display the enhanced therapeutic efficacy of T_Es cultured continuously for the full 12 d in MS *(24)*. The challenge of optimizing culture conditions to preserve or enhance T_Es performance independent of repertoire modulations is ideally accomplished in preclinical mouse models, where individual culture parameters can be assessed primarily by their impact on therapeutic performance, rather than by their impacts on incompletely predictive in vitro properties.

6. CONCLUSIONS

Several advances previously feared unattainable in aggressive mouse tumor models are now well accepted and the starting point for further preclinical advances. Both CD4+ and CD8+ antitumor T_Es with a relatively high degree of subset independence can now be isolated and anti-CD3 activated from mice bearing aggressive, advanced tumors. Although administration of adjunct cytokines can often enhance the therapeutic outcome of AIT, no adjunct to date has proved consistently as effective as optimally prepared and dosed T_Es alone. Administration of combined CD4+ and CD8+ T_Es appears to have synergistic benefits, based on the capacity of CD4+ T_Es to sustain proliferative and host recruiting effects, and the capacity of CD8+ T-cells to secure and accelerate the rejection process even against large tumors. The possibility not only of augmenting T_E dosing, but also of maintaining or even enhancing enhanced therapeutic efficacy, will likely be a consequence of improved cell culture. The recent recognition that culture can positively impact fundamental T-cell functions, such as trafficking capacity and resistance to apoptosis, underscores the possibility of inducing additional, previously unimaginable improvements in T_E characteristics, including true CD4+ or CD8+ subset independence. Recognizing that T_E therapeutic failure can be because of features other than an inadequate T_E repertoire, including passenger T_Ss and negative impacts of culture on trafficking or apoptotic susceptibility, provides the incentive to monitor such insidious events and to prevent or correct them prospectively. Finally, understanding the mechanism(s) by which nonmyeloablative chemotherapy or radiation markedly facilitate AIT will allow for optimization of this major effect, as well as the development of less-toxic surrogate treatments that accomplish the same end.

REFERENCES

1. Cohen PA, Peng L, Plautz GE, et al. CD4+ T cells in adoptive immunotherapy and the indirect mechanism of tumor rejection. *Crit Rev Immunol* 2000; 20:17–56.
2. Cohen PA, Peng L, Kjaergaard J, et al. T-cell adoptive therapy of tumors: mechanisms of improved therapeutic performance. *Crit Rev Immunol* 2001; 21:215–248.
3. Fernandez-Cruz E, Halliburton B, Feldman JD. In vivo elimination by specific effector cells of an established syngeneic rat moloney virus-induced sarcoma. *J Immunol* 1979; 123:1772–1777.

4. Fernandez-Cruz E, Woda BA, Feldman JD. Elimination of syngeneic sarcomas in rats by a subset of T lymphocytes. *J Exp Med* 1980; 152:823–841.

5. Fernandez-Cruz E, Gilman SC, Feldman JD. Immunotherapy of a chemically-induced sarcoma in rats: characterization of the effector T cell subset and nature of suppression. *J Immunol* 1982; 128:1112–1117.

6. Cheever MA, Greenberg PD, Fefer A. Specificity of adoptive chemoimmunotherapy of established syngeneic tumors. *J Immunol* 1980; 125:711–714.

7. Cheever MA, Greenberg PD, Fefer A, Gillis S. Augmentation of the anti-tumor therapeutic efficacy of long-term cultured T lymphocytes by in vivo administration of purified interleukin 2. *J Exp Med* 1982; 155:968–980.

8. Greenberg PD, Cheever MA, Fefer A. Eradication of disseminated murine leukemia by chemoimmunotherapy with cyclophosphamide and adoptively transferred immune syngeneic Lyt-1+2- lymphocytes. *J Exp Med* 1981; 154:952–963.

9. Shu S, Steerenberg PA, Hunter JT, Evans CH, Rapp HJ. Adoptive immunity to the guinea pig line 10 hepatoma and the nature of in vitro lymphoid-tumor cell interactions. *Cancer Res* 1981; 41(9 Pt 1): 3499–3506.

10. Shu S, Hunter JT, Rapp HJ, Fonseca LS. Mechanisms of immunologic eradication of a syngeneic guinea pig tumor. I. Quantitative analysis of adoptive immunity. *J Natl Cancer Inst* 1982; 68:673–680.

11. Greenberg PD, Kern DE, Cheever MA. Therapy of disseminated murine leukemia with cyclophosphamide and immune Lyt-1+,2- T cells. Tumor eradication does not require participation of cytotoxic T cells. *J Exp Med* 1985; 161:1122–1134.

12. Klarnet JP, Kern DE, Dower SK, Matis LA, Cheever MA, Greenberg PD. Helper-independent CD8+ cytotoxic T lymphocytes express IL-1 receptors and require IL-1 for secretion of IL-2. *J Immunol* 1989; 142:2187–2191.

13. Shu S, Rosenberg SA. Adoptive immunotherapy of a newly induced sarcoma: Immunologic characteristics of effector cells. *J Immunol* 1985; 135:2895–2903.

14. Matis LA, Shu S, Groves ES, et al. Adoptive immunotherapy of a syngeneic murine leukemia with a tumor-specific cytotoxic T cell clone and recombinant human interleukin 2: correlation with clonal IL 2 receptor expression. *J Immunol* 1986; 136:3496–3501.

15. Mule JJ, Yang JC, Afreniere RL, Shu SY, Rosenberg SA. Identification of cellular mechanisms operational in vivo during the regression of established pulmonary metastases by the systemic administration of high-dose recombinant interleukin 2. *J Immunol* 1987; 139:285–294.

16. Kagamu H, Touhalisky JE, Plautz GE, Krauss JC, Shu S. Isolation based on L-selectin expression of immune effector T cells derived from tumor-draining lymph nodes. *Cancer Res* 1996; 56:4338–4342.

17. Cohen PA, Cohen PJ, Rosenberg SA, Mule JJ. CD4+ T-cells from mice immunized to syngeneic sarcomas recognize distinct, non-shared tumor antigens. *Cancer Res* 1994; 54:1055–1058.

18. Peng L, Kjaergaard J, Weng DE, Plautz GE, Shu S, Cohen PA. Helper-independent CD8+/CD62L low T cells with broad anti-tumor efficacy are naturally sensitized during tumor progression. *J Immunol* 2000; 165:5738–5749.

19. Dudley ME, Wunderlich JR, Robbins PF, et al. Cancer regression and autoimmunity in patients after clonal repopulation with antitumor lymphocytes. *Science* 2002; 298:850–854.

20. Kagamu H, Shu S. Purification of L-selectinlow cells promotes the generation of highly potent CD4 anti-tumor effector T lymphocytes. *J Immunol* 1998; 160:3444–3452.

21. Knutson KL, Disis ML. IL-12 enhances the generation of tumour antigen-specific Th1 CD4 T cells during ex vivo expansion. *Clin Exp Immunol* 2004; 135:322–329.

22. Wang L-X, Huang W-X, Graor H, et al. Adoptive immunotherapy of cancer with polyclonal, 108-fold hyperexpanded, CD4+ and CD8+ T cells. *J Transl Med* 2004; 2:41.

23. Cohen PA, Kim H, Fowler DH, et al. Use of interleukin-7, interleukin-2, and interferon-gamma to propagate CD4+ T cells in culture with maintained antigen specificity. *J Immunother* 1993; 14:242–252.

24. Awad M, Kjaergaard J, Peng L, et al. In vitro correlates of anti-tumor T cell adoptive therapy: Culture conditions can dictate therapeutic outcome and T cell apoptotic susceptibility independent of detectable repertoire shifts. *Am Assoc Cancer Res 2004 Proc* 2004; (abstract no. 4693).

25. Shu SY, Rosenberg SA. Adoptive immunotherapy of newly induced murine sarcomas. *Cancer Res* 1985; 45:1657–1662.

26. Rosenberg SA, Spiess P, Lafreniere R. A new approach to the adoptive immunotherapy of cancer with tumor- infiltrating lymphocytes. *Science* 1986; 233:1318–1321.

27. Spiess PJ, Yang JC, Rosenberg SA. In vivo antitumor activity of tumor-infiltrating lymphocytes expanded in recombinant interleukin-2. *J Natl Cancer Inst* 1987; 79:1067–1075.

28. Chang AE, Shu S, Chou T, Lafreniere R, Rosenberg SA. Differences in the effects of host suppression on the adoptive immunotherapy of subcutaneous and visceral tumors. *Cancer Res* 1986; 46:3426–3430.

29. Chou T, Bertera S, Chang AE, Shu S. Adoptive immunotherapy of microscopic and advanced visceral metastases with in vitro sensitized lymphoid cells from mice bearing progressive tumors. *J Immunol* 1988; 141:1775–1781.

30. Shu S, Chou T, Rosenberg SA. In vitro sensitization and expansion with viable tumor cells and interleukin 2 in the generation of specific therapeutic effector cells. *J Immunol* 1986; 136:3891–3898.

31. Correa MR, Ochoa AC, Ghosh P, Mizoguchi H, Harvey L, Longo DL. Sequential development of structural and functional alterations in T cells from tumor-bearing mice. *J Immunol* 1997; 158:5292–5296.

32. Liu J, Finke J, Krauss JC, Shu S, Plautz GE. Ex vivo activation of tumor-draining lymph node T cells reverses defects in signal transduction molecules. *Cancer Immunol Immunother* 1998; 46:268–276.

33. Mizoguchi H, O'Shea JJ, Longo DL, Loeffler CM, McVicar DW, Ochoa AC. Alterations in signal transduction molecules in T lymphocytes from tumor-bearing mice [*see* comments]. *Science* 1992; 258:1795–1798.

34. Wang Q, Stanley J, Kudoh S, Myles J, Kolenko V, Yi T, et al. T cells infiltrating non-Hodgkin's B cell lymphomas show altered tyrosine phosphorylation pattern even though T cell receptor/CD3- associated kinases are present. *J Immunol* 1995; 155:1382–1392.

35. Speiser DE, Miranda R, Zakarian A, et al. Self-antigens expressed by solid tumors Do not efficiently stimulate naive or activated T cells: implications for immunotherapy. *J Exp Med* 1997; 186:645–653.

36. Kammula US, Lee K-H, Riker AI, et al. Functional analysis of antigen-specific T lymphocytes by serial measurement of gene expression in peripheral blood mononuclear cells and tumor specimens. *J Immunol* 1999; 163:6867–6875.

37. Deeths MJ, Kedl RM, Mescher MF. CD8+ T cells become nonresponsive (anergic) following activation in the presence of costimulation. *J Immunol* 1999; 163:102–110.

38. Shrikant P, Mescher MF. Control of syngeneic tumor growth by activation of CD8+ T cells: efficacy is limited by migration away from the site and induction of nonresponsiveness. *J Immunol* 1999; 162:2858–2866.

39. Shrikant P, Khoruts A, Mescher MF. CTLA-4 blockade reverses CD8+ T cell tolerance to tumor by a CD4+ T cell- and IL-2-dependent mechanism. *Immunity* 1999; 11:483–493.

40. Marzo AL, Kinnear BF, Lake RA, et al. Tumor-specific CD4+ T cells have a major "post-licensing" role in CTL mediated anti-tumor immunity. *J Immunol* 2000; 165:6047–6055.

41. Marzo AL, Lake RA, Lo D, et al. Tumor antigens are constitutively presented in the draining lymph nodes. *J Immunol* 1999; 162:5838–5845.

42. Stephenson KR, Perry-Lalley D, Griffith KD, Shu S, Chang AE. Development of antitumor reactivity in regional draining lymph nodes from tumor-immunized and tumor-bearing murine hosts. *Surgery* 1989; 105:523–528.

43. Peng L, Kjaergaard J, Plautz GE, et al. Tumor-induced L selectin high suppressor T cells mediate potent effector T cell blockade and cause failure of otherwise curative adoptive immunotherapy. *J Immunol* 2002; 169:4811–4821.

44. Cruz PD, Bergstresser PR. Antigen processing and presentation by epidermal langerhans cells, induction of immunity or unresponsiveness. *Dermatol Clin* 1990; 8:633–646.

45. Girolomoni G, Simon JC, Bergstresser PR, Cruz PD. Freshly isolated spleen dendritic cells and epidermal langerhans cells undergo similar phenotypic and functional changes during short-term culture. *J Immunol* 1990; 145:2820–2826.

46. Caux C, Massacrier C, Vanbervliet B, et al. Activation of human dendritic cells through CD40 cross-linking. *J Exp Med* 1994; 180:1263–1272.

47. Toes REM, Schoenberger SP, van der Voort EIH, Offringa R, Melief CJM. CD40-CD40 ligand interactions and their role in cytotoxic T lymphocyte priming and anti-tumor immunity. *Semin Immunol* 1998; 10:443–448.

48. Ridge JP, Di Rosa F, Matzinger P. A conditioned dendritic cell can be a temporal bridge between a CD4+ T- helper and a T-killer cell. *Nature* 1998; 393:474–478.

49. Lu Z, Yuan L, Zhou X, Sotomayor E, Levitsky HI, Pardoll DM. CD40-independent pathways of T cell help for priming of CD8(+) cytotoxic T lymphocytes. *J Exp Med* 2000; 191:541–550.

50. Wick M, Dubey P, Koeppen H, et al. Antigenic cancer cells grow progressively in immune hosts without evidence for T cell exhaustion or systemic anergy. *J Exp Med* 1997; 186:229–238.

51. Chou T, Chang AE, Shu SY. Generation of therapeutic T lymphocytes from tumor-bearing mice by in vitro sensitization. Culture requirements and characterization of immunologic specificity. *J Immunol* 1988; 140:2453–2461.

52. Barth RJ Jr, Mule JJ, Asher AL, Sanda MG, Rosenberg SA. Identification of unique murine tumor associated antigens by tumor infiltrating lymphocytes using tumor specific secretion of interferon-gamma and tumor necrosis factor. *Methods* 1991; 140:269–279X.

53. Wang LX, Kjaergaard J, Cohen PA, Shu S, Plautz GE. Memory T cells originate from adoptively transferred effectors and reconstituting host cells after sequential lymphodepletion and adoptive immunotherapy. *J Immunol* 2004; 172:3462–3468.

54. Lou Y, Wang G, Lizee G, et al. Dendritic cells strongly boost the antitumor activity of adoptively transferred T cells in vivo. *Cancer Res* 2004; 64:6783–6790.

55. Arca MJ, Krauss JC, Aruga A, Cameron MJ, Shu S, Chang AE. Therapeutic efficacy of T cells derived from lymph nodes draining a poorly immunogenic tumor transduced to secrete granulocyte-macrophage colony-stimulating factor. *Cancer Gene Ther* 1996; 3:39–47.

56. Chang AE, Aruga A, Cameron MJ, et al. Adoptive immunotherapy with vaccine-primed lymph node cells secondarily activated with anti-CD3 and interleukin-2. *J Clin Oncol* 1997; 15:796–807.

57. Geiger JD, Wagner PD, Shu S, Chang AE. A novel role for autologous tumour cell vaccination in the immunotherapy of the poorly immunogenic B16-BL6 melanoma. *Surg Oncol* 1992; 1:199–208.

58. Geiger JD, Wagner PD, Cameron MJ, Shu S, Chang AE. Generation of T-cells reactive to the poorly immunogenic B16-BL6 melanoma with efficacy in the treatment of spontaneous metastases. *J Immunother* 1993; 13:153–165.

59. Inoue M, Plautz GE, Shu S. Treatment of intracranial tumors by systemic transfer of superantigen-activated tumor-draining lymph node T cells. *Cancer Res* 1996; 56:4702–4708.

60. Krauss JC, Strome SE, Chang AE, Shu S. Enhancement of immune reactivity in the lymph nodes draining a murine melanoma engineered to elaborate interleukin-4. *J Immunother Emphasis Tumor Immunol* 1994; 16:77–84.

61. Krauss JC, Shu S. Secretion of biologically active superantigens by mammalian cells. *J Hematother* 1997; 6:41–51.

62. Matsumura T, Krinock RA, Chang AE, Shu S. Cross-reactivity of anti-CD3/IL-2 activated effector cells derived from lymph nodes draining heterologous clones of a murine tumor. *Cancer Res* 1993; 53: 4315–4321.

63. Matsumura T, Sussman JJ, Krinock RA, Chang AE, Shu S. Characteristics and in vivo homing of long-term T-cell lines and clones derived from tumor-draining lymph nodes. *Cancer Res* 1994; 54:2744–2750.

64. Plautz GE, Inoue M, Shu S. Defining the synergistic effects of irradiation and T-cell immunotherapy for murine intracranial tumors. *Cell Immunol* 1996; 171:277–284.

65. Plautz GE, Touhalisky JE, Shu S. Treatment of murine gliomas by adoptive transfer of ex vivo activated tumor-draining lymph node cells. *Cell Immunol* 1997; 178:101–107.

66. Plautz GE, Barnett GH, Miller DW, et al. Systemic T cell adoptive immunotherapy of malignant gliomas. *J Neurosurg* 1998; 89:42–51.

67. Shu S, Sussman JJ, Chang AE. In vivo antitumor efficacy of tumor-draining lymph node cells activated with nonspecific T-cell reagents. *J Immunother* 1993; 14:279–285.

68 Shu S, Krinock RA, Matsumura T, Sussman JJ, et al. Stimulation of tumor-draining lymph node cells with superantigenic staphylococcal toxins leads to the generation of tumor-specific effector T cells. *J Immunol* 1994; 152:1277–1288.

69. Shu S, Krinock RA, Matsumura T, et al. Stimulation of tumor-draining lymph node cells with superantigenic staphylococcal toxins leads to the generation of tumor-specific effector T cells. *J Immunol* 1994; 152:1277–1288.

70. Sondak VK, Tuck MK, Shu S, Yoshizawa H, Chang AE. Enhancing effect of interleukin 1 alpha administration on antitumor effector T-cell development. *Arch Surg* 1991; 126:1503–1508; discussion 1508–1509.

71. Sussman JJ, Shu S, Sondak VK, Chang AE. Activation of T lymphocytes for the adoptive immunotherapy of cancer. *Ann Surg Oncol* 1994; 1:296–306.

72. Wahl WL, Sussman JJ, Shu S, Chang AE. Adoptive immunotherapy of murine intracerebral tumors with anti- CD3/interleukin-2-activated tumor-draining lymph node cells. *J Immunother Emphasis Tumor Immunol* 1994; 15:242–250.

73. Wahl WL, Strome SE, Nabel GJ, et al. Generation of therapeutic T-lymphocytes after in vivo tumor transfection with an allogeneic class I major histocompatibility complex gene. *J Immunother Emphasis Tumor Immunol* 1995; 17:1–11.

74. Yoshizawa H, Chang AE, Shu S. Specific adoptive immunotherapy mediated by tumor-draining lymph node cells sequentially activated with anti-CD3 and IL-2. *J Immunol* 1991; 147:729–737.

75. Peng L, Shu S, Krauss JC. Treatment of subcutaneous tumor with adoptively transferred T cells. *Cell Immunol* 1997; 178:24–32.

76. Mitchell MS. Relapse in the central nervous system in melanoma patients successfully treated with biomodulators. *J Clin Oncol* 1989; 7:1701–1709.

77. Cohen PJ, Cohen PA, Rosenberg SA, Katz SI, Mule JJ. Murine epidermal Langerhans cells and splenic dendritic cells present tumor-associated antigens to primed T cells. *Eur J Immunol* 1994; 24:315–319.

78. Greenberg P, Klarnet J, Kern D, Okuno K, Riddell S, Cheever M. Requirements for T cell recognition and elimination of retrovirally-transformed cells. *Princess Takamatsu Symp* 1988; 19:287–301.

79. Kjaergaard J, Peng L, Cohen PA, Drazba JA, Weinberg AD, Shu S. Augmentation vs inhibition: effects of conjunctional OX-40 receptor monoclonal antibody and IL-2 treatment on adoptive immunotherapy of advanced tumor. *J Immunol* 2001; 167:6669–6677.

80. Cohen PA, Fowler DJ, Kim H, et al. Propagation of murine and human T cells with defined antigen specificity and function. In: Frazer I, Chadwick D, Marsh J, eds. *Ciba Foundation Symposium No 187: Vaccines Against Virally Induced Cancers.* Chichester, UK: Wiley. 1994: pp. 179–193.

81. Cohen PA. CD4+ T cells in tumor rejection: past evidence and current prospects. In: Chang AE, Shu S, eds. *Immunotherapy of Cancer with Sensitized-Lymphocytes.* Philadelphia: Lippincott. 1994.

82. Kjaergaard J, Shu S. Tumor infiltration by adoptively transferred T cells is independent of immunologic specificity but requires down-regulation of L-selectin expression. *J Immunol* 1999; 163:751–759.

83. Kjaergaard J, Peng L, Cohen PA, Shu S. Therapeutic efficacy of adoptive immunotherapy is predicated on in vivo antigen-specific proliferation of donor T cells. *Clin Immunol* 2003; 108:8–20.

84. Mukai S, Kjaergaard J, Shu S, Plautz GE. Infiltration of tumors by systemically transferred tumor-reactive T lymphocytes is required for antitumor efficacy. *Cancer Res* 1999; 59:5245–5249.

85. Sallusto F, Lenig D, Forster R, Lipp M, Lanzavecchia A. Two subsets of memory T lymphocytes with distinct homing potentials and effector functions. *Nature* 1999; 401:708–712.

86. Masopust D, Vezys V, Marzo AL, Lefrancois L. Preferential localization of effector memory cells in nonlymphoid tissue. *Science* 2001; 291:2413–2417.

87. Tussey L, Speller S, Gallimore A, Vessey R. Functionally distinct CD8+ memory T cell subsets in persistent EBV infection are differentiated by migratory receptor expression. *Eur J Immunol* 2000; 30: 1823–1829.

88. Bradley LM, Duncan DD, Tonkonogy S, Swain SL. Characterization of antigen-specific CD4+ effector T cells in vivo: immunization results in a transient population of MEL-14-, CD45RB- helper cells that secretes interleukin 2 (IL-2), IL-3, IL- 4, and interferon gamma. *J Exp Med* 1991; 174:547–559.

89. Bradley LM, Yoshimoto K, Swain SL. The cytokines IL-4, IFN-gamma, and IL-12 regulate the development of subsets of memory effector helper T cells in vitro. *J Immunol* 1995; 155:1713–1724.

90. Mule JJ, Ettinghausen SE, Spiess PJ, Shu S, Rosenberg SA. Antitumor efficacy of lymphokine-activated killer cells and recombinant interleukin-2 in vivo: survival benefit and mechanisms of tumor escape in mice undergoing immunotherapy. *Cancer Res* 1986; 46:676–683.

91. Wallace PK, Morahan PS. Role of macrophages in the immunotherapy of Lewis lung peritoneal carcinomatosis. *J Leukoc Biol* 1994; 56:41–51.

92. Peng L, Krauss JC, Plautz GE, Mukai S, Shu S, Cohen PA. T-cell mediated rejection of established tumors displays a varied requirement for perforin and IFN-gamma expression which is not predicted by in vitro lytic capacity. *J Immunol* 2000; 165:7116–7124.

93. Plautz GE, Mukai S, Cohen PA, Shu S. Cross presentation of tumor antigens to effector T cells is sufficient to mediate effective immunotherapy of established intracranial tumors. *J Immunol* 2000; 165: 3656–3662.

94. Mukai S, Kagamu H, Shu S, Plautz GE. Critical role of CD11a (LFA-1) in therapeutic efficacy of systemically transferred antitumor effector T cells. *Cell Immunol* 1999; 192:122–132.

95 Winter H, Hu HM, Urba WJ, Fox BA. Tumor regression after adoptive transfer of effector T cells is independent of perforin or Fas ligand (APO-1L/CD95L). *J Immunol* 1999; 163:4462–4472.

96. Surman DR, Dudley ME, Overwijk WW, Restifo NP. CD4+ T cell control of CD8+ T cell reactivity to a model tumor antigen. *J Immunol* 2000; 164:562–565.

97. Ksander BR, Acevedo J, Streilein JW. Local T helper cell signals by lymphocytes infiltrating intraocular tumors. *J Immunol* 1992; 148:1955–1963.

98. Thivolet C, Bendelac A, Bedossa P, Bach JF, Carnaud C. CD8+ T cell homing to the pancreas in the nonobese diabetic mouse is CD4+ T cell-dependent. *J Immunol* 1991; 146:85–88.

99. Nishimura T, Iwakabe K, Sekimoto M, et al. Distinct role of antigen-specific T helper type 1 (Th1) and Th2 cells in tumor eradication in vivo. *J Exp Med* 1999; 190:617–627.

100. Hung K, Hayashi R, Lafond-Walker A, Lowenstein C, Pardoll D, Levitsky H. The central role of CD4(+) T cells in the antitumor immune response. *J Exp Med* 1998; 188:2357–2368.

101. Roszkowski JJ, Yu DC, Rubinstein MP, McKee MD, Cole DJ, Nishimura MI. CD8-independent tumor cell recognition is a property of the T cell receptor and not the T cell. *J Immunol* 2003; 170:2582–2589.

102. Nishimura MI, Avichezer D, Custer MC, et al. MHC class I-restricted recognition of a melanoma antigen by a human CD4+ tumor infiltrating lymphocyte. *Cancer Res* 1999; 59:6230–6238.

103. Asher AL, Mule JJ, Rosenberg SA. Recombinant human tumor necrosis factor mediates regression of a murine sarcoma in vivo via Lyt-2+ cells. *Cancer Immunol Immunother* 1989; 28:153–156.

104. Asher AL, Mule JJ, Kasid A, et al. Murine tumor cells transduced with the gene for tumor necrosis factor-alpha. Evidence for paracrine immune effects of tumor necrosis factor against tumors. *J Immunol* 1991; 146:3227–3234.

105. Mule JJ, Asher A, McIntosh J, et al. Antitumor effect of recombinant tumor necrosis factor-alpha against murine sarcomas at visceral sites: tumor size influences the response to therapy. *Cancer Immunol Immunother* 1988; 26:202–208.

106. Poehlein CH, Hu HM, Yamada J, et al. TNF plays an essential role in tumor regression after adoptive transfer of perforin/IFN-gamma double knockout effector T cells. *J Immunol* 2003; 170:2004–2013.

107. Berke G. The CTL's kiss of death. *Cell* 1995; 81:9–12.

108. Berke G. The Fas-based mechanism of lymphocytotoxicity. *Hum Immunol* 1997; 54:1–7.

109. Henkart PA. Lymphocyte-mediated cytotoxicity: two pathways and multiple effector molecules. *Immunity* 1994; 1:343–346.

110. Nagata S, Golstein P. The Fas death factor. *Science* 1995; 267:1449–1456.

111. Rosen D, Li J-H, Keidar S, Markon I, Orda R, Berke G. Tumor immunity in perforin-deficient mice: a role for CD95 (Fas/APO-1). *J Immunol* 2000; 164:3229–3235.

112. Frey AB, Cestari S. Killing of rat adenocarcinoma 13762 *in situ* by adoptive transfer of CD4+ antitumor T cells requires tumor expression of cell surface MHC class II molecules. *Cell Immunol* 1997; 178:79–90.

113. Miki S, Ksander B, Streilein JW. Studies on the minimum requirements for in vitro "cure" of tumor cells by cytotoxic T lymphocytes. *Reg Immunol* 1992; 4:352–362.

114. Bachmann MF, Kundig TM, Freer G, et al. Induction of protective cytotoxic T cells with viral proteins. *Eur J Immunol* 1994; 24:2228–2236.

115. Mayordomo JI, Tjandrawan T, DeLeo AB, Clarke MR, Lotze MT, Storkus WJ. Therapy of murine tumors with tumor peptide-pulsed dendritic cells: dependence on T cells, B7 costimulation, and T helper cell 1-associated cytokines. *J Exp Med* 1996; 183:87–97.

116. Rosenberg SA, Yang JC, Schwartzentruber DJ, et al. Immunologic and therapeutic evaluation of a synthetic peptide vaccine for the treatment of patients with metastatic melanoma [*see* comments]. *Nat Med* 1998; 4:321–327.

117. Silla S, Fallarino F, Boon T, Uyttenhove C. Enhancement by IL-12 of the cytolytic T lymphocyte (CTL) response of mice immunized with tumor-specific peptides in an adjuvant containing QS21 and MPL. *Eur Cytokine Netw* 1999; 10:181–190.

118. Walter EA, Greenberg PD, Gilbert MJ, et al. Reconstitution of cellular immunity against cytomegalovirus in recipients of allogeneic bone marrow by transfer of T-cell clones from the donor [*see* comments]. *N Engl J Med* 1995; 333:1038–1044.

119. Klarnet JP, Matis LA, Kern DE, et al. Antigen-driven T cell clones can proliferate in vivo, eradicate disseminated leukemia, and provide specific immunologic memory. *J Immunol* 1987; 138:4012–4017.

120. Shrikant P, Mescher MF. Control of syngeneic tumor growth by activation of CD8+ T cells: efficacy is limited by migration away from the site and induction of nonresponsiveness. *J Immunol* 1999; 162:2858–2866.

121. Chambers CA, Allison JP. Costimulatory regulation of T cell function. *Curr Opin Cell Biol* 1999; 11:203–210.

122. Diehl L, den Boer AT, Schoenberger SP, et al. CD40 activation in vivo overcomes peptide-induced peripheral cytotoxic T-lymphocyte tolerance and augments anti-tumor vaccine efficacy. *Nat Med* 1999; 5:774–779.

123. French RR, Chan HT, Tutt AL, Glennie MJ. CD40 antibody evokes a cytotoxic T-cell response that eradicates lymphoma and bypasses T-cell help. *Nat Med* 1999; 5:548–553.

124. Gajewski TF, Renauld JC, Van Pel A, Boon T. Costimulation with B7-1, IL-6, and IL-12 is sufficient for primary generation of murine antitumor cytolytic T lymphocytes in vitro. *J Immunol* 1995; 154: 5637–5648.

125. Sotomayor EM, Borrello I, Tubb E, Allison JP, Levitsky HI. In vivo blockade of CTLA-4 enhances the priming of responsive T cells but fails to prevent the induction of tumor antigen- specific tolerance. *Proc Natl Acad Sci USA* 1999; 96:11,476–11,481.

126. Bando Y, Ksander BR, Streilein JW. Characterization of specific T helper cell activity in mice bearing alloantigenic tumors in the anterior chamber of the eye. *Eur J Immunol* 1991; 21:1923–1931.

127. Ridge JP, Di Rosa F, Matzinger P. A conditioned dendritic cell can be a temporal bridge between a CD4$^+$ T- helper and a T-killer cell. *Nature* 1998; 393:474–478.

128. Thivolet C, Bendelac A, Bedossa P, Bach JF, Carnaud C. CD8$^+$ T cell homing to the pancreas in the nonobese diabetic mouse is CD4$^+$ T cell-dependent. *J Immunol* 1991; 146:85–88.

129. Plautz GE, Inoue M, Shu S. Defining the synergistic effects of irradiation and T-cell immunotherapy for murine intracranial tumors. *Cell Immunol* 1996; 171:277–284.

130. Peng L, Krauss JC, Plautz GE, Mukai S, Shu S, Cohen PA. T cell-mediated tumor rejection displays diverse dependence upon perforin and IFN-gamma mechanisms that cannot be predicted from in vitro T cell characteristics. *J Immunol* 2000; 165:7116–7124.

131. Mihalyo MA, Doody AD, McAleer JP, et al. In vivo cyclophosphamide and IL-2 treatment impedes self-antigen-induced effector CD4 cell tolerization: implications for adoptive immunotherapy. *J Immunol* 2004; 172:5338–5345.

132. Peng L, Awad M, Kjaergaard J, et al. Nonmyeloablative radiation enables successful antitumor adoptive immunotherapy by an abscopal (remote) mechanism associated with activation and mobilization of CD34^{pos} stem cells. *Am Assoc Cancer Res 2004 Proc* 2004; (abstract no. 2473).

133. Childs R, Chernoff A, Contentin N, et al. Regression of metastatic renal-cell carcinoma after nonmyeloablative allogeneic peripheral-blood stem-cell transplantation. *N Engl J Med* 2000; 343:750–758.

134. Winter H, Hu HM, McClain K, Urba WJ, Fox BA. Immunotherapy of melanoma: a dichotomy in the requirement for IFN-gamma in vaccine-induced antitumor immunity versus adoptive immunotherapy. *J Immunol* 2001; 166:7370–7380.

135. Rosenberg SA, Yannelli JR, Yang JC, et al. Treatment of patients with metastatic melanoma with autologous tumor-infiltrating lymphocytes and interleukin2. *J Natl Cancer Inst* 1994; 86:1159–1166.

136. Uzzo RG, Rayman P, Kolenko V, et al. Mechanisms of apoptosis in T cells from patients with renal cell carcinoma. *Clin Cancer Res* 1999; 5:1219–1229.

137. Gastman BR, Johnson DE, Whiteside TL, Rabinowich H. Tumor-induced apoptosis of T lymphocytes: elucidation of intracellular apoptotic events. *Blood* 2000; 95:2015–2023.

138. Whiteside TL. Immune cells in the tumor microenvironment. Mechanisms responsible for functional and signaling defects. *Adv Exp Med Biol* 1998; 451:167–171.

139. Childs RW. Nonmyeloablative blood stem cell transplantation as adoptive allogeneic immunotherapy for metastatic renal cell carcinoma. *Crit Rev Immunol* 2001; 21:91–203.

140. Dudley ME, Wunderlich J, Nishimura MI, et al. Adoptive transfer of cloned melanoma-reactive T lymphocytes for the treatment of patients with metastatic melanoma. *J Immunother* 2001; 24:363 373.

141. Dudley ME, Wunderlich JR, Yang JC, et al. A phase I study of nonmyeloablative chemotherapy and adoptive transfer of autologous tumor antigen-specific T lymphocytes in patients with metastatic melanoma. *J Immunother* 2002; 25:243–251.

142. Aebersold P, Hyatt C, Johnson S, et al. Lysis of autologous melanoma cells by tumor-infiltrating lymphocytes: association with clinical response. *J Natl Cancer Inst* 1991; 83:932–937.

143. Schwartzentruber DJ, Hom SS, Dadmarz R, et al. In vitro predictors of therapeutic response in melanoma patients receiving tumor-infiltrating lymphocytes and interleukin-2. *J Clin Oncol* 1994; 12:1475–1483.

144. Barth RJ Jr, Mule JJ, Spiess PJ, Rosenberg SA. Interferon gamma and tumor necrosis factor have a role in tumor regressions mediated by murine CD8$^+$ tumor-infiltrating lymphocytes. *J Exp Med* 1991; 173: 647–658X.

145. Shrikant P, Mescher MF. Opposing effects of IL-2 in tumor immunotherapy: promoting CD8 T cell growth and inducing apoptosis. *J Immunol* 2002; 169:1753–1759.
146. Tanaka H, Tanaka J, Kjaergaard J, Shu S. Depletion of CD4+CD25+ regulatory cells aguments the generation of specific immune T cells in tumor-draining lymph nodes. *J Immunother* 2002; 25:207–217.
147. Pockaj BA, Sherry RM, Wei JP, et al. Localization of 111indium-labeled tumor infiltrating lymphocytes to tumor in patients receiving adoptive immunotherapy. Augmentation with cyclophosphamide and correlation with response. *Cancer* 1994; 73:1731–1737.
148. Yee C, Gilbert MJ, Riddell SR, et al. Isolation of tyrosinase-specific CD8+ and CD4+ T cell clones from the peripheral blood of melanoma patients following in vitro stimulation with recombinant vaccinia virus. *J Immunol* 1996; 157:4079–4086.
149. Yee C, Thompson JA, Byrd D, et al. Adoptive T cell therapy using antigen-specific CD8+ T cell clones for the treatment of patients with metastatic melanoma: in vivo persistence, migration, and antitumor effect of transferred T cells. *Proc Natl Acad Sci USA* 2002; 99:16,168–16,173.
150. Knutson KL, Schiffman K, Disis ML. Immunization with a HER-2/*neu* helper peptide vaccine generates HER-2/*neu* CD8 T-cell immunity in cancer patients. *J Clin Invest* 2001; 107:477–484.
151. Disis ML, Grabstein KH, Sleath PR, Cheever MA. Generation of immunity to the HER-2/*neu* oncogenic protein in patients with breast and ovarian cancer using a peptide-based vaccine. *Clin Cancer Res* 1999; 5:1289–1297.
152. Knutson KL, Disis ML. Clonal diversity of the T-cell population responding to a dominant HLA-A2 epitope of HER-2/*neu* after active immunization in an ovarian cancer patient. *Hum Immunol* 2002; 63:547–557.

13 Retroviral-Mediated Gene Transfer for Engineering Tumor-Reactive T-Cells

*Jeffrey J. Roszkowski
and Michael I. Nishimura*

SUMMARY

Immunotherapy for cancer has taken several approaches including vaccinating patients to elicit T-cell responses to tumor antigens and adoptive transfer of tumor-reactive T-cells to patients. Vaccination has historically been ineffective in generating objective clinical responses. Whereas adoptive cell transfer therapy has shown some promise, the difficulties in obtaining the large number of requisite tumor-reactive T-cells warrant investigation into alternate models of immunotherapy. A novel approach is the retroviral-mediated transfer of genes encoding recognition of tumor antigens into peripheral blood T-cells. By cloning genes for T-cell receptors that mediate antitumor reactivity and introducing them into a patient's own T-cells, we can rapidly generate the large number of T-cells necessary for adoptive transfer therapy for any patient, regardless of the patient's immune status.

Key Words: Cancer; gene therapy; T-cell receptor; melanoma; immunotherapy.

1. INTRODUCTION

Because of the discovery that tumor cells can elicit both humoral and cell-mediated immune responses, medical researchers have been attempting to use the immune system to fight cancer. Investigators have tried to identify the immunological properties of cancer cells and the ways in which the immune system responds to the presence of these cells. Immune responses are typically because of the presence of tumor-associated antigens (TAAs) expressed by tumor cells *(1,2)*. Multiple methods of targeting TAAs have been explored with varied levels of success. In this chapter, following an initial discussion of some basic principles of cancer immunology and current immunotherapeutic approaches, we discuss a novel approach to immunotherapy whereby retroviral vectors are used to genetically engineer T-cells to recognize cancer cells. T-cells have been engineered to express various receptors that target TAAs with varied results. The nature of these receptors, their introduction into normal T-cells, and their biological function are reviewed.

From: *Cancer Drug Discovery and Development: Immunotherapy of Cancer*
Edited by: M. L. Disis © Humana Press Inc., Totowa, NJ

1.1. Tumor Antigens

TAAs may be recognized by both the cellular and humoral components of the immune system. One class of TAAs is normal proteins expressed by tumor cells that can be recognized by antibodies *(3)*. Antibodies are generated by B-cells and are an intricate component of the humoral immune response. Antibody binding to tumor cells can lead to antibody-dependent cell-mediated cytotoxicity and complement-mediated lysis *(4)*. Antibodies targeting TAAs can also serve to block the cell surface receptors they target, thereby impairing cellular function in tumor cells *(5)*.

Some TAAs may also be degraded during normal cellular function and appear as peptide fragments that are "presented" to immune cells, resulting in T-cell-mediated immune responses. These antigenic peptides are bound to molecules of the major histocompatibility complex (MHC) on the surface of either tumor cells or antigen-presenting cells (APCs), such as dendritic cells (DCs), which are then recognized by T-cells *(6,7)*. This recognition occurs through the T-cell receptor (TCR), a heterodimer consisting of α- and β-chains that, when co-expressed, recognize a specific peptide bound to a particular MHC molecule. T-cells and T-cell epitopes are recognized as a critical component of antitumor immunity, with most immunotherapies designed to elicit or enhance T-cell responses. T-cell epitopes are peptide fragments bound to either class I or class II MHC molecules (human leukocyte antigen [HLA] in humans), which are recognized by $CD8^+$ cytotoxic T-lymphocytes (CTLs) and $CD4^+$ T-cells or T-helper (Th) cells, respectively.

The proteins from which T-cell-recognized antigens are derived may be normal proteins that are aberrantly expressed or overexpressed by tumor cells, or may be the result of genetic mutations or an alternate open reading frame *(1,2)*. As a result, TAAs recognized by T-cells fall into one of several classifications based on their pattern of expression.

One category of TAAs, called the cancer/testis antigens (so named for their expression on histologically different human tumors, as well as normal testis tissues), includes the first reported TAA, melanoma-associated antigen (MAGE)-1, as well as several others (B melanoma antigen, G antigen, NY-ESO-1) *(8,9)*.

Differentiation antigens are a second group of TAAs found in both tumors and the normal tissues from which those tumors were derived. Melanoma antigen recognized by T-cells (MART)-1, gp100, and tyrosinase are all TAAs of melanoma-containing epitopes that elicit T-cell responses *(10–14)*. This category also includes the prostate-specific antigen *(15,16)*.

A third class of TAAs is the widely expressed antigens that are found in both normal tissues and a variety of histologically distinct tumor types. These "self" proteins may become antigenic by their overexpression in tumor cells as compared to normal tissues, thereby breaking immunological tolerance. These include Her-2/*neu*, which is commonly associated with breast cancer, and carcinoembryonic antigen (CEA), often expressed by colon carcinoma, as well as others tumors *(5,17,18)*.

Yet another group includes the tumor-specific antigens, which result from point mutations in normal genes; hence, they are unique to the tumors from which they are derived. Still other T-cell-recognized TAAs are the result of fusion proteins derived through the process of carcinogenesis, and are not found in normal tissue.

The vast majority of known TAA T-cell epitopes are class I MHC-restricted and therefore, recognized by CTLs. However, a smaller number of class II MHC-restricted epitopes recognized by Th cells have been identified. (For a complete review of T-cell-recognized TAAs, *see* Renkvist et al. *[16]*.)

1.2. Strategies for Immunotherapy

Various approaches for immune targeting of TAAs have been developed and include monoclonal antibody (MAb) therapy, vaccination, and adoptive T-cell transfer therapy. Several MAbs targeting TAAs are in clinical use *(19–21)*. Trastuzumab (Herceptin®), an antibody used to treat breast cancer patients, inhibits the cellular proliferation of breast cancer cells expressing the Her-2/*neu* antigen *(5,22)*. Edrecolomab (Panorax®) is an antibody targeting the antigen gp17-1A in colorectal cancer *(23)*. Several antibodies have been developed to target B-cell antigens for the treatment of non-Hodgkin's lymphoma *(19,24–26)*. However, the low efficacy rate and toxicity that can often accompany the use of antibody therapy has led some to search for alternative forms of immunotherapy that utilize cell-mediated immune responses.

Vaccination strategies are generally designed to elicit B- and T-cell responses to tumor antigens. Vaccinating with irradiated tumor cells, tumor-cell lysates, antigenic peptide, or peptide-loaded DCs have been employed, most often in melanoma patients *(27–30)*. Although an increase in the presence of melanoma-reactive CTLs has been observed, there has been little or no correlation between the induction of these CTL and clinical responses *(31–38)*. Vaccination strategies for other forms of cancer have proven particularly ineffective at increasing TAA-reactive CTL, with even fewer clinical responses. The general ineffectiveness of vaccination to date has led to the use of yet another form of immunotherapy, adoptive T-cell transfer.

Adoptive T-cell transfer therapy, which involves infusing a cancer patient with autologous tumor-reactive T-cells, has led to tumor regression in some patients *(39–43)*. Adoptive T-cell transfer requires large-scale expansion of T-cells with antitumor reactivity in vitro (reviewed by Dudley and Rosenberg *[44]*). Providing for a source of these reactive T-cells is a difficult process. Early efforts included lymphokine-activated killer cells or anti-CD3 antibody-activated peripheral blood lymphocytes (PBLs) *(45–48)*. Other methods have included isolating T-cells from the draining lymph nodes of tumor vaccine recipients or using peptide-loaded DCs to stimulate PBLs isolated from patients *(49–51)*. However, the latter process can be lengthy and is often unsuccessful.

Another source of T-cells for adoptive transfer has been tumor-infiltrating lymphocytes (TILs) isolated from tumor lesions, expanded ex vivo, and screened for antitumor reactivity before reinfusion into the patient *(52)*. TILs have been generated from renal cell carcinoma, glioma, and melanoma. Melanoma is particularly conducive to isolating TILs because of the access to cutaneous tumor lesions *(43,53,54)*. Autologous TILs combined with interleukin (IL)-2 administration has been used to treat melanoma patients, with some tumor regressions observed *(41,42)*. Although clinical responses in melanoma patients have occurred using TIL, persistence of the transferred cells was short-lived *(55)*. Isolating tumor-reactive CTLs from the TILs of other tumor types has proven very difficult and often fruitless.

Although adoptive T-cell transfer has clearly shown promise for some forms of cancer, the problem of generating a response of sufficient strength and persistence for complete or even partial tumor regression of most tumor types, including melanoma, remains a hurdle. Therefore, new ways must be found to generate a significant and lasting source of tumor-reactive T-cells. A relatively new proposal for generating large numbers of tumor-reactive T-cells is to use gene therapy methods to generate artificially T-cells that are reactive to TAAs. Transferring genes encoding reactivity to TAAs into normal T-cells isolated from the blood of cancer patients may provide the means to quickly generate a large

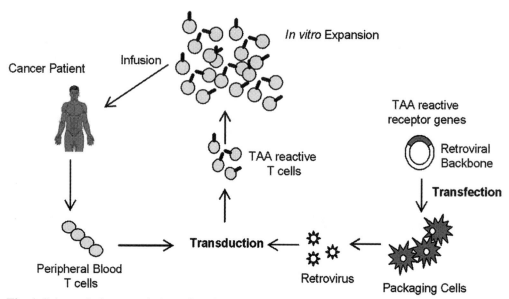

Fig. 1. Schematic for retroviral-mediated T-cell gene transfer therapy for cancer. Genes encoding a tumor-associated antigen (TAA)-reactive receptor are inserted into a retroviral vector. The vector is transfected into packaging cells for generation of retroviral supernatants. Peripheral blood T-cells from a cancer patient are isolated and transduced with a retrovirus-encoding receptor gene for TAA recognition. The resulting T-cells express the TAA-reactive receptor and may be expanded in vitro. Following confirmation of TAA reactivity in vitro the transduced T-cells are adoptively transferred back to the patient.

population of reactive cells for use in adoptive transfer. The most widely utilized method of gene transfer to T-cells employs retroviral vectors to transduce T-cell populations with the cancer-reactive receptor of choice.

2. GENE TRANSFER TO T-CELLS

The rationale of retroviral-mediated gene transfer to T-cells is outlined in Fig. 1. Essentially, genes encoding for cell-surface receptors specific for TAAs are inserted into a retroviral backbone. These constructs are then transfected into cell lines that produce replication-defective, infectious retroviral particles. These retroviral supernatants are used to transduce PBLs isolated from a cancer patient. The resulting T-cell cultures express the receptor encoding TAA reactivity. These cells may then be expanded in vitro and are adoptively transferred back into the patient providing a large pool of T-cells that can react to the patient's tumor cells. The receptors displaying TAA reactivity may take different forms including chimeric antibody-based receptors, full-length TCRs, or chimeric TCRs (cTCRs).

2.1. Tumor-Specific Chimeric Antibody Receptors

One class of cell surface receptors capable of transferring antitumor reactivity to T-cells is chimeric antibody receptors (cAbRs). cAbRs have been constructed that have an extracellular antibody domain (scFv), a single chain consisting of the antibody variable heavy, and light-chain fragments connected with a linker, which is then fused to an intracellular

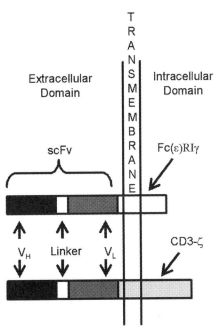

Fig. 2. Typical structure of chimeric antibody receptors. A single-chain antibody domain consisting of the variable heavy and light chain immunoglobulin fragments connected with a linker makes up the extracellular domain providing for antigen recognition. A intracellular domain, typically from the Fc receptor γ-chain or CD3-ζ chain, is then fused to the extracellular domain to provide for receptor signaling.

signaling domain *(56–58)*. The signaling molecules commonly used are from CD3-ζ, a component of the TCR complex, or the FcεRI-γ chain (Fig. 2). These cAbRs, when expressed on T-cells, show similar binding specificity and affinity for TAAs as the original MAb from which they were derived. Additionally, cAbRs mediate specific immune function, including cytokine release and target cell lysis, by cells on which they are expressed including CTL, natural-killer cells, TILs, and normal T-cells *(59–64)*. cAbr-expressing T-cells were shown to lyse specifically melanoma cells by targeting the ganglioside GD3, or the high-molecular-weight melanoma-associated antigen *(65–67)*. Her-2/*neu*-expressing tumor cells were recognized by T-cells expressing a Her-2-specific cAbR, and T-cells expressing a cAbR against the G250 antigen were able kill renal cell carcinoma cells *(68,69)*. MAGE-1-reactive cAbRs have also been successfully transferred to human T-cells *(70,71)*.

Mouse tumor models have been used to evaluate the in vivo efficacy of cAbRs. Established tumors expressing Her-2/*neu* were completely rejected on treatment of mice with normal T-cells expressing a Her-2-specific cAbR *(72)*. T-cells expressing a cAbR specific for CEA-mediated control or rejection of human colon carcinoma in severe combined immunodeficiency mice or mouse colon adenocarcinoma in C57BL/6 mice *(73)*. The CTLs expressing these cAbR produced both perforin and interferon (IFN)-γ, both believed to be critical for antitumor effects. In yet another study, nude mice implanted with human ovarian cancer were treated with adoptively transferred TILs expressing a cAbR specific for folate-binding protein *(74)*. Mice treated with these TILs had significantly longer survival rates than those treated with TIL expressing an irrelevant receptor.

Potential benefits of cAbRs include the ability to engineer expression in cells of the immune system other than classical α-/β-TCR$^+$ T-cells. Antitumor effects in mice treated with bone marrow cells retrovirally transduced with a cAbR in which α-/β-TCR$^+$ T-cells were depleted before transfer have been reported *(75)*. Other advantages include recognition of TAAs in an MHC-independent manner. The fact that cAbRs recognize antibody-defined antigens, such as normal cell surface receptors, gangliosides, or carbohydrates, means that any given receptor has the potential to treat a large number of patients, independent of their expressed MHC phenotype. However, there may be drawbacks to using cAbRs. Conflicting studies have shown that antigen recognition by T-cells and their subsequent cell signaling and effector function is a complex process that may not be accurately reflected by the artificial nature of these chimeric molecules *(57,76)*. Because cAbRs bind to TAAs with as much as 1000-fold-higher affinity than TCRs to MHC-bound peptides, T-cells expressing cAbRs may be incapable of recycling their lytic capacity following initial antigen encounter *(77)*. The temporal length of these interactions may hinder optimal activation and function of the T-cells *(78,79)*. The strong binding interaction may also induce activation induced cell death in the T-cells *(80)*. Investigators have attempted to address these concerns by modifying cAbRs to contain the signaling domain of CD28. CD28 is a co-stimulatory molecule on T-cells that binds to CD80 on target cells. This interaction serves to promote T-cell proliferation and immune function while protecting against T-cell death on antigen recognition by T-cells *(81)*. In vitro data suggests that employing CD28 signaling domains on cAbRs may overcome the problems associated with strong receptor–ligand interactions otherwise occurring independent of CD28 *(82–84)*. However, in vivo data are still unavailable. Finally, the fusion of different protein domains to create cAbRs may result in immunogenic structures that can elicit an immune response against cells bearing these receptors. These concerns have led others and us to employ full-length TCR genes to engineer tumor reactive T-cells.

2.2. Tumor-Specific TCRs

A second class of cell surface receptors that can transfer reactivity to TAAs into T-cells are full-length TCRs. As stated earlier, the TCR consists as a heterodimer, made up of unique α- and β-chains. The α-chain is composed of variable (V), joining (J), and constant segments, whereas an additional diversity region is located between the V and J segments of the β-chain. Germline rearrangements of these regions coupled with random nucleotide deletions or insertions between the V/J (α) and J/diversity (β) during receptor formation lead to an immense diversity in the TCR repertoire. A TCR recognizes a specific peptide bound to a particular MHC molecule (peptide–MHC complex). T-cells reactive to tumor-specific peptide/MHC complex have been isolated and cloned *(85–91)*. Determining the immune function of these clones combined with genetic analysis of their TCRs by polymerase chain reaction and DNA sequencing of the J regions revealed that multiple V regions were employed in functional recognition of a single antigen *(92)*. Therefore, several different TCR genes may be utilized in gene transfer to direct T-cell specificity towards a single antigen.

2.2.1. Transfer of a MART-1-Reactive TCR

As stated previously, MART-1 is a melanocyte differentiation antigen and is expressed by most melanoma tumors. In particular, the MART-1 peptide consisting of amino acids 27–35 is presented to T-cells in the context of *HLA-A2 (93)*. *HLA-A2* is the predominant

MHC allele expressed in the United States, occurring in approx 50% of the Caucasian population. Identifying a TCR specific for MART-1$_{27-35}$ to use in gene transfer would provide the ability to treat the widest potential patient pool. We therefore undertook studies to determine if wild-type T-cells could functionally express a MART-1-specific TCR in the presence of the endogenous TCR.

Jurkat cells, a T-cell lymphoma line, were co-transfected with plasmids containing the individual α- and β-chain genes identified for a MART-1$_{27-35}$-reactive T-cell clone (TIL-5) derived from a TIL culture isolated from a melanoma patient (86). TIL-5 TCR expression by transfected clones was confirmed indirectly by antibody treatment of the cells. No antibodies exist for the specific α- and β-chains (Vα1, Vβ7.3) that compose the TIL-5 TCR. However, the endogenous TCR of Jurkat cells utilizes the Vβ8 gene and becomes downregulated on ligation with anti-Vβ8 antibody. CD3, which is expressed in conjunction with TCRs, becomes downregulated as well. Therefore, the level of TCR and/or CD3 on the surface of the transfected clones treated with Vβ8 antibody correlated to the level of the transferred MART-1-reactive TCR. The functional capacity of transfected clones with varied levels of TCR expression was determined by co-culturing the clones with T2 cells, an HLA-A2-restricted APC line, loaded with MART-1$_{27-35}$ peptide. Transfected Jurkat clones secreted IL-2 in response to culture with MART-1-loaded T2 cells, but not T2 cells loaded with an irrelevant peptide. Furthermore, the functional avidity of the transfected clones correlated with the level of TIL-5 TCR on their surface. Clones expressing higher levels of the transferred TCR required less peptide to stimulate IL-2 secretion and secreted more total IL-2 as the peptide concentration increased. Wild-type Jurkats did not secrete IL-2 in response to MART-1 peptide. This was the first demonstration of functionally transferring a TAA-specific TCR to alternate T-cells. Since these studies, Jurkat cells have been used to evaluate the transfer of other TCRs, including an HLA-A2-restricted TCR specific for MAGE-3 (94,95).

2.2.2. REDIRECTING SPECIFICITY OF NORMAL PERIPHERAL BLOOD T-CELLS FOR MART-1

The preceding study led us to attempt to transfer the TIL-5 TCR to primary human T-cells obtained from PBLs. A retroviral vector encoding the TIL-5 TCR was used to transduce PBLs (96). PBLs were first activated with anti-CD3 antibody to stimulate T-cell proliferation, which is required for incorporation of retrovirus into the target-cell genome (97). As with Jurkat cells, transduction of primary T-cells resulted in cultures that responded to stimulation with MART-1-loaded T2 cells by secreting cytokines. Some cultures also secreted cytokines when cultured with HLA-A2$^+$ melanoma cells but not HLA-A2$^-$ melanoma lines, indicating direct recognition of tumor cells in an MHC-restricted manner. This study verified that one could generate a culture of tumor-reactive T-cells by TCR gene transfer that could potentially be expanded for adoptive transfer to cancer patients.

Clones generated from these cultures had varied effector functions in response to co-culture with target cells. Some clones were capable of both significant IFN-γ secretion and effective lysis of both peptide-loaded APCs and melanoma cells. Others only lysed targets, whereas still others only secreted IFN-γ. Further analysis of these clones revealed that only those that expressed the CD8 coreceptor were capable of recognizing tumor cells with subsequent effector function. Clones that expressed only the CD4 coreceptor could produce IFN-γ only in response to MART-1$_{27-35}$-loaded T2 cells or tumor cells loaded with an excess of exogenous peptide. The TIL-5 TCR-expressing Jurkat T-cells

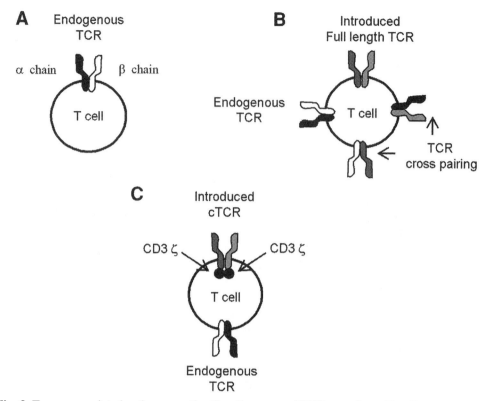

Fig. 3. Tumor associated antigen-reactive T-cell receptor (TCR) transfer to T-cells may result in receptors with unknown specificity. (**A**) T-cells used for TCR gene transfer express an endogenous TCR consisting of α- and β-chains. (**B**) Introduction of a full-length TCR can result in crosspairing of the endogenous α-chain with the introduced β-chain and vice versa. (**C**) Chimeric TCRs contain a signaling domain, often CD3-ζ, fused to the TCR α- and β-chains. This can eliminate TCR cross-pairing as the two chains of the chimeric TCRs can only pair with each other.

described earlier also lack the CD8 co-receptor, and similar to the above CD4⁺ clones, were unable to recognize tumor cells unless they were loaded with exogenous peptide. These results demonstrated that the MHC class I-restricted, MART-$1_{27–35}$-reactive TIL-5 TCR is dependent on CD8 for full receptor function. The CD8 co-receptor both enhances the stability of the TCR/peptide/MHC complex by binding to class I MHC molecules and promotes signal transduction through the recruitment of the protein kinase lck to the TCR/CD3 complex *(98)*. Lack of TCR function in the absence of CD8 may imply that the TCR is of low affinity for the peptide/MHC ligand.

2.3. Chimeric TCRs

Whereas some investigators have continued to explore the retroviral transfer of various full-length TCRs, others have explored genetically modifying the TCR genes in attempts to increase the effective function of retrovirally modified T-cells. cTCR genes have been generated to increase the stable expression of introduced TCR α- and β-chains. When full-length TCR genes are introduced into normal T-cells, the native TCR α- and β-chains may pair with the exogenous TCR β- and α-chains respectively (Fig. 3). This serves to dilute the number of functionally paired TCRs on the cell surface *(99,100)*. It also raises the concern of generating TCRs with unknown specificity, which may lead to an autoimmune response. One group attempted to circumvent this problem by fusing the cytoplasmic signaling domain of CD3-ζ to MAGE-1-reactive TCR α and β genes *(101)*. These genes were shown to pair exclusively to each other following retroviral transfer to T-cells, preventing both dilution of functional transferred TCR and generation of TCRs with unknown specificity (Fig. 3). It also increased the stability of TCR α-chain expression, which can be less stable in unmodified TCRs. Furthermore, the gene-modified T-cells conferred MAGE-1-reactive function following retroviral transfer. This group has also created a single-chain version of this chimeric MAGE-1 TCR, whereby a single-gene construct consisted of the αV region fused to the βV chain and again fused with CD3ζ. This single-gene construct maintained MAGE-1 reactivity following retroviral transfer to T-cells. This circumvents the concerns of generating unknown specificities using full-length TCR genes, and allows a smaller, simpler viral vector to enhance gene expression. Other signaling domains from CD28, CD3-ε, and FcεRI-γ-chain have been used in efforts to increase the efficacy of the transferred receptor. cTCRs thus appear to have benefits over unmodified TCRs, but also share some of the concerns cited with regard to cAbRs. Regardless of the choice to use cTCRs or unmodified full-length TCRs, results of work performed to date, including results of transfer of the MART-1-specific TCR described in Subheading 2.2.2., have led to questions about the properties of a TCR that are important when selecting it for use in TCR gene transfer.

2.4. TCR Properties

The antigen specificity of a TCR is certainly the first consideration in choosing a TCR for gene transfer. Since the first functional transfer of a tumor-specific TCR to primary T-cells, TCRs specific for a number of TAAs, as well as viral antigens associated with tumor development, have been successfully introduced into T-cells via retroviral gene transfer. These include TCRs specific for melanoma antigens MAGE-3, gp100, tyrosinase, and CTL-recognized antigen on melanoma; the widely expressed oncoprotein MDM2; and the Epstein-Barr virus protein latent membrane protein-2, expressed by Hodgkin's lymphoma *(94,95,102–107)*. It will be important to continue to identify potential target antigens for various tumor types, because immune evasion mechanisms can result in antigen loss by the tumor or in T-cell unresponsiveness *(108–111)*. It may therefore become necessary to treat patients with T-cells targeting multiple antigens, either in combination or in serial treatments. Another possibility is to use T-cells engineered to express multiple receptors to confer multiple specificities. Recently, the transfer of a TCR into T-cells with known specificity has been shown to result in individual cells reactive to both antigens *(112,113)*. It is therefore conceivable to introduce multiple TAA-specific TCRs into T-cells.

In conjunction with antigen specificity, MHC restriction will dictate the patient population that can be treated with a given TCR. As stated previously, our laboratory has focused on HLA-A2-restricted epitopes because of the prevalence of this allele in the US population. However, populations with different genetic backgrounds would require TCRs restricted to alternate MHC alleles. For instance, *HLA-A24* is the predominant allele in Japan, and epitopes for a number of other MHC alleles have been identified *(16)*.

Although the antigen specificity of a tumor-specific TCR is its most fundamental property, several genetically distinct TCRs can lead to recognition of a given peptide–MHC complex, as mentioned in Subheading 2.2. Thus, given single-epitope specificity, what may make one TCR more effective than the next? Avidity of T-cells, or sensitivity to antigen, is important to consider because high avidity has been shown to correlate with tumor recognition in vitro and tumor regression in vivo (114,115). It is reasonable to conclude that TCRs expressed by high-avidity T-cells would be superior to those expressed by low-avidity T-cells. Others and we have demonstrated that transferring a TCR into alternate T-cells can result in cells with comparable avidity to the original T-cell from which the TCR was isolated (102–104).

Another factor in considering a TCR is the dependence on CD8 for antigen recognition. It has been suggested that CD8-independent antigen recognition by T-cells indicates expression of a high-affinity TCR (116). However, the vast majorities of MHC class I-restricted T-cells are CD8-dependent and would therefore have intermediate- to low-affinity TCRs. The TIL-5 TCR reviewed earlier may represent a low-affinity TCR because of the fact that only $CD8^+$ T-cells could recognize tumor cells directly. A more recent study described the retroviral transfer of a gp100:$_{209-217}$-reactive TCR to normal T-cells (103). The resulting $CD8^+$ T-cells had high avidity for peptide-loaded APCs and recognized tumor cells. The $CD4^+$ T-cells also recognized peptide-loaded APCs with high avidity, but the authors presented no evidence of tumor cell recognition, suggesting that the TCR was similar to the TIL-5 TCR that lacks sufficient affinity to activate T-cells on encountering physiological levels of antigen on tumor cells in the absence of CD8.

In work previously done in our laboratory, we isolated and transferred a TCR specific for an HLA-A2-restricted epitope of the melanoma antigen tyrosinase (104). This class I MHC-restricted TCR is unusual in that it was cloned from $CD4^+$ TILs (TIL 1383I [117]). We hypothesized that this TCR, which recognized tumor cells in the absence of CD8, was of high affinity and could function following transfer to $CD8^-$ T-cells.

We first modified the TCR gene sequence to allow expression in a mouse T-cell line BW58 α^-/β^-, which lacks expression of an endogenous TCR and does not contain the human CD8 molecule. Cells transduced with a retrovirus encoding the TIL 1383I TCR expressed TCR on their surface and secreted IL-2 in response to both peptide-loaded T2 cells as well as HLA-A2$^+$ melanoma cells. Clones generated from these cultures had functional avidity comparable to the original TIL 1383I, and avidity correlated with the level of TCR expression. Therefore, full CD8-independent function of a class I MHC- restricted TCR was established following genetic transfer, implying the TIL 1383I TCR is a high-affinity T-cell receptor.

As stated previously, the vast majority of TAA epitopes described thus far are class I MHC-restricted. This is partly because of the extreme diversity of class II MHC genes in humans. It is far less likely that TCRs that are class II-restricted would be capable of treating a large number of patients. We have recently demonstrated the transfer of the TIL 1383I TCR into normal, PBLs (105). The resulting cultures contained both $CD8^+$ and $CD4^+$ T-cells that displayed reactivity to melanoma cell lines by releasing cytokines and/or lysing tumor cell targets. These results demonstrate the potential to generate $CD4^+$ T-cell help against class I MHC-restricted antigen on tumor cells. The lack of shared class II MHC epitopes has made studying cancer-specific T-cell help in humans difficult, but in vitro studies and animal models have demonstrated the importance of T-cell help in combating malignancies (118–121). Th cells secrete cytokines and aid in the activation of $CD8^+$ T-cells to make them functionally more effective (119,122,123). One clinical trial has shown the importance of T-cell help in viral clearance. T-cells specific for a cytomegalovirus antigen (CMV) that were adoptively transferred to patients persisted longer in the periphery in those patients with detectable levels of anti-CMV T-cell help *(124)*. Therefore, TCRs with CD8-independent TAA recognition may enable us to provide for a key component of T-cell-mediated immune function while targeting the more prevalent class I MHC TAA epitopes.

All of the above characteristics of T-cells and their receptors (antigen specificity, MHC restriction, affinity, and functional avidity) will factor into the development of tumor-reactive TCR gene transfer. The goal is to find TCRs with properties resulting in the most effective gene-modified T-cells that can treat the largest numbers of patients.

3. OPTIMAL VECTOR DESIGN

3.1. Retroviruses

Another critical consideration for gene modification of T-cells is the design of the vectors to deliver the genes. Adenovirus and pox viruses were early vectors used in the development of gene therapy because of their ability to infect both dividing and nondividing cells with high efficiency, and their ability to generate very high-titer viral stocks *(125)*. However, these vectors lack the ability to provide long-term transgene expression and are highly immunogenic *(126)*. The viral vector of choice for many gene therapy studies, particularly in hematopoietic cells, is the retrovirus. Retroviruses infect only dividing cells and incorporate into the host cell genome, providing for long-term transgene expression. They also have low immunogenicity, providing a combination of beneficial properties for their use in gene therapies. (For a complete review of vectors for gene therapy, *see* Gould and Favorov *[125]*.)

Retroviral vectors have frequently been based on the Moloney murine leukemia virus (MMLV) *(127,128)*. Traditionally, MMLV-based vectors, as well as other retroviral vectors have been modified to remove or inactivate the protein coding regions of the viral genome. Removal or inactivation of the genes *gag* (structural), *pol* (nucleic acid metabolism), and *env* (envelope) serves to prevent self-replication of the retrovirus following infection of target cells. The functions of these genes are provided by transfecting the retroviral backbone into packaging cells expressing the *gag, pol*, and *env* genes, which act in trans to enable the production of infectious retroviral particles *(129–131)*.

The genetic structure of the vectors can have an impact on both the titer of infectious retroviral particles produced by packaging cells and, more importantly, the efficiency of expression of the transgenes. The simplest MMLV vectors consist of 5' and 3' long terminal repeats (LTRs) that drive gene expression, a ψ-packaging signal, a multiple cloning site for insertion of a transgene, and sometimes, a selectable marker gene (Fig. 4). Generation of retroviral particles in transiently transfected packaging cells is under control of the 5' LTR. Transgenes in transduced cells are under control of the 3' LTR, which is reverse-transcribed to the 5' end during incorporation of the virus into the target cell genome. However, a reduction in gene transcription levels over time both in vitro, and particularly in vivo, as a result of methylation of the LTR has been demonstrated *(132–134)*. Multiple strategies have been designed to increase the activity of both LTRs, including replacing them with the LTR of other viral species, such as the murine embryonic stem cell virus *(135,136)*. Our laboratory now employs a vector in which segments of the LTR have been replaced with elements of the CMV immediate early gene promoter. This hybrid promoter allows higher transcription levels in transiently transfected packaging cells, leading

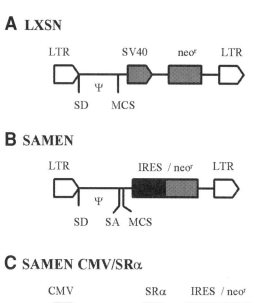

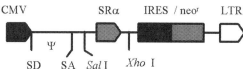

Fig. 4. Recombinant retroviral vectors for gene transfer. Moloney murine leukemia virus (MMLV)-based vectors include 5' and 3' long terminal repeats (LTRs), RNA splice donor, and splice acceptor sites, the Ψ-packaging signal, and multiple cloning sites for insertion of foreign genes. **(A)** The LXSN vector contains a multiple cloning site downstream of the LTR and an internal simian virus (SV)40 promoter to drive expression of a neomycin resistance gene (*neo*^{r}) for selection of transduced cells with G418. **(B)** The SAMEN cytomegalovirus (CMV)/SRα vector uses an internal ribosomal entry site downstream of the multiple cloning site to facilitate translation of the *neo*^{r} gene. **(C)** The SAMEN CMV/SRα vector employs a hybrid CMV/MMLV promoter in place of the 5' LTR to drive high-level transcription in transiently-transfected packaging cells for high-titer retroviral production. Unique restriction sites (*Sal*I and *Xho*I) and an internal SRα promoter allow for expression of two introduced genes (e.g., TCR α and β) whereas *neo*^{r} is translated via an internal ribosome entry site downstream of the SRα promoter.

to higher retroviral titer. Replacement of the 3' LTR with LTRs from other viral species, such as spleen focus forming virus, may afford higher gene expression in certain target cell types following genetic transfer *(135)*. Vectors based on the murine stem-cell virus have been shown to be less susceptible to methylation *(137)*. Many retroviral vectors incorporate molecular elements including leader sequences and RNA splicing signals to enhance the expression of the transgenes. Other *cis*-acting DNA elements can lead to increased transgene expression in both activated and quiescent T-cells, which is important for the long-term expression and function of gene-modified T-cells *(104,135,136,138–141)*.

Multiple promoters may be necessary if multiple genes are to be inserted into T-cells. Whereas cAbRs consist of a single gene, a selectable marker for enriching gene-modified T-cells may be employed. This marker may be a gene for resistance to a selection agent, such as G-418, or may be a gene for a cell surface protein not normally found in the target cell, such as the nerve growth factor receptor *(142,143)*. In either case, the presence of a second gene requires a transcriptional element. This may be a second promoter within the viral construct, which, like the LTR, could be chosen for optimal activity in the target cells. In the case of TCR transfer, two TCR genes, α and β, are introduced to T-cells. A selectable marker would therefore provide a third gene to be expressed. A second internal promoter can be used to transcribe one of the TCR genes, with the other transcribed by the viral LTR.

Another option is an internal ribosomal entry site (IRES), a nucleic acid sequence that allows initiation of protein translation from within a sequence of transcribed RNA with the second transgene downstream of the IRES sequence *(144)*. Our current retroviral vector (SAMEN CMV/SRα) employs both an internal promoter, as well as an IRES to allow for transcription of both TCR genes, as well as a selectable marker *(see* Fig. 4). However, multiple promoters can interfere with each other, leading to lower transcription levels, and transcription from an IRES may be less efficient as well. Some have attempted to use separate viral vectors for each TCR gene with some success.

All of these modifications are made to the viral backbone itself in an effort to maximize the molecular control elements to achieve the highest level of viral production and transgene expression. This is in contrast to modifying the transgenes, as in the case of chimeric TCRs discussed previously.

3.2. Lentiviruses

Lentiviruses are a subset of retroviruses that are more genetically complex than retroviruses like MMLV. (The human immunodeficiency virus is a thoroughly studied example of a lentivirus.) Their low immunogenic properties coupled with the capability of infecting nondividing cells have made them a candidate for use in gene therapy *(125)*. The development of lentiviral vectors for gene therapy includes modifications similar to MMLV-based retroviral vectors in removal of structural and packaging genes to prevent self-replication, as well as addition or deletion of regulatory control elements as described in Subheading 3.1. Studies have resulted in the ex vivo transduction of hematopoietic stem cells with long-term engraftment in nonobese diabetic/severe combined immunodeficiency mice *(145–147)*. Recently, several groups have demonstrated lentiviral-based gene transfer to primary human T-cells *(148–151)*. Whereas transduction of nondividing T-cells is possible, it has been shown repeatedly that T-cell activation is still necessary for high-level transfer and expression of the transgene *(151,152)*. T-cells activated by anti-CD3 antibody or exposure to homeostatic cytokines progressed from the G_0 to the G_1 phase of the cell cycle, facilitating higher transduction frequency but maintaining resting cell phenotypes *(148,149)*. Most of these studies have been preliminary in nature, with only one group thus far demonstrating the generation of tumor-reactive T-cells by transfer of a cAbR specific for CEA *(151)*. We have seen no reports of full-length TCR gene transfer via lentiviral transduction at the time of writing this review. Furthermore, whereas the use of retroviral-based gene therapy is clinically established, lentiviral-based therapies are not yet approved for clinical use.

4. CONCLUSIONS

Adoptive transfer of autologous T-cells genetically modified to express genes encoding reactivity to tumor antigens represents a novel approach to the immunotherapy of cancer. This method could circumvent the present difficulties in isolating and/or generating tumor-reactive T-cells for adoptive transfer. This modification has centered on three approaches

Table 1
Quick Reference of Reviewed Tumor-Associated
Antigen-Reactive Receptors for Gene Modification of T-Cells

Antigen	Tumor type	Receptor type	Reference
GD3	Melanoma	cAbR	65
HMW-MAA	Melanoma	cAbR	66,67
Her-2/*neu*	Adenocarcinoma	cAbR	68,72
CEA	Colon carcinoma	cAbR	73
FBP	Ovarian adenocarcinoma	cAbR	74,75
G250	Renal cell carcinoma	cAbR	69
MAGE-1	Melanoma	cAbR	70,71
MAGE-1	Melanoma	cTCR	101
MAGE-3	Melanoma	Full-length TCR	94
MART-1	Melanoma	Full-length TCR	96,153
Tyrosinase	Melanoma	Full-length TCR	104,105
gp100	Melanoma	Full-length TCR	102,103
CAMEL	Melanoma	Full-length TCR	95
LMP2	Hodgkin's lymphoma	Full-length TCR	107
MDM2	Various	Full-length TCR	106

cAbR, chimeric antibody receptors; HMW-MAA, high-molecular-weight melanoma-associated antigen; CEA, carcinoembryonic antigen; FBP, folate-binding protein; MAGE-1, melanoma-associated antigen 1; cTCR, chimeric T-cell receptor genes; MART-1, melanoma antigen recognized by T-cells-1; CAMEL, cytotoxic T-lymphocyte-recognized antigen on melanoma; LMP2, latent membrane protein 2.

thus far: cAbRs consisting of an antibody-derived recognition domain coupled to intracellular signaling molecules, full-length TCR gene transfer, and chimeric TCR-like molecules. Each has distinct advantages over the other systems as well as drawbacks. cAbRs recognize non-MHC-restricted antigens and could therefore treat a more diverse patient population, but they may not best reflect the complexity of T-cell activation and effector function, and they may be undesirably immunogenic. Full-length TCR transfer results in more physiological T-cells, but hybrid TCRs resulting from exogenous and endogenous TCR chain crosspairing may yield TCRs with unknown specificities, which could lead to an autoimmune response. Chimeric TCRs have been shown to eliminate full-length TCR crosspairing with the endogenous TCR, but the same concerns raised by cAbRs are present. However, the demonstrated potential of all three approaches warrants continued investigation into both the methods of delivering these genes to T-cells with high efficiency, as well as which genes may best confer strong antitumor reactivity to T-cells. The studies described in this review (Table 1) clearly demonstrate the ability to redirect the specificity of T-cells to recognize tumor antigens. In addition to the clinical application, these techniques offer invaluable experimental tools to understand better the process of immune recognition of cancer cells.

REFERENCES

1. Boon T, Old LJ. Cancer tumor antigens. *Curr Opin Immunol* 1997; 9:681–683.
2. Rosenberg SA, Yang JC, White DE, Steinberg SM. Durability of complete responses in patients with metastatic cancer treated with high-dose interleukin-2: identification of the antigens mediating response. *Ann Surg* 1998; 228:307–319.

3. White CA, Weaver RL, Grillo-Lopez AJ. Antibody-targeted immunotherapy for treatment of malignancy. *Annu Rev Med* 2001; 52:125–145.

4. Glennie MJ, Johnson PW. Clinical trials of antibody therapy. *Immunol Today* 2000; 21:403–410.

5. Menard S, Tagliabue E, Campiglio M, Pupa SM. Role of *HER2* gene overexpression in breast carcinoma. *J Cell Physiol* 2000; 182:150–162.

6. Bjorkman PJ, Saper MA, Samraoui B, Bennett WS, Strominger JL, Wiley DC. The foreign antigen binding site and T cell recognition regions of class I histocompatibility antigens. *Nature* 1987; 329:512–518.

7. Rotzschke O, Falk K, Deres K, et al. Isolation and analysis of naturally processed viral peptides as recognized by cytotoxic T cells. *Nature* 1990; 348:252–254.

8. van der Bruggen BP, Traversari C, Chomez P, et al. A gene encoding an antigen recognized by cytolytic T lymphocytes on a human melanoma. *Science* 1991; 254:1643–1647.

9. Traversari C, van der Bruggen P, Luescher, IF, et al. A nonapeptide encoded by human gene MAGE-1 is recognized on HLA-A1 by cytolytic T lymphocytes directed against tumor antigen MZ2-E. *J Exp Med* 1992; 176:1453–1457.

10. Coulie PG, Lehmann F, Lethe B, et al. A mutated intron sequence codes for an antigenic peptide recognized by cytolytic T lymphocytes on a human melanoma. *Proc Natl Acad Sci USA* 1995; 92:7976–7980.

11. Kawakami Y, Eliyahu S, Delgado CH, et al. Cloning of the gene coding for a shared human melanoma antigen recognized by autologous T cells infiltrating into tumor. *Proc Natl Acad Sci USA* 1994; 91: 3515–3519.

12. Kawakami Y, Eliyahu S, Delgado CH, et al. Identification of a human melanoma antigen recognized by tumor-infiltrating lymphocytes associated with in vivo tumor rejection. *Proc Natl Acad Sci USA* 1994; 91:6458–6462.

13. Cox AL, Skipper J, Chen Y, et al. Identification of a peptide recognized by five melanoma-specific human cytotoxic T cell lines. *Science* 1994; 264:716–719.

14. Wolfel T, Van Pel A, Brichard V, et al. Two tyrosinase nonapeptides recognized on HLA-A2 melanomas by autologous cytolytic T lymphocytes. *Eur J Immunol* 1994; 24:759–764.

15. Correale P, Walmsley K, Nieroda C, et al. In vitro generation of human cytotoxic T lymphocytes specific for peptides derived from prostate-specific antigen. *J Natl Cancer Inst* 1997; 89:293–300.

16. Renkvist N, Castelli C, Robbins PF, Parmiani G. A listing of human tumor antigens recognized by T cells. *Cancer Immunol Immunother* 2001; 50:3–15.

17. Agus DB, Bunn PA Jr, Franklin W, Garcia M, Ozols RF. HER-2/*neu* as a therapeutic target in non-small cell lung cancer, prostate cancer, and ovarian cancer. *Semin Oncol* 2000; 27(Suppl 11):53–63.

18. Ras E, van der Burg SH, Zegveld ST, et al. Identification of potential HLA-A *0201-restricted CTL epitopes derived from the epithelial cell adhesion molecule (Ep-CAM) and the carcinoembryonic antigen (CEA). *Hum Immunol* 1997; 53:81–89.

19. Johnson PW. The therapeutic use of antibodies for malignancy. *Transfus Clin Biol* 2001; 8:255–259.

20. Baselga J, Tripathy D, Mendelsohn J, et al. Phase II study of weekly intravenous recombinant humanized anti-p185HER2 monoclonal antibody in patients with HER2/*neu*-overexpressing metastatic breast cancer. *J Clin Oncol* 1996; 14:737–744.

21. Cobleigh MA, Vogel CL, Tripathy D, et al. Multinational study of the efficacy and safety of humanized anti-HER2 monoclonal antibody in women who have HER2-overexpressing metastatic breast cancer that has progressed after chemotherapy for metastatic disease. *J Clin Oncol* 1999; 17:2639–2648.

22. Stebbing J, Copson E, O'Reilly S. Herceptin (trastuzamab) in advanced breast cancer. *Cancer Treat Rev* 2000; 26:287–290.

23. Riethmuller G, Holz E, Schlimok G, et al. Monoclonal antibody therapy for resected Dukes' C colorectal cancer: seven-year outcome of a multicenter randomized trial. *J Clin Oncol* 1998; 16:1788–1794.

24. Coiffier B, Haioun C, Ketterer N, et al. Rituximab (anti-CD20 monoclonal antibody) for the treatment of patients with relapsing or refractory aggressive lymphoma: a multicenter phase II study. *Blood* 1998; 92:1927–1932.

25. Nitschke L, Floyd H, Crocker PR. New functions for the sialic acid-binding adhesion molecule CD22, a member of the growing family of Siglecs. *Scand J Immunol* 2001; 53:227–234.

26. Kaminski MS, Estes J, Zasadny KR, et al. Radioimmunotherapy with iodine (131)I tositumomab for relapsed or refractory B-cell non-Hodgkin lymphoma: updated results and long-term follow-up of the University of Michigan experience. *Blood* 2000; 96:1259–1266.

27. Acres B, Paul S, Haegel-Kronenberger H, Calmels B, Squiban P. Therapeutic cancer vaccines. *Curr Opin Mol Ther* 2004; 6:40–47.

28. Campoli M, Ferrone S. T-cell-based immunotherapy of melanoma: what have we learned and how can we improve? *Expert Rev Vaccines* 2004; 3:171–187.

29. Brichard VG, Rard G. Melanoma vaccines: achievements and perspectives. *Forum (Genova)* 2003; 13: 144–157.

30. Ridgway D. The first 1000 dendritic cell vaccinees. *Cancer Invest* 2003; 21:873–886.

31. Arienti F, Sule-Suso J, Belli F, et al. Limited antitumor T cell response in melanoma patients vaccinated with interleukin-2 gene-transduced allogeneic melanoma cells. *Hum Gene Ther* 1996; 7:1955–1963.

32. Chakraborty NG, Sporn JR, Tortora AF, et al. Immunization with a tumor-cell-lysate-loaded autologous-antigen-presenting-cell-based vaccine in melanoma. *Cancer Immunol Immunother* 1998; 47:58–64.

33. Marchand M, van Baren N, Weynants P, et al. Tumor regressions observed in patients with metastatic melanoma treated with an antigenic peptide encoded by gene MAGE-3 and presented by HLA-A1. *Int J Cancer* 1999; 80:219–230.

34. Moller P, Sun Y, Dorbic T, et al. Vaccination with IL-7 gene-modified autologous melanoma cells can enhance the anti-melanoma lytic activity in peripheral blood of patients with a good clinical performance status: a clinical phase I study. *Br J Cancer* 1998; 77:1907–1916.

35. Morton DL, Foshag LJ, Hoon DS, et al. Prolongation of survival in metastatic melanoma after active specific immunotherapy with a new polyvalent melanoma vaccine. *Ann Surg* 1992; 216:463–482.

36. Nestle FO, Alijagic S, Gilliet M, et al. Vaccination of melanoma patients with peptide- or tumor lysate-pulsed dendritic cells. *Nat Med* 1998; 4:328–332.

37. Rosenberg SA, Yang JC, Schwartzentruber DJ, et al. Immunologic and therapeutic evaluation of a synthetic peptide vaccine for the treatment of patients with metastatic melanoma. *Nat Med* 1998; 4:321–327.

38. Soiffer R, Lynch T, Mihm M, et al. Vaccination with irradiated autologous melanoma cells engineered to secrete human granulocyte-macrophage colony-stimulating factor generates potent antitumor immunity in patients with metastatic melanoma. *Proc Natl Acad Sci USA* 1998; 95:13,141–13,146.

39. Rooney CM, Smith CA, Ng CY, et al. Use of gene-modified virus-specific T lymphocytes to control Epstein-Barr-virus-related lymphoproliferation. *Lancet* 1995; 345:9–13.

40. Comoli P, Labirio M, Basso S, et al. Infusion of autologous Epstein-Barr virus (EBV)-specific cytotoxic T cells for prevention of EBV-related lymphoproliferative disorder in solid organ transplant recipients with evidence of active virus replication. *Blood* 2002; 99:2592–2598.

41. Rosenberg SA, Yannelli JR, Yang JC, et al. Treatment of patients with metastatic melanoma with autologous tumor-infiltrating lymphocytes and interleukin 2. *J Natl Cancer Inst* 1994; 86:1159–1166.

42. Dudley ME, Wunderlich JR, Robbins PF, et al. Cancer regression and autoimmunity in patients after clonal repopulation with antitumor lymphocytes. *Science* 2002; 298:850–854.

43. Figlin RA, Pierce WC, Kaboo R, et al. Treatment of metastatic renal cell carcinoma with nephrectomy, interleukin-2 and cytokine-primed or CD8(+) selected tumor infiltrating lymphocytes from primary tumor. *J Urol* 1997; 158(3 Pt 1):740–745.

44 Dudley ME, Rosenberg SA. Adoptive-cell-transfer therapy for the treatment of patients with cancer. *Nat Rev Cancer* 2003; 3:666–675.

45. Mule JJ, Shu S, Schwarz SL, Rosenberg SA. Adoptive immunotherapy of established pulmonary metastases with LAK cells and recombinant interleukin-2. *Science* 1984; 225:1487–1489.

46. Grimm EA, Mazumder A, Zhang HZ, Rosenberg SA. Lymphokine-activated killer cell phenomenon. Lysis of natural killer-resistant fresh solid tumor cells by interleukin 2-activated autologous human peripheral blood lymphocytes. *J Exp Med* 1982; 155:1823–1841.

47. Lum LG, LeFever AV, Treisman JS, Garlie NK, Hanson JP Jr. Immune modulation in cancer patients after adoptive transfer of anti-CD3/anti-CD28-costimulated T cells-phase I clinical trial. *J Immunother* 2001; 24:408–419.

48. Curti BD, Ochoa AC, Powers GC, et al. Phase I trial of anti-CD3-stimulated CD4+ T cells, infusional interleukin-2, and cyclophosphamide in patients with advanced cancer. *J Clin Oncol* 1998; 16:2752–2760.

49. Chang AE, Li Q, Jiang G, Sayre DM, Braun TM, Redman BG. Phase II trial of autologous tumor vaccination, anti-CD3-activated vaccine-primed lymphocytes, and interleukin-2 in stage IV renal cell cancer. *J Clin Oncol* 2003; 21:884–890.

50. Plautz GE, Bukowski RM, Novick AC, et al. T-cell adoptive immunotherapy of metastatic renal cell carcinoma. *Urology* 1999; 54:617–623.

51. Meidenbauer N, Marienhagen J, Laumer M, et al. Survival and tumor localization of adoptively transferred Melan-A-specific T cells in melanoma patients. *J Immunol* 2003; 170:2161–2169.

52. Rosenberg SA, Packard BS, Aebersold PM, et al. Use of tumor-infiltrating lymphocytes and inter-leukin-2 in the immunotherapy of patients with metastatic melanoma. A preliminary report. *N Engl J Med* 1988; 319:1676–1680.

53. Quattrocchi KB, Miller CH, Cush S, et al. Pilot study of local autologous tumor infiltrating lympho-cytes for the treatment of recurrent malignant gliomas. *J Neurooncol* 1999; 45:141–157.

54. Bakker AB, Schreurs MW, de Boer AJ, et al. Melanocyte lineage-specific antigen gp100 is recognized by melanoma-derived tumor-infiltrating lymphocytes. *J Exp Med* 1994; 179:1005–1009.

55. Rosenberg SA, Aebersold P, Cornetta K, et al. Gene transfer into humans—immunotherapy of patients with advanced melanoma, using tumor-infiltrating lymphocytes modified by retroviral gene transduc-tion. *N Engl J Med* 1990; 323:570–578.

56. Eshhar Z. Tumor-specific T-bodies: towards clinical application. *Cancer Immunol Immunother* 1997; 45:131–136.

57. Brocker T. Chimeric Fv-zeta or Fv-epsilon receptors are not sufficient to induce activation or cytokine production in peripheral T cells. *Blood* 2000; 96:1999–2001.

58. Weijtens ME, Willemsen RA, Valerio D, Stam K, Bolhuis RL. Single chain Ig/gamma gene-redirected human T lymphocytes produce cytokines, specifically lyse tumor cells, and recycle lytic capacity. *J Immunol* 1996; 157:836–843.

59. Stancovski I, Schindler DG, Waks T, Yarden Y, Sela M, Eshhar Z. Targeting of T lymphocytes to Neu/HER2-expressing cells using chimeric single chain Fv receptors. *J Immunol* 1993; 151:6577–6582.

60. Moritz D, Wels W, Mattern J, Groner B. Cytotoxic T lymphocytes with a grafted recognition speci-ficity for ERBB2-expressing tumor cells. *Proc Natl Acad Sci USA* 1994; 91:4318–4322.

61. Hwu P, Shafer GE, Treisman J, et al. Lysis of ovarian cancer cells by human lymphocytes redirected with a chimeric gene composed of an antibody variable region and the Fc receptor gamma chain. *J Exp Med* 1993; 178:361–366.

62. Fitzer-Attas CJ, Schindler DG, Waks T, Eshhar Z. Harnessing Syk family tyrosine kinases as signaling domains for chimeric single chain of the variable domain receptors: optimal design for T cell activation. *J Immunol* 1998; 160:145–154.

63 Tran AC, Zhang D, Byrn R, Roberts MR. Chimeric zeta-receptors direct human natural killer (NK) effec-tor function to permit killing of NK-resistant tumor cells and HIV-infected T lymphocytes. *J Immunol* 1995; 155:1000–1009.

64. Roberts MR, Qin L, Zhang D, et al. Targeting of human immunodeficiency virus-infected cells by CD8+ T lymphocytes armed with universal T-cell receptors. *Blood* 1994; 84:2878–2889.

65. Yun CO, Nolan KF, Beecham EJ, Reisfeld RA, Junghans RP. Targeting of T lymphocytes to melanoma cells through chimeric anti-GD3 immunoglobulin T-cell receptors. *Neoplasia* 2000; 2:449–459.

66. Reinhold U, Liu L, Ludtke-Handjery HC, et al. Specific lysis of melanoma cells by receptor grafted T cells is enhanced by anti-idiotypic monoclonal antibodies directed to the scFv domain of the receptor. *J Invest Dermatol* 1999; 112:744–750.

67. Abken H, Hombach A, Heuser C, Reinhold U. A novel strategy in the elimination of disseminated mela-noma cells: chimeric receptors endow T cells with tumor specificity. *Recent Results Cancer Res* 2001; 158:249–264.

68. Turatti F, Figini M, Alberti P, Willemsen RA, Canevari S, Mezzanzanica D. Highly efficient redirected anti-tumor activity of human lymphocytes transduced with a completely human chimeric immune recep-tor. *J Gene Med* 2004; 7:158–170.

69. Weijtens ME, Willemsen RA, van Krimpen BA, Bolhuis RL. Chimeric scFv/gamma receptor-mediated T-cell lysis of tumor cells is coregulated by adhesion and accessory molecules. *Int J Cancer* 1998; 77:181–187.

70. Willemsen RA, Debets R, Hart E, Hoogenboom HR, Bolhuis RL, Chames P. A phage display selected fab fragment with MHC class I-restricted specificity for MAGE-A1 allows for retargeting of primary human T lymphocytes. *Gene Ther* 8:1601–1608.

71. Chames P, Willemsen RA, Rojas G, et al. TCR-like human antibodies expressed on human CTLs medi-ate antibody affinity-dependent cytolytic activity. *J Immunol* 2002; 169:1110–1118.

72. Altenschmidt U, Kahl R, Moritz D, et al. Cytolysis of tumor cells expressing the Neu/erbB-2, erbB-3, and erbB-4 receptors by genetically targeted naive T lymphocytes. *Clin Cancer Res* 1996; 2:1001–1008.

73. Darcy PK, Haynes NM, Snook MB, et al. Redirected perforin-dependent lysis of colon carcinoma by ex vivo genetically engineered CTL. *J Immunol* 2000; 164:3705–3712.

74. Hwu P, Yang JC, Cowherd R, et al. In vivo antitumor activity of T cells redirected with chimeric anti-body/T-cell receptor genes. *Cancer Res* 1995; 55:3369–3373.

75. Wang G, Chopra RK, Royal RE, Yang JC, Rosenberg SA, Hwu P. A T cell-independent antitumor response in mice with bone marrow cells retrovirally transduced with an antibody/Fc-gamma chain chimeric receptor gene recognizing a human ovarian cancer antigen. *Nat Med* 1998; 4:168–172.

76. Geiger TL, Leitenberg D, Flavell RA. The TCR zeta-chain immunoreceptor tyrosine-based activation motifs are sufficient for the activation and differentiation of primary T lymphocytes. *J Immunol* 1999; 162:5931–5939.

77. Shinkai Y, Ma A, Cheng HL, Alt FW. CD3 epsilon and CD3 zeta cytoplasmic domains can independently generate signals for T cell development and function. *Immunity* 1995; 2:401–411.

78. Viola A, Lanzavecchia A. T cell activation determined by T cell receptor number and tunable thresholds. *Science* 1996; 273:104–106.

79. Kalergis AM, Boucheron N, Doucey MA, et al. Efficient T cell activation requires an optimal dwell-time of interaction between the TCR and the pMHC complex. *Nat Immunol* 2001; 2:229–234.

80. Davis MM, Boniface JJ, Reich Z, et al. Ligand recognition by alpha beta T cell receptors. *Annu Rev Immunol* 1998; 16:523–544.

81. Jenkins MK. The ups and downs of T cell costimulation. *Immunity*1994; 1:443–446.

82. Beecham EJ, Ma Q, Ripley R, Junghans RP. Coupling CD28 co-stimulation to immunoglobulin T-cell receptor molecules: the dynamics of T-cell proliferation and death. *J Immunother* 2000; 23:631–642.

83. Finney HM, Lawson AD, Bebbington CR, Weir AN. Chimeric receptors providing both primary and costimulatory signaling in T cells from a single gene product. *J Immunol* 1998; 161:2791–2797.

84. Krause A, Guo HF, Latouche JB, Tan C, Cheung NK, Sadelain M. Antigen-dependent CD28 signaling selectively enhances survival and proliferation in genetically modified activated human primary T lymphocytes. *J Exp Med* 1998; 188:619–626.

85. Aruga A, Yamauchi K, Takasaki K, Furukawa T, Hanyu F. Induction of autologous tumor-specific cytotoxic T cells in patients with liver cancer. Characterizations and clinical utilization. *Int J Cancer* 1991; 49:19–24.

86. Cole DJ, Weil DP, Shilyansky J, et al. Characterization of the functional specificity of a cloned T-cell receptor heterodimer recognizing the MART-1 melanoma antigen. *Cancer Res* 1995; 55:748–752.

87. Hom SS, Rosenberg SA, Topalian SL. Specific immune recognition of autologous tumor by lymphocytes infiltrating colon carcinomas: analysis by cytokine secretion. *Cancer Immunol Immunother* 1993; 36: 1–8.

88. Ioannides CG, Fisk B, Tomasovic B, Pandita R, Aggarwal BB, Freedman RS. Induction of interleukin-2 receptor by tumor necrosis factor alpha on cultured ovarian tumor-associated lymphocytes. *Cancer Immunol Immunother* 1992; 35:83–91.

89. Schwartzentruber DJ, Solomon D, Rosenberg SA, Topalian SL. Characterization of lymphocytes infiltrating human breast cancer: specific immune reactivity detected by measuring cytokine secretion. *J Immunother* 1992; 12:1–12.

90. Schwartzentruber DJ, Stetler-Stevenson M, Rosenberg SA, Topalian SL. Tumor-infiltrating lymphocytes derived from select B-cell lymphomas secrete granulocyte-macrophage colony-stimulating factor and tumor necrosis factor-alpha in response to autologous tumor stimulation. *Blood* 1993; 82:1204–1211.

91. Wahab ZA, Metzgar RS. Human cytotoxic lymphocytes reactive with pancreatic adenocarcinoma cells. *Pancreas* 1991; 6:307–317.

92. Shilyansky J, Nishimura MI, Yannelli JR, et al. T-cell receptor usage by melanoma-specific clonal and highly oligoclonal tumor-infiltrating lymphocyte lines. *Proc Natl Acad Sci USA* 1994; 91:2829–2833.

93. Kawakami Y, Eliyahu S, Sakaguchi K, et al. Identification of the immunodominant peptides of the MART-1 human melanoma antigen recognized by the majority of HLA-A2-restricted tumor infiltrating lymphocytes. *J Exp Med* 1994; 180:347–352.

94. Calogero A, Hospers GA, Kruse KM, et al. Retargeting of a T cell line by anti MAGE-3/HLA-A2 alpha beta TCR gene transfer. *Anticancer Res* 2000; 20:1793–1799.

95. Aarnoudse CA, Kruse M, Konopitzky R, Brouwenstijn N, Schrier PI. TCR reconstitution in Jurkat reporter cells facilitates the identification of novel tumor antigens by cDNA expression cloning. *Int J Cancer* 2002; 99:7–13.

96. Clay TM, Custer MC, Sachs J, Hwu P, Rosenberg SA, Nishimura MI. Efficient transfer of a tumor antigen-reactive TCR to human peripheral blood lymphocytes confers anti-tumor reactivity. *J Immunol* 1999; 163:507–513.

97. Miller DG, Adam MA, Miller AD. Gene transfer by retrovirus vectors occurs only in cells that are actively replicating at the time of infection. *Mol Cell Biol* 1990; 10:4239–4242.

98. Veillette A, Bookman MA, Horak EM, Bolen JB. The CD4 and CD8 T cell surface antigens are associated with the internal membrane tyrosine-protein kinase p56lck. *Cell* 1988; 55:301–308.

99. Blichfeldt E, Munthe LA, Rotnes JS, Bogen B. Dual T cell receptor T cells have a decreased sensitivity to physiological ligands due to reduced density of each T cell receptor. *Eur J Immunol* 1996; 26:2876–2884.

100. Munthe LA, Blichfeldt E, Sollien A, Dembic Z, Bogen B. T cells with two Tcrbeta chains and reactivity to both MHC/idiotypic peptide and superantigen. *Cell Immunol* 1996; 170:283–290.

101. Willemsen RA, Weijtens ME, Ronteltap C, et al. Grafting primary human T lymphocytes with cancer-specific chimeric single chain and two chain TCR. *Gene Ther* 2000; 7:1369–1377.

102. Schaft N, Willemsen RA, de Vries J, et al. Peptide fine specificity of anti-glycoprotein 100 CTL is preserved following transfer of engineered TCR alpha beta genes into primary human T lymphocytes. *J Immunol* 2003; 170:2186–2194.

103. Morgan RA, Dudley ME, Yu YY, et al. High efficiency TCR gene transfer into primary human lymphocytes affords avid recognition of melanoma tumor antigen glycoprotein 100 and does not alter the recognition of autologous melanoma antigens. *J Immunol* 2003; 171:3287–3295.

104. Roszkowski JJ, Yu DC, Rubinstein MP, McKee MD, Cole DJ, Nishimura MI. CD8-independent tumor cell recognition is a property of the T cell receptor and not the T cell. *J Immunol* 2003; 170:2582–2589.

105. Roszkowski JJ, Eiben GE, Kast WM, Yee C, Van Besien K, Nishimura MI. Simultaneous generation of CD8+ and CD4+ melanoma-reactive T cells by retroviral mediated transfer of a single T cell receptor. *Cancer Res* 2005; 15:1570–1576.

106. Stanislawski T, Voss RH, Lotz C, et al. Circumventing tolerance to a human MDM2-derived tumor antigen by TCR gene transfer. *Nat Immunol* 2001; 2:962–970.

107. Orentas RJ, Roskopf SJ, Nolan GP, Nishimura MI. Retroviral transduction of a T cell receptor specific for an Epstein-Barr virus-encoded peptide. *Clin Immunol* 2001; 98:220–228.

108. Gilboa E. How tumors escape immune destruction and what we can do about it. *Cancer Immunol Immunother* 1999; 48:382–385.

109. Medema JP, de Jong J, Peltenburg LT, et al. Blockade of the granzyme B/perforin pathway through overexpression of the serine protease inhibitor PI-9/SPI-6 constitutes a mechanism for immune escape by tumors. *Proc Natl Acad Sci USA* 2001; 98:11,515–11,520.

110 Medema JP, de Jong J, van Hall T, Melief CJ, Offringa R. Immune escape of tumors in vivo by expression of cellular FLICE-inhibitory protein. *J Exp Med* 1999; 190:1033–1038.

111. Khong HT, Wang QJ, Rosenberg SA. Identification of multiple antigens recognized by tumor-infiltrating lymphocytes from a single patient: tumor escape by antigen loss and loss of MHC expression. *J Immunother* 2004; 27:184–190.

112. Heemskerk MH, Hoogeboom M, Hagedoorn R, Kester MG, Willemze R, Falkenburg JH. Reprogramming of virus-specific T cells into leukemia-reactive T cells using T cell receptor gene transfer. *J Exp Med* 2004; 199:885–894.

113. Langerman A, Callender GG, Nishimura MI. Retroviral transduction of peptide stimulated T cells can generate dual T cell receptor-expressing (bifunctional) T cells reactive with two defined antigens. *J Transl Med* 2:42.

114 Zeh HJ III, Perry-Lalley D, Dudley ME, Rosenberg SA, Yang JC. High-avidity CTLs for two self-antigens demonstrate superior in vitro and in vivo antitumor efficacy. *J Immunol* 1999; 162:989–994.

115. Dudley ME, Nishimura MI, Holt AK, Rosenberg SA. Antitumor immunization with a minimal peptide epitope (G9-209-2M) leads to a functionally heterogeneous CTL response. *J Immunother* 1999; 22:288–298.

116. Kerry SE, Buslepp J, Cramer LA, et al. Interplay between TCR affinity and necessity of coreceptor ligation: high-affinity peptide-MHC/TCR interaction overcomes lack of CD8 engagement. *J Immunol* 2003; 171:4493–4503.

117. Nishimura MI, Avichezer D, Custer MC, et al. MHC class I-restricted recognition of a melanoma antigen by a human CD4+ tumor infiltrating lymphocyte. *Cancer Res* 1999; 59:6230–6238.

118. Marzo AL, Kinnear BF, Lake RA, et al. Tumor-specific CD4+ T cells have a major "post-licensing" role in CTL mediated anti-tumor immunity. *J Immunol* 2000; 165:6047–6055.

119. Mattes J, Hulett M, Xie W, et al. Immunotherapy of cytotoxic T cell-resistant tumors by T helper 2 cells: an eotaxin and STAT6-dependent process. *J Exp Med* 2003; 197:387–393.

120. Ossendorp F, Mengede E, Camps M, Filius R, Melief CJ. Specific T helper cell requirement for optimal induction of cytotoxic T lymphocytes against major histocompatibility complex class II-negative tumors. *J Exp Med* 1998; 187:693–702.

121 Lu Z, Yuan L, Zhou X, Sotomayor E, Levitsky HI, Pardoll DM. CD40-independent pathways of T cell help for priming of CD8(+) cytotoxic T lymphocytes. *J Exp Med* 2000; 191:541–550.

122 Yu P, Spiotto MT, Lee Y, Schreiber H, Fu YX. Complementary role of CD4+ T cells and secondary lymphoid tissues for cross-presentation of tumor antigen to CD8+ T cells. *J Exp Med* 2003; 197:985–995.

123. Hung K, Hayashi R, Lafond-Walker A, Lowenstein C, Pardoll D, Levitsky H. The central role of CD4(+) T cells in the antitumor immune response. *J Exp Med* 1998; 188:2357–2368.

124. Walter EA, Greenberg PD, Gilbert MJ, et al. Reconstitution of cellular immunity against cytomegalovirus in recipients of allogeneic bone marrow by transfer of T-cell clones from the donor. *N Engl J Med* 1995; 333:1038–1044.

125. Gould DJ, Favorov P. Vectors for the treatment of autoimmune disease. *Gene Ther* 2003; 10:912–927.

126. Yang Y, Li Q, Ertl HC, Wilson JM. Cellular and humoral immune responses to viral antigens create barriers to lung-directed gene therapy with recombinant adenoviruses. *J Virol* 1995; 69:2004–2015.

127 Miller AD, Rosman GJ. Improved retroviral vectors for gene transfer and expression. *Biotechniques* 1989; 7:980–986, 989.

128. Treisman J, Hwu P, Minamoto S, et al. Interleukin-2-transduced lymphocytes grow in an autocrine fashion and remain responsive to antigen. *Blood* 1995; 85:139–145.

129. Markowitz D, Goff S, Bank A. A safe packaging line for gene transfer: separating viral genes on two different plasmids. *J Virol* 1988; 62:1120–1124.

130. Miller AD, Buttimore C. Redesign of retrovirus packaging cell lines to avoid recombination leading to helper virus production. *Mol Cell Biol* 1986; 6:2895–2902.

131 Miller AD, Garcia JV, von Suhr N, Lynch CM, Wilson C, Eiden MV. Construction and properties of retrovirus packaging cells based on gibbon ape leukemia virus. *J Virol* 1991; 65:2220–2224.

132. Jahner D, Stuhlmann H, Stewart CL, et al. De novo methylation and expression of retroviral genomes during mouse embryogenesis. *Nature* 1982; 298:623–628.

133. Challita PM, Kohn DB. Lack of expression from a retroviral vector after transduction of murine hematopoietic stem cells is associated with methylation in vivo. *Proc Natl Acad Sci USA* 1994; 91:2567–2571.

134. Svoboda J, Hejnar J, Geryk J, Elleder D, Vernerova Z. Retroviruses in foreign species and the problem of provirus silencing. *Gene* 261:181–188.

135. Ketteler R, Glaser S, Sandra O, Martens UM, Klingmuller U. Enhanced transgene expression in primitive hematopoietic progenitor cells and embryonic stem cells efficiently transduced by optimized retroviral hybrid vectors. *Gene Ther* 2002; 9:477–487.

136. Agarwal M, Austin TW, Morel F, Chen J, Bohnlein E, Plavec I. Scaffold attachment region-mediated enhancement of retroviral vector expression in primary T cells. *J Virol* 1998; 72:3720–3728.

137 Hawley RG, Lieu FH, Fong AZ, Hawley TS. Versatile retroviral vectors for potential use in gene therapy. *Gene Ther* 1994; 1:136–138.

138. Dang Q, Auten J, Plavec I. Human beta interferon scaffold attachment region inhibits de novo methylation and confers long-term, copy number-dependent expression to a retroviral vector. *J Virol* 2000; 74:2671–2678.

139. Emery DW, Yannaki E, Tubb J, Stamatoyannopoulos G. A chromatin insulator protects retrovirus vectors from chromosomal position effects. *Proc Natl Acad Sci USA* 2000; 97:9150–9155.

140. Zufferey R, Donello JE, Trono D, Hope TJ. Woodchuck hepatitis virus posttranscriptional regulatory element enhances expression of transgenes delivered by retroviral vectors. *J Virol* 1999; 73:2886–2892.

141. Schambach A, Wodrich H, Hildinger M, Bohne J, Krausslich HG, Baum C. Context dependence of different modules for posttranscriptional enhancement of gene expression from retroviral vectors. *Mol Ther* 2000; 2:435–445.

142. Koehne G, Gallardo HF, Sadelain M, O'Reilly RJ. Rapid selection of antigen-specific T lymphocytes by retroviral transduction. *Blood* 2000; 96:109–117.

143. Abad JL, Serrano F, San Roman AL, Delgado R, Bernad A, Gonzalez MA. Single-step, multiple retroviral transduction of human T cells. *J Gene Med* 2002; 4:27–37.

144. Vagner S, Galy B, Pyronnet S. Irresistible IRES. Attracting the translation machinery to internal ribosome entry sites. *EMBO Rep* 2001; 2:893–898.

145. Sirven A, Pflumio F, Zennou V, et al. The human immunodeficiency virus type-1 central DNA flap is a crucial determinant for lentiviral vector nuclear import and gene transduction of human hematopoietic stem cells. *Blood* 2000; 96:4103–4110.

146. Woods NB, Fahlman C, Mikkola H, et al. Lentiviral gene transfer into primary and secondary NOD/SCID repopulating cells. *Blood* 2000; 96(12):3725–3733.

147. Scherr M, Battmer K, Blomer U, et al. Lentiviral gene transfer into peripheral blood-derived CD34$^+$ NOD/SCID-repopulating cells. *Blood* 2002; 99:709–712.
148 Cavalieri S, Cazzaniga S, Geuna M, et al. Human T lymphocytes transduced by lentiviral vectors in the absence of TCR activation maintain an intact immune competence. *Blood* 2003; 102:497–505.
149. Maurice M, Verhoeyen E, Salmon P, Trono D, Russell SJ, Cosset FL. Efficient gene transfer into human primary blood lymphocytes by surface-engineered lentiviral vectors that display a T cell-activating polypeptide. *Blood* 2002; 99:2342–2350.
150 Zhou X, Cui Y, Huang X, et al. Lentivirus-mediated gene transfer and expression in established human tumor antigen-specific cytotoxic T cells and primary unstimulated T cells. *Hum Gene Ther* 2003; 14: 1089–1105.
151. Gyobu H, Tsuji T, Suzuki Y, et al. Generation and targeting of human tumor-specific Tc1 and Th1 cells transduced with a lentivirus containing a chimeric immunoglobulin T-cell receptor. *Cancer Res* 2004; 64:1490–1495.
152. Korin YD, Zack JA. Progression to the G1b phase of the cell cycle is required for completion of human immunodeficiency virus type 1 reverse transcription in T cells. *J Virol* 1998; 72:3161–3168.
153. Chao NJ, Rosenberg SA, Horning SJ. CEPP(B): an effective and well-tolerated regimen in poor-risk, aggressive non-Hodgkin's lymphoma. *Blood* 1990; 76:1293–1298.

14

Harnessing the Potential
of Graft-vs-Tumor

Nancy M. Hardy and Michael R. Bishop

Summary

The curative potential of allogeneic hematopoietic stem cell transplantation in treating cancer is derived in large part from the donor immune system reacting against host or tumor cell antigens to generate a graft-vs-tumor (GVT) effect. Whereas early animal models suggested this allogeneic immune response, evidence for its role in human transplantation was not realized until the late 1970s and early 1980s, when the association between graft-vs-host disease and tumor response became clear. In this chapter, the animal and human data that established the GVT effect as the major therapeutic component of allogeneic hematopoietic stem cell transplantation are reviewed, and ongoing efforts to understand and build on GVT as a therapeutic modality for other tumor types are described. The current thinking on the biology of the effectors and modulators of GVT are discussed. The progress that has been made in clinical application of immunotherapy in the autologous setting and of solid tumor therapy in the allogeneic setting is reviewed. Finally, the potential for continued advances in the efficacy and safety of immunotherapy for cancer is explored, as reflected in recent and ongoing efforts to apply the growing understanding of alloreactivity toward fulfillment of the potential for targeted antitumor therapies.

Key Words: Graft-vs-tumor; allogeneic; hematopoietic stem cell transplantation; adoptive cell therapy; alloreactivity.

1. INTRODUCTION

Identification of the role of the graft-vs-leukemia or graft-vs-tumor (GVT) effect in the success of bone marrow transplantation *(1,2)* was a turning point for the fields of tumor immunology and hematopoietic stem cell transplantation (HSCT). Broader application of allogeneic HSCT has been limited, however, by the availability of suitable donors, by the acute toxicity of the early myeloablative preparative regimens and the graft-vs-host disease (GVHD) that often accompanies GVT, and the relative unresponsiveness of lymphoid and other solid tumors as compared with chronic myelogenous leukemia (CML), to the GVT effect. It is the basis for ongoing efforts to bring the success seen in CML to other hematological and solid tumors and to develop effective, less toxic preparative regimens that can be administered to a broader range of patients. Efforts to harness GVT

From: *Cancer Drug Discovery and Development: Immunotherapy of Cancer*
Edited by: M. L. Disis © Humana Press Inc., Totowa, NJ

and differentiate it from GVHD have yielded major contributions to our understanding of immune effectors and tolerance. Allogeneic HSCT is increasingly used as a platform from which immunotherapeutic interventions can be launched, taking advantage of the power of alloreactivity to overcome the limitations of autologous tumor immunity and autologous immunotherapy in the treatment of established cancer.

2. HISTORY OF IMMUNOTHERAPY IN THE TREATMENT OF CANCER

Barnes and Loutit opened the field of cellular immunotherapy with experiments following the observation that, contrary to what was understood at the time regarding the principles of tissue transplantation and rejection, allogeneic bone marrow or (infant) spleen cells were capable of repopulating lethally irradiated mice (3,4). Their seminal work tested two hypotheses. First, if myeloablative doses of radiation alone could cure murine leukemia, then mice rescued with "isologous" bone marrow or infant spleen would survive. Second, if leukemia could not be eliminated by myeloablative doses of radiation, then mice rescued with "homologous" bone marrow might still be cured by "the reaction of immunity" of the reconstituting donor cells. Their experiments suggested that both myeloablation and immunity against tumor have potential therapeutic roles in the treatment of leukemia. Of interest, in animals given homologous marrow, survival was limited by development of a wasting syndrome, characterized by weight loss and diarrhea (5). Medical science continues to grapple with the two hypotheses put forth by Barnes and Loutit, which remain the theoretical bases for autologous and allogeneic HSCT. In addition, as was the case with the initial experiments, the challenge of "wasting syndrome," or GVHD, remains a major hurdle in the broad application of allogeneic immunotherapy in cancer treatment.

2.1. Early Human Trials

The first attempts to administer allogeneic bone marrow in man were reported in the late 1950s (6–10). Subsequently, successful engraftment was achieved in syngeneic transplants using supralethal doses of irradiation (11), and in allogeneic transplantation for leukemia (12). The latter, however, was limited by mortality secondary to complications from GVHD (13). The first successful allogeneic HSCT was for severe combined immunodeficiency. This was important in demonstrating the tolerability of the procedure of marrow transplantation (14), and subsequent reports of syngeneic transplantation were encouraging. However, by the late 1960s, there had been sufficient negative experience with allogeneic HSCT in humans to have the procedure proclaimed to be of limited clinical value in the treatment of leukemia (15,16). Whereas the field made progress in animal models of allogeneic transplantation (17–21,22), clinical efforts were limited (23,24).

During this period, building on the growing understanding in the field of tissue compatibility, particularly the major histocompatibility complex (MHC), work with murine and canine models established the role of the human leukocyte antigen (HLA) system in human bone marrow rejection and GVHD. The HLA complex on chromosome 6 encodes more than 200 genes. About 20 of these are class I genes encoding α-chains of the class I molecule, including the three class Ia genes, *HLA-A, -B*, and *-C*. The class II genes encode the α- and β-chains of the class II molecules, including HLA-DR, DP, and DQ. Class I genes are expressed, to a variable degree, by most somatic cells and class II gene expression is, in humans, limited to antigen-presenting cells (APCs), activated T-cells, and thymic epi-thelial cells. T-cells are selected in the thymus to recognize "self" HLA molecules. When presented with allogeneic HLA, the resulting alloreactivity is a form of crossreactivity in which large numbers of T-cells become activated resulting in cell, and ultimately tissue, destruction. In transplantation, this recognition is either of HLA on donor APCs (direct presentation) or the donor's processed HLA molecules in the context of recipient APC presentation (indirect presentation). Knowledge of the HLA system allowed for better donor selection, so that siblings that were identical for selected HLA class I and class II molecules, or "matches," were selected, resulting in less alloreactivity and GVHD *(25–27)*. Now, more sophisticated molecular HLA screening methods permit "high-resolution" typing, thereby improving donor selection from among unrelated volunteers.

2.2. Early Evidence for Antitumor Immune Responses

The theory of immune surveillance, which first appeared in the 1950s, gained support in the 1960s, following the observations of murine tumor formation induced by polyoma virus and the increased incidence of tumors in patients who were immunosuppressed after renal transplantation. The clinical observation that sporadic cases of malignant mela-noma and renal cell carcinoma could resolve spontaneously also contributed to the belief that the immune system is capable of detecting and eradicating established tumor, and formed the basis of the immunosurveillance hypothesis put forth by Burnet and Thomas in the 1950s *(17)*. When Stutman *(28–30)* and others *(31,32)* published experiments with the athymic nude mouse model, finding no differences in the incidence or natural history of nonviral tumors, the theory was abandoned. This theory has regained attention because of increasing numbers of individuals that are chronically immunosuppressed because of iatrogenic and pathological causes and the incidence of malignancy in these populations, and the development of more sophisticated animal models that permit examination of specific immune defects. Recent modifications of the theory have expanded it to a more general process of cancer immunoediting, ascribing to the immune system both host pro-tection against cancer and exertion of selective pressure resulting in tumor escape from immune destruction *(33)*. Efforts to capitalize on the power of the immune system have had two major emphases: circumventing mechanisms of tumor escape in the autologous setting and channeling donor immunity toward GVT in the allogeneic setting.

3. THE EVIDENCE FOR TUMOR IMMUNITY

3.1. Tumor Escape

The growth and metastatic spread of tumors depends on their ability to evade the host immune system. Whereas expression of antigens that are recognized by the immune sys-tem characterizes most tumors, in established tumors the immune response elicited is obviously inadequate. Effective cytotoxic T-cell immunity requires that tumor antigens be presented in the context of MHC class I complexes on the tumor cell or MHC class II complexes on APCs that are capable of inducing tumor-specific cytotoxic T-lympho-cytes. The presence of costimulatory molecules, such as B7-1 and B7-2, on APCs and the secretion of interleukin (IL)-2 promote the differentiation of recruited CD8+ T-lympho-cytes into cytotoxic T-lymphocytes capable of eradicating tumor cells. Failure of antigen processing or binding to MHC molecules, inadequate or low-affinity binding of MHC complexes to T-cell receptors, or inadequate expression of co-stimulatory molecules in conjunction with the antigen-presenting MHC complex are all factors that lead to poor immunogenicity of tumor antigens, impaired antitumor responses, and tumor immune escape *(34)*. Each of these factors can be exploited in efforts to augment the immune response to tumor.

3.2. Autologous or Syngeneic Immunotherapy

3.2.1. MURINE LEUKEMIA MODELS

There are reports of antitumor effects of adoptive cell therapy using syngeneic cell sources for a variety of effector cells, including tumor-associated antigen (TAA)-specific T-cells, natural-killer (NK) cells, T-cells that have been activated with anti-CD3 antibody, or activated with IL-2 lymphokine-activated killer (LAK) cells and NK T-cells. Whereas efficacy is limited in the setting of established tumor, this is markedly improved if immunoablative chemotherapy is administered before cell therapy *(35–42)*. From these studies, successful syngeneic immunotherapy appears to require TAA specificity in the context of MHC, and proliferation and persistence of the effector cell population *(43)*.

3.2.2. CLINICAL CELL THERAPY TRIALS

Early work with IL-2 suggested a potential role for the cytokine in tumor immunotherapy. Murine splenocytes or human lymphocytes from tumor-bearing and normal hosts could be incubated in IL-2 to generate a cell population capable of lysing syngeneic and autologous tumor, respectively, while sparing normal cells in vitro *(44–46)*. Adoptive transfer experiments using the murine B16 melanoma model demonstrated an antitumor effect in animals with established metastatic tumors *(47,48)*. Clinical trials followed *(49, 50)*, including a prospective randomized trial comparing LAK cells plus IL-2 to IL-2 alone, which revealed no survival difference in patients with metastatic melanoma or renal cell carcinoma *(51)*.

The same investigators also isolated lymphocytes from tumor and expanded them in vitro with IL-2, finding that these tumor-infiltrating lymphocytes (TILs) had 50- to 100-fold greater potency than LAK cells in mediating regression of established micrometastases in a murine cancer model. In LAK-resistant tumors, they found that animals that were first immunosuppressed and then treated with TILs had regression of large metastases as well *(52)*. In humans, TAA-reactive TILs can be generated from virtually all tumor types *(53)*. The most recent iteration of TIL therapy in humans has produced impressive clinical responses in refractory, metastatic melanoma *(54)*. In this protocol, melanoma antigen-specific TILs were administered following immune-depleting chemotherapy in conjunction with high-dose IL-2. These findings suggest that, in the autologous setting, clinically relevant antitumor effects resulting from antigen-specific, adoptively transferred T-cells might require or be greatly augmented by host T-cell depletion and/or posttransfer cytokine support. These studies and others *(55,56)* have made the interesting observation that antitumor responses were associated with the development of vitiligo, an autoimmune condition characterized by loss of dermal melanocytes. Relatively few studies have evaluated adoptive T-cell therapy against malignancies other than melanoma, although recent studies have involved patients with head and neck cancer, Hodgkin's and non-Hodgkin's lymphomas, including Epstein-Barr virus-related lymphoma and malignant glioma *(57–65)*.

Other means of T-cell activation to augment tumor immunity have included in vitro and in vivo approaches. June and colleagues have developed a technique for generating co-stimulated, activated T-cells using an artificial dendritic cell (DC) system based on anti-

CD3/anti-CD28 antibody-coated magnetic beads *(57,58,65–68)*. Another approach being tried is the administration of in vitro-generated DCs loaded with tumor antigen. Initial studies using carcinoembryonic antigen peptide have demonstrated the feasibility of this form of cell therapy, with some patient responses *(69–71)*. As methods improve to generate antigen-specific T-cells of enhanced effector function, future trials will focus on defining relevant TAAs. Antigen targeting of the immune T-cell response may be directed against molecules present on multiple tumor types, such as NY-ESO, Wilms' tumor 1, or telomerase, or against antigens with a relatively restricted tumor cell expression, such as PR1 in myeloid malignancy or HER-2/*neu* in breast and prostate cancer *(72–82)*.

3.3. The "Homologous"/Allogeneic System: GVT

After the work of Barnes and Loutit opened the field of allogeneic cell therapy, subsequent study of adoptive immunotherapy established the validity of the GVT effect using increasingly sophisticated animal models *(3,5,83–87)*. Early evidence for its relevance in humans was noted following the first successful transplants for leukemia *(12)*.

Allogeneic HSCT is currently used to treat a variety of hematological malignancies and an increasing spectrum of nonmalignant diseases *(88)*. The curative potential of allogeneic HSCT appears to be derived from donor immune T-cells that react against host or tumor cell antigens to generate a GVT effect *(2,89,90)*. Evidence supporting the existence of an allogeneic GVT effect includes an increased relapse rate in recipients of T-cell-depleted allografts *(91–94)*, an inverse correlation between relapse and GVHD severity *(19)*, and an increased relapse rate after syngeneic *(1,2,18)* or autologous HSCT *(18,19,92, 95–98)*. A retrospective study of data collected by the International Bone Marrow Transplant Registry demonstrated an increased leukemia relapse rate among patients receiving syngeneic bone marrow or T-cell-depleted, allogeneic marrow *(2)*. These data suggested that alloreactive T-cells within the allograft were directly involved in eradicating leukemia. Reports of tumor regression following cessation of immunosuppression are also suggestive *(99)*. Interestingly, however, recipients of syngeneic or autologous bone marrow transplants can develop GVHD while taking cyclosporin A. The mechanism for cyclosporin A-induced GVHD is not clear, but it probably involves dysregulation of self-tolerance during a critical period of immune system reconstitution. This loss of tolerance may result in some GVT effect as well *(100–105)*. Finally, the most compelling evidence for an immune T-cell-mediated GVT effect originates from the observation that infusion of allogeneic lymphocytes, a donor lymphocyte infusion (DLI), at a time remote from the transplant preparative regimen can successfully treat leukemia relapse post-HSCT *(106–110)*.

In an initial report, DLI therapy was given to three patients with CML whose disease had recurred after an allogeneic HSCT *(106)*. The DLI, without any additional cytotoxic therapy, resulted in sustained cytogenetic and molecular remission. Evidence of a GVT effect has also been observed against other hematological malignancies including multiple myeloma and lymphomas *(111–113)*.

3.4. Mechanisms/Effectors of GVT

With recent advances in immunology, the biological bases for antitumor immunity are beginning to unfold. $CD8^+$ and $CD4^+$ T-lymphocytes can respond to tumor antigens presented as peptides in association with MHC molecules on tumor cells (class I) or on "professional" APCs, such as DCs (class II), respectively *(34)*. Although antitumor-specific T-cell immune responses can be readily demonstrated in vitro and in vivo, such responses typically do not eliminate established tumor. Alloreactivity is highly unpredictable and can dramatically alter the balance between the immune response to tumor and mechanisms of tumor escape. HLA mismatch and minor histocompatibility antigens influence of the establishment of both GVHD and GVT *(114)*. The roles of the regulatory T-cell subsets, including $CD4^+CD25^+$ T-cells and NK T-cells, in GVT and their potential to separate the antitumor immune response from more general immune reactions characteristic of GVHD are areas of active exploration.

In patients undergoing allogeneic transplantation for malignancy, the GVT effector populations, target antigens, and the relationship to GVHD are also quite variable, and likely depend on several factors acting interdependently: the degree of HLA and minor antigen histocompatibility, the type of tumor, and the history of selective pressures affecting immunogenicity that have been exerted on the tumor at the time of transplant.

4. T-CELLS

In animal models, the effectors of GVT vary with the model used. In an MHC-mismatched murine model, DLI enriched for either $CD4^+$ or $CD8^+$ T-cells exhibited some GVT, although $CD8^+$ T-cells had the more potent GVT effect, and unselected DLI showed the greatest antitumor activity. In contrast, when naive MHC-matched cells were given as DLI, depletion of either $CD8^+$ or $CD4^+$ T-cells resulted in elimination of the GVT effect. Host alloantigen-primed $CD8^+$ T-cells from MHC-matched donors, however, mediated a $CD4^+$ T-independent GVT reaction *(115)*.

4.1. Minor Histocompatibility Antigens

The existence of histocompatibility loci in addition to MHC accounts for the development of GVHD in the setting of HLA-identical allogeneic HSCT. Alloantigens encoded by histocompatibility loci outside of MHC, the minor histocompatibility antigens, contribute not only to GVHD but also to the GVT effect. Whereas some minor antigens are universally expressed on cells of a given individual, some are tissue-specific to the lympho-hematopoietic system or to epithelial cells, for example. In any one donor–recipient pair, it appears that alloreactivity is limited to a few minor histocompatibility antigens; thus, as our understanding of these antigens increases it may become possible to better predict, measure, and manipulate the immune response after allogeneic HSCT *(116–119)*.

4.2. Tumor-Specific Clones and TAAs

Whereas alloreactivity is a major component in the GVT effect, there is evidence that TAAs play a role in the allogeneic setting as well. In a recent study using an allogeneic parent-into-F1 murine transplant model, tumors derived from either parental strain were used to evaluate tumor-specific GVT effects. $CD8^+$ T-cell-mediated GVT effects occurred in both allogeneic HSCT models, even when the absence of histoincompatibility between donor cells and host tumor precluded allorecognition, indicating that TAAs were the target of the immune response. In this model, MHC disparity between donor cells and normal host tissue resulted in GVHD, and its development was associated with both TAA-specific and allospecific GVT effects. Adoptive transfer of the effector cells into secondary tumor-bearing recipients confirmed sustained antitumor activity, and the absence of GVHD in these secondary recipients demonstrated the specificity of the T-cell antitumor response *(120)*. Whereas TAA-specific T-cell responses are thought to play a major role in immunity in the autologous setting *(121–125)*, their role in allogeneic cell therapy is a recent observation.

4.3. NK Cells

The role of donor NK cells in GVHD and GVT is under active investigation. Early studies seemed to indicate that donor NK cells played a limited role, if any, in these graft-mediated immune reactions *(126,127)*. More recently, however, a role for NK cells in the MHC-mismatched setting has been elucidated. The interaction of killer cell immunoglobu-lin-like receptor with MHC inhibits the cytotoxic activity of NK cells *(128–130)*. Recent work examined the impact of donor-vs-recipient NK cell alloreactivity on relapse, rejection, GVHD, and survival in the HLA-mismatched, or haploidentical, allogeneic HSCT setting. It was found that donor–recipient pairs with killer cell immunoglobulin-like receptor ligand incompatibility in the graft-vs-host direction experienced less leukemia relapse, graft rejection, and GVHD. In mice, pretransplant infusion of alloreactive NK cells similarly enhanced engraftment and protected against GVHD, the latter by ablation of host APCs *(128,131)*. Work is ongoing to understand better the mechanisms involved and how to exploit NK cell receptor mismatch in the clinic *(132–136)*. Although these multiple benefits of NK alloreactivity were found in haploidentical HSCT, there have been conflicting data relative to this benefit in the setting of allogeneic HSCT from HLA-matched, unrelated donors *(137,138)*.

4.4. Antigen-Presenting Cells

It has long been recognized that an optimal GVT effect requires efficient antigen presentation by APCs, such as DCs, and appropriate costimulatory signals to T-cells *(139–141)*. The observation in a murine model for allogeneic BMT that, despite the presence of numerous donor APCs, only host-derived APCs initiated GVHD suggests a possible point of separation between GVHD and GVT *(142)*. In support of this, the same investigators found that donor APCs were not required for CD8[+] T-cell-mediated GVT against a murine model of chronic-phase CML *(143,144)*. It follows, then, that one strategy for improving GVT without getting GVHD is to eliminate the host APCs before administration of donor effector cells. Observations that NK-receptor mismatch in allogeneic HSCT result in enhanced GVT without an increase in GVHD may be related; early clearance of host APCs by alloreactive NK cells may result in lower rates of GVHD without impairing the GVT effect. This may explain the lower incidence of GVHD when donor lymphocytes are administered after a delay following the preparative regimen *(145)*.

5. IMMUNOMODULATORS OF GVT

There is tremendous variability relative to the clinical effectiveness of GVT against different hematological malignancies after allogeneic HSCT. Factors that affect GVT after allogeneic HSCT include the presence of mixed T-cell chimerism, the development of donor–host tolerance, the susceptibility of the hematological malignancy to the GVT effect, and suboptimal GVT reactivity *(146)*.

The expression of surface or intracellular molecules is essential for recognition or elimination by effector lymphocytes. Tumor cells may directly suppress effector cells through secretion of inhibitory cytokines, such as transforming growth factor-β *(147)*. Tumor cells may also downregulate HLA class I and class II molecules, may have low or missing expression of co-stimulatory molecules, such as CD80, CD83, CD86, CD40, and intercellular adhesion molecule or alter the presentation of antigenic peptide sequences *(148–151)*. The cytotoxic effects of effector cells are primarily mediated through fatty acid synthase or tumor necrosis factor (TNF) receptors or through direct binding of perforin and activation of granzyme B *(152)*. Decreased fatty acid synthase ligand expression or reduced perforin binding can impair the potency of the GVT effect *(153–155)*.

Tumor burden is a clinical factor negatively affecting GVT activity. This often coincides with chemotherapy-insensitive tumors. In extremely chemotherapy-refractory patients, the GVT effect may not be sufficiently potent to be clinically detectable, because the tumor growth rate exceeds the ability of the immune effect to eliminate disease. Patients with chemotherapy-sensitive disease also tend to have less of a disease burden, and the greatest efficacy of the GVT effect has been observed in minimal residual disease states. Specifically, relapse is higher among patients who are not in remission at the time of allogeneic HSCT or DLI. If one looks specifically at chronic phase CML, the efficacy of DLI is inversely related to the disease burden, with greatest efficacy observed when disease is only detectable by polymerase chain reaction methods and the lowest efficacy among patients with hematological relapses.

The failure to detect clinical evidence of GVT after allogeneic HSCT can be attributed to the biological characteristics of the disease, such as histology and chemotherapy sensitivity *(156)*. There are different significant differences in the GVT susceptibility of different hematological malignancies, and there can be significant differences in GVT responsiveness among the histological subtypes of many hematological malignancies *(109,157)*. For example, evidence of a GVT effect and the efficacy of DLI in non-Hodgkin's lymphoma have been primarily limited to follicular or "low-grade" histologies, with only anecdotal cases in patients with diffuse large B-cell or more aggressive histologies *(157,158)*. This may reflect the biological characteristics, such as growth rate or antigen expression, of the respective histologies. The hematological malignancy can also localize to privileged sites where effector cells have difficulty reaching tumor cells, such as the central nervous system *(159)*.

5.1. T-Cell Cytokine Profile Phenotype

CD4+ and CD8+ T-cells, which can exist in T-helper (Th)1/Th2 or cytotoxic T-cell (Tc) 1/Tc2 states of cytokine polarity *(160,161)*, appear to differentially influence GVHD *(162)*. In murine models, GVHD has been characterized primarily as a type I cytokine-driven response resulting in an IL-1α- and TNF-α-based "cytokine storm" *(160,163–165)*. Fowler et al. hypothesized and demonstrated that adoptively transferred donor Th2-type CD4+ T-cells could ameliorate GVHD in a murine parent-into-F1 model *(166)*, and subsequently, others and we found that administration of either Th2 or Tc2 cells resulted in reduced GVHD *(167–170)*. Importantly, whereas donor Tc2 cells are modestly less potent in the induction of GVT than their Tc1 counterparts, they maintain a significant capacity to kill tumors *(169,171)*. These results are consistent with Tc1 or Tc2 cell administration in syngeneic models, where Tc1 cells are typically more potent in mediating tumor regression *(172)*.

5.2. Co-Stimulation

Separation of GVHD from the GVT effect is an important objective in developing safe and effective allogeneic immunotherapy of cancer. Interruption of T-cell co-stimulation via in vivo CD28/B7 blockade can reduce GVHD lethality *(173)*, and forced B7 ligand expression can augment an antitumor immune response in mice *(174,175)*. In a murine allogeneic transplant model of the GVT effect of DLI, in which the GVHD:GVT balance is a function of the splenocyte cell dose:tumor inoculum ratio, anti-B7 monoclonal antibody infusion abrogated the GVT response to C1498-induced acute myelogenous leukemia. In contrast, using the same transplant model, EL4 cell-induced T-acute lymphocytic leukemia elicited a more modest GVT effect. The forced expression of B7-1 on EL4 cells markedly augmented the GVT effect of DLI, in contrast to the forced expression of B7-2 on EL4 cells. From this, it was concluded that the administration of anti-B7 monoclonal antibodies may impair the GVT effect of DLI, and that the forced expression of B7-1 ligands stimulates a GVT effect without adversely affecting the GVHD lethality effect of DLI *(176,177)*.

5.3. DLI Manipulations

5.3.1. TIMING

T-cell-depleted allogeneic HSCT as a strategy to reduce GVHD is limited by higher incidences of both graft rejection and relapse. However, delayed infusion of donor lymphocytes after T-depleted allogeneic HSCT can establish full-donor chimerism, reduce GVHD, and reestablish the GVT effect that is lost during the mixed chimeric state *(145,178)*. Efforts to carry this observation into the clinic have yielded mixed results *(94,179–181)*.

5.3.2. CHIMERISM

The relationship between chimerism and relapse has been extensively investigated, and whereas findings are not in complete agreement, perhaps because of differences in response rates for different types of malignancy, it does seem that the state of mixed chimerism is associated with failure of GVT, both in the initial control of disease and in a higher incidence of relapse *(182–184)*. An early study looked prospectively at 32 patients with CML after CD34+ cell-selected allogeneic HSCT for T-cell chimerism and minimal residual disease using polymerase chain reaction, and found a strong association with loss of T-cell chimerism and molecular relapse, as well as with clinical and hematological relapse *(184)*. A larger prospective study of patients with a range of hematological malignancies also found an association between relapse and mixed chimerism *(185)*. Data on chimerism after nonmyeloablative and reduced-intensity preparative regimens are becoming available, and whereas comparisons are complicated by differences in the conditioning regimens and tumor type, the relationship between T-cell chimerism and disease control appears the same as observed in allogeneic HSCT after myeloablative preparative regimens *(186–188)*.

Not all studies agree on the requirement for full-donor chimerism for the GVT effect. After observations in the mouse revealed that DLI administered to mixed chimeras resulted in GVH reaction that was limited to the lymphohematopoietic system, a clinical trial attempted to establish a state of mixed chimerism as a platform for DLI. The study showed clinically significant responses to DLI in the patients that successfully achieved a state of mixed chimerism after nonmyeloablative bone marrow transplantation. A comparison of mixed and full-donor chimerism as a platform for DLI in a murine EL4 leukemia model showed that DLI administration to mixed chimeras produced enhanced leukemia-free survival compared with full-donor chimeras. The same study also found that DLI converted mixed chimeras to full chimeras without causing GVHD, and that the magnitude of the GVT effect was dependent on the level of MHC class I expression on recipient hematopoietic cells in mixed chimeras *(189–192)*. Given the fact that mixed T-cell chimeras are converted to full donor in these models, the reported findings are not necessarily at odds with other reported studies. Whereas differences in murine models and clinical preparative regimens preclude direct comparison, the role of chimerism dynamics in the GVT response remains intriguing.

5.3.3. Dose

A prospective study looked at the relationship of DLI cell dose to GVT and GVHD in patients with CML at different stages. In this study, each patient received escalating doses of DLI. In the 19 of 22 patients who achieved remission, nearly half responded at a dose of 10^7 cells/kg, although a significant minority of patients did not respond until reaching a dose of 5×10^8 cells/kg. The incidence of GVHD correlated with the dose of T-cells administered, and of note, only one of the eight patients who achieved remission at a T-cell dose of 10^7/kg developed GVHD. Also of note, most of the patients who obtained a GVT effect were mixed T-cell chimeras before treatment and became full-donor T-cell chimeras at the time of remission *(193)*.

Whereas lymphocyte dose appears to strengthen GVT, it is associated with increased toxicity in the form of GVHD *(194,195)*. A retrospective analysis of 298 patients with CML treated with DLI sought to identify a DLI dose that might provide a GVT effect with limited GVHD *(194)*. Patients were classified into three groups: receiving less than 0.20×10^8, $0.21–2.0 \times 10^8$, or greater than 2.0×10^8 mononuclear cells/kg. Because recipients of the lower DLI dose had a lower incidence of GVHD, a similar response rate, and better overall and failure-free survival, the authors concluded that, at least in the setting of CML, an initial DLI dose of approx 0.2×10^8 mononuclear cells/kg might provide the best ratio of GVT to GVHD effects.

5.4. Cytokines

The role of various cytokines in separating GVT from GVHD has been an area of long and intensive investigation. Some of the earliest work involved IL-2 *(196–202)*. Administration of IL-2 was first shown to augment the antitumor response of allogeneic T-cell therapy *(202)* and to reduce the incidence of acute and chronic GVHD in murine models of T-cell depleted bone marrow transplants *(201)*. Its effects, however, appeared to be model-specific: in a fully MHC-mismatched plus minor histocompatibility antigen-mismatched murine GVHD model, the protective effect of IL-2 administration was found to be through inhibition of CD4[+] T-cell-mediated GVHD *(203)*. In contrast, the exclusively CD8[+] T-cell-mediated GVT effect observed in the EL4 leukemia/lymphoma model was not inhibited by IL-2 treatment *(203–205)*. In a different model, administration of fully allogeneic spleen cells and T-cell-depleted marrow led to a significant delay in leukemic mortality in IL-2-treated mice that was entirely mediated by donor CD4[+] and CD8[+] T-cells. IL-2 administration did not diminish the magnitude of the GVT effect of either T-cell subset. Of interest, the investigators noted that CD4[+] T-cell-mediated GVHD was inhibited in the same animals in which CD4[+] T-cell-mediated GVT effects were not reduced by IL-2 treatment. In retrospect, it seems likely that these findings were the result of in vivo expansion of a CD4[+]CD25[+] regulatory T-cell population in IL-2 treated animals, leading to reduced GVHD.

In clinical studies, treatment with in vitro IL-2-activated donor lymphocytes and in vivo IL-2 therapy resulted in responses in some patients with hematological tumors that relapsed after allogeneic HSCT and DLI *(206)*. These investigators used the same IL-2 activation protocol to administer activated allogeneic lymphocytes to patients with metastatic breast cancer following autologous transplantation. Whereas GVT could not be verified in the setting of concurrent high-dose chemotherapy, the cells were administered with minimal toxicity *(207)*.

In mice, TNF-α but not IL-1 has been shown to be required for T-cell cytotoxicity-mediated GVT *(165)*; keratinocyte growth factor, apparently through reduction of lipopolysaccharide and TNFα, *(208)*; and IL-11 can significantly reduce CD4+ T-cell-dependent GVHD without impairing cytolytic function or subsequent GVT activity of CD8+ T-cells *(209)*. Whereas there is some evidence in murine models that IL-12 can separate GVT effect from GVHD, the IL-12 effect on T-cell-mediated GVT is likely primarily because of driving the undifferentiated T-cell population to a type 1 cytokine profile, which has been shown to augment both the GVT and GVH response *(168)*. More recent investigations, however, have focused on the role of IL-12 and IL-18 in NK cell cytotoxicity-mediated GVT *(133)*, and selective killing by NK cells may account for some of the GVT/GVHD discrimination observed in earlier work using these cytokines.

Granulocyte colony-stimulating factor ([G-CSF] filgrastim) has also been identified as a potential modulator of GVT. In murine models, transplantation with G-CSF-mobilized peripheral blood progenitor cells resulted in reduced GVHD without loss of GVT. GVT appeared to be mediated by cytotoxic T-cell activity via a perforin pathway *(210)*. These effects seem to be the result of activity on donor rather than host cells *(211)*. There have also been clinical observations of G-CSF administration resulting in leukemic remission in patients that relapse after allogeneic HSCT *(212,213)*. Additionally, it has been reported that administration of G-CSF postallogeneic HSCT drives T-cells toward a Th2 phenotype in the haploidentical allogeneic HSCT setting *(214)*. Whereas this may be consistent with the GVT observations described in the above paragraph, it may also result in immune dysfunction, with abnormal APC functions and T-cell reactivity.

5.5. Regulatory T-Cells

From murine models, it has been shown that donor-derived CD4+CD25+ regulatory T-cells inhibit lethal GVHD after allogeneic bone marrow transplantation across MHC class I and II barriers *(215,216)* and in a minor histocompatibility antigen-disparate model *(217)*. In recipient mice with leukemia and lymphoma, CD4+CD25+ regulatory T-cells suppress the early expansion of alloreactive donor T-cells, their IL-2-receptor α-chain expression, and their capacity to induce GVHD without abrogating their GVT effector function, mediated primarily by the perforin lysis pathway *(218)*. These same investigators have recently reported in vitro expansion of human, polyclonal CD4+CD25+ regulatory cells, a requisite first step in using these cells as part of a GVT immunotherapeutic strategy *(219)*. In a murine model, this regulatory T-cell population was expanded ex vivo using stimulation with allogeneic APCs, resulting in a cell population that could control GVHD and favored immune reconstitution *(220)*.

5.6. NK T-Cells

NK T-lymphocytes are a subset of regulatory lymphocytes with important immunomodulatory effects. The inhibitory NK cell receptors on NK cells that negatively regulate NK cell functions through their binding to MHC class I molecules can be found on CD8+ memory T-cells. These NK T-cells have been shown, in murine studies, to be important in GVHD *(221,222)*. There is a growing body of evidence that these cells also play a role in GVT. It has been demonstrated that NK-like activity and T-cell receptor-mediated killing activity of cytotoxic NK T-cells were suppressed by HLA class I recognition by the

NK receptors. However, these same cells may induce a GVT effect against tumor cells that have mismatched or decreased expression of HLA class I molecules and do not cause GVHD against host cells that have normal expression of HLA class I molecules (223). Ex vivo-activated and expanded NK T-cells can be generated from patients with malignancies. These cells mediate cytotoxicity against autologous malignant cells in vitro. In murine allogeneic HSCT experiments, large numbers of expanded CD8+ NK T-cells could be transplanted across MHC barriers without causing severe GVHD, and GVT effects were retained (221).

6. CLINICAL EXPLOITATION OF GVT

Given the potent antitumor effects associated with allogeneic HSCT for hematological malignancy, and potentially for solid tumors, expansion of efforts in allogeneic cellular immunotherapy is warranted. However, this approach is associated with significant morbidity and mortality, which primarily stems from GVHD mediated by donor CD4+ and CD8+ T-cells (224). As such, allogeneic GVT effects must be balanced by an acceptable pattern of GVHD.

6.1. "Nonmyeloablative" or "Reduced-Intensity" Allogeneic HSCT

The recognition that donor T-lymphocytes mediate curative GVT effects led to the hypothesis that the myeloablative conditioning component of allogeneic HSCT may be eliminated without impairment of tumor eradication. To avoid the toxicity associated with myeloablative preparative regimens, investigators developed nonmyeloablative and reduced-intensity preparative regimens primarily intended to provide adequate suppression of the host immune system to allow engraftment of donor hematopoietic stem cells and use of allogeneic T-cells as adoptive cellular therapy. Several trials using a variety of these nonmyeloablative and reduced-intensity regimens have demonstrated that engraftment of donor hematopoietic stem cells can occur (186,225–228). However, the degree of donor engraftment is quite variable, and graft rejection was observed with some regimens. In these studies, the attainment of complete donor lymphoid engraftment, which likely permits an optimal GVT effect, often did not occur without posttransplant maneuvers, such as early removal of GVHD chemoprophylaxis or administration DLI therapy. Whereas often effective in establishing of full-donor chimerism and obtaining GVT (229), not unexpectedly, such maneuvers have been associated with a significant incidence of lethal GVHD (226,228). As such, although nonmyeloablative and reduced-intensity allogeneic HSCT reduces early treatment-related mortality and thereby allows transplantation of older patients or individuals with impaired organ function, the same obstacles associated with myeloablative allogeneic HSCT, most notably GVHD, persist and will have to be addressed in future clinical trials.

6.2. Solid Tumor Immunotherapy

A better understanding of the contribution of the GVT effect to allogeneic HSCT and the evolution of less toxic preparative regimens paved the way for application of allogeneic immunotherapy to other solid tumors. Allogeneic HSCT utilizing reduced-intensity preparative regimens has primarily been used to treat leukemia, lymphoma, and multiple myeloma (226,227,230–233). Similar to results with myeloablative allogeneic HSCT, antitumor response appears to be associated with disease sensitivity and bulk before transplant *(230,231)*. Given the reduced toxicity and maintained GVT effect of reduced-intensity preparative regimens, investigators have begun to evaluate whether solid tumors with a history of responding to immune therapies, such as renal cell carcinoma and malignant melanoma, might be responsive to allogeneic adoptive T-cell therapy. Investigators at the National Institutes of Health National Heart Lung and Blood Institute treated patients with metastatic renal cell cancer with allogeneic HSCT after a fludarabine- and cyclophosphamide-conditioning regimen *(187)*. Ten of 19 patients responded, with three complete and seven partial remissions. Responses were delayed and occurred a median of 129 d post-HSCT and coincident with establishment of complete donor T-cell chimerism. Allogeneic GVT responses to renal cell carcinoma have been reported by other investigators; further research will need to evaluate whether these responses translate into significant clinical improvements or cures *(187,234–237)*.

Reduced-intensity allogeneic HSCT is also being evaluated in other solid tumors, including breast, ovarian, lung, and colon cancer, malignant melanoma, and sarcoma *(234–236, 238–253)*. We are evaluating allogeneic T-cell therapy in patients with metastatic and refractory breast cancer. In the initial protocol, allografts were T-cell-depleted, so that any antitumor effect mediated by the preparative regimen could be dissociated from that mediated by a GVT effect. Donor T-cell immunotherapy was administered as a DLI beginning on day 42. Seven of 17 evaluable patients that received transplants achieved a clinical disease response after day 28+ that could be attributed to the allogeneic cell therapy *(252)*. These initial results provided a proof-of-principle that clinically significant allogeneic GVT effects against metastatic breast cancer can be generated after reduced-intensity allogeneic HSCT, and serve as the basis for ongoing efforts to augment the GVT effect, through the administration of donor Tc2 cells at the time of stem cell infusion.

6.3 Donor Th2/Tc2 Graft Augmentation

Based on murine results, we have initiated clinical trials to evaluate allograft augmentation with cytokine-defined donor T-cell subsets in order to enhance GVT while limiting GVHD *(162)*. In initial studies, we found that extensive host immune depletion before allogeneic PBSCT resulted in rapid donor chimerism, a potent GVT effect, and significant GVHD *(230)*. Subsequently, the safety and feasibility of allograft supplementation with in vitro expanded donor Th2 cells was established. Early clinical results demonstrate that Th2 cells, which are generated by CD3 and CD28 co-stimulation under Th2 polarizing conditions, can be feasibly generated and safely administered *(254)*. More recent clinical trial data indicate that Th2 cells appear to promote allogeneic T-cell expansion and activation early post-HSCT, without an apparent increase in GVHD *(255)*. We are also conducting clinical trials involving allogeneic stem cell graft augmentation with both Th2-type CD4+ T-cells and CD8+ T-cells of Tc2 phenotype. Because murine studies indicate that Tc2 cells can mediate a GVT or GVT effect with reduced GVHD, allogeneic HSCT with adoptive transfer of allogeneic CD8+ Tc2 cells may offer a beneficial GVT effect with reduced GVHD.

6.4. Improving the Therapeutic Window of Donor Lymphocyte Infusions

The efficacy of DLI for therapy of recurrent malignancy postallogeneic HSCT is influenced by tumor histology, disease status, and lymphocyte dose *(109,110,115,193,207, 256,257)*. CML is particularly responsive to DLI, with remission rates of 60–80% for patients in cytogenetic or molecular relapse, respectively. In cases of more extensive

CML relapse, response rates for DLI therapy are lower (10–30%) and typically, not durable *(110)*. Furthermore, although DLI can mediate significant clinical responses in other hematological diseases, response rates are generally less than 50% in non-CML diagnoses, with particularly disappointing results in acute myelogenous leukemia and acute lymphocytic leukemia. Strategies to improve the antitumor specificity of DLI include donor immunization with host tumor *(258,259)*, IL-2 augmented DLI following autologous HSCT *(260)*, and gene-modified DLI *(64,261–263)*.

6.5. Vaccines

6.5.1. TUMOR OR TAA VACCINES

TAAs provide an attractive target for vaccine development, but may be limited in efficacy in the autologous setting by host tolerance. Efforts to circumvent this through augmentation with adjuvant and exogenous cytokine have had considerable success *(264, 265)*. Taking advantage of alloreactivity is another strategy to strengthen immunogenicity of tumor antigens. Postallogeneic HSCT vaccination with tumor cell vaccines has shown promise in enhancing GVT without exacerbating GVHD in murine models *(266–270)*. After demonstrating that donor immunization with anti-idiotype vaccine derived from recipient tumor pre-HSCT could result in the transfer of idiotype-specific T-cell responses in a patient with multiple myeloma *(271)*, the National Cancer Institute is currently evaluating the administration of patient tumor-derived vaccine to donors prestem cell collection and of patients in the post-HSCT period in the reduced-intensity setting *(272)*.

Another approach is to take advantage of alloreactivity without attempting to single out a specific TAA while augmenting the GVT effect further with the administration of cytokine. This has been done in a murine model using irradiated B16 melanoma cells that were genetically altered to secrete granulocyte-macrophage colony-stimulating factor (sargramostim). Vaccination was effective in stimulating potent and long-lasting antitumor activity in recipients of T-cell-depleted allogeneic bone marrow without eliciting GVHD *(268)*.

6.5.2. ALLOGENEIC DCs

Allogeneic APC therapy represents another vaccine strategy. A phase I/II study evaluating the administration of allogeneic DCs, with or without cyclophosphamide, in the treatment of patients with metastatic renal cell carcinoma found that allogeneic immunotherapy with DCs is feasible and well tolerated. Whereas the immunogenicity of allogeneic DCs was weak as assessed in vitro, there were two mixed responses and three patients with disease stabilization *(273)*.

7. CONCLUSIONS

Adoptive T-cell immunotherapy represents a promising approach to the treatment of cancer. In the autologous setting, advances in the science of T-cell therapy have led successful clinical application. These scientific advances, which include identification of immunogenic cancer antigens and an increased ability to identify and expand T-cells with tumor reactivity, will likely translate into future clinical progress. Hopefully, such progress will apply to common tumor types that to date have been relatively refractory to immunomodulatory approaches, such as breast, lung, colon, and prostate cancers. In the allogeneic setting, the situation with adoptive T-cell immunotherapy is somewhat reversed, as clinical applications and success at treating malignancy lead the scientific understanding of the biology of these tumor regressions. To this extent, efforts are underway to elucidate the mechanism(s) of curative allogeneic GVT effects. This understanding is of significant importance, as it may allow the identification of the mechanisms of GVT that are distinct from GVHD, and may enhance our ability to generate allogeneic GVT responses against solid tumors. Future strategies of enlarging the therapeutic window of GVT will likely include targeting the allogeneic immune T-cell repertoire toward TAAs or toward tissue-restricted minor histocompatibility antigens, which appear to be present on both hemato-poietic cells and epithelial tumor cells *(116, 117)*, and taking advantage of the specificity of the alloresponse of NK cell receptor mismatch *(129, 274, 275)*. With these thoughts in mind, it is apparent that the fields of autologous and allogeneic T-cell therapy conceptually overlap, with each application attempting to focus an immune T-cell response against can-cer cells with relatively reduced toxicity against normal host tissue, specifically, reduced GVHD in allogeneic T-cell therapy and a reasonable degree of autoimmunity in autologous T-cell therapy. Future opportunity and success will likely take advantage of what we have learned from both fields of study, harnessing the potential of alloreactivity with increased tumor specificity to achieve optimal antitumor immune responses.

REFERENCES

1. Fefer A, Sullivan KM, Weiden P, et al. Graft versus leukemia effect in man: the relapse rate of acute leukemia is lower after allogeneic than after syngeneic marrow transplantation. *Prog Clin Biol Res* 1987; 244:401–408.
2. Horowitz MM, Gale RP, et al. Graft-versus-leukemia reactions after bone marrow transplantation. *Blood* 1990; 75:555–562.
3. Barnes DW, Corp MJ, Loutit JF, Neal FE. Treatment of murine leukaemia with X rays and homologous bone marrow; preliminary communication. *Br Med J* 1956; 32:626–627.
4. Barnes DW, Loutit JF. Protective effects of implants of splenic tissue. *Proc R Soc Med* 1953; 46: 251–252.
5. Barnes DW, Loutit JF. Treatment of murine leukaemia with x-rays and homologous bone marrow. II. *Br J Haematol* 1957; 3:241–452.
6. Thomas ED, Lochte HL Jr, Lu WC, Ferrebee JW. Intravenous infusion of bone marrow in patients receiving radiation and chemotherapy. *N Engl J Med* 1957; 257:491–496.
7. Mathe G, Hartmann L, Loverdo A, Bernard J. Attempt at protection against radiogold-induced mortal-ity by injection of isologous or homologous bone marrow cells (in French). *Rev Fr Etud Clin Biol* 1958; 3:1086–1087.
8. Mathe G, Bernard J, Schwarzenberg L, et al. Trial treatment of patients afflicted with acute leukemia in remission with total irradiation followed by homologous bone marrow transfusion (in French). *Rev Fr Etud Clin Biol* 1959; 4:675–704.
9. Mathe G, Jammet H, Pendic B, et al. Transfusions and grafts of homologous bone marrow in humans after accidental high dosage irradiation (in French). *Rev Fr Etud Clin Biol* 1959; 4:226–238.
10. Mathe G, Bernard J. Trial of treatment of experimental leukemia by the graft of normal hematopoietic cells (in French). *Sangre (Barc)* 1959; 30:789–801.
11. Thomas ED, Lochte HL Jr, Cannon JH, Sahler OD, Ferrebee JW. Supralethal whole body irradiation and isologous marrow transplantation in man. *J Clin Invest* 1959; 38:1709–1716.
12. Mathe G, Amiel JL, Schwarzenberg L, et al. Successful allogenic bone marrow transplantation in man: chimerism, induced specific tolerance and possible anti-leukemic effects. *Blood* 1965; 25:179–196.
13. Mathe G, Amiel JL, Schwarzenberg L, Cattan A, Schneider M. Adoptive immunotherapy of acute leukemia: experimental and clinical results. *Cancer Res* 1965; 25:1525–1531.
14. Gatti RA, Meuwissen HJ, Allen HD, Hong R, Good RA. Immunological reconstitution of sex-linked lymphopenic immunological deficiency. *Lancet* 1968; 2:1366–1369.
15. Bortin MM. A compendium of reported human bone marrow transplants. *Transplantation* 1970; 9: 571–587.
16. Thomas ED, Blume KG. Historical markers in the development of allogeneic hematopoietic cell trans-plantation. *Biol Blood Marrow Transplant* 1999; 5:341–346.
17. Burnet FM. Immunological surveillance in neoplasia. *Transplant Rev* 1971; 7:3–25.

18. Weiden PL, Flournoy N, Thomas ED, et al. Antileukemic effect of graft-versus-host disease in human recipients of allogeneic-marrow grafts. *N Engl J Med* 1979; 300:1068–1073.

19. Weiden PL, Sullivan KM, Flournoy N, Storb R, Thomas ED. Antileukemic effect of chronic graft-versus-host disease: contribution to improved survival after allogeneic marrow transplantation. *N Engl J Med* 1981; 304:1529–1533.

20. Thomas ED, Storb R, Clift RA, et al. Bone-marrow transplantation (second of two parts). *N Engl J Med* 1975; 292:895–902.

21. Thomas E, Storb R, Clift RA, et al. Bone-marrow transplantation (first of two parts). *N Engl J Med* 1975; 292:832–843.

22. McGovern JJ Jr, Russell PS, Atkins L, Webster EW. Treatment of terminal leukemic relapse by total-body irradiation and intravenous infusion of stored autologous bone marrow obtained during remission. *N Engl J Med* 1959; 260:675–683.

23. Fefer A, Einstein AB, Thomas ED, et al. Bone-marrow transplantation for hematologic neoplasia in 16 patients with identical twins. *N Engl J Med* 1974; 290:1389–1393.

24. Fefer A, Buckner CD, Clift RA, et al. Marrow grafting in identical twins with hematologic malignancies. *Transplant Proc* 1973; 5:927–931.

25. Klein J, Sato A. The HLA system. First of two parts. *N Engl J Med* 2000; 343:702–709.

26. Klein J, Sato A. The HLA system. Second of two parts. *N Engl J Med* 2000; 343:782–786.

27. Amos DB. Human histocompatibility locus HL-A. *Science* 1968; 159:659–660.

28. Stutman O. Tumor development after 3-methylcholanthrene in immunologically deficient athymic-nude mice. *Science* 1974; 183:534–546.

29. Stutman O. Delayed tumour appearance and absence of regression in nude mice infected with murine sarcoma virus. *Nature* 1975; 253:142–144.

30. Stutman O. Tumor development after polyoma infection in athymic nude mice. *J Immunol* 1975; 114: 1213–1217.

31. De Clercq E. Tumor induction by Moloney sarcoma virus in athymic nude mice. *J Natl Cancer Inst* 1975; 54:473–477.

32. Martin WJ, Martin SE. Naturally occurring cytotoxic anti-tumour antibodies in sera of congenitally athymic (nude) mice. *Nature* 1974; 249:564–565.

33. Dunn GP, Bruce AT, Ikeda H, Old LJ, Schreiber RD. Cancer immunoediting: from immunosurveillance to tumor escape. *Nat Immunol* 2002; 3:991–998.

34. Foss FM. Immunologic mechanisms of antitumor activity. *Semin Oncol* 2002; 29:5–11.

35. Fass L, Fefer A. Factors related to therapeutic efficacy in adoptive chemoimmunotherapy of a Friend virus-induced lymphoma. *Cancer Res* 1972; 32:2427–2431.

36. Fass L, Fefer A. Studies of adoptive chemoimmunotherapy of a Friend virus-induced lymphoma. *Cancer Res* 1972; 32:997–1001.

37. Fefer A, Einstein AB, Cheever MA. Adoptive chemoimmunotherapy of cancer in animals: a review of results, principles, and problems. *Ann NY Acad Sci* 1976; 277:492–504.

38. Cheever MA, Kempf RA, Fefer A. Tumor neutralization, immunotherapy, and chemoimmunotherapy of a Friend leukemia with cells secondarily sensitized in vitro. *J Immunol* 1977; 119:714–718.

39. Cheever MA, Greenberg PD, Fefer A. Tumor neutralization, immunotherapy, and chemoimmuno-therapy of a Friend leukemia with cells secondarily sensitized in vitro: II. Comparison of cells cultured with and without tumor to noncultured immune cells. *J Immunol* 1978; 121:2220–2227.

40. Fefer A, Einstein AB Jr, Cheever MA, Berenson JR. Models for syngeneic adoptive chemoimmuno-therapy of murine leukemias. *Ann NY Acad Sci* 1976; 276:573–583.

41. Greenberg PD, Cheever MA, Fefer A. Eradication of disseminated murine leukemia by chemoimmuno-therapy with cyclophosphamide and adoptively transferred immune syngeneic Lyt-1+2- lymphocytes. *J Exp Med* 1981; 154:952–963.

42. Greenberg PD, Cheever MA, Fefer A. Specific adoptive immunotherapy: experimental basis and future potential. *Surv Immunol Res* 1982; 1:85–90.

43. Fefer A, Blume KG, Forman SJ, Appelbaum FR, eds. *Thomas' Hematopoietic Cell Transplantation.* Malden, MA: Blackwell. 2004: pp. 369–379.

44. Yron I, Wood TA Jr, Spiess PJ, Rosenberg SA. In vitro growth of murine T cells. V. The isolation and growth of lymphoid cells infiltrating syngeneic solid tumors. *J Immunol* 1980; 125:238–245.

45. Grimm EA, Mazumder A, Zhang HZ, Rosenberg SA. Lymphokine-activated killer cell phenomenon. Lysis of natural killer-resistant fresh solid tumor cells by interleukin 2-activated autologous human peripheral blood lymphocytes. *J Exp Med* 1982; 155:1823–1841.

46. Lotze MT, Grimm EA, Mazumder A, Strausser JL, Rosenberg SA. Lysis of fresh and cultured autologous tumor by human lymphocytes cultured in T-cell growth factor. *Cancer Res* 1981; 41:4420–4405.

47. Mazumder A, Rosenberg SA. Successful immunotherapy of natural killer-resistant established pulmonary melanoma metastases by the intravenous adoptive transfer of syngeneic lymphocytes activated in vitro by interleukin 2. *J Exp Med* 1984; 159:495–507.

48. Mule JJ, Shu S, Schwarz SL, Rosenberg SA. Adoptive immunotherapy of established pulmonary metastases with LAK cells and recombinant interleukin-2. *Science* 1984; 225, 1487–1489.

49. Rosenberg SA, Lotze MT, Muul LM, et al. Observations on the systemic administration of autologous lymphokine-activated killer cells and recombinant interleukin-2 to patients with metastatic cancer. *N Engl J Med* 1985; 313:1485–1492.

50. Rosenberg SA, Lotze MT, Muul LM, et al. A progress report on the treatment of 157 patients with advanced cancer using lymphokine-activated killer cells and interleukin-2 or high-dose interleukin-2 alone. *N Engl J Med* 1987; 316:889–897.

51. Rosenberg SA, Lotze MT, Yang JC, et al. Prospective randomized trial of high-dose interleukin-2 alone or in conjunction with lymphokine-activated killer cells for the treatment of patients with advanced cancer. *J Natl Cancer Inst* 1993; 85:622–632.

52. Rosenberg SA, Spiess P, Lafreniere R. A new approach to the adoptive immunotherapy of cancer with tumor-infiltrating lymphocytes. *Science* 1986; 233:1318–1321.

53. Balch CM, Riley LB, Bae YJ, et al. Patterns of human tumor-infiltrating lymphocytes in 120 human cancers. *Arch Surg* 1990; 125:200–205.

54. Dudley ME, Wunderlich JR, Robbins PF, et al. Cancer regression and autoimmunity in patients after clonal repopulation with antitumor lymphocytes. *Science* 2002; 298:850–854.

55. Yee C, Savage PA, Lee PP, Davis MM, Greenberg PD. Isolation of high avidity melanoma-reactive CTL from heterogeneous populations using peptide-MHC tetramers. *J Immunol* 1999; 162:2227–2234.

56. Yee C, Thompson JA, Roche P, et al. Melanocyte destruction after antigen-specific immunotherapy of melanoma: direct evidence of T cell-mediated vitiligo. *J Exp Med* 2000; 192:1637–1644.

57. Garlie NK, Siebenlist RE, Lefever AV. T-cells activated in vitro as immunotherapy for renal cell carcinoma: characterization of 2 effector T-cell populations. *J Urol* 2001; 166:299–303.

58. Garlie NK, LeFever AV, Siebenlist RE, Levine BL, June CH, Lum LG. T cells coactivated with immobilized anti-CD3 and anti-CD28 as potential immunotherapy for cancer. *J Immunother* 1999; 22:336–345.

59. Schultze JL, Anderson KC, Gilleece MH, Gribben JG, Nadler LM. A pilot study of combined immunotherapy with autologous adoptive tumour-specific T-cell transfer, vaccination with CD40-activated malignant B cells and interleukin 2. *Br J Haematol* 2001; 113:455–460.

60. Rooney CM, Smith CA, Ng CY, et al. Infusion of cytotoxic T cells for the prevention and treatment of Epstein-Barr virus-induced lymphoma in allogeneic transplant recipients. *Blood* 1998; 92:1549–1555.

61. Plautz GE, Miller DW, Barnett GH, et al. T cell adoptive immunotherapy of newly diagnosed gliomas. *Clin Cancer Res* 2000; 6:2209–2218.

62. Gottschalk S, Heslop HE, Rooney CM. Adoptive immunotherapy for EBV-associated malignancies. *Leuk Lymphoma* 2005; 46:1–10.

63. Savoldo B, Huls MH, Liu Z, et al. Autologous Epstein-Barr virus (EBV)-specific cytotoxic T cells for the treatment of persistent active EBV infection. *Blood* 2002; 100:4059–4066.

64. Wagner HJ, Bollard CM, Vigouroux S, et al. A strategy for treatment of Epstein-Barr virus-positive Hodgkin's disease by targeting interleukin 12 to the tumor environment using tumor antigen-specific T cells. *Cancer Gene Ther* 2004; 11:81–91.

65. Lum LG, LeFever AV, Treisman JS, Garlie NK, Hanson JP Jr. Immune modulation in cancer patients after adoptive transfer of anti-CD3/anti-CD28-costimulated T cells-phase I clinical trial. *J Immunother* 2001; 24:408–419.

66. Laport GG, Levine BL, Stadtmauer EA, et al. Adoptive transfer of costimulated T cells induces lymphocytosis in patients with relapsed/refractory non-Hodgkin's lymphoma following CD34+-selected hematopoietic cell transplantation. *Blood* 2003; 102:2004–2013.

67. Levine BL, Bernstein WB, Aronson NE, et al. Adoptive transfer of costimulated CD4+ T cells induces expansion of peripheral T cells and decreased CCR5 expression in HIV infection. *Nat Med* 2002; 8: 47–53.

68. Rapoport AP, Levine BL, Badros A, et al. Molecular remission of CML after autotransplantation followed by adoptive transfer of costimulated autologous T cells. *Bone Marrow Transplant* 2004; 33:53–60.

69. Nair SK, Hull S, Coleman D, Gilboa E, Lyerly HK, Morse MA. Induction of carcinoembryonic antigen (CEA)-specific cytotoxic T-lymphocyte responses in vitro using autologous dendritic cells loaded with

CEA peptide or CEA RNA in patients with metastatic malignancies expressing CEA. *Int J Cancer* 1999; 82:121–124.

70. Morse MA, Nair SK, Boczkowski D, et al. The feasibility and safety of immunotherapy with dendritic cells loaded with CEA mRNA following neoadjuvant chemoradiotherapy and resection of pancreatic cancer. *Int J Gastrointest Cancer* 2002; 32:1–6.

71. Morse MA, Deng Y, Coleman D, et al. A Phase I study of active immunotherapy with carcinoembryonic antigen peptide (CAP-1)-pulsed, autologous human cultured dendritic cells in patients with metastatic malignancies expressing carcinoembryonic antigen. *Clin Cancer Res* 1999; 5:1331–1338.

72. Molldrem JJ, Lee PP, Wang C, Champlin RE, Davis MM. A PR1-human leukocyte antigen-A2 tetramer can be used to isolate low-frequency cytotoxic T lymphocytes from healthy donors that selectively lyse chronic myelogenous leukemia. *Cancer Res* 1999; 59:2675–2681.

73. Vonderheide RH, Schultze JL, Anderson KS, et al. Equivalent induction of telomerase-specific cytotoxic T lymphocytes from tumor-bearing patients and healthy individuals. *Cancer Res* 2001; 61:8366–8370.

74. Vonderheide RH. Telomerase as a universal tumor-associated antigen for cancer immunotherapy. *Oncogene* 2002; 21:674–679.

75. Oka Y, Elisseeva OA, Tsuboi A, et al. Human cytotoxic T-lymphocyte responses specific for peptides of the wild-type Wilms' tumor gene (WT1) product. *Immunogenetics* 2000; 51:99–107.

76. Zeng G, Wang X, Robbins PF, Rosenberg SA, Wang RF. CD4(+) T cell recognition of MHC class II-restricted epitopes from NY-ESO-1 presented by a prevalent HLA DP4 allele: association with NY-ESO-1 antibody production. *Proc Natl Acad Sci USA* 2001; 98:3964–3969.

77. Zeng G, Touloukian CE, Wang X, Restifo NP, Rosenberg SA, Wang RF. Identification of CD4+ T cell epitopes from NY-ESO-1 presented by HLA-DR molecules. *J Immunol* 2000; 165:1153–1159.

78. Knutson KL, Schiffman K, Disis ML. Immunization with a HER-2/*neu* helper peptide vaccine generates HER-2/*neu* CD8 T-cell immunity in cancer patients. *J Clin Invest* 2001; 107:477–484.

79. Knutson KL, Disis ML. Clonal diversity of the T-cell population responding to a dominant HLA-A2 epitope of HER-2/*neu* after active immunization in an ovarian cancer patient. *Hum Immunol* 2002; 63: 547–557.

80. Disis ML, Schiffman K, Guthrie K, et al. Effect of dose on immune response in patients vaccinated with an her-2/*neu* intracellular domain protein-based vaccine. *J Clin Oncol* 2004; 22:1916–1925.

81. Knutson KL, Schiffman K, Cheever MA, Disis ML. Immunization of cancer patients with a HER-2/*neu*, HLA-A2 peptide, p369-377, results in short-lived peptide-specific immunity. *Clin Cancer Res* 2002; 8:1014–1018.

82. Knutson KL, Disis ML. Expansion of HER2/*neu*-specific T cells ex vivo following immunization with a HER2/neu peptide-based vaccine. *Clin Breast Cancer* 2001; 2:73–79.

83. Bortin MM, Rimm AA, Saltzstein EC, Rodey GE. Graft versus leukemia. 3. Apparent independent antihost and antileukemia activity of transplanted immunocompetent cells. *Transplantation* 1973; 16: 182–188.

84. Bortin MM, Rimm AA, Saltzstein EC. Graft versus leukemia: quantification of adoptive immunotherapy in murine leukemia. *Science* 1973; 179:811–813.

85. Saltzstein EC, Glasspiegel JS, Rimm AA, Giller RH, Bortin MM. Graft versus leukemia for "cell cure" of long-passage AKR leukemia after chemoradiotherapy. *Cancer Res* 1972; 32:1658–1662.

86. Bortin MM, Rimm AA, Rose WC, Saltzstein EC. Graft-versus-leukemia. V. Absence of antileukemic effect using allogeneic h-2-identical immunocompetent cells. *Transplantation* 1974; 18:280–283.

87. Boranic M. Delayed mortality in sublethally irradiated mice treated with allogeneic lymphoid and myeloid cells. *J Natl Cancer Inst* 1968: 41:439–450.

88. Armitage JO. Bone marrow transplantation. *N Engl J Med* 1994; 330:827–838.

89. Sullivan KM, Storb R, Buckner CD, et al. Graft-versus-host disease as adoptive immunotherapy in patients with advanced hematologic neoplasms. *N Engl J Med* 1989; 320:828–834.

90. Buckner CD, Clift RA, Fefer A, et al. Marrow transplantation for the treatment of acute leukemia using HL-A-identical siblings. *Transplant Proc* 1974; 6:365–356.

91. Goldman JM, Gale RP, Horowitz MM, et al. Bone marrow transplantation for chronic myelogenous leukemia in chronic phase. Increased risk for relapse associated with T-cell depletion. *Ann Intern Med* 1988; 108:806–814.

92. Maraninchi D, Gluckman E, Blaise D, et al. Impact of T-cell depletion on outcome of allogeneic bone-marrow transplantation for standard-risk leukaemias. *Lancet* 1987; 2:175–178.

93. Markiewicz M, Holowiecki J, Wojnar J, et al. Allogeneic transplantation of selected peripheral CD34+ cells with controlled CD3+ cells add-back in high-risk patients. *Transplant Proc* 2004; 36:3194–3199.

94. Elmaagacli AH, Peceny R, Steckel N, et al. Outcome of transplantation of highly purified peripheral blood CD34+ cells with T-cell add-back compared with unmanipulated bone marrow or peripheral blood stem cells from HLA-identical sibling donors in patients with first chronic phase chronic myeloid leukemia. *Blood* 2003; 101:446–453.

95. Zittoun RA, Mandelli F, Willemze R, et al. Autologous or allogeneic bone marrow transplantation compared with intensive chemotherapy in acute myelogenous leukemia. European Organization for Research and Treatment of Cancer (EORTC) and the Gruppo Italiano Malattie Ematologiche Maligne dell'Adulto (GIMEMA) Leukemia Cooperative Groups. *N Engl J Med* 1995; 332:217–223.

96. van Besien K, Sobocinski KA, Rowlings PA, et al. Allogeneic bone marrow transplantation for low-grade lymphoma. *Blood* 1998: 92:1832–1836.

97. Levine JE, Harris RE, Loberiza FR Jr, et al. A comparison of allogeneic and autologous bone marrow transplantation for lymphoblastic lymphoma. *Blood* 2003; 101:2476–2482.

98. Fefer A, Cheever MA, Greenberg PD. Identical-twin (syngeneic) marrow transplantation for hematologic cancers. *J Natl Cancer Inst* 1986; 76:1269–1273.

99. Collins RH Jr, Rogers ZR, Bennett M, Kumar V, Nikein A, Fay JW. Hematologic relapse of chronic myelogenous leukemia following allogeneic bone marrow transplantation: apparent graft-versus-leukemia effect following abrupt discontinuation of immunosuppression. *Bone Marrow Transplant* 1992; 10:391–395.

100. Vogelsang GB, Jones RJ, Hess AD, Geller R, Schucter L, Santos GW. Induction of autologous graft-versus-host disease. *Transplant Proc* 1989; 21:2997–2998.

101. Hess AD, Vogelsang GB, Silanskis M, Friedman KA, Beschorner WE, Santos GW. Syngeneic graft-versus-host disease after allogeneic bone marrow transplantation and cyclosporine treatment. *Transplant Proc* 1988; 20:487–492.

102. Hess AD, Vogelsang GB, Heyd J, Beschorner WE. Cyclosporine-induced syngeneic graft-versus-host disease: assessment of T cell differentiation. *Transplant Proc* 19:2683–2686.

103. Hess AD, Fischer AC, Beschorner WE. Effector mechanisms in cyclosporine A-induced syngeneic graft-versus-host disease. Role of CD4+ and CD8+ T lymphocyte subsets. *J Immunol* 1990; 145:526–533.

104. Hess AD, Fischer AC, Beschorner WE. Regulation of syngeneic graft-versus-host disease by auto-suppressor mechanisms. *Transplant Proc* 1989; 21:3013–3015.

105. Hess AD, Fischer AC. Immune mechanisms in cyclosporine-induced syngeneic graft-versus-host disease. *Transplantation* 1989; 48:895–900.

106. Kolb HJ, Mittermuller J, Clemm C, et al. Donor leukocyte transfusions for treatment of recurrent chronic myelogenous leukemia in marrow transplant patients. *Blood* 1990; 76:2462–2465.

107. Porter DL, Roth MS, McGarigle C, Ferrara JL, Antin JH. Induction of graft-versus-host disease as immunotherapy for relapsed chronic myeloid leukemia. *N Engl J Med* 1994; 330:100–106.

108. Porter DL, Roth MS, Lee SJ, McGarigle C, Ferrara JL, Antin JH. Adoptive immunotherapy with donor mononuclear cell infusions to treat relapse of acute leukemia or myelodysplasia after allogeneic bone marrow transplantation. *Bone Marrow Transplant* 1996; 18:975–980.

109. Collins RH Jr, Shpilberg O, Drobyski WR, et al. Donor leukocyte infusions in 140 patients with relapsed malignancy after allogeneic bone marrow transplantation. *J Clin Oncol* 1997; 15:433–444.

110. Porter DL, Collins RH Jr, Shpilberg O, et al. Long-term follow-up of patients who achieved complete remission after donor leukocyte infusions. *Biol Blood Marrow Transplant* 1999; 5:253–261.

111. Badros A, Barlogie B, Morris C, et al. High response rate in refractory and poor-risk multiple myeloma after allotransplantation using a nonmyeloablative conditioning regimen and donor lymphocyte infusions. *Blood* 2001; 97:2574–2579.

112. Tricot G, Vesole DH, Jagannath S, et al. Graft-versus-myeloma effect: proof of principle. *Blood* 1996; 87:1196–1198.

113. Jones RJ, Ambinder RF, Piantadosi S, Santos GW. Evidence of a graft-versus-lymphoma effect associated with allogeneic bone marrow transplantation. *Blood* 1991; 77:649–653.

114. Fabre JW. The allogeneic response and tumor immunity. *Nat Med* 2001; 7:649–652.

115. Johnson BD, Becker EE, Truitt RL. Graft-vs.-host and graft-vs.-leukemia reactions after delayed infusions of donor T-subsets. *Biol Blood Marrow Transplant* 1999; 5:123–132.

116. Klein CA, Wilke M, Pool J, et al. The hematopoietic system-specific minor histocompatibility antigen HA-1 shows aberrant expression in epithelial cancer cells. *J Exp Med* 2002; 196:359–368.

117. Warren EH, Greenberg PD, Riddell SR. Cytotoxic T-lymphocyte-defined human minor histocompatibility antigens with a restricted tissue distribution. *Blood* 1998; 91:2197–2207.

118. Chao NJ. Minors come of age: minor histocompatibility antigens and graft-versus-host disease. *Biol Blood Marrow Transplant* 2004; 10:215–223.

119. de la Selle V, Miconnet I, Gilbert D, Bruley-Rosset M. Peripheral tolerance to host minor histocompatibility antigens in radiation bone marrow chimeras abrogates lethal GVHD while preserving GVL effect. *Bone Marrow Transplant* 1995; 16:111–118.

120. Stelljes M, Strothotte R, Pauels HG, et al. Graft-versus-host disease after allogeneic hematopoietic stem cell transplantation induces a CD8+ T cell-mediated graft-versus-tumor effect that is independent of the recognition of alloantigenic tumor targets. *Blood* 2004; 104:1210–1216.

121. Schiltz PM, Beutel LD, Nayak SK, Dillman RO. Characterization of tumor-infiltrating lymphocytes derived from human tumors for use as adoptive immunotherapy of cancer. *J Immunother* 1997; 20: 377–386.

122. Huang J, El-Gamil M, Dudley ME, Li YF, Rosenberg SA, Robbins PF. T cells associated with tumor regression recognize frameshifted products of the CDKN2A tumor suppressor gene locus and a mutated HLA class I gene product. *J Immunol* 2004; 172:6057–6064.

123. Zhou J, Dudley ME, Rosenberg SA, Robbins PF. Selective growth, in vitro and in vivo, of individual T cell clones from tumor-infiltrating lymphocytes obtained from patients with melanoma. *J Immunol* 2004; 173:7622–7629.

124. Zhou J, Dudley ME, Rosenberg SA, Robbins PF. Persistence of multiple tumor-specific T-cell clones is associated with complete tumor regression in a melanoma patient receiving adoptive cell transfer therapy. *J Immunother* 2005; 28:53–62.

125. Rosenberg SA, Dudley ME. Cancer regression in patients with metastatic melanoma after the transfer of autologous antitumor lymphocytes. *Proc Natl Acad Sci USA* 2004; 101(Suppl 2):14,639–14,645.

126. Johnson BD, Truitt RL. A decrease in graft-vs.-host disease without loss of graft-vs.-leukemia reactivity after MHC-matched bone marrow transplantation by selective depletion of donor NK cells in vivo. *Transplantation* 1992; 54:104–112.

127. Johnson BD, Dagher N, Stankowski WC, Hanke CA, Truitt RL. Donor natural killer (NK1.1+) cells do not play a role in the suppression of GVHD or in the mediation of GVL reactions after DLI. *Biol Blood Marrow Transplant* 2001; 7:589–595.

128. Ruggeri L, Capanni M, Casucci M, et al. Role of natural killer cell alloreactivity in HLA-mismatched hematopoietic stem cell transplantation. *Blood* 1999: 94:333–339.

129. Farag SS, Fehniger TA, Ruggeri L, Velardi A, Caligiuri MA. Natural killer cell receptors: new biology and insights into the graft-versus-leukemia effect. *Blood* 2002; 100:1935–1947.

130. Gao JX, Liu X, Wen J, et al. Two-signal requirement for activation and effector function of natural killer cell response to allogeneic tumor cells. *Blood* 2003; 102:4456–4463.

131. Ruggeri L, Capanni M, Urbani E, et al. Effectiveness of donor natural killer cell alloreactivity in mismatched hematopoietic transplants. *Science* 2002; 295:2097–2100.

132. Zhao Y, Ohdan H, Manilay JO, Sykes M. NK cell tolerance in mixed allogeneic chimeras. *J Immunol* 2003; 170:5398–5405.

133. Leung W, Iyengar R, Turner V, et al. Determinants of antileukemia effects of allogeneic NK cells. *J Immunol* 2004; 172:644–650.

134. Hsu KC, Keever-Taylor CA, Wilton A, et al. Improved outcome in HLA-identical sibling hematopoietic stem cell transplantation for acute myelogenous leukemia (AML) predicted by KIR and HLA genotypes. *Blood* 2005; 105:4878–4884.

135. Beelen DW, Ottinger H, Ferencik S, et al. Genotypic inhibitory killer immunoglobulin-like receptor ligand incompatibility enhances the long-term antileukemic effect of unmodified allogeneic hematopoietic stem cell transplantation in patients with myeloid leukemias. *Blood* 2004; 105:2594–2600.

136. Igarashi T, Wynberg J, Srinivasan R, et al. Enhanced cytotoxicity of allogeneic NK cells with killer immunoglobulin-like receptor ligand incompatibility against melanoma and renal cell carcinoma cells. *Blood* 2004; 104:170–177.

137. Davies SM, Ruggieri L, DeFor T, et al. Evaluation of KIR ligand incompatibility in mismatched unrelated donor hematopoietic transplants. Killer immunoglobulin-like receptor. *Blood* 2002; 100: 3825–3827.

138. Giebel S, Locatelli F, Lamparelli T, et al. Survival advantage with KIR ligand incompatibility in hematopoietic stem cell transplantation from unrelated donors. *Blood* 2003; 102:814–819.

139. Gimmi CD, Freeman GJ, Gribben JG, Gray G, Nadler LM. Human T-cell clonal anergy is induced by antigen presentation in the absence of B7 costimulation. *Proc Natl Acad Sci USA* 1993; 90:6586–6590.

140. Avigan D. Dendritic cells: development, function and potential use for cancer immunotherapy. *Blood Rev* 1999; 13:51–64.

141. Appleman LJ, Boussiotis VA. T cell anergy and costimulation. *Immunol Rev* 2003; 192:161–180.

142. Shlomchik WD, Couzens MS, Tang CB, et al. Prevention of graft versus host disease by inactivation of host antigen-presenting cells. *Science* 1999; 285:412–415.

143. Matte CC, Liu J, Cormier J, et al. Donor APCs are required for maximal GVHD but not for GVL. *Nat Med* 2004; 10:987–992.

144. Anderson BE, McNiff JM, Jain D, Blazar BR, Shlomchik WD, Shlomchik MJ. Distinct roles for donor-and host-derived antigen-presenting cells and costimulatory molecules in murine chronic graft-versus-host disease: requirements depend on target organ. *Blood* 2005; 105:2227–2234.

145. Johnson BD, Drobyski WR, Truitt RL. Delayed infusion of normal donor cells after MHC-matched bone marrow transplantation provides an antileukemia reaction without graft-versus-host disease. *Bone Marrow Transplant* 1993; 11:329–336.

146. Truitt RL, Johnson BD. Principles of graft-vs.-leukemia reactivity. *Biol Blood Marrow Transplant* 1995; 1:61–68.

147. Bergmann L, Schui DK, Brieger J, Weidmann E, Mitrou PS, Hoelzer D. The inhibition of lymphokine-activated killer cells in acute myeloblastic leukemia is mediated by transforming growth factor-beta 1. *Exp Hematol* 1995; 23:1574–1580.

148. Kolb HJ, Schmid C, Barrett AJ, Schendel DJ. Graft-versus-leukemia reactions in allogeneic chimeras. *Blood* 2004; 103:767–776.

149. Brouwer RE, van der Heiden P, Schreuder GM, et al. Loss or downregulation of HLA class I expression at the allelic level in acute leukemia is infrequent but functionally relevant, and can be restored by interferon. *Hum Immunol* 2002; 63:200–210.

150. Brouwer RE, Hoefnagel J, Borger van Der Burg B, et al. Expression of co-stimulatory and adhesion molecules and chemokine or apoptosis receptors on acute myeloid leukaemia: high CD40 and CD11a expression correlates with poor prognosis. *Br J Haematol* 2001; 115:298–308.

151. Dermime S, Mavroudis D, Jiang YZ, Hensel N, Molldrem J, Barrett AJ. Immune escape from a graft-versus-leukemia effect may play a role in the relapse of myeloid leukemias following allogeneic bone marrow transplantation. *Bone Marrow Transplant* 1997; 19:989–999.

152. Schimmer AD, Hedley DW, Penn LZ, Minden MD. Receptor- and mitochondrial-mediated apoptosis in acute leukemia: a translational view. *Blood* 2001; 98:3541–3553.

153. Hsieh MH, Korngold R. Differential use of FasL- and perforin-mediated cytolytic mechanisms by T-cell subsets involved in graft-versus-myeloid leukemia responses. *Blood* 2000; 96:1047–1055.

154. Tsukada N, Kobata T, Aizawa Y, Yagita H, Okumura K. Graft-versus-leukemia effect and graft-versus-host disease can be differentiated by cytotoxic mechanisms in a murine model of allogeneic bone marrow transplantation. *Blood* 1999; 93:2738–2747.

155. Lehmann C, Zeis M, Schmitz N, Uharek L. Impaired binding of perforin on the surface of tumor cells is a cause of target cell resistance against cytotoxic effector cells. *Blood* 2000; 96:594–600.

156. Bishop MR. The graft-versus-lymphoma effect: fact, fiction, or opportunity? *J Clin Oncol* 2003; 21:3713–3715.

157. Bierman PJ, Sweetenham JW, Loberiza FR Jr, et al. Syngeneic hematopoietic stem-cell transplantation for non-Hodgkin's lymphoma: a comparison with allogeneic and autologous transplantation—The Lymphoma Working Committee of the International Bone Marrow Transplant Registry and the European Group for Blood and Marrow Transplantation. *J Clin Oncol* 2003; 21:3744–3753.

158. Grigg A, Ritchie D. Graft-versus-lymphoma effects: clinical review, policy proposals, and immunobiology. *Biol Blood Marrow Transplant* 2004; 10:579–590.

159. Salutari P, Sica S, Micciulli G, Rutella S, Di Mario A, Leone G. Extramedullary relapse after allogeneic bone marrow transplantation plus buffy-coat in two high risk patients. *Haematologica* 1996; 81:182–185.

160. Mosmann TR, Cherwinski H, Bond MW, Giedlin MA, Coffman RL. Two types of murine helper T cell clone. I. Definition according to profiles of lymphokine activities and secreted proteins. *J Immunol* 1986; 136:2348–2357.

161. Sad S, Marcotte R, Mosmann TR. Cytokine-induced differentiation of precursor mouse CD8+ T cells into cytotoxic CD8+ T cells secreting Th1 or Th2 cytokines. *Immunity* 1995; 2:271–279.

162. Fowler DH, Bishop MR, Gress RE. Immunoablative reduced-intensity stem cell transplantation: potential role of donor Th2 and Tc2 cells. *Semin Oncol* 2004; 31:56–67.
163. Nestel FP, Price KS, Seemayer TA, Lapp WS. Macrophage priming and lipopolysaccharide-triggered release of tumor necrosis factor alpha during graft-versus-host disease. *J Exp Med* 1992; 175:405–413.
164. Croft M, Carter L, Swain SL, Dutton RW. Generation of polarized antigen-specific CD8 effector populations: reciprocal action of interleukin (IL)-4 and IL-12 in promoting type 2 versus type 1 cytokine profiles. *J Exp Med* 1994; 180:1715–1728.
165. Hill GR, Teshima T, Gerbitz A, et al. Differential roles of IL-1 and TNF-alpha on graft-versus-host disease and graft versus leukemia. *J Clin Invest* 1999; 104:459–467.
166. Fowler DH, Kurasawa K, Smith R, Eckhaus MA, Gress RE. Donor CD4-enriched cells of Th2 cytokine phenotype regulate graft-versus-host disease without impairing allogeneic engraftment in sublethally irradiated mice. *Blood* 1994; 84:3540–3549.
167. Fowler DH, Kurasawa K, Husebekk A, Cohen PA, Gress RE. Cells of Th2 cytokine phenotype prevent LPS-induced lethality during murine graft-versus-host reaction. Regulation of cytokines and CD8$^+$ lymphoid engraftment. *J Immunol* 1994; 152:1004–1013.
168. Fowler DH, Breglio J, Nagel G, Eckhaus MA, Gress RE. Allospecific CD8$^+$ Tc1 and Tc2 populations in graft-versus-leukemia effect and graft-versus-host disease. *J Immunol* 1996; 157:4811–4821.
169. Fowler DH, Breglio J, Nagel G, Hirose C, Gress RE. Allospecific CD4$^+$, Th1/Th2 and CD8$^+$, Tc1/Tc2 populations in murine GVL: type I cells generate GVL and type II cells abrogate GVL. *Biol Blood Marrow Transplant* 1996; 2:118–125.
170. Krenger W, Snyder KM, Byon JC, Falzarano G, Ferrara JL. Polarized type 2 alloreactive CD4$^+$ and CD8$^+$ donor T cells fail to induce experimental acute graft-versus-host disease. *J Immunol* 1995; 155: 585–593.
171. Fuzak J, Jung US, Foley J, Eckhaus MA, Fowler DH. Allospecific Tc2 cells mediate a graft-vs.-tumor effect without inducing ongoing GVHD in a murine model of metastatic breast cancer. *Blood* 2000; 96: 2367.
172. Dobrzanski MJ, Reome JB, Dutton RW. Type 1 and type 2 CD8$^+$ effector T cell subpopulations promote long-term tumor immunity and protection to progressively growing tumor. *J Immunol* 2000; 164: 916–925.
173. Blazar BR, Sharpe AH, Taylor PA, et al. Infusion of anti-B7.1 (CD80) and anti-B7.2 (CD86) monoclonal antibodies inhibits murine graft-versus-host disease lethality in part via direct effects on CD4$^+$ and CD8$^+$ T cells. *J Immunol* 1996; 157:3250–3259.
174. Chen L, McGowan P, Ashe S, Johnston JV, Hellstrom I, Hellstrom KE. B7-1/CD80-transduced tumor cells elicit better systemic immunity than wild-type tumor cells admixed with Corynebacterium parvum. *Cancer Res* 1994; 54:5420–5423.
175. Li Y, McGowan P, Hellstrom I, Hellstrom KE, Chen L. Costimulation of tumor-reactive CD4+ and CD8+ T lymphocytes by B7, a natural ligand for CD28, can be used to treat established mouse melanoma. *J Immunol* 1994; 153:421–428.
176. Blazar BR, Kwon BS, Panoskaltsis-Mortari A, Kwak KB, Peschon JJ, Taylor PA. Ligation of 4-1BB (CDw137) regulates graft-versus-host disease, graft-versus-leukemia, and graft rejection in allogeneic bone marrow transplant recipients. *J Immunol* 2001; 166:3174–3183.
177. Blazar BR, Taylor PA, Boyer MW, Panoskaltis-Mortari A, Allison JP, Vallera DA. CD28/B7 interactions are required for sustaining the graft-versus-leukemia effect of delayed post-bone marrow transplantation splenocyte infusion in murine recipients of myeloid or lymphoid leukemia cells. *J Immunol* 1997; 159:3460–3473.
178. Billiau AD, Fevery S, Rutgeerts O, Landuyt W, Waer M. Crucial role of timing of donor lymphocyte infusion in generating dissociated graft-versus-host and graft-versus-leukemia responses in mice receiving allogeneic bone marrow transplants. *Blood* 2002; 100:1894–1902.
179. Drobyski WR, Hessner MJ, Klein JP, et al. T-cell depletion plus salvage immunotherapy with donor leukocyte infusions as a strategy to treat chronic-phase chronic myelogenous leukemia patients undergoing HLA-identical sibling marrow transplantation. *Blood* 1999; 94:434–441.
180. Chakrabarti S, MacDonald D, Hale G, et al. T-cell depletion with Campath-1H "in the bag" for matched related allogeneic peripheral blood stem cell transplantation is associated with reduced graft-versus-host disease, rapid immune constitution and improved survival. *Br J Haematol* 2003; 121:109–118.
181. Naparstek E, Or R, Nagler A, et al. T-cell-depleted allogeneic bone marrow transplantation for acute leukaemia using Campath-1 antibodies and post-transplant administration of donor's peripheral blood lymphocytes for prevention of relapse. *Br J Haematol* 1995; 89:506–515.

182. Huss R, Deeg HJ, Gooley T, et al. Effect of mixed chimerism on graft-versus-host disease, disease recurrence and survival after HLA-identical marrow transplantation for aplastic anemia or chronic myelogenous leukemia. *Bone Marrow Transplant* 1996; 18:767–776.

183. Nakamura R, Bahceci E, Read EJ, et al. Transplant dose of CD34(+) and CD3(+) cells predicts outcome in patients with haematological malignancies undergoing T cell-depleted peripheral blood stem cell transplants with delayed donor lymphocyte add-back. *Br J Haematol* 2001; 115:95–104.

184. Mackinnon S, Barnett L, Heller G, O'Reilly RJ. Minimal residual disease is more common in patients who have mixed T-cell chimerism after bone marrow transplantation for chronic myelogenous leukemia. *Blood* 1994; 83:3409–3416.

185. Wasch R, Bertz, H, Kunzmann R, Finke J. Incidence of mixed chimaerism and clinical outcome in 101 patients after myeloablative conditioning regimens and allogeneic stem cell transplantation. *Br J Haematol* 2000; 109:743–750.

186. Childs R, Clave E, Contentin N, et al. Engraftment kinetics after nonmyeloablative allogeneic peripheral blood stem cell transplantation: full donor T-cell chimerism precedes alloimmune responses. *Blood* 1999; 94:3234–3241.

187. Childs R, Chernoff A, Contentin N, et al. Regression of metastatic renal-cell carcinoma after nonmyeloablative allogeneic peripheral-blood stem-cell transplantation. *N Engl J Med* 2000; 343:750–758.

188. Peggs KS, Thomson K, Hart DP, et al. Dose-escalated donor lymphocyte infusions following reduced intensity transplantation: toxicity, chimerism, and disease responses. *Blood* 2004; 103:1548–1556.

189. Kim YM, Mapara MY, Down JD, et al. Graft-versus-host-reactive donor CD4 cells can induce T cell-mediated rejection of the donor marrow in mixed allogeneic chimeras prepared with nonmyeloablative conditioning. *Blood* 2004; 103:732–739.

190. Mapara MY, Kim YM, Marx J, Sykes M. Donor lymphocyte infusion-mediated graft-versus-leukemia effects in mixed chimeras established with a nonmyeloablative conditioning regimen: extinction of graft-versus-leukemia effects after conversion to full donor chimerism. *Transplantation* 2003; 76:297–305.

191. Rubio MT, Kim YM, Sachs T, Mapara M, Zhao G, Sykes M. Antitumor effect of donor marrow graft rejection induced by recipient leukocyte infusions in mixed chimeras prepared with nonmyeloablative conditioning: critical role for recipient-derived IFN-gamma. *Blood* 2003; 102:2300–2307.

192. Mapara MY, Kim YM, Wang SP, Bronson R, Sachs DH, Sykes M. Donor lymphocyte infusions mediate superior graft-versus-leukemia effects in mixed compared to fully allogeneic chimeras: a critical role for host antigen-presenting cells. *Blood* 2002; 100:1903–1909.

193. Mackinnon S, Papadopoulos EB, Carabasi MH, et al. Adoptive immunotherapy evaluating escalating doses of donor leukocytes for relapse of chronic myeloid leukemia after bone marrow transplantation: separation of graft-versus-leukemia responses from graft-versus-host disease. *Blood* 1995; 86:1261–1268.

194. Guglielmi C, Arcese W, Dazzi F, et al. Donor lymphocyte infusion for relapsed chronic myelogenous leukemia: prognostic relevance of the initial cell dose. *Blood* 2002; 100:397–405.

195. Dazzi F, Szydlo RM, Cross NC, et al. Durability of responses following donor lymphocyte infusions for patients who relapse after allogeneic stem cell transplantation for chronic myeloid leukemia. *Blood* 2000; 96:2712–2716.

196. Rosenberg SA, Spiess PJ, Schwarz S. In vivo administration of Interleukin-2 enhances specific alloimmune responses. *Transplantation* 1983; 35:631–634.

197. Sykes M. Dissociating graft-vs-host disease from the graft-vs-leukemia effect of allogeneic T cells: the potential role of IL-2. *Bone Marrow Transplant* 1992; 10(Suppl 1):1–4.

198. Abraham VS, Sachs DH, Sykes M. Mechanism of protection from graft-versus-host disease mortality by IL-2. III. Early reductions in donor T cell subsets and expansion of a CD3$^+$CD4$^-$CD8$^-$ cell population. *J Immunol* 1992; 148:3746–3752.

199. Ackerstein A, Kedar E, Slavin S. Use of recombinant human interleukin-2 in conjunction with syngeneic bone marrow transplantation in mice as a model for control of minimal residual disease in malignant hematologic disorders. *Blood* 1991; 78:1212–1215.

200. Abraham VS, Sykes M. Mechanism of the anti-GVHD effect of IL-2. I. Protective host-type cell populations are not induced by IL-2 treatment alone. *Bone Marrow Transplant* 1991; 7(Suppl 1): 29–32.

201. Sykes M, Romick ML, Hoyles KA, Sachs DH. In vivo administration of interleukin 2 plus T cell-depleted syngeneic marrow prevents graft-versus-host disease mortality and permits alloengraftment. *J Exp Med* 1990; 171:645–658.

202. Slavin S, Ackerstein A, Kedar E, Weiss L. IL-2 activated cell-mediated immunotherapy: control of minimal residual disease in malignant disorders by allogeneic lymphocytes and IL-2. *Bone Marrow Transplant* 1990; 6(Suppl 1):86–90.

203. Sykes M, Abraham VS, Harty MW, Pearson DA. IL-2 reduces graft-versus-host disease and preserves a graft-versus-leukemia effect by selectively inhibiting CD4+ T cell activity. *J Immunol* 1993; 150:197–205.

204. Sykes M, Harty MW, Szot GL, Pearson DA. Interleukin-2 inhibits graft-versus-host disease-promoting activity of CD4+ cells while preserving CD4− and CD8-mediated graft-versus-leukemia effects. *Blood* 1994; 83:2560–2569.

205. Yang YG, Sergio JJ, Pearson DA, Szot GL, Shimizu A, Sykes M. Interleukin-12 preserves the graft-versus-leukemia effect of allogeneic CD8 T cells while inhibiting CD4-dependent graft-versus-host disease in mice. *Blood* 1997; 90:4651–4660.

206. Slavin S, Naparstek E, Nagler A, et al. Allogeneic cell therapy with donor peripheral blood cells and recombinant human interleukin-2 to treat leukemia relapse after allogeneic bone marrow transplantation. *Blood* 1996; 87:2195–2204.

207. Or R, Ackerstein A, Nagler A, et al. Allogeneic cell-mediated immunotherapy for breast cancer after autologous stem cell transplantation: a clinical pilot study. *Cytokines Cell Mol Ther* 1998: 4:1–6.

208. Krijanovski OI, Hill GR, Cooke KR, et al. Keratinocyte growth factor separates graft-versus-leukemia effects from graft-versus-host disease. *Blood* 1999; 94:825–831.

209. Teshima T, Hill GR, Pan L, et al. IL-11 separates graft-versus-leukemia effects from graft-versus-host disease after bone marrow transplantation. *J Clin Invest* 1999; 104:317–325.

210. Pan L, Teshima T, Hill GR, et al. Granulocyte colony-stimulating factor-mobilized allogeneic stem cell transplantation maintains graft-versus-leukemia effects through a perforin-dependent pathway while preventing graft-versus-host disease. *Blood* 1999; 93:4071–4078.

211. Reddy V, Hill GR, Pan L, et al. G-CSF modulates cytokine profile of dendritic cells and decreases acute graft-versus-host disease through effects on the donor rather than the recipient. *Transplantation* 2000; 69:691–693.

212. Bishop MR, Tarantolo SR, Pavletic ZS, et al. Filgrastim as an alternative to donor leukocyte infusion for relapse after allogeneic stem-cell transplantation. *J Clin Oncol* 2000; 18:2269–2272.

213. Giralt S, Escudier S, Kantarjian H, et al. Preliminary results of treatment with filgrastim for relapse of leukemia and myelodysplasia after allogeneic bone marrow transplantation. *N Engl J Med* 1993; 329: 757–761.

214. Volpi I, Perruccio K, Tosti A, et al. Postgrafting administration of granulocyte colony-stimulating factor impairs functional immune recovery in recipients of human leukocyte antigen haplotype-mismatched hematopoietic transplants. *Blood* 2001; 97:2514–2521.

215. Hoffmann P, Ermann J, Edinger M, Fathman CG, Strober S. Donor-type CD4(+)CD25(+) regulatory T cells suppress lethal acute graft-versus-host disease after allogeneic bone marrow transplantation. *J Exp Med* 2002; 196:389–399.

216. Cohen JL, Trenado A, Vasey D, Klatzmann D, Salomon BL. CD4(+)CD25(+) immunoregulatory T cells: new therapeutics for graft-versus-host disease. *J Exp Med* 2002; 196:401–406.

217. Jones SC, Murphy GF, Korngold R. Post-hematopoietic cell transplantation control of graft-versus-host disease by donor CD425 T cells to allow an effective graft-versus-leukemia response. *Biol Blood Marrow Transplant* 2003; 9:243–256.

218. Edinger M, Hoffmann P, Ermann J, et al. CD4+CD25+ regulatory T cells preserve graft-versus-tumor activity while inhibiting graft-versus-host disease after bone marrow transplantation. *Nat Med* 2003; 9:1144–1150.

219. Hoffmann P, Eder R, Kunz-Schughart LA, Andreesen R, Edinger M. Large-scale in vitro expansion of polyclonal human CD4(+)CD25high regulatory T cells. *Blood* 2004; 104:895–903.

220. Trenado A, Charlotte F, Fisson S, et al. Recipient-type specific CD4+CD25+ regulatory T cells favor immune reconstitution and control graft-versus-host disease while maintaining graft-versus-leukemia. *J Clin Invest* 2003; 112:1688–1696.

221. Verneris MR, Baker J, Edinger M, Negrin RS. Studies of ex vivo activated and expanded CD8+ NK-T cells in humans and mice. *J Clin Immunol* 2002; 22:131–136.

222. Margalit M, Ilan Y, Ohana M, et al. Adoptive transfer of small numbers of DX5+ cells alleviates graft-versus-host disease in a murine model of semiallogeneic bone marrow transplantation: a potential role for NKT lymphocytes. *Bone Marrow Transplant* 2005; 35:191–197.

223. Tanaka J, Toubai T, Tsutsumi Y, et al. Cytolytic activity and regulatory functions of inhibitory NK cell receptor-expressing T cells expanded from granulocyte colony-stimulating factor-mobilized peripheral blood mononuclear cells. *Blood* 2004; 104:768–774.

224. Korngold R, Sprent J. Graft-versus-host disease in experimental allogeneic bone marrow transplantation. *Proc Soc Exp Biol Med* 1991; 197:12–18.

225. Giralt S, Estey E, Albitar M, et al. Engraftment of allogeneic hematopoietic progenitor cells with purine analog-containing chemotherapy: harnessing graft-versus-leukemia without myeloablative therapy. *Blood* 1997; 89:4531–4536.

226. McSweeney PA, Niederwieser D, Shizuru JA, et al. Hematopoietic cell transplantation in older patients with hematologic malignancies: replacing high-dose cytotoxic therapy with graft-versus-tumor effects. *Blood* 2001; 97:3390–3400.

227. Spitzer TR, McAfee S, Sackstein R, et al. Intentional induction of mixed chimerism and achievement of antitumor responses after nonmyeloablative conditioning therapy and HLA-matched donor bone marrow transplantation for refractory hematologic malignancies. *Biol Blood Marrow Transplant* 2000; 6:309–320.

228. Slavin S, Nagler A, Naparstek E, et al. Nonmyeloablative stem cell transplantation and cell therapy as an alternative to conventional bone marrow transplantation with lethal cytoreduction for the treatment of malignant and nonmalignant hematologic diseases. *Blood* 1998; 91:756–763.

229. Bethge WA, Hegenbart U, Stuart MJ, et al. Adoptive immunotherapy with donor lymphocyte infusions after allogeneic hematopoietic cell transplantation following nonmyeloablative conditioning. *Blood* 2004; 103:790–795.

230. Bishop MR, Hou JW, Wilson WH, et al. Establishment of early donor engraftment after reduced-intensity allogeneic hematopoietic stem cell transplantation to potentiate the graft-versus-lymphoma effect against refractory lymphomas. *Biol Blood Marrow Transplant* 2003; 9:162–169.

231. Robinson SP, Goldstone AH, Mackinnon S, et al. Chemoresistant or aggressive lymphoma predicts for a poor outcome following reduced-intensity allogeneic progenitor cell transplantation: an analysis from the Lymphoma Working Party of the European Group for Blood and Bone Marrow Transplantation. *Blood* 2002; 100:4310–4316.

232. Giralt S, Thall PF, Khouri I, et al. Melphalan and purine analog-containing preparative regimens: reduced-intensity conditioning for patients with hematologic malignancies undergoing allogeneic progenitor cell transplantation. *Blood* 2001; 97:631–637.

233. Nagler A, Slavin S, Varadi G, Naparstek E, Samuel S, Or R. Allogeneic peripheral blood stem cell transplantation using a fludarabine-based low intensity conditioning regimen for malignant lymphoma. *Bone Marrow Transplant* 2000; 25:1021–1028.

234. Appelbaum FR, Sandmaier B. Sensitivity of renal cell cancer to nonmyeloablative allogeneic hematopoietic cell transplantations: unusual or unusually important? *J Clin Oncol* 2002; 20:1965–1967.

235. Rini BI, Zimmerman T, Stadler WM, Gajewski TF, Vogelzang NJ. Allogeneic stem-cell transplantation of renal cell cancer after nonmyeloablative chemotherapy: feasibility, engraftment, and clinical results. *J Clin Oncol* 2002; 20:2017–2024.

236. Bregni M, Dodero A, Peccatori J, et al. Nonmyeloablative conditioning followed by hematopoietic cell allografting and donor lymphocyte infusions for patients with metastatic renal and breast cancer. *Blood* 2002; 99:4234–4236.

237. Childs RW, Clave E, Tisdale J, Plante M, Hensel N, Barrett J. Successful treatment of metastatic renal cell carcinoma with a nonmyeloablative allogeneic peripheral-blood progenitor-cell transplant: evidence for a graft-versus-tumor effect. *J Clin Oncol* 1999; 17:2044–2049.

238. Childs RW. Nonmyeloablative allogeneic peripheral blood stem-cell transplantation as immunotherapy for malignant diseases. *Cancer J* 2000; 6:179–187.

239. Moscardo F, Martinez JA, Sanz GF, et al. Graft-versus-tumour effect in non-small-cell lung cancer after allogeneic peripheral blood stem cell transplantation. *Br J Haematol* 2000; 111:708–710.

240. Barkholt L, Hentschke P, Zetterquist H, et al. An allogeneic anti-cancer effect after hematopoietic stem cell transplantation. *Transplant Proc* 2001; 33:1862–1864.

241. Carella AM, Corsetti MT, Beltrami G, et al. (2002) Autografting and non-myeloablative allogeneic stem cell transplantation in metastatic breast cancer. *Haematologica* 2002; 87:10–11.

242. Blaise D, Bay JO, Faucher C, et al. Reduced-intensity preparative regimen and allogeneic stem cell transplantation for advanced solid tumors. *Blood* 2004; 103:435–441.

243. Siena S, Giorgiani G, et al. Allogeneic hematopoietic stem cell transplantation for solid tumors other than renal cell cancer. *Haematologica* 2002; 87:17–20.

244. Pedrazzoli P, Da Prada GA, Giorgiani G, et al. Allogeneic blood stem cell transplantation after a reduced-intensity, preparative regimen: a pilot study in patients with refractory malignancies. *Cancer* 2002; 94: 2409–2415.

245. Kurokawa T, Fischer K, Bertz H, et al. In vitro and in vivo characterization of graft-versus-tumor responses in melanoma patients after allogeneic peripheral blood stem cell transplantation. *Int J Cancer* 2002; 101:52–60.

246. Kasow KA, Handgretinger R, Krasin MJ, Pappo AS, Leung W. Possible allogeneic graft-versus-tumor effect in childhood melanoma. *J Pediatr Hematol Oncol* 2003; 25:982–986.

247. Bay JO, Choufi B, Pomel C, et al. Potential allogeneic graft-versus-tumor effect in a patient with ovarian cancer. *Bone Marrow Transplant* 2000; 25:681–682.

248. Bay JO, Fleury J, Choufi B, et al. Allogeneic hematopoietic stem cell transplantation in ovarian carcinoma: results of five patients. *Bone Marrow Transplant* 2002; 30:95–102.

249. Eibl B, Schwaighofer H, Nachbaur D, et al. Evidence for a graft-versus-tumor effect in a patient treated with marrow ablative chemotherapy and allogeneic bone marrow transplantation for breast cancer. *Blood* 1996; 88:1501–1508.

250. Ueno NT, Rondon G, Mirza NQ, et al. Allogeneic peripheral-blood progenitor-cell transplantation for poor-risk patients with metastatic breast cancer. *J Clin Oncol* 1998; 16:986–993.

251. Ueno NT, Shpall EJ, Champlin RE, Jones RB. Graft–versus–breast cancer effect by allogeneic hematopoietic stem-cell transplantation: a possible new frontier. *J Clin Oncol* 2004; 22:3846–3847.

252. Bishop MR, Fowler DH, Marchigiani D, et al. Allogeneic lymphocytes induce tumor regression of advanced metastatic breast cancer. *J Clin Oncol* 2004; 22:3886–3892.

253. Ben-Yosef R, Or R, Nagler A, Slavin S. Graft-versus-tumour and graft-versus-leukaemia effect in patient with concurrent breast cancer and acute myelocytic leukaemia. *Lancet* 1996; 348:1242–1243.

254. Fowler D, Hou J, Foley J, et al. Phase I clinical trial of donor T-helper type-2 cells after immunoablative, reduced intensity allogeneic PBSC transplant. *Cytotherapy* 2002; 4:429–430.

255. Fowler DH, Odom D, Castro K, et al. Co-stimulated Th2 cells for modulation of acute GVHD: Phase I clinical trial results. *Blood* 2002; 100:804.

256. Kolb HJ, Schattenberg A, Goldman JM, et al. Graft-versus-leukemia effect of donor lymphocyte transfusions in marrow grafted patients. European Group for Blood and Marrow Transplantation Working Party Chronic Leukemia. *Blood* 1995; 86:2041–2050.

257. Porter DL, Connors JM, Van Deerlin VM, et al. Graft-versus-tumor induction with donor leukocyte infusions as primary therapy for patients with malignancies. *J Clin Oncol* 1999; 17:1234.

258. Ji YH, Weiss L, Zeira M, et al. Allogeneic cell-mediated immunotherapy of leukemia with immune donor lymphocytes to upregulate antitumor effects and downregulate antihost responses. *Bone Marrow Transplant* 2003; 32:495–504.

259. Slavin S, Ackerstein A, Morecki S, Gelfand Y, Cividalli G. Immunotherapy of relapsed resistant chronic myelogenous leukemia post allogeneic bone marrow transplantation with alloantigen pulsed donor lymphocytes. *Bone Marrow Transplant* 2001; 28:795–798.

260. Ballester OF, Fang T, Raptis A, et al. Adoptive immunotherapy with donor lymphocyte infusions and interleukin-2 after high-dose therapy and autologous stem cell rescue for multiple myeloma. *Bone Marrow Transplant* 2004; 34:419–423.

261. Parker LL, Do MT, Westwood JA, et al. Expansion and characterization of T cells transduced with a chimeric receptor against ovarian cancer. *Hum Gene Ther* 2000; 11:2377–2387.

262. Morgan RA, Dudley ME, Yu YY, et al. High efficiency TCR gene transfer into primary human lymphocytes affords avid recognition of melanoma tumor antigen glycoprotein 100 and does not alter the recognition of autologous melanoma antigens. *J Immunol* 2003; 171:3287–3295.

263. Burt RK, Drobyski WR, Traynor AE, Link CJ Jr. Herpes simplex thymidine kinase (HStk) transgenic donor lymphocytes. *Bone Marrow Transplant* 1999; 24:1043–1051.

264. Hsu FJ, Caspar CB, Czerwinski D, et al. Tumor-specific idiotype vaccines in the treatment of patients with B-cell lymphoma—long-term results of a clinical trial. *Blood* 1997; 89:3129–3135.

265. Bendandi M, Gocke CD, Kobrin CB, et al. Complete molecular remissions induced by patient-specific vaccination plus granulocyte-monocyte colony-stimulating factor against lymphoma. *Nat Med* 1999; 5:1171–1177.

266. Zoller M. Tumor vaccination after allogeneic bone marrow cell reconstitution of the nonmyeloablatively conditioned tumor-bearing murine host. *J Immunol* 2003; 171:6941–6953.

267. Teshima T, Liu C, Lowler KP, Dranoff G, Ferrara JL. Donor leukocyte infusion from immunized donors increases tumor vaccine efficacy after allogeneic bone marrow transplantation. *Cancer Res* 2002; 62: 796–800.

268. Teshima T, Mach N, Hill GR, et al. Tumor cell vaccine elicits potent antitumor immunity after allogeneic T-cell-depleted bone marrow transplantation. *Cancer Res* 2001; 61:162–171.

269. Rosenberg SA, Yang JC, Schwartzentruber DJ, et al. Immunologic and therapeutic evaluation of a synthetic peptide vaccine for the treatment of patients with metastatic melanoma. *Nat Med* 1998; 4:321–327.

270. Anderson LD Jr, Savary CA, Mullen CA. Immunization of allogeneic bone marrow transplant recipients with tumor cell vaccines enhances graft-versus-tumor activity without exacerbating graft-versus-host disease. *Blood* 2000; 95:2426–2433.

271. Kwak LW, Taub DD, Duffey PL, et al. Transfer of myeloma idiotype-specific immunity from an actively immunised marrow donor. *Lancet* 1995; 345:1016–1020.

272. Kwak LW, Neelapu SS, Bishop MR. Adoptive immunotherapy with antigen-specific T cells in myeloma: a model of tumor-specific donor lymphocyte infusion. *Semin Oncol* 2004; 31:37–46.

273. Hšltl L, Ramoner R, Zelle-Rieser C, et al. Allogeneic dendritic cell vaccination against metastatic renal cell carcinoma with or without cyclophosphamide. *Cancer Immunol Immunother* 2004; 54:663–670.

274. Farag SS, Fehniger TA, Becknell B, Blaser BW, Caligiuri MA. New directions in natural killer cell-based immunotherapy of human cancer. *Expert Opin Biol Ther* 2003; 3:237–250.

275. Miller JS, Soignier Y, Panoskaltsis-Mortari A, et al. Successful adoptive transfer and in vivo expansion of human haploidentical NK cells in cancer patients. *Blood* 2005; 105:3051–3057.

15

Tumor-Induced Immune Suppression and Immune Escape

Mechanisms and Impact on the Outcome of Immunotherapy of Malignant Disease

Michael Campoli and Soldano Ferrone

SUMMARY

A large body of evidence supports the notion that both the adaptive and nonadaptive immune systems play an important role in the control of tumor progression in patients with malignant disease. These findings have provided the rationale for the development of active specific immunotherapy for the treatment of malignant disease. The enthusiastic application of active specific immunotherapy in a large number of patients has conclusively shown that:

1. Several of the immunization strategies used elicit a tumor antigen (TA)-specific immune response.
2. The results of immunomonitoring assays in patients treated with active specific immunotherapy have poor, if any, predictive value of clinical responses.
3. Irrespective of the TA or immunization strategy used, clinical responses have only occasionally been observed.
4. Disease frequently progresses and recurs in spite of induction and/or persistence of TA-specific immune responses.

These disappointing findings are likely to reflect, at least in part, the ability of tumor cells to manipulate the ongoing TA-specific immune response as well as evade immune recognition and destruction, utilizing multiple mechanisms. The latter include tumor cell-induced qualitative and/or quantitative defects in the generation and maintenance of TA-specific immune responses, tumor cell-induced immune suppression, and/or changes in the antigenic profile of tumor cells because of their genetic instability. These topics are reviewed in this chapter, following a brief description of the essential components of a TA-specific immune response. Lastly, potential strategies to counteract tumor immune suppression and immune escape mechanisms are discussed, because these approaches may improve the outcome of immunotherapy in patients with malignant disease.

Key Words: CTL; dendritic cells; HLA class I antigens; immune escape; immune suppression; NK cells; tumor antigens.

From: *Cancer Drug Discovery and Development: Immunotherapy of Cancer*
Edited by: M. L. Disis © Humana Press Inc., Totowa, NJ

1. INTRODUCTION

During the last three decades, a large body of evidence has accumulated to provide support for the concept that the host immune system interacts with developing tumors and, in some cases, may be responsible for the arrest of tumor growth and for tumor regression *(1–3)*. Tumor antigen (TA)-specific T-cells have been shown to play an active role in eliminating tumors and metastases, as well as in inducing TA-specific T-cell memory responses in a wide range of animal tumor models *(1)*. Similarly, in vitro studies employing human peripheral blood lymphocytes isolated from patients with malignant diseases have been reported to contain TA-specific CD8+ and CD4+ T-cell precursors *(4–7)*, as well as natural-killer (NK) cells *(8)* and macrophages *(9)* that are capable of killing tumor cell targets after appropriate in vitro activation. These findings, along with (a) the lack of effective treatment for advanced stage malignancies by conventional therapies *(10,11)*; (b) the identification and molecular characterization of TA *(12)*; (c) the development of highly specific probes, i.e., monoclonal antibodies (MAbs) *(13)* and cytotoxic T-lymphocytes (CTLs) *(14)*; and (d) the development of effective immunization strategies *(15,16)* have provided the rationale for the development and application of immunotherapy for the treatment of malignant disease.

A large number of active-specific immunotherapy trials have been conducted in patients with malignant disease to date *(7,17)*. It is clear from these studies that vaccines are able to induce and/or augment already established TA-specific immunity, that the immune responses generated against the tumor are far more specific than those elicited by cytokines alone, and that the various types of vaccines have limited or no toxicity. However, clinical responses have been the exception more than the rule. In fact, the general evidence has been that the results of immunomonitoring assays in patients receiving TA-specific vaccines have poor, if any, predictive value, and that lack of clinical response and/or recurrence of disease occurs frequently, in spite of induction and/or persistence of TA-specific immune responses *(7)*. It is worth noting that a majority of the immunomonitoring assays utilized in patients treated with active specific immunotherapy have primarily made use of assays that quantify and characterize the T-cell response to immunizations and have not made any attempt to assess the effect of microenvironment on TA-specific immune responses and to monitor tumor cell susceptibility to TA-specific T-cell immune responses *(18)*. It still remains to be determined when and how patients' immune response should be assessed and whether ex vivo functional evaluation of peripheral T-cells provides an accurate representation of what is occurring at the tumor site. In retrospect, the lack of correlation between immune response and clinical response observed in patients treated with active specific immunotherapy is not surprising, because the results of these assays do not take into account a patient's tumor cell susceptibility to recognition by T-cells and to lysis by T-cells. In addition, the in vitro expansion of epitope-specific CD8+ T-cells may not accurately reflect in vivo immune responsiveness, because their in vitro expansion is dependent on their exposure to arbitrarily high concentrations of antigen and exogenous cytokines. The latter may exaggerate the extent of the immune responses ongoing in vivo.

During the past 10 yr, it has become apparent that, in vivo, tumor cells have evolved multiple means to resist and/or hide from immune effector mechanisms *(19–23)*. The latter include tumor cell-induced qualitative and/or quantitative defects in the generation and maintenance of TA-specific immune responses, changes in the antigenic profile of tumor cells because of their genetic instability and/or the potential negative impact of the tumor cell microenvironment on the interaction between host immune cells and tumor cells. Therefore, one of the major challenges facing tumor immunologists is the characterization of the molecular mechanisms by which tumor cells evade immune recognition and destruction and the development of strategies to counteract these escape mechanisms. In this chapter, we first provide a brief summary of the characteristics and components required to generate and maintain an effective TA-specific immune response. Second, we discuss the immune escape mechanisms utilized by tumor cells to avoid a TA-specific immune response. Lastly, we discuss potential approaches to counteract tumor immune suppression and immune escape mechanisms, because they may improve the outcome of immunotherapy in patients with malignant disease.

2. COMPONENTS OF AN EFFECTIVE TA-SPECIFIC IMMUNE RESPONSE

A number of components are necessary for the generation and maintenance of an effective TA-specific immune response including TA, antigen-presenting cells (APCs), immune effectors, and cytokines (Figs. 1 and 2). For the purpose of this chapter, we focus on the generation and maintenance of a TA-specific T-cell-based immune response owing to the general belief that T-cells play a major role in tumor growth control (1). However, it should be noted that antibody responses are a requisite component of effective antitumor immune responses in murine systems (24) and are associated with the clinical course of the disease in several human antitumor vaccine protocols (25,26). Therefore, it should be stressed that B-cells may also play a role in the establishment of an effective TA-specific immune response by secreting immunostimulatory cytokines and acting as APCs (27). Moreover, both non-specific and specific components of the host immune response play a role in the control of tumor growth and metastasis, with some components, e.g., macrophages (9), NK cells (8) and polymorphonuclear cells (28), thought to participate in the early phase of the response, before the appearance of T- or B-cells. It is noteworthy that at particular stages of tumor development, NK cells may also play a role in the elimination of tumor cells, which fail to express major histocompatibility complex (MHC) antigens, and thus are not recognized by TA-specific CTLs (8).

Tumor cell recognition by CTLs is mediated by the interaction of T-cell receptors (TCRs) with class I human leukocyte antigens (HLAs) complexed to TA-derived peptides (i.e., HLA class I antigen–TA peptide complexes) generated by the antigen-processing machinery (APM) (see Fig. 1; [29]). These complexes can be presented to T-cells directly by tumor cells through a process defined as *direct priming*; however, the tumor cell itself is not considered a major player in the presentation of HLA class I antigen TA peptide complexes to activate T-cells. Alternatively, TA can be captured by professional APCs and processed for indirect priming of CTL via T-helper (Th) cells (30). Tumor cells can also transfer TA to APCs via apoptotic or necrotic tumor cells, tumor-derived exosomes and/or tumor-derived heat shock proteins. TA-derived peptides are then presented to T-cells through a process defined as *crosspriming (31,32)*. The most potent APCs are represented by dendritic cells (DCs), which have a high surface density of MHC antigens and of co-stimulatory molecules and can produce immunostimulatory cytokines and chemokines (33). DCs are very efficient at processing exogenous antigens, presenting HLA class I and class II antigen–TA peptide complexes and stimulating cells of the adaptive immune system (i.e., CD4+ and CD8+ T-cells, as well as B-cells), and innate immune system (i.e., NK

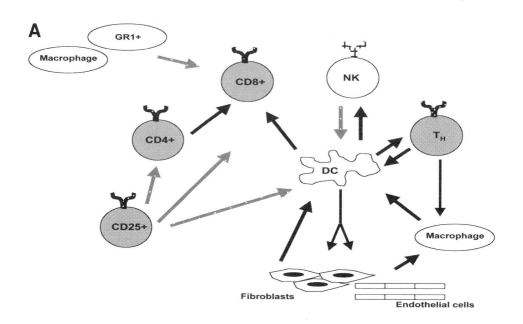

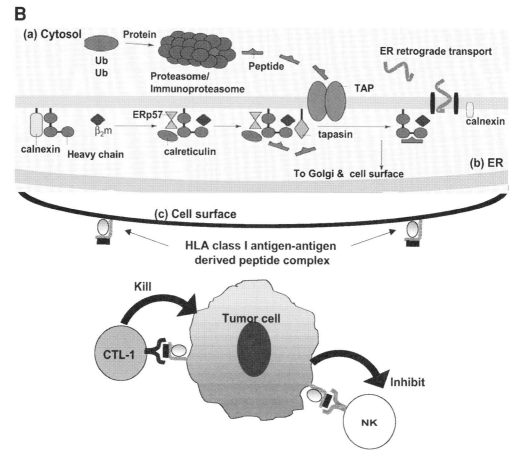

and NK T-cells) *(33–39)*. After internalizing TA at the tumor site, DCs may traffic to tumor-draining lymph nodes to activate naïve CD8$^+$ T-cells or remain at the tumor site where they are referred to as tumor-associated DC (TADCs). TADCs crosspresent TA to recruited CD8$^+$ T-cells, potentially inducing their activation, proliferation, and maturation into TA-specific effector cells *(40)*. Interaction of TCRs with HLA class I antigen–peptide complexes on APCs, together with help from activated CD4$^+$ T-cells, leads to activation and clonal expansion of TA-specific CD8$^+$ T-cells. CTLs are expected to induce programmed cell death of malignant cells that express targeted HLA class I antigen–peptide complexes, through the perforin-granzyme mechanism and/or the fatty acid synthase (Fas)/Fas ligand (FasL) pathway *(41)*. The latter requires the expression of Fas receptor on target cells and FasL on effector CTLs.

Cytokines and chemokines play a significant role in shaping functional attributes and survival of both T-cells and DCs in the tumor microenvironment. Based on our current understanding, CD8$^+$ and CD4$^+$ T-lymphocytes, as well as DCs, can be categorized into at least three functional subsets, depending on the cytokines they produce *(42–45)*. These subsets include:

1. Cytotoxic T-cells (Tc)1/Th1 or DC1 (type 1) cells that produce interferon (IFN)-γ, interleukin (IL)-2, and tumor necrosis factor-α.
2. Tc2/Th2 or DC2 (type 2) cells that produce IL-4, -5, -6, and -10.
3. Th3/T-regulatory (Treg) or DC3 cells that produce IL-10 and/or transforming growth factor-β (TGF-β).

Fig. 1. *(Opposite page)* **(A)** Schematic representation of the interactions between immune cells in the generation of an effective tumor antigen (TA)-specific immune response. TAs are captured by professional antigen-presenting cells, i.e., dendritic cells (DCs), and processed for direct and indirect priming of naïve CD8$^+$ T-cells via helper T-cells (Th). Th cells in turn further activate DCs, fibroblasts, endothelial cells, and macrophages, resulting in the release of proinflammatory cytokines. This proinflammatory environment helps DCs to activate both CD8$^+$ T-cells as well as natural-killer (NK) cells. The process of CD8$^+$ T-cell activation can be inhibited by CD4$^+$CD25$^+$ regulatory T-cells, GR1$^+$ myeloid cells, macrophage, and NK cells. (Black arrows indicate activation; gray arrows indicate inhibition). **(B)** Generation of human leukocyte antigen (HLA) class I antigen-TA peptide complexes. Intracellular protein antigens, which are mostly endogenous, are marked for ubiquitination within the cytosol and subsequently, degraded into peptides by the proteasome. Peptides are then transported into the endoplasmic reticulum (ER) through transporter associated with antigen processing protein (TAP). Nascent, HLA class I antigen heavy chains are synthesized in the ER and associate with the chaperone immunoglobulin heavy-chain binding protein, a universal ER chaperone involved in the translation and insertion of proteins into the ER. Following insertion into the ER, the HLA class I heavy chain associates with the chaperone calnexin and the thiol-dependent reductase ERp57. Calnexin dissociation is followed by HLA class I heavy chain association with β$_2$ microglobulin, tapasin, and the chaperone calreticulin. Calnexin, calreticulin, and ERp57 play a role in folding of the HLA class I heavy chain. Tapasin brings the HLA class I heavy chain–β$_2$ microglobulin–chaperone complex into association with TAP. Both TAP and tapasin play a role in quantitative and qualitative peptide selection. The trimeric HLA class I–β$_2$ microglobulin–peptide complex is then transported to the plasma membrane, where it plays a major role in the interactions between target cells and activation of peptide-specific cytotoxic T-lymphocytes through T-cell receptors or inhibition of NK cell-mediated killing through killer immunoglobulin-like receptors.

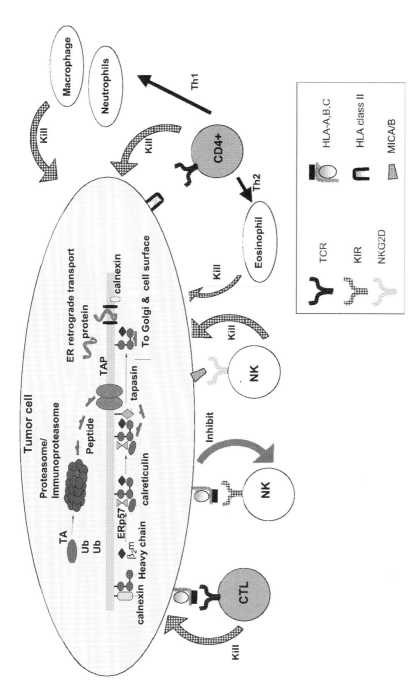

Fig. 2. Schematic representation of interactions between immune effector cells and tumor cells. Classical human leukocyte antigen (HLA) class I antigens play a major role in the interactions between target cells and (1) activation of peptide-specific cytotoxic T-lymphocytes (CTLs) through T-cell receptor and (2) inhibition of natural-killer (NK) cell-mediated killing through killer immunoglobulin-like receptors. NK cell activating ligands major histocompatibility complex class I-related chains A/B play a major role in the interactions between target cells and activation of NK cells through NKG2D. HLA class II antigens play a major role in the interaction between CD4⁺T-helper (Th) cells and target cells and (1) activation of macrophage through release of Th1 cytokines, (2) activation of eosinophils through release of Th2 cytokines, and (3) activation of CTLs through release of Th1 cytokines.

268

Table 1
Tumor Cell-Induced Immune Suppression

1. Signaling defects in TIL and PBL-T
   a. NFκB abnormalities
   b. ζ chain defects: either low expression or absence
   c. Ca++ flux alterations
2. Cytokine expression: absent/decreased Th1-type cytokines
3. Inhibition of lymphocyte proliferation, cytotoxic activity, or cytokine production
4. Inhibition of leukocyte migration
5. Induction of T-cell and/or DC apoptosis
6. Expansion of immunosuppressive CD25+ T-cells, GR1+ cells, and/or macrophages
7. DC dysfunction

TIL, tumor-infiltrating lymphocytes; PBL-T, peripheral blood T-cells; NF, nuclear factor; Th, T-helper cell; DC, dendritic cell.

Type 1-biased immune responses are strongly supported by IL-12p70 *(42–45)* and generally mediate the cellular immune response through the activities of CTLs, macrophages, and NK cells, and are associated with the host's ability to control and eliminate intracellular pathogens and tumors. On the other hand, type 2-biased immune responses enhance immune reactions mediated by antibodies and do not favor the development of cellular tumor immunity. Type 3-biased immune responses assume an overall down-regulatory activity. It is noteworthy that type 1- and type 2-biased immune responses can be crossinhibitory of one another; type 2 responses exert anti-inflammatory effects, which suppress the activity of type 1 responses.

3. MECHANISMS UNDERLYING THE LACK OF CORRELATION BETWEEN CLINICAL AND IMMUNE RESPONSES

The major unanswered question in human tumor immunology today is why the presence of TA-specific immune responses, which can be detected in a variable percentage of patients, is not paralleled by a clinical response in the majority of immunized patients despite the presence of all the necessary components (i.e., TA, APCs, immune effector cells, and cytokines), for the successful development of these responses *(7)*. In the following section, we review the available information regarding the possible mechanisms underlying the lack of correlation between immunological and clinical responses in immunized patients. They include qualitative and/or quantitative defects in the generation and maintenance of TA-specific immune responses and/or changes in the antigenic profile of tumor cells because of their genetic instability.

3.1. Tumor Cell-Induced Immune Suppression

A large body of evidence has clearly demonstrated immune suppression in cancer patients and tumor-bearing animals. Table 1 summarizes the types of immune system defects observed in patients with malignant disease. Many studies have demonstrated that a high percentage of T-cells undergo apoptosis in patients with cancer *(21,23,46)*. Furthermore, apoptosis of T-cells is not limited to the tumor site because an increased percentage of apoptotic T-cells are also found in the peripheral blood of patients with head and neck squamous cell cancer, breast carcinoma, and melanoma *(21,23,47,48)*. This apoptosis appears to be preferential for TA-specific CD8+ T-cells in patients with cancer

(T. Whiteside, personal communication). Immune effector cells have also been found to be unresponsive in patients with malignant disease. In comparison to autologous blood lymphocytes or T-cells isolated from tissues distant from the tumor, tumor infiltrating lymphocytes (TILs) have been consistently found to be poorly responsive or unresponsive to traditional T-cell-activating stimuli *(49,50)*. In addition, alterations in systemic TA-specific T-cell immunity also occur in patients with malignant disease. T-cells and NK cells from approximately half of the patients with carcinoma of the head and neck *(46,49,51)*, breast *(46,49,52)*, stomach *(46,49)*, colon *(46,49,53,54)*, kidney *(46,49,55,56)*, ovary *(46,49,57)*, and prostate *(46,49)*; with Hodgkin's lymphoma *(46,49,58)*; with acute myelocytic leukemia *(46,49)*; and with melanoma *(46,49,59)* demonstrate a decreased in vitro response to antigens or mitogens and a decreased level of CD3ζ chain expression. The latter is associated with the TCR–CD3 complex in T-lymphocytes and the Fcγ RIII in NK cells and functions as a transmembrane signaling molecule in lymphocytes *(60)*. Circulating T-cells have also been shown to be biased in their cytokine profile *(49,51,61–64)*. Furthermore, alterations in circulating T-cell function, as determined by CD3ζ-chain expression, proliferative index or nuclear factor-κB activity, are associated with the extent of alterations in TIL function and with tumor stage *(49,51,61–64)*. These observations suggest that CD3ζ-chain expression may be a marker of immune competence in patients with malignant disease and that individuals who have normal CD3ζ-chain expression are most likely to respond favorably to biotherapy *(49,50)*. It is noteworthy that changes in signal transduction molecules are not limited to CD3ζ chain, because Jak-3, a tyrosine kinase associated with the γ-chain and a common element to IL-2, IL-4, IL-7, and IL-15 cytokine receptors, is also decreased in T-cells from renal cell carcinoma (RCC) patients *(65)*. Moreover, T-cells from RCC patients also have a diminished ability to translocate nuclear factor-κBp65 *(55,56,63,66)*. Regardless of the specific defect, the presence of such systemic alterations may explain, in part, the lack of correlation between immune and clinical responses in patients treated with active specific immunotherapy.

It is noteworthy that functional defects in systemic immunity, as well as TILs, appear to be clinically significant. Alterations in T-cell signal transduction are associated with advanced tumor stage in colon carcinoma *(54)* and RCC *(61)*. Moreover, the level of CD3ζ-chain expression in TILs from patients with oral carcinoma is an independent predictive parameter of 5-yr survival rate in patients with advanced stage disease *(67)*. Notably, abnormalities in T-cell signal transduction might also occur early in disease, as diminished CD3ζ-chain expression has been found in patients with *in situ* cervical carcinoma *(68,69)*.

Functional impairments have also been noted for alternate effector cells that accumulate within tumor sites. A large body of evidence indicating that DC maturation is impaired in patients with malignant disease has been collected *(70)*. Moreover, TADCs have been shown to be functionally defective, especially in their antigen-presenting capacity in several malignant diseases *(70,71)*. Lastly, tumor-associated macrophages also exhibit functional defects relative to their counterparts obtained from tumor-uninvolved inflammatory sites in the same patient *(71,72)*. However, the functional consequences of these impairments have not yet been elucidated.

3.1.1. MECHANISMS OF TUMOR CELL-INDUCED IMMUNE SUPPRESSION

Inflammatory and/or lytic molecules produced by tumor cells may play a role in modulating the host immune response within the tumor microenvironment. In fact, early experiments dating back more than 30 yr provided evidence that tumor-derived factors

Table 2
Tumor Cell-Associated Immunosuppressive Factors[a]

1. TNF family ligands (FasL/Fas, TRAIL/TRAIL-Rs, TNF/TNFR1)
2. Small molecules
    a. Prostaglandin E2 (PGE2)
    b. Histamine
    c. Epinephrine
    d. Free radicals (H_2O_2)
    e. VEGF
    f. Soluble MIC
3. Cytokines
    a. TGF-β
    b. IL-10
    c. IL-8

[a]A partial list of immunosuppressive factors selected to demonstrate their diversity.
TNF, tumor necrosis factor; FasL, fatty acid synthase ligand; TRAIL; TRAIL-R, TRAIL receptor; VEGF, vascular endothelial growth factor; MIC; TGF, transforming growth factor; IL, interleukin.

can alter the normal functions of immune cells in vitro *(73)*. More recently, serum derived from patients with malignant disease has been shown to interfere with DC differentiation and T-cell activation and to induce apoptosis in activated T-cells *(70,74–76)*. Over the years, a number of tumor-derived factors with immunosuppressive activity have been identified (Table 2). The unresponsiveness of the immune system in patients with cancer has been attributed to paucity of Th1 cytokines (i.e., IFN-γ, IL-2, and IL-12) at the tumor site or tumor-draining lymph node, as well as the prevalence of Treg cytokines (i.e., IL-10 or TGF-β), to condition evolving TA-specific T-cells toward the less efficacious Th2 or Treg functional phenotypes. In fact, in patients with malignant disease, TILs have been shown to display a predominant type 2 or/Treg functional phenotype associated with the local production of IL-4 or IL-10 rather than the mixed type 1/type 2 responsiveness observed in normal donors *(77)*. IL-10 also inhibits differentiation, maturation, and functional status of DCs *(70)*, thus interfering with the induction of TA-specific immune responses. It is noteworthy that in parallel, IL-10 may suppress T-cell recognition of tumor cells by downregulating APM components, thereby reducing HLA class I antigen expression *(21)*. Tumor cell-secreted TGF-β has been shown to inhibit TA-specific T-cells and reverse the immune stimulating properties of IL-2 *(78)*. Furthermore, TGF-β is often found at high levels in malignancies and is associated with poor prognosis and lack of response to immunotherapy *(78)*. Prostaglandin E2 has also been implicated in tumor cell immune escape, because it plays a role in the suppression of Th1-type immune responses while enhancing Th2-type immune responses *(78)*. In addition, IL-8 *(79)*, soluble MHC class I chain-related molecule *(80–82)*, and vascular endothelial growth factor *(70,83)* production has been implicated as a potential means of tumor cell escape by modulating immune effector cell function. It should be stressed that tumor cells vary in their ability to express and produce inhibitory molecules.

Different mechanisms may account for the high frequency of T-cell apoptosis observed in patients with cancer. Malignant cells have been shown to escape immune recognition by developing resistance to Fas-mediated apoptosis and acquiring expression of FasL that they may use for eliminating activated Fas$^+$ lymphocytes (74–76,84,85). On the other hand, chronically stimulated T-cells are likely to undergo activation-induced cell death mediated by the Fas–FasL pathway, or they may die because appropriate cytokines are not secreted (86). In this regard, TILs, lymph node lymphocytes, or peripheral T-cells in patients with cancer experience chronic or repeated antigenic stimulation with TA and often express CD95 on the cell surface (46,47). Therefore, the chronic or acute systemic dissemination of TA may result in an excess of antigen and "high-dose" tolerance of specific T- and B-cells, making them particularly susceptible to activation-induced cell death. More recently, the co-inhibitory molecules of the B7-CD28 family, in particular B7-H1, which plays a role in the deletion of peripheral effector T-cells, has been found to be expressed on a variety of tumor cell types (87). It has been suggested that B7-H1 expression by tumor cells may provide an additional mechanism to induce T-cell apoptosis, because administration of B7-H1-specific antagonistic MAbs can enhance the therapeutic efficacy of adoptive immunotherapy with polyclonal T-cells (88).

Dysfunction, and ultimately, death of T-cells *in situ* might also result from impaired TADC functions (70,71). TADCs not only process and present TA, but are important sources of IFN-α, IL-1, IL-12, IL-15, IL-18, IL-23, and IL-27, among other cytokines. They are also rich in co-stimulatory molecules (CD80, CD86, OX40, 4-1BBL) necessary as second signals or growth factors for T-cell differentiation, proliferation, and memory development (89). Therefore, if TADCs are dysfunctional, as suggested by data in the literature (70,71), or if they also undergo apoptosis *in situ*, then TADC–TIL interactions are not likely to be optimal for productive TA-specific immunity. Elimination of DCs or DC precursors in the tumor microenvironment may, in part, contribute to an ineffective TA-specific T-cell immune response in patients with malignant disease (70,71). The mechanisms involved in the induction of apoptosis and protection of different DC subpopulations, as well as DC precursors from death signals include the following:

1. Downregulation of the anti-apoptotic B-cell leukemia (Bcl)-2 family proteins in DCs (90).
2. Accumulation of ceramides that may interfere with phosphatidylinositol-3 kinase-mediated survival signals.
3. Production of nitric oxide (NO) species by tumor cells that suppresses expression of cellular inhibitors of apoptosis proteins (IAPs) or inhibitor of caspase 8-cellular Fas-associated death domain-like IL-1β-converting enzyme (FLICE) inhibitory protein (cFLIP) (91).

Analysis of gene and protein expression in DCs and DC precursors in the tumor microenvironment has demonstrated that expression of several intracellular signaling molecules is reproducibly altered in DC co-incubated with tumor cells, including IL-2Rγ, interferon regulatory factor 2, Mcl-1, and small Rho guanosine triphosphatases among others (70). It appears that both intrinsic and extrinsic apoptotic pathways are involved in tumor-induced apoptosis of DC, as determined by an increased resistance to apoptosis of DC genetically modified to overexpress Bcl-xL, caspase 8, FLIP, or X-linked IAP.

It is noteworthy that crosstalk between NK cells and DC may be important in regulation of an effective immune response. In this regard, DCs play a crucial role in the activation of NK cells (35,92). Once activated, NK cells are able to kill immature DCs because of their low MHC class I molecule expression (35,92), as well as mature DCs that do not express optimal surface densities of MHC class I molecules (33). The interactions between NK cells and DCs provide a coordinated mechanism that is involved not only in the regulation of innate immunity, but also in the promotion of appropriate downstream adaptive immune response. Therefore, alterations in the communication between DCs and NK cells may provide an alternative means of immune deviation in the tumor microenvironment.

3.1.2. MYELOID SUPPRESSOR CELLS

A group of CD11b$^+$, GR1$^+$ cells known as myeloid suppressor cells (MSCs), are also thought to play an important role in tumor unresponsiveness by suppressing TA-specific T-cell immune responses (93–96). MSCs represent a heterogeneous population that includes mature granulocytes, monocytes, and immature cells of the myelomonocytic lineage. There is ample evidence that tumor growth in patients with all types of malignant disease, as well as in tumor-bearing mice, is associated with an accumulation of MSCs (93–96). In vitro studies indicate that MSCs purified from tumor-bearing mice, but not from naïve mice, can suppress CD8$^+$ T-cells. This suppression is NO-independent, antigen-specific, requires direct cell–cell contact through TCR and MHC class I antigen interactions. Whereas the molecular mechanisms underlying this phenomenon are unclear, several studies indicate that reactive oxygen species (ROS) may play a significant role. In this regard, many human tumors and cell lines are capable of secreting cytokines not limited to, but including, granulocyte-macrophage colony-stimulating factor, IL-3, IL-6, macrophage colony-stimulating factor, and vascular endothelial growth factor. These cytokines are capable of expanding the myeloid cell pool and may also lead to an increase in ROS production and arginase activity in MSCs (93–96). The latter enzyme indirectly increases the ROS level by decreasing L-arginine concentrations. Constant production of these factors could lead to the different levels of ROS observed in MSCs derived from tumor-bearing and tumor-free mice. In fact, the ROS level has been found to be threefold greater in MSCs derived from tumor-bearing mice than in tumor-free mice (93–96). The main target for ROS on T-cells has been shown to be CD3ζ, ultimately resulting in the suppression of CD3ζ and IFN-γ expression in CD8$^+$ T-cells present in advanced cancer patients. ROS are short-lived substances, and therefore, the antigen-specific nature of their inhibition may be explained by the need for direct MSC–T-cell contact (93–96). In this regard, antigen-specific interactions between T-cells and APCs are much more stable and last longer than interactions in the absence of antigen. MSCs express MHC class I molecules, but have low or undetectable levels of MHC class II antigens; this phenotype may explain the lack of CD4$^+$ T-cell suppression by MSCs (93–96).

3.1.3. CD25$^+$ TREG CELLS

Accumulating evidence indicates that a population of CD4$^+$CD25$^+$ Treg cells may at least be partially responsible for T-cell dysfunction. CD4$^+$CD25$^+$ T-cells prevent the induction of a variety of autoimmune diseases in murine models (97). CD4$^+$CD25$^+$ regulatory T-cells dramatically suppress the function and proliferation of CD4$^+$CD25$^-$ and CD8$^+$ T-cells (97). The immune regulatory function of these cells has been attributed to their capacity to secrete immune-suppressive cytokines, such as IL-10 and TGF-β, which inhibit CTL responses. Therefore, it has been suggested that these cells play a role in the regulation of immune responses to TA, because tumor immunity can be thought of as an autoimmune process.

In this regard, in vivo studies performed in murine models have shown that CD4$^+$CD25$^+$ T-cells, which comprise 5–10% of CD4$^+$ T-cells in naïve mice, can inhibit the generation of TA-specific T-cell immune responses (97). Depletion of CD4$^+$CD25$^+$ T-cells has been shown to promote rejection of several tumors in mice *(97)*. This rejection is dependent on CD8$^+$ or CD4$^+$ T-cells alone or in combination, depending on the murine strain and tumor model. In vitro studies suggest that CD25$^+$ T-cells may suppress CD8$^+$ and CD4$^+$ T-cells in an antigen-nonspecific fashion through the production of TGF-β *(97)*. In humans, CD4$^+$CD25$^+$ T-cells are found at a higher frequency in the peripheral blood of cancer patients and may induce peripheral ignorance of tumor cells, facilitating metastatic spread of the disease *(98)*. Moreover, CD4$^+$CD25$^+$ T-cells have been shown to be present in several types of tumors including breast, lung, pancreas, and ovarian *(98,99)*. However, their functional role in the modulation of TA-specific immune responses has yet to be elucidated.

3.2. Tumor-Cell Escape From Immune Recognition and Killing

Multiple immune escape mechanisms may be utilized by tumor cells to evade the host's immune response as well as recognition and destruction by host CTL (Fig. 3). Because of their genetic instability *(100)*, tumor cells may change in the expression of molecules such as TA, HLA class I antigens and/or components of the APM, each of which plays a crucial role in the generation of the HLA class I antigen–TA peptide complex *(20,21)*. The latter mediates the recognition of tumor cells by host CTLs. Abnormalities in TA expression, as well as a variable degree of inter- and intralesional heterogeneity, characterize many tumors *(21,101–104)*. As a result, peptides may not be generated from TA or may be formed in very low amounts. Therefore, the corresponding HLA class I antigen–TA peptide complexes are not formed, in spite of the expression of the relevant HLA class I allospecificity. Furthermore, malignant cells may present TA-derived peptide analogs with antagonist activity resulting in suboptimal T-cell activation *(78)*. These defects render malignant cells ineffective targets for TA-specific T-cells.

As reviewed elsewhere *(21,105)*, the frequency of HLA class I antigen loss or downregulation has been found to range from 16 to 80% of the various types of tumors stained with MAb-recognizing monomorphic determinants. It is likely that multiple reasons contribute to the differences in the frequency of classical HLA class I antigen defects in various types of tumors. Some of them are technical in nature and include the sensitivity of the immunohistochemical (IHC) reaction used, the characteristics of the MAbs used in the IHC reactions, and the subjective evaluation of IHC staining. Additional important variables that play a role in the different frequency of HLA class I antigen abnormalities observed in tumors of different histotype include the extent of immune selective pressure imposed on tumor cell populations, their genetic instability, the time length between onset of tumor and diagnosis, the characteristics of the patient population investigated, and the histological classification of the type of tumor analyzed.

Abnormalities in HLA class I antigen expression are caused by distinct mechanisms. They include both structural and functional defects in β$_2$-microglobulin, HLA class I antigen and/or APM component expression *(21,105)*. The latter plays a crucial role in the generation of TA-derived peptides, their loading onto HLA class I antigens, and the presentation of HLA class I antigen–peptide complexes on the surface of cells. It is noteworthy that defects in APM expression and/or function may result in alterations in the repertoire of peptides presented by HLA class I antigens while not affecting the actual level of HLA class I antigen expression. This possibility provides a mechanism for resistance to CTL-mediated lysis of tumor cells without detectable defects in HLA class I antigen expression, such as head and neck squamous cell carcinoma cells *(21,105)*. The role of HLA class I antigen defects in the clinical course of the disease is highlighted by the increased

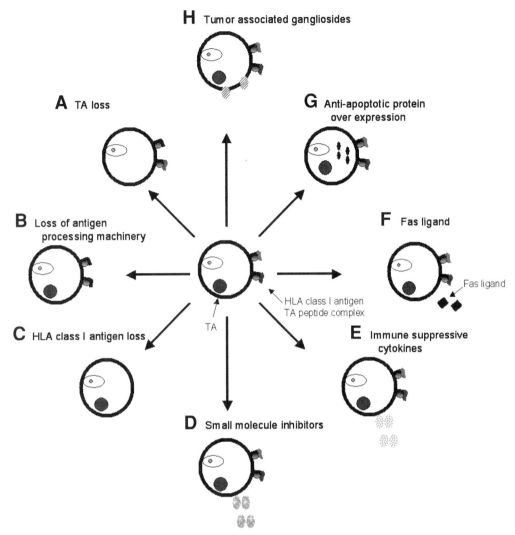

Fig. 3. Immune escape and immune suppression mechanisms utilized by tumor cells. Escape mechanisms utilized by tumor cells include human leukocyte antigen (HLA) class I antigen-tumor-associated-derived peptide complex loss that can result from loss of **(A)** tumor antigen, **(B)** antigen-processing machinery components, or **(C)** HLA class I antigens; **(D)** release of immune suppressive small molecules such as prostaglandin 2, inducible nitric oxide synthase, and/or H_2O_2; **(E)** release of immune suppressive cytokines resulting in altered immune cell function; **(F)** fatty acid synthase (Fas) ligand expression resulting in the killing of Fas+ lymphocytes **(G)** overexpression of antiapoptotic proteins in melanoma cells, resulting in apopotitic resistance; and **(H)** expression of tumor associated gangliosides which can inhibit interleukin-2-dependent lymphocyte proliferation, as well as induce apoptotic signals.

frequency of HLA class I antigen abnormalities in malignant lesions in patients treated with T-cell-based immunotherapy *(21)*. Furthermore, HLA class I antigen loss has been frequently found in lesions that have recurred in patients who had experienced clinical responses following T-cell-based immunotherapy *(21)*. It is noteworthy that in some of these cases, HLA class I antigen expression can be restored by cytokines *(22)*. Therefore, these patients, in contrast to those whose lesions possess structural defects in HLA class I antigen-encoding genes, are likely to benefit by combining T-cell-based immunotherapy with administration of cytokines.

As discussed in Section 2, CTLs are expected to induce programmed cell death of malignant cells via the Fas/FasL pathway. However, malignant cells themselves can become resistant to apoptosis through a variety of mechanisms. The mechanisms identified include the overexpression of key antiapoptotic proteins, such as two members of the inhibitor of aptosis (IAP) family (survivin and melanoma-IAP), bcl2, cFLIP, and NO synthetases (84). Tumors also display loss of Fas expression, which renders them resistant to apoptosis (106). Alternately, alterations may appear further downstream in the death receptor signaling pathway, including functional impairment of Fas-associated death domain protein and caspase 10 by inactivation mutations (107). Lastly, another way for tumor cells to escape recognition by CTLs, as well as NK cells, is by overexpressing protease inhibitor (PI)-9 (in mice known as SPI-6) (108). PI-9 is a serine PI that inactivates granzyme B. The latter is one of the important components of granule-mediated CTL killing (109).

4. TOWARD IMPROVING IMMUNOTHERAPY

Clinical trials have convincingly shown that active immunotherapy can generate TA-specific immune responses in patients with minimal side effects and, in a minor subset of patients, induce tumor regression (7,17). Despite these encouraging findings, no study has demonstrated that immunotherapy can improve on the currently available treatment modalities for malignant disease. In fact, the lack of convincing and reproducible associations between immune response and objective clinical responses to immunotherapies in patients with malignant disease has cast a doubt regarding the utility of biological therapies in general, as well as the ability of an optimal host immune response to control tumor growth. However, during the last decade, our understanding of how the immune system interacts with tumor cells has greatly improved. It is now clear that tumor cell-induced immune suppression and tumor immune escape both represent major obstacles in the successful application of immunotherapy in patients with malignant disease. Therefore, in the future, it will be important to develop strategies to counteract tumor cell-induced immune suppression and tumor immune escape in order to enhance the efficacy of immunotherapeutic strategies. In the remaining part of this section, we review several potential strategies that may counteract the multiple escape mechanisms utilized by tumor cells.

Recent progress into our understanding of the mechanisms underlying immune effector cell proliferation and death, cytokine and growth factor biology, the role of DCs in antigen presentation, as well as regulation of target-cell killing in the tumor microenvironment, provides support for the concept that tumor cells may directly and/or indirectly lead to dysfunction and/or death of T-cells, as well as DCs. Therefore, it is unlikely that active specific immunotherapy of malignant disease will be successful in the setting of tumor cell-induced immune suppression. Novel therapeutic strategies that protect immune effector cells from tumor cell-induced dysfunction in the tumor microenvironment must be developed in order to improve the efficacy of active specific immune therapy. Unfortunately, the question of how to best protect immune effector cells from tumor cell-induced immune suppression has yet to be adequately addressed. Based on preliminary results from various laboratories, it appears that biotherapy with cytokines and/or DCs is the most effective and practical way of providing protection from apoptosis to immune effector cells (110–112). Although the mechanisms responsible for this protection are not clear, it is now recognized that DCs play a crucial role in T-cell survival. The therapeutic implications of this finding are profound. In effect, this concept shifts the emphasis from the well-recognized role of DCs as APCs to their additional role as T-cell protectors from signals mediated by the tumor necrosis factor family of receptors/ligands or other apoptosis-inducing signals. Enhancing both the number and function of DC may become the primary objective of biological therapies in patients with cancer, where premature death of TA-specific CD8[+] and CD4[+] T-cell effectors occurs.

To achieve adequate protection of T-cells from apoptosis in the tumor microenvironment, it will also be necessary to investigate mechanisms of tumor cell-induced DC immune suppression and formulate strategies for inhibition of this process, perhaps by using cytokines, such as IL-7 and IL-12. In parallel, new strategies for cytokine delivery and perhaps new cytokines themselves (e.g., IL-15) are likely to be necessary to rescue dying cells or, better, to protect viable cells from death-inducing signals. These studies are viewed as essential for defining mechanisms responsible for T-cell protection from tumor cell-induced DC immune suppression and for the subsequent design of therapies, which are most likely to result in the reinforcement of protective, and inhibition of suppressive, molecular pathways in T-cells functioning within the tumor microenvironment. It is noteworthy that although therapy with cytokines, such as IFN-γ, IL-2, or IL-12 has been used by many investigators to treat patients with malignant disease (113), cytokine therapy has never been specifically directed toward preventing the death of immune effector cells or toward repairing defective antigen-processing and -presentation pathways in tumor cells. On the contrary, the rationale behind cytokine therapies has been the predicted upregulation of antitumor effector functions, especially those associated with TA-specific T-cells. In retrospect, attempts to upregulate the functionality of dying cells are not likely to succeed. New strategies for cytokine delivery, as well as new cytokines themselves (e.g., IL-15), are likely to be necessary to rescue dying cells or, better, to protect viable cells from death-inducing signals. Such therapeutic strategies based on creative and novel use of cytokines are both rational and practical. Whereas the precedent exists for clinical applications of these cytokines in humans, the novelty of the suggested approach is that it targets biotherapy to the specific pathways or even affected molecules and is designed to carefully evaluate the impact of these corrective measures on tumor-specific functions of immune cells in treated patients.

More recently, attempts have been made to boost TA-specific T-cell activity and overcome immune suppression by the administration of anticytotoxic T-lymphocyte-associated antigen (CTLA)-4 MAbs. CTLA-4 is an immunoregulatory molecule expressed on activated T-cells and a subset of regulatory T-cells (114). This molecule is capable of downregulating T-cell activation (114). Blockade of its function has been shown to enhance TA-specific responses and potentiate the activity of cancer vaccines in animal models (114). Immunization of melanoma patients with a gp100-derived peptide-based vaccine along with anti-CTLA-4 MAbs resulted in cancer regression in 3 of 14 patients (115), suggesting a potential role for CTLA-4 blockade in melanoma immunotherapy. However, 6 of 14 patients, including the three responders, developed severe grade III/IV autoimmunity. Therefore, it remains to be determined whether side effects will be a major obstacle to the use of this strategy.

Patients' tumor cell susceptibility to immune recognition and destruction must also become a major focus of investigations in order to improve the outcome of immunotherapy. During the last few years, defects in TA, APM components, and HLA class I antigen expression have been convincingly documented in malignant lesions. Although not con-clusive, the available evidence suggests that these defects may be clinically relevant. This information has been useful to focus investigators' attention on the potential role of TA, APM components, and HLA antigen defects in tumor cell escape. To date, a majority of the immunotherapy clinical trials conducted have targeted only one HLA class I anti-gen–TA peptide complex. Clearly, abnormalities in the expression of TA, APM compo-nents, and/or HLA class I antigens will lead to alterations in HLA class I antigen–TA peptide complex expression and ultimately, impair CTL recognition of tumor cells. In this regard, polyvalent vaccines, which utilize more than one TA, may be preferable to the widely used strategy to immunize patients with one TA, in order to counteract the neg-ative impact of the selective loss of the TA used as a target on the outcome of immunother-apy. The presence of multiple TA in these vaccines also increases their potential to induce effective T-cell responses to multiple HLA class I antigen–TA peptide complexes that is expected to counteract the multiple escape mechanisms utilized by tumor cells (e.g., TA loss, HLA class I allospecificity loss, APM component loss). The multiple TA epi-topes present in polyvalent vaccines may lead to the activation of CD4+ T-lymphocytes, which are important immune components in the eradication of tumor cells (116). The choice of polyvalent vaccines is also supported by the reports of beneficial effects on the clinical course of the disease in the trials conducted with polyvalent vaccines (117–121). Lastly, the observation that tumors can preferentially downregulate the expression of particular HLA class I allospecificities (20,21) emphasizes the need to utilize vaccines that target multiple HLA class I allospecificity TA–peptide complexes. The types of TAs currently being utilized in clinical trials should also be reexamined. In this regard, most of the currently used TAs are selected on the basis of their immunogenicity and tissue dis-tribution, without paying much attention to their function in tumor cell biology. In the future, targeting TAs that play crucial roles in tumor cell biology may prove more useful in active specific immunotherapy, because loss of the functional TA itself may lead to tumor cell death. In addition, the concomitant targeting of antigens present in normal cells, which are crucial for malignant cell survival and proliferation, may counteract the negative impact of tumor cell genetic instability on the outcome of immunotherapy.

It should be noted that the types of patients currently being enrolled in clinical trials as well as the criteria to evaluate clinical responses may also need to be reevaluated. Because of ethical considerations, T-cell-based immunotherapy trials have been performed in patients who have failed to respond to all conventional means of treatment and usually have advanced disease. These patients are often immune suppressed and not as responsive to immunization (122,123). Moreover, a patient's pretreatment tumor burden has been shown to be of critical importance for the induction of a maximum TA-specific immune response (124). These findings suggest that the use of active specific immunotherapy may only be successful when administered early during the course of the disease and/or in the adjuvant setting. In addition, the potential effect of the HLA phenotype on the clinical response to active specific immunotherapy (125) suggests that a patient's genetic make-up plays a crucial role in determining the nature of their immune response. Future studies directed at identifying genetic algorithm(s) responsible for successful tumor rejection in response to immunization may help in the selection of patients likely to benefit from specific immu-nization strategies. Lastly, the possible role played by immune selective pressure in the generation of malignant lesions with HLA class I antigen defects suggests that the use of T-cell-based immunotherapy for the treatment of malignant disease may only be successful in a limited number of cases. Even when successful, it is likely that the selective pressure imposed by T-cell-based immunotherapy will facilitate the emergence and expansion of tumor cell populations with HLA class I antigen defects and eventually the recurrence of malignant lesions. Therefore, it will be important to combine T-cell-based immunotherapy with other types of immunological and nonimmunological strategies, which utilize distinct mechanisms to control tumor growth.

5. CONCLUSION

Our understanding of how the immune system interacts with tumor cells has greatly improved during the last decade. It is now evident that tumor cells have evolved multiple means to induced qualitative and/or quantitative defects in the generation and maintenance of TA-specific immune responses. Furthermore, tumor cell genetic instability gives them the ability to alter their antigenic profile and avoid immune destruction. Both of these phenomena remain important obstacle for the treatment of human malignancies through active specific immunotherapy. Understanding the molecular mechanisms behind tumor cell-induced immune suppression and tumor cell immune escape will provide valuable insight in designing effective immunotherapeutic strategies for the treatment of malignant diseases.

REFERENCES

1. Restifo NP, Wunderlich JR. Principles of tumor immunity: biology of cellular immune responses. In: DeVita VT, Hellman S, Rosenderg SA, eds. *Biologic Therapy of Cancer*. Philadelphia: Lippincott. 1996: pp. 3–21.
2. Dunn GP, Bruce AT, Ikeda H, Old LJ, Schreiber RD. Cancer immunoediting: from immunosurveillance to tumor escape. *Nat Immunol* 2002; 3:991–998.
3. Dunn GP, Old LJ, Schreiber RD. The three Es of cancer immunoediting. *Annu Rev Immunol* 2004; 22: 329–360.
4. Marchand M, Weynants P, Rankin E, et al. Tumor regression responses in melanoma patients treated with a peptide encoded by gene MAGE-3. *Int J Cancer* 1995; 63:883–885.
5. Jaeger E, Bernhard H, Romero P, et al. Generation of cytotoxic T-cell responses with synthetic melanoma-associated peptides in vivo: implications for tumor vaccines with melanoma-associated antigens. *Int J Cancer* 1996; 66:162–169.
6. Pittet MJ, Valmori D, Dunbar PR, et al. High frequencies of naïve Melan-A/MART-1-specific CD8$^+$ T cells in a large proportion of human histocompatibility leukocyte antigen HLA-A2 individuals. *J Exp Med* 1999; 190: 705–715.
7. Parmiani G, Castelli C, Dalerba P, et al. Cancer immunotherapy with peptide-based vaccines: what have we achieved? Where are we going? *J Natl Cancer Inst* 2002; 94:805–818.
8. Wu J, Lanier LL. Natural killer cells and cancer. *Adv Cancer Res* 2003; 90:127–156.
9. Ohno S, Suzuki N, Ohno Y, Inagawa H, Soma G, Inoue M. Tumor-associated macrophages: foe or accomplice of tumors? *Anticancer Res* 2003; 23:4395–4409.
10. Fojo T, Bates S. Strategies for reversing drug resistance. *Oncogene* 2003; 22:7512–7523.
11. Pommier Y, Sordet O, Antony S, Hayward RL, Kohn KW. Apoptosis defects and chemotherapy resistance: molecular interaction maps and networks. *Oncogene* 2004; 23:2934–2949.
12. Renkvist N, Castelli C, Robbins PF, Parmiani G. A listing of human tumor antigens recognized by T cells. *Cancer Immunol Immunother* 2001; 50:3–15.
13. Trikha M, Yan L, Nakada MT. Monoclonal antibodies as therapeutics in oncology. *Curr Opin Biotechnol* 2002; 13:609–614.
14. Panelli MC, Wang E, Monsurro V, et al. Vaccination with T cell-defined antigens. *Expert Opin Biol Ther* 2004; 4:697–707.
15. Naftzger C, Takechi Y, Kohda H, Hara I, Vijayasaradhi S, Houghton AN. Immune response to a differentiation antigen induced by altered antigen: a study of tumor rejection and autoimmunity. *Proc Natl Acad Sci USA* 1996; 93:14,809–14,814.

16. Egen JG, Kuhns MS, Allison JP. CTLA-4: new insights into its biological function and use in tumor immunotherapy. *Nat Immunol* 2002; 3:611–618.

17. Durrant LG, Spendlove I. Cancer vaccines entering Phase III clinical trials. *Expert Opin Emerg Drugs* 2003; 8:489–500.

18. Romero P, Cerottini JC, Speiser DE. Monitoring tumor antigen specific T-cell responses in cancer patients and phase I clinical trials of peptide-based vaccination. *Cancer Immunol Immunother* 2004; 53:249–255.

19. Sogn JA. Tumor immunology: the glass is half full. *Immunity* 1998; 9:757–763.

20. Marincola FM, Jaffee EM, Hicklin DJ, Ferrone S. Escape of human solid tumors from T-cell recognition: molecular mechanisms and functional significance. *Adv Immunol* 2000; 74:181–273.

21. Ferrone S. Tumour immune escape. *Semin Cancer Biol* 2002; 12:1–86.

22. Khong HT, Restifo NP. Natural selection of tumor variants in the generation of "tumor escape" phenotypes. *Nat Immunol* 2002; 3:999–1005.

23. Whiteside TL. Apoptosis of immune cells in the tumor microenvironment and peripheral circulation of patients with cancer: implications for immunotherapy. *Vaccine* 2002; 20(Suppl 4):46–51.

24. Reilly RT, Machiels JP, Emens LA, et al. The collaboration of both humoral and cellular HER-2/*neu*-targeted immune responses is required for the complete eradication of HER-2/*neu*-expressing tumors. *Cancer Res* 2001; 61:880–883.

25. DiFronzo LA, Gupta RK, Essner R, et al. Enhanced humoral immune response correlates with improved disease-free and overall survival in American Joint Committee on Cancer stage II melanoma patients receiving adjuvant polyvalent vaccine. *J Clin Oncol* 2002; 20:3242–3248.

26. Chung MH, Gupta RK, Hsueh E, et al. Humoral immune response to a therapeutic polyvalent cancer vaccine after complete resection of thick primary melanoma and sentinel lymphadenectomy. *J Clin Oncol* 2003; 21:313–319.

27. Noorchashm H, Greeley SA, Naji A. The role of t/b lymphocyte collaboration in the regulation of autoimmune and alloimmune responses. *Immunol Res* 2003; 27:443–450.

28. Di Carlo E, Forni G, Musiani P. Neutrophils in the antitumoral immune response. *Chem Immunol Allergy* 2003; 83:182–203.

29. Yewdell J. Generating peptide ligands for MHC class I molecules. *Mol Immunol* 2002; 39:125–259.

30. Velders MP, Markiewicz MA, Eiben GL, Kast WM. CD4$^+$ T cell matters in tumor immunity. *Int Rev Immunol* 2003; 22:113–140.

31. Heath WR, Carbone FR. Cross-presentation, dendritic cells, tolerance and immunity. *Annu Rev Immunol* 2001; 19:47–64.

32. Li Z, Menoret A, Srivastava P. Roles of heat-shock proteins in antigen presentation and cross-presentation. *Curr Opin Immunol* 2002; 14:45–51.

33. Thery C, Amigorena S. The cell biology of antigen presentation in dendritic cells. *Curr Opin Immunol* 2001; 13:45–51.

34. Gretz JE, Anderson AO, Shaw S. Cords, channels, corridors and conduits: critical architectural elements facilitating cell interactions in the lymph node cortex. *Immunol Rev* 1997; 156:11–24.

35. Cooper MA, Fehniger TA, Fuchs A, Colonna M, Caligiuri MA. NK cell and DC interactions. *Trends Immunol* 2004; 25:47–52.

36. Foti M, Granucci F, Ricciardi-Castagnoli P. A central role for tissue-resident dendritic cells in innate responses. *Trends Immunol* 2004; 25:650–654.

37. Ikeda H, Chamoto K, Tsuji T, et al. The critical role of type-1 innate and acquired immunity in tumor immunotherapy. *Cancer Sci* 2004; 95:697–703.

38. Raulet DH. Interplay of natural killer cells and their receptors with the adaptive immune response. *Nat Immunol* 2004; 5:996–1002.

39. Jego G, Pascual V, Palucka AK, Banchereau J. Dendritic cells control B cell growth and differentiation. *Curr Dir Autoimmun* 2005; 8:124–139.

40. Allison JP, Hurwitz AA, Leach DR. Manipulation of costimulatory signals to enhance anti-tumor T cell responses. *Curr Opin Immunol* 1995; 7:682–686.

41. Barry M, Bleackley RC. Cytotoxic T lymphocytes: all roads lead to death. *Nat Rev Immunol* 2002; 2:401–409.

42. Creusot RJ, Mitchison NA. How DCs control cross-regulation between lymphocytes. *Trends Immunol* 2004; 25:126–131.

43. Heath WR, Belz GT, Behrens GM, et al. Cross-presentation, dendritic cell subsets, and the generation of immunity to cellular antigens. *Immunol Rev* 2004; 199:9–26.

44. Pulendran B. Modulating TH1/TH2 responses with microbes, dendritic cells, and pathogen recognition receptors. *Immunol Res* 2004; 29:187–196.

45. Mazzoni A, Segal DM. Controlling the Toll road to dendritic cell polarization. *J Leukoc Biol* 2004; 75: 721–730.

46. Reichert TE, Rabinowich H, Johnson JT, Whiteside TL. Human immune cells in the tumor microenvironment: mechanisms responsible for signaling and functional defects. *J Immunother* 1998; 21:295–306.

47. Hoffmann TK, Dworacki G, Tsukihiro T, et al. Spontaneous apoptosis of circulating T lymphocytes in patients with head and neck cancer and its clinical importance. *Clin Cancer Res* 2002; 8:2553–2562.

48. Saito T, Dworacki G, Gooding W, Lotze MT, Whiteside TL. Spontaneous apoptosis of CD8$^+$ T lymphocytes in peripheral blood of patients with advanced melanoma. *Clin Cancer Res* 2000; 6:1351–1364.

49. Whiteside TL. Signaling defects in T lymphocytes of patients with malignancy. *Cancer Immunol Immunother* 1999; 48:346–352.

50. Whiteside TL. Down-regulation of zeta-chain expression in T cells: a biomarker of prognosis in cancer? *Cancer Immunol Immunother* 2004; 53:865–878.

51. Kuss I, Saito T, Johnson JT, Whiteside TL. Clinical significance of decreased zeta chain expression in peripheral blood lymphocytes of patients with head and neck cancer. *Clin Cancer Res* 1999; 5:329–334.

52. Kurt RA, Urba WJ, Smith JW, Schoof DD. Peripheral T lymphocytes from women with breast cancer exhibit abnormal protein expression of several signaling molecules. *Int J Cancer* 1998; 78:16–20.

53. Nakagomi H, Petersson M, Magnusson I, et al. Decreased expression of the signal-transducing ζ chains in tumor-infiltrating T-cell and NK cells of patients with colorectal carcinoma. *Cancer Res* 1993; 53: 5610–5612.

54. Matsuda M, Petersson M, Lenkei R, et al. Alterations in the signal-transducing molecules of T cells and NK cells in colorectal tumor-infiltrating gut mucosal and peripheral lymphocytes: correlation with the stage of the disease. *Int J Cancer* 1995; 61:765–772.

55. Finke JH, Zea AH, Stanley J, et al. Loss of T-cell receptor ζ chain and p56lck in T-cell infiltrating human renal cell carcinoma. *Cancer Res* 1993; 53:5613–5616.

56. Li X, Liu J, Park J-K, Hamilton TA, et al. T cells from renal cell carcinoma patients exhibit an abnormal pattern of NFκB specific DNA binding activity. *Cancer Res* 1994; 54:5424–5429.

57. Lai P, Rabinowich H, Crowley-Nowick PA, Bell MC, Mantovani G, Whiteside TL. Alterations in expression and function of signal transduction proteins in tumor associated NK and T lymphocytes from patients with ovarian carcinoma. *Clin Cancer Res* 1996; 2:161–173.

58. Wang Q, Stanley J, Kudoh S, et al. T cells infiltrating non-Hodgkin's B cell lymphomas show altered tyrosine phosphorylation pattern even though T cell receptor/CD3-associated kinases are present. *J Immunol* 1995; 155:1382–1392.

59. Zea AH, Cutri BD, Longo DL, et al. Alterations in T cell receptor and signal transduction molecules in melanoma patients. *Clin Cancer Res* 1995; 1:1327–1335.

60. Kersh EN, Shaw AS, Allen PM. Fidelity of T cell activation through multistep T cell receptor zeta phosphorylation. *Science* 1998; 281:572–575.

61. Bukowski RM, Rayman P, Uzzo R, et al. Signal transduction abnormalities in T lymphocytes from patients with advanced renal cell carcinoma: clinical relevance and effects of cytokine therapy. *Clin Cancer Res* 1998; 4:2337–2347.

62. Uzzo R, Rayman P, Kolenko V, et al. Renal cell carcinoma-derived gangliosides suppress nuclear factor-κB activation in T cells. *J Clin Invest* 1999; 104:769–776.

63. Reichert TE, Strauss L, Wagner EM, Gooding W, Whiteside TL. Signaling abnormalities and reduced proliferation of circulating and tumor-infiltrating lymphocytes in patients with oral carcinoma. *Clin Cancer Res* 2002; 8:3137–3145.

64. Bauernhofer T, Kuss I, Henderson B, Baum AS, Whiteside TL. Preferential apoptosis of CD56^{dim} natural killer cell subset in patients with cancer. *Eur J Immunol* 2003; 33:119–124.

65. Kolenko V, Wang Q, Riedy MC, et al. Tumor-induced suppression of T lymphocyte proliferation coincides with inhibition of Jak3 expression and IL-2 receptor signaling: role of soluble products from human renal cell carcinomas. *J Immunol* 1997; 159:3057–3067.

66. Uzzo RG, Clark PE, Rayman P, et al. Evidence that tumor inhibits NFκB activation in T lymphocytes of patients with renal cell carcinoma. *J Natl Cancer Inst* 1999; 91:718–721.

67. Reichert TE, Day R, Wagner E, Whiteside TL. Absent or low expression of the ζ chain in T cells at the tumor site correlates with poor survival in patients with oral carcinoma. *Cancer Res* 1998; 58:5344–5347.

68. Kono K, Ressing ME, Brandt RM, et al. Decreased expression of signal-transducing zeta chain in peripheral T cells and natural killer cells in patients with cervical cancer. *Clin Cancer Res* 1996; 2:1825–1828.

69. de Gruijl TD, Bontkes HJ, Peccatori F, et al. Expression of CD3-zeta on T-cells in primary cervical carcinoma and in metastasis-positive and -negative pelvic lymph nodes. *Br J Cancer* 1999; 79:1127–1132.

70. Yang L, Carbone DP. Tumor-host immune interactions and dendritic cell dysfunction. *Adv Cancer Res* 2004; 92:13–27.

71. Mantovani A, Allavena P, Sozzani S, Vecchi A, Locati M, Sica A. Chemokines in the recruitment and shaping of the leukocyte infiltrate of tumors. *Semin Cancer Biol* 2004; 14:155–160.

72. Mantovani A, Bottazzi B, Colotta F, Sozzani S, Ruco L. The origin and function of tumor-associated macrophages. *Immunol Today* 1992; 13:265–270.

73. Whiteside TL, Rabinowich H. The role of Fas/FasL in immunosuppression induced by human tumors. *Cancer Immunol Immunother* 1998; 46:175–184.

74. Andreola G, Rivoltini L, Castelli C, et al. Induction of lymphocyte apoptosis by tumor cell secretion of FasL-bearing microvesicles. *J Exp Med* 2002; 195:1303–1316.

75. Abrahams VM, Straszewski SL, Kamsteeg M, et al. Epithelial ovarian cancer cells secrete Fas ligand. *Cancer Res* 2003; 63:5573–5581.

76. Taylor DD, Gercel-Taylor C, Lyons KS, Stanson J, Whiteside TL. T-cell apoptosis and suppression of T-cell receptor/CD3-ζ by Fas ligand-containing membrane vesicles shed from ovarian tumors. *Clin Cancer Res* 2003; 9:5113–5119.

77. Shurin MR, Lu L, Kalinski P, Stewart-Akers AM, Lotze MT. Th1/Th2 balance in cancer, transplantation and pregnancy. *Springer Semin Immunopathol* 1999; 21:339–359.

78. Rivoltini L, Carrabba M, Huber V, et al. Immunity to cancer: attack and escape in T lymphocyte-tumor cell interaction. *Immunol Rev* 2002; 188:97–113.

79. Singh RK, Varney ML. IL-8 expression in malignant melanoma: implications in growth and metastasis. *Histol Histopathol* 2000; 15:843–849.

80. Groh V, Wu J, Yee C, Spies T. Tumour-derived soluble MIC ligands impair expression of NKG2D and T-cell activation. *Nature* 2002; 419:734–738.

81. Doubrovina ES, Doubrovin MM, Vider E, et al. Evasion from NK cell immunity by MHC class I chain-related molecules expressing colon adenocarcinoma. *J Immunol* 2003; 171:6891–6899.

82. Wu JD, Higgins LM, Steinle A, Cosman D, Haugk K, Plymate SR. Prevalent expression of the immunostimulatory MHC class I chain-related molecule is counteracted by shedding in prostate cancer. *J Clin Invest* 2004; 114:560–568.

83. Streit M, Detmar M. Angiogenesis, lymphangiogenesis, and melanoma metastasis. *Oncogene* 2003; 22:3172–3179.

84. Finke J, Ferrone S, Frey A, Mufson A, Ochoa A. Where have all the T cells gone? Mechanisms of immune evasion by tumors. *Immunol Today* 1999; 20:158–160.

85. Ivanov VN, Bhoumik A, Ronai Z. Death receptors and melanoma resistance to apoptosis. *Oncogene* 2003; 22:3152–3161.

86. Van Parijs L, Ibrahimov A, Abbas AK. The roles of costimulation and Fas in T cell apoptosis and peripheral tolerance. *Immunity* 1996; 93:951–955.

87. Carreno BM, Collins M. The B7 family of ligands and its receptors: new pathways for costimulation and inhibition of immune responses. *Annu Rev Immunol* 2002; 20:29–53.

88. Chen L. Co-inhibitory molecules of the B7-CD28 family in the control of T-cell immunity. *Nat Rev Immunol* 2004; 4:336–347.

89. Shurin MR, Gabrilovich DI. Regulation of dendritic cell system by tumor. *Cancer Res Ther Control* 2001; 11:65–78.

90. Pirtskhalaishvili G, Shurin GV, Esche C, Salup RR, Lotze MT, Shurin MR. Cytokine-mediated protection of human dendritic cells from prostate cancer-induced apoptosis is regulated by the Bcl-2 family of proteins. *Br J Cancer* 2000; 83:506–513.

91. Esche C, Shurin GV, Kirkwood JM, et al. TNF-α-promoted expression of Bcl-2 and inhibition of mitochondrial cytochrome *c* release mediated resistance of mature dendritic cells to melanoma-induced apoptosis. *Clin Cancer Res* 2001; 7:974–979.

92. Moretta L, Ferlazzo G, Mingari MC, Melioli G, Moretta A. Human natural killer cell function and their interactions with dendritic cells. *Vaccine* 2003; 21(Suppl 2):S38–S42.

93. Gabrilovich DI, Velders MP, Sotomayor EM, Kast WM. Mechanism of immune dysfunction in cancer mediated by immature Gr-1[+] myeloid cells. *J Immunol* 2001; 166:5398–5406.

94. Terabe M, Matsui S, Park JM, et al. Transforming growth factor-beta production and myeloid cells are an effector mechanism through which CD1d-restricted T cells block cytotoxic T lymphocyte-mediated tumor immunosurveillance: abrogation prevents tumor recurrence. *J Exp Med* 2003; 198:1741–1752.

95. Kusmartsev S, Nefedova Y, Yoder D, Gabrilovich DI. Antigen-specific inhibition of CD8+ T cell response by immature myeloid cells in cancer is mediated by reactive oxygen species. *J Immunol* 2004; 172:989–999.

96. Serafini P, De Santo C, Marigo I, et al. Derangement of immune responses by myeloid suppressor cells. *Cancer Immunol Immunother* 2004; 53:64–72.

97. Terabe M, Berzofsky JA. Immunoregulatory T cells in tumor immunity. *Curr Opin Immunol* 2004; 16: 157–162.

98. Liyanage UK, Moore TT, Joo HG, et al. Prevalence of regulatory T cells is increased in peripheral blood and tumor microenvironment of patients with pancreas or breast adenocarcinoma. *J Immunol* 2002; 169:2756–2761.

99. Woo EY, Chu CS, Goletz TJ, et al. Regulatory CD4(+)CD25(+) T cells in tumors from patients with early-stage non-small cell lung cancer and late-stage ovarian cancer. *Cancer Res* 2001; 61:4766–4772.

100. Onyango P. Genomics and cancer. *Curr Opin Oncol* 2002; 14:79–85.

101. Riker A, Cormier J, Panelli M, et al. Immune selection after antigen-specific immunotherapy of melanoma. *Surgery* 1999; 126:112–120.

102. Hoffmann TK, Nakano K, Elder EM, et al. Generation of T cells specific for the wild-type sequence p53(264–272) peptide in cancer patients: implications for immunoselection of epitope loss variants. *J Immunol* 2000; 165:5938–5944.

103. Slingluff CL Jr, Colella TA, Thompson L, et al. Melanomas with concordant loss of multiple melanocytic differentiation proteins: immune escape that may be overcome by targeting unique or undefined antigens. *Cancer Immunol Immunother* 2000; 48:661–672.

104. Saleh FH, Crotty KA, Hersey P, Menzies SW, Rahman W. Autonomous histopathological regression of primary tumours associated with specific immune responses to cancer antigens. *J Pathol* 2003; 200: 383–395.

105. Chang CC, Campoli M, Ferrone S. HLA class I antigens and malignant disease. *Adv Cancer Res* 2005; 93:189–234.

106. Landowski TH, Qu N, Buyuksal I, Painter JS, Dalton WS. Mutations in the Fas antigen in patients with multiple myeloma. *Blood* 1997; 90:4266–4270.

107. Shin MS, Park WS, Kim SY, et al. Alterations of Fas (Apo-1/CD95) gene in cutaneous malignant melanoma. *Am J Pathol* 1999; 154:1785–1791.

108. Medema JP, de Jong J, Peltenburg LT, et al. Blockade of the granzyme B/perforin pathway through overexpression of the serine protease inhibitor PI-9/SPI-6 constitutes a mechanism for immune escape by tumors. *Proc Natl Acad Sci USA* 2001; 98:11,515–11,520.

109. Trapani JA, Sutton VR, Smyth MJ. CTL granules: evolution of vesicles essential for combating virus infections. *Immunol Today* 1999; 20:351–356.

110. Mailliard RB, Egawa S, Cai Q, et al. Complementary dendritic cell-activating function of CD8+ and CD4+ cells: helper role of CD8+ T cells in the development of T helper type 1 responses. *J Exp Med* 2002; 195:473–483.

111. Mailliard RB, Son Y-I, Redlinger R, et al. Dendritic cells mediate NK cell help for Th1 and CTL responses: two-signal requirement for the induction of NK cell helper function. *J Immunol* 2003; 171: 2366–2373.

112. Tatsumi T, Kierstead LS, Ranieri E, et al. MAGE-6 encodes DRβ1*0401-presented epitopes recognized by CD4+ T cells derived from patients with melanoma or renal cell carcinoma. *Clin Cancer Res* 2003; 9:947–954.

113. Lotze MT. Cytokines and the treatment of cancer. In: Weir DM, Herzenberg LA, Herzenberg LA, Blackwell CC, eds. *The Handbook of Experimental Immunology, 5th Edition*. Cambridge, MA: Blackwell Sciences. 1996: pp. 199.1–199.25.

114. Chambers CA, Kuhns MS, Egen JG, Allison JP. CTLA-4-mediated inhibition in regulation of T cell responses: mechanisms and manipulation in tumor immunotherapy. *Annu Rev Immunol* 2001; 19: 565–594.

115. Phan GQ, Yang JC, Sherry RM, et al. Cancer regression and autoimmunity induced by cytotoxic T lymphocyte-associated antigen 4 blockade in patients with metastatic melanoma. *Proc Natl Acad Sci USA* 2003; 100:8372–8377.

116. Yu Z, Restifo NP. Cancer vaccines: progress reveals new complexities. *J Clin Invest* 2002; 110:289–294.

117. Bystryn JC, Zeleniuch-Jacquotte A, Oratz R, Shapiro RL, Harris MN, Roses DF. Double-blind trial of a polyvalent, shed-antigen, melanoma vaccine. *Clin Cancer Res* 2001; 7:1882–1887.

118. Belli F, Testori A, Rivoltini L, et al. Vaccination of metastatic melanoma patients with autologous tumor-derived heat shock protein gp96-peptide complexes: clinical and immunologic findings. *J Clin Oncol* 2002; 20:4169–4180.

119. Berd D. M-Vax: an autologous, hapten-modified vaccine for human cancer. *Expert Opin Biol Ther* 2002; 2:335–342.

120. Ward S, Casey D, Labarthe MC, et al. Immunotherapeutic potential of whole tumour cells. *Cancer Immunol Immunother* 2002; 51:351–357.

121. Rivoltini L, Castelli C, Carrabba M, et al. Human tumor-derived heat shock protein 96 mediates in vitro activation and in vivo expansion of melanoma- and colon carcinoma-specific T cells. *J Immunol* 2003; 171:3467–3474.

122. Kiessling R, Wasserman K, Horiguchi S, et al. Tumor-induced immune dysfunction. *Cancer Immunol Immunother* 1999; 48:353–362.

123. Pawelec G, Heinzel S, Kiessling R, Muller L, Ouyang Q, Zeuthen J. Escape mechanisms in tumor immunity: a year 2000 update. *Crit Rev Oncog* 2000; 11:97–133.

124. Morton DL, Hsueh EC, Essner R, et al. Prolonged survival of patients receiving active immunotherapy with Canvaxin therapeutic polyvalent vaccine after complete resection of melanoma metastatic to regional lymph nodes. *Ann Surg* 2002; 236:438–448.

125. Sosman JA, Unger JM, Liu PY, et al. Adjuvant immunotherapy of resected, intermediate-thickness, node-negative melanoma with an allogeneic tumor vaccine: impact of HLA class I antigen expression on outcome. *J Clin Oncol* 2002; 20:2067–2075.

16 The Tumor Microenvironment

Regulation of Antitumor Immunity and Implications for Immunotherapy

George Coukos and Jose-Ramon Conejo-Garcia

SUMMARY

After more than 30 yr of crusading against cancer, targeting mostly the tumor cell cycle, the need for novel therapeutic strategies has become increasingly clear. Survival and expansion of tumor cells cannot be achieved in the absence of a favorable microenvironment, the main components of which are leukocytes, vascular cells, and fibroblasts. This tumor microenvironment critically provides growth factors and survival signals for tumor cell proliferation, secretes angiogenic factors that control tumor vascularization, and directs invasion and metastasis through adhesion molecule interactions. In addition, a successful antitumor immune response is prevented by multiple mechanisms of evasion orchestrated by nontumor cells. Understanding how the tumor microenvironment modulates the immune response is vital to designing new potential ways of boosting anticancer immunity. This chapter is focused on providing a rationale for new prospects of manipulating the tumor microenvironment to minimize escape from natural anticancer immune response and targeted immunotherapies.

Key Words: Neoplasm; vascular endothelial growth factor A; lymphocytes; tumor infiltrating; cytokines; immunotherapy.

1. INTRODUCTION

It is now generally accepted that tumor cells express unique antigens that are recognized by the immune system *(1–3)*. These can be differentiation antigens, also expressed by embryonal cells but not by adult normal cells; overexpression/amplification antigens, also expressed by normal cells but at levels that are too low to induce an immune response under physiological conditions; and newly acquired mutational antigens, resulting from mutations associated with the oncogenic process. In addition, select tumors express viral xenoantigens. CD45$^+$ leukocyte infiltration is detectable in most tumors. The presence of tumor-infiltrating T-lymphocytes has been shown to correlate with clinical outcome in vertical-growth-phase melanoma, as well as in ovarian, breast, prostate, renal cell, esophageal, and colorectal carcinomas *(4–10)*. In ovarian cancer, for example, CD45$^+$ cells represent up to 45% of total cells in many specimens *(11)*, and T-cells are detectable

From: *Cancer Drug Discovery and Development: Immunotherapy of Cancer*
Edited by: M. L. Disis © Humana Press Inc., Totowa, NJ

within tumor cell islets, in surrounding stroma, or both *(4)*. Yet, established cancers represent failures of immune surveillance *(12)*. A number of soluble, as well as membrane-bound, molecules have been isolated by tumor cells and have been postulated to mediate immune evasion, including immunosuppressive growth factors and cytokines such as vascular endothelial growth factor (VEGF)-A, transforming growth factor (TGF)-β, interleukin (IL)-10, prostaglandin E2, death ligands to the tumor necrosis factor (TNF) receptor family, such as Fas (CO95) ligand and TNF-related apoptosis-inducing ligand (TRAIL), ligands to the negative regulator cytotoxic T-lymphocyte-associated molecule (CTLA)-4, and the programmed death receptor ligand 1 (DD-L1) *(12,13)*.

In addition to the presence of tumor cells, solid cancers are composed of host cells including inflammatory leukocytes, a variety of stroma cells, and vascular endothelial cells and pericytes. This microenvironment influences in a critical manner tumor growth, invasion, and metastasis. Emerging evidence indicates that it also plays a central role in regulating immune recognition and attack of tumors.

As tumors establish themselves, complex interactions are developed between tumor cells and the host. It has been proposed that antitumor immune mechanisms edit the tumor *(12)*, promoting the expansion of tumor clones that can survive—and benefit—from the surrounding inflammation. In turn, tumor cells edit their microenvironment by influencing the expression of growth factors, cytokines, and chemokines that establish combinatorial signals in the tumor, which ultimately regulates the pattern of infiltration of inflammatory cell subtypes and endothelial cell precursors. Tumor cells also modify the function of host cells, inducing the production of factors that promote tolerance and angiogenesis. Until recently, "nontumor" host cells were thought to be normal diploid cells that do not acquire mutations. This concept has been recently challenged by reports showing the presence of the same chromosomal aberrations in endothelial cells and surrounding tumor cells in lymphomas *(14)*, as well as loss of heterozygosity in stromal cells from solid tumors *(15–17)*. These new findings, together with a revival of the immunosurveillance theory and the failure of anticancer therapies focused exclusively on inhibiting the proliferation of tumor cells, have made the role of the tumor microenvironment the subject of intensive research in the last few years. Understanding how the tumor microenvironment modulates the immune response is vital to designing new potential ways of boosting anticancer immunity. This chapter is focused on new prospects of manipulating the tumor microenvironment to minimize tumor escape from anticancer immune response.

2. EFFECTS OF THE TUMOR MICROENVIRONMENT ON ANTIGEN PRESENTATION

Dendritic cells (DCs) are viewed as critical regulators of adaptive immune responses, including those against tumors. DCs take up, process, and present antigens to naïve T-cells in major histocompatibility complex (MHC) class I- and/or class II-restricted fashion *(18)*. DCs are now recognized as a diverse population of cells with remarkable plasticity, which exhibit different phenotypes that can elicit potent type 1 T-cell stimulation, promote type 2 responses, or induce T-cell tolerance, depending on lineage and environmental instructions *(18–20)*. Although DC-based vaccine therapies are generally viewed as systemic, it is now understood that the antigen-presenting function of DCs is severely compromised in patients with cancer, not only within the tumor microenvironment, but also systemically *(21–23)*.

2.1. The Tumor Microenvironment Retains Immature DCs Within The Tumor, Preventing Adaptive Immune Response

The number and activation state of intratumoral DCs are critical factors in regulating host response to tumors *(24)*. To trigger effective immune responses, DCs should be recruited into solid tumors, engulf tumor antigen, and then undergo maturation and consequently, migrate to lymphoid organs, where they present antigen to lymphocytes. Immature DCs are attracted by select inflammatory chemokines *(25)* and are known to infiltrate tumors *(26)* through the action of chemokines, such as the CXC chemokine receptor 4 ligand stroma-derived factor (SDF)-1/CXCL12 *(27)* or the CCR6 ligand macrophage inflammatory protein (MIP)-3α/CCL20 *(28)*. β-Defensins are antimicrobial peptides that also recruit immature DCs through CCR6 *(29)*. β-Defensins are expressed by monocytes, macrophages, and DCs *(30)*, whereas we demonstrated that tumor cells also express β-defensins in ovarian cancer *(31)*. High levels of β-defensins have been described in many tumors including squamous cell head and neck tumors *(32)*, *Helicobacter pylori*-associated gastric cancer *(33,34)*, renal cancer *(35)*, colon cancer *(36)*, bladder cancer *(37)*, ovarian cancer *(31)*, oral cancer with opportunistic *Candida* infections *(38)*, and leukemia *(39)*.

Most DCs detected in tumors have an immature phenotype, and it has been proposed that such cells are retained within the tumor, a mechanism that may prevent efficient T-cell priming *(28)*. Lack of maturation in the tumor microenvironment may be one of the reasons DCs are unable to migrate to secondary lymphoid organs, as they lack expression of the CCR7 receptor, which makes them responsive to MIP-3β/CCL19 and secondary lymphoid organ/CCL21 chemokines expressed in lymph nodes. Similarly, poorly matured DCs maintain a higher expression of CXCR1, CCR1, CCR2, and CCR5 *(25)*, as well as CCR6, remaining sensitive to inflammatory chemokines expressed by the tumor.

Tumor-associated DCs express low levels of co-stimulatory molecules *(40)*, a mechanism that has been implicated in induction of tolerance *(41,42)*. Thus, immature or partially mature DCs retained in tumors may provide a constant supply of tolerogenic signals.

2.2. The Tumor Microenvironment Induces Phenotype Switch in DCs to Promote Tumor Immune Evasion, Angiogenesis, and Growth

Immunosuppressive molecules produced by tumors, such as IL-10, and TGF-β inhibit DC maturation and IL-12 production, and induce T-helper (Th)2 or regulatory T-cell responses *(43–46)*. VEGF-A, a critical mediator of the angiogenic switch in most tumors, is also a critical mediator of tumor-associated immunodeficiency. VEGF-A inhibits the differentiation of hematopoietic progenitor cells into DCs *(47)* and the maturation of DCs *(48,49)*. High levels of VEGF-A in blood result in decreased numbers of competent DCs and accumulation of immature hematopoietic cells *(50)*. Antibodies to VEGF-A enhance the efficacy of cancer immunotherapy by improving endogenous DC function *(51)*. In ovarian carcinoma, VEGF-A is a strong predictor of the absence of intratumoral T-cells *(4)*. VEGF-A may therefore affect the behavior of cancer not only by promoting angiogenesis, but also by reducing the numbers of T-cells.

In addition to the inhibition of DC maturation, we have described a novel mechanism by which VEGF-A promotes tumor vasculogenesis *(31)*. Our data indicate that tumor or host cell-derived β-defensins recruit DC precursors via CCR6 into the tumor, where VEGF-A induces them to acquire endothelial-like phenotype. These endothelial-like DCs engage in vasculogenesis and function as co-conspirators of tumor progression. This process can be blocked in vivo by targeting VEGF receptor 2, which is functionally expressed by tumor-infiltrating and bone marrow-derived DCs. Similar cooperation in the tumor is expected between VEGF-A and bona fide chemokines that recruit DC precursors via CCR6, such as MIP-3α/CCL20. We confirmed the existence of the same population of leukocytes coexpressing endothelial and DC markers in human ovarian carcinoma, where these cells were detected at remarkably high frequency in many specimens analyzed *(52)*. This new subset, named vascular leukocytes because of their mixed phenotype, has the capacity to generate functional blood vessels. Vascular leukocytes express high levels of matrix metalloproteinases 2 and 9 and VEGF-A (our unpublished observations). Their retention within the tumor therefore further contributes to angiogenesis and tumor metastasis. Although the relative contribution of β-defensins to different histological types of tumors needs to be evaluated, as many as 27 human β-defensins have been recently reported, warranting research in the context of physiological or pathological angiogenesis. Depletion of CCR6[+] cells through an immunotoxin decreases tumor growth more than 20-fold in a murine ovarian cancer model *(31)*, providing new therapeutic strategies against tumor angiogenesis.

Lineage-negative CD1a[-]CD4[+]CD11c[-]DR[+] plasmacytoid DCs (PDCs) expressing CD123, the IL-3 receptor α-chain, have been identified in tumors. High frequencies of PDCs have been detected in malignant human ovarian cancer ascites, where they are recruited by SDF-1α through CXC chemokine receptor-4 *(27)*. Tumor PDCs were found to induce significant T-cell IL-10 and inhibit T-cell activation. Importantly, tumor-associated PDCs were also recently reported to induce angiogenesis in vivo through production of TNF-α and IL-8. By contrast, bona fide myeloid DCs derived in vitro suppressed angiogenesis in vivo through production of IL-12 *(53)*.

2.3. Implications for DC Vaccine Therapies

The impairment of antigen presentation by the tumor microenvironment affects several factors regarding the production and delivery of anticancer DC vaccines. The first lesson painfully learned from clinical trials is that mature DCs are superior to immature DCs in the induction of immunological responses. A direct comparison of peptide-loaded immature and mature DCs in patients with metastatic melanoma has shown that only mature DCs induce antigen-specific cytolytic effector responses *(54)*, whereas analysis of published vaccine trials for melanoma showed that mature DCs correlated with favorable clinical outcomes *(55)*. In fact, immature DCs might rather induce tolerance to presented antigens in the context of therapeutic vaccination *(54,56)*. Therefore, DCs loaded with tumor antigen need to be matured ex vivo before injection into patients. However, in vivo matured DCs might have superior migratory and immunostimulatory capacities when compared with DCs matured ex vivo *(57)*, rendering the use of "less-than-fully" matured DCs attractive. Because tumor-derived factors can induce systemic suppression of DC differentiation and/or maturation, the level and stability of DC maturation are critical factors that may affect the efficacy of vaccine therapy. Immature DCs could revert to a phagocyte/macrophage phenotype, whereas partly mature DCs might fail to undergo full maturation, losing their antigen-presenting function *(47,51,58)*. Tumor-induced paralysis of DC function is reversible *(59,60)*. Thus, DC preparation methods become crucial in this context *(61)*. DCs with partial but irreversible maturation might be best positioned to achieve efficient vaccination. For example, genetic manipulation of DCs ex vivo to confer expression of cytokine transgenes or CD40 ligand has been shown to maintain the therapeutic potency of DC vaccines (*see* following paragraphs). Alternatively, blockade of systemic immunosuppressive factors might permit proper maturation of DCs in vivo (*62*).

One important variable affecting the efficacy of DC vaccines relates to the route of administration. Intravenous administration allows delivering large amounts of DCs, but it may not allow optimal homing of DCs to lymph nodes. Intralymphatic injection delivers DCs directly to the desired location, but requires cannulating lymphatic vessels in the feet under lymphangiography. Alternatively, intranodal vaccines are administered directly into unaltered nodes under ultrasound control. Although technically more demanding, these are the most efficient means to deliver DCs to lymph nodes, the site where T-cell priming occurs, and may augment tumor responses with respect to other routes (*63*). A far more convenient alternative for the induction of cytotoxic lymphocytes may be the commonly used subcutaneous or the emerging intradermal administration (*64–66*).

The effects of the tumor microenvironment become highly relevant in the case of intratumoral injection of DCs (*67–71*). This approach offers the distinct advantage that DCs may induce vaccination by capturing antigen available *in situ*, obviating the need of preparing tumor antigen ex vivo (*72*). Ex vivo manipulation of DCs to ensure maturation *in situ* via transfection with inflammatory cytokines, such as IL-7, IL-12, IL-18, or CD40 ligand, has facilitated tumor immune rejection (*73–78*). Alternatively, timed administration of chemotherapy or radiation therapy may provide similar benefits, possibly through the combined production of massive tumor cell death and manipulation of the tumor microenvironment (*79–83*). Similar concepts may be applicable to vaccination via systemic routes. For example, timed administration of select chemotherapy agents before vaccination has been shown to dramatically enhance the efficacy of tumor vaccines (*84, 85*), partly through the suppression of regulatory cell populations (*86*).

3. EFFECTS OF THE TUMOR MICROENVIRONMENT ON EFFECTOR MECHANISMS

3.1. Cytokine-Mediated Tumor Immune Evasion

Tumors play an important role in mediating antigen-specific immune evasion through at least three mechanisms: functional suppression through switch of the cytokine milieu from Th1 to Th2 or Th3 (regulatory), deletion of tumor antigen-specific T-cells, and induction of tolerance through expansion of T-regulatory (Treg) cells (*41*). The tumor microenvironment may induce myeloid DCs to acquire a type 2 cytokine profile through the production of IL-4 and IL-10 (*87*), as well as the production of prostaglandin E2 (*88,89*), resulting in a change from Th1 to Th2 responses, which is believed to be less efficient at tumor rejection (*90*). Type 2 cytokine polarization of the tumor microenvironment further affects the phenotype of effector cells, as chemokines tend to reproduce the Th1/Th2 dichotomy applied to cytokines. Thus, Th2 cells produce preferentially type 2 chemokines, which in turn attract more Th2 cells (*see* Subheading 3.5).

IL-10 and TGF-β are powerful immunosuppressive factors that can block activation and function of effector T-cells. IL-10 inhibits CD28 tyrosine phosphorylation, the initial step of the CD28 signaling pathway, and consequently, the phosphatidylinositol 3-kinase p85 binding to CD28. IL-10 only inhibits T-cells stimulated by low numbers of triggered T-cell receptors, which therefore depend on CD28 co-stimulation. T-cells receiving a strong signal from the T-cell receptor alone, and thus not requiring CD28 co-stimulation, are not affected by IL-10. Thus, IL-10-induced selective inhibition of the CD28 co-stimulatory pathway acts as a decisive mechanism in determining whether a T-cell will contribute to an immune response or become anergic *(91)*. TGF-β also directly inhibits activation and interferon (IFN)-γ or IL-2 production by T-cells and counters the ability of IL-12 to activate T-cell Janus kinase–signal transducing and activators of transcription pathway signaling. The critical nature of the TGF-β signaling pathway in regulating effector T-cell function has been documented in transgenic mice in which expression of a dominant-negative TGF-β receptor II under a T-cell-specific promoter culminates in spontaneous T-cell activation, Th1 and Th2 cytokine release, and autoimmune, inflammatory disease affecting the lung, colon, stomach, pancreas, and/or kidney *(92)*. Vice versa, administration of TGF-β can prevent or inhibit experimental autoimmune diseases *(93)*.

3.2. Apoptotic Depletion of Effector T-Cells

The mechanism of deletion of antigen-specific T-cell clones is not precisely understood. Activated lymphocytes express death receptors and become susceptible to "fratricide" killing by lymphocytes *(94,95)* and/or by nonlymphoid cells expressing the cognate ligands *(96,97)*. Fas/CD95 mediates rapid apoptosis through recruitment and activation of caspase 8 *(98,99)*. Its cognate ligand, Fas ligand (FasL), has been implicated in the control of autoimmunity *(100)* and establishment of immune privilege in reproductive organs *(100–102)*. In the context of cancer, FasL expressed at the surface of tumor cells has been related to the organization of an "immune privilege" in the tumor by inducing Fas-mediated apoptosis of antitumor T-cells *(103)*. However, this role has been questioned because of the lack of specificity of the antibodies employed to detect FasL *(104)*. Although it is possible that only a small proportion of tumor cells express membrane-bound FasL, intracellular FasL secreted in the context of microvesicles released by tumor cells may induce Fas-mediated lymphocyte apoptosis *(105)*. In addition, DCs expressing FasL have been associated with the induction of apoptosis of T-cells during antigen presentation, thus inducing antigen-specific tolerance *(4)*.

Ligands for programmed cell death (PD)-1, B7-H1/PD-L1 and PD-L2, expressed by tumor cells or leukocytes (including DCs), are responsible for inducing tumor immune evasion, in part trough contact-dependent apoptosis of effector tumor-infiltrating lymphocytes (TILs) *(106–108)*. Virtually all myeloid DCs isolated from ovarian carcinomas or draining lymph nodes express B7-H1, which is upregulated in DCs by IL-10 and VEGF-A *(109)*. In a murine model, forced expression of B7-H1 in highly immunogenic tumors expressing B7-1 induced dramatic tumor progression by abrogating tumor immunity. On the contrary, tumors expressing only B7-1 could induce vigorous T-cell activation and underwent complete regression after injection into syngeneic mice *(106)*. These results demonstrate that expression of B7-H1 evades tumor immunity, abrogating CD28 co-stimulation.

Lastly, tumor cells and select leukocyte subsets including CD123+CCR6+ PDCs produce indolamine 2,3-dioxygenase (IDO), which profoundly inhibits T-cell proliferation *(110,111)* and can induce Fas-independent T-cell apoptosis by degrading tryptophan *(112, 113)*. Tryptophan metabolites in the kynurenine pathway, such as 3-hydroxyanthranilic and quinolinic acids, induce selective apoptosis of Th1, but not Th2 cells. T-cell apoptosis requires relatively low concentrations of kynurenines and is associated with the activation of casapase 8 and the release of cytochrome *c* from mitochondria *(114)*. The finding that a subset of PDCs constitutively expresses immunosuppressive levels of IDO selectively in tumor-draining (but not in normal) lymph nodes suggests a very early role of IDO in apoptotic depletion or anergy of tumor-specific T-cells. Despite comprising only 0.5% of lymph nodes cells, these PDCs in vitro potently suppressed T-cell responses to antigens presented by the PDCs themselves and, in a dominant fashion, suppressed T-cell responses to third-party antigens presented by nonsuppressive antigen-presenting cells (APCs). Importantly, anergy was prevented by targeted disruption of the IDO gene in the DCs or by administration of the IDO inhibitor L-methyl-D-tryptophan to recipient mice (111).

3.3. Regulatory T-Cells

A critical mechanism of peripheral immune tolerance is mediated by CD4$^+$CD25$^+$ Tregs. Tregs represent a heterogeneous population: One subset is naturally occurring, developing during the normal process of T-cell maturation in the thymus as polyclonal populations that recognize a variety of self-antigens. Although Tregs represent 5–10% of the CD25$^+$ population, the Treg TCR repertoire is as diverse as the CD25$^-$ repertoire (115). Interestingly, there is only limited overlap, and Tregs exhibit a high frequency of T-cell receptors (TCRs) directed against self-antigens presented by APCs through MHC class II molecules. This implies that at least a fraction of naturally arising Tregs is chronically stimulated. Because many tumor antigens represent molecules expressed at very low levels by normal cells, Tregs showing a TCR directed against those antigens might be specifically expanded during tumor progression. Other "adaptive" Tregs are induced on antigenic stimulation (116,117), apparently by activation of mature T-cells under conditions of suboptimal antigen exposure or co-stimulation. Tumor VEGF and macrophage-secreted IL-10 induce tumor-infiltrating DCs to express inhibitory B7-H1. The T-cells induced by these tumor-conditioned DCs display many properties of Tregs, suffer programmed cell death, and IL-10 is produced during priming (109). The first direct in vivo evidence that human Tregs play an immunopathological role in human cancer has been recently provided (118). Treg accumulation predicted a remarkable decrease in patient survival, providing the final proof linking Tregs and the immunopathogenesis of human ovarian cancer.

Tregs prevent specific T-cell immunity against tumor-associated antigens by suppressing effector T-cell activation, secretion of IL-2 and IFN-γ, and inhibiting specific cytotoxicity in a contact-dependent fashion. Tregs in tumors are generally in the proximity of CD8$^+$ T-cells and spontaneously express CTLA-4. Another part of the suppressive phenomena can be attributed to secretion of immunosuppressive cytokines, such as IL-10 and TGF-β (119,120). Interestingly, in human ovarian carcinomas Tregs migrate preferentially to tumor mass and associated malignant ascites, rather than to the draining lymph nodes. Given that T-cell priming probably takes place mainly in lymph nodes, CD4$^+$CD25$^+$ Tregs in cancer may primarily work by inhibiting the extranodal effector cell function of cytotoxic CD8$^+$ cells. Why Tregs are more represented in tumors than in the draining node is not entirely clear, although tumor Tregs express functional CCR4, the receptor for monocyte-derived chemokine (MDC)/CCL22. The source of this chemoattractant CCL22 may be ovarian cancer cells (4) or tumor macrophages. Notably, Tregs functionally respond to MIP-3α/CCL20 (121), which specifically interact with CCR6.

Treg depletion by anti-CD25 monoclonal antibody-induced effective immune responses against syngeneic tumors in mice that did not previously respond to immune therapy (122, 123). Targeting of Tregs is currently undergoing clinical testing using anti-CTLA-4 monoclonal antibody (124,125) or DAB(389)/IL-2 diphtheria toxin fusion protein (denileukin diftitox, ONTAK® directed against IL-2 receptor/CD25 (126), with promising results. The idea that elimination of Tregs by lymphoablative chemotherapy possibly contributed to regression of metastatic melanoma and clonal repopulation of adoptively transferred tumor-specific T-cells in a recent study is certainly tantalizing *(127)*. If these initial data are confirmed, suppression of Tregs will certainly become an important component of tumor immunotherapy strategies. A better understanding about the generation, function, and migratory capacities of Tregs will assist in the development of novel combinatorial immune-boosting strategies based on removing this suppressive subset.

3.4. Natural-Killer Group 2D-Dependent Immune Responses

Although tumors represent failures of immune surveillance, evidence that tumors are kept in check by cell-mediated immunity continues to accumulate in humans. For example, we have demonstrated that the presence of intratumoral T-cells in ovarian carcinoma denotes ongoing activation of antitumor immune response (unpublished observations) and associates with significantly longer survival *(4)*. Critical to an antitumor immune response are the balance between inhibitory and activating signals in tumor-specific CTLs. CTLs recognizing tumor antigens presented in the context of MHC class I complexes. Thus, vigorous expression of MHC I by tumors favors immune recognition, whereas loss of MHC I allows evasion *(12)*.

Natural-killer group 2D (NKG2D) is an activating receptor expressed on most NK cells, CD8+ T-cells, and $\gamma\delta$ T-cells. It binds to the adaptor molecule DNAX-activation protein 10, and interacts with phosphoinositide-3 kinases on phosphorylation *(128–130)*. There is evidence that ligands for NKG2D mark tumor cells for cell-mediated killing. Thus, ectopic expression of murine ligands results in cell-mediated rejection of tumor cells *(131)*. Furthermore, skin-associated $\gamma\delta$ T-cells can mediate destruction of carcinoma cells utilizing a mechanism dependent on NKG2D receptor engagement *(132)*.

Several human and murine molecules related to class I MHC molecules have been identified as ligands for NKG2D. In humans, the ligands for NKG2D fall into either the MHC I-related chain (MIC) group or the UL-16 binding protein (ULBP) group. The MIC group consists of MICA and MICB, which are encoded within the human MHC, and are expressed on a wide range of epithelial tumors *(128)*. MICA and MICB are stress-inducible molecules that trigger NK cell target cytotoxicity and function as a costimulatory molecule that can substitute for B7 ligand *(133)*. The ULBP group consists of ULBP1, ULBP2, and ULBP3, identified based on their ability to bind to the human cytomegalovirus glycoprotein UL-16 *(134,135)*. We reported the discovery of a new MHC I-related ligand for the NKG2D receptor that we named lymphocyte effector cell toxicity activation ligand (Letal) *(11, 136)*. Letal was shown to afford co-stimulation in CD8+ CTLs, inducing their expansion and activation; increased glycolytic influx; downregulated Fas; and protected CD8+ lymphocytes from FasL-induced programmed cell death or apoptosis induced by cytotoxic drugs *(136)*. Most advanced stage ovarian cancers expressing NKG2D ligand Letal also express MHC I. Therefore, tumor cells coexpressing MHC I and Letal are able to present efficiently their specific antigens to competent cytotoxic T-cells, providing both signal 1 and signal 2. Importantly, a significant proportion of CD8+ TILs are CD28[neg/low] in ovarian cancer, indicating that they are sensitive to NKG2D ligands but not CD28 ligands for co-stimulation *(11)*. We found that Letal was upregulated in advanced ovarian carcinomas with intratumoral T-cells, in spite of FasL expression in vivo. These results suggest an important role for Letal in the homeostasis of peripheral CD8+ effector T-cells and the immune defense against tumors in the human.

A variation of a method for the expansion of T-cells through APCs *(137)* has been described based on expression of Letal *(11)*. Thus, the stimulatory effects of NKG2D ligands could be used to expand in vitro tumor-reactive T-cells for adoptive transfer. The efficacy of adoptive transfer of ex vivo expanded tumor-infiltrating lymphocytes has been recently documented in chemoresistant melanoma *(138)*. NKG2D ligands could accelerate the generation of clinically relevant amounts of effector T-cells derived from CD8+ CD28$^{neg/low}$ TILs. Furthermore, CD8+ cytotoxic lymphocytes expanded through costimulation of NKG2D could prove resistant to apoptosis in vivo and thus, have improved engraftment capability.

Given the above, how do tumors evade NKG2D-supported immune surveillance mechanisms? One mechanism may relate to the action of metalloproteases, which may release soluble MICA fragments or phospholipase C and which may cleave phophastidyl-inositol glycane-anchored molecules, such as ULBP1-3, in the tumor microenvironment. Shedding of NKG2D ligands may not only abrogate activation, but may also attenuate the expression of NKG2D on host immune CD8+ T-cells *(139)*. Thus, it has been suggested that the immunological competence of patients with cancer may be compromised, rather than enhanced, by NKG2D ligands. However, because engagement of NKG2D in the absence of TCR signaling increases glucose metabolism and survival of CD8+ lymphocytes *(136)*, the effect of shedding of NKG2D ligands warrants further investigation in the context of cancer.

3.5. Cytokine–Chemokine Networks

During the orchestration of the immune response, Th cells, DCs, and other leukocytes express cytokines that define Th1/Th2 dominance. Accordingly, Th1 cells trigger cellular immunity to combat intracellular pathogens, such as viruses, allotransplants, and tumor cells, whereas Th2 cells drive humoral immunity and upregulate antibody production to fight extracellular organisms. Because either pathway can downregulate the other, Th1 responses would be responsible for protective anticancer immunity, whereas Th2 responses would drive nonprotective responses. In human tumors, this model is probably too simplistic, because cytokines are seldom restricted to pure Th1 or Th2 patterns. Humoral immunity may in fact cooperate with cellular immunity in coordinated immunity programs to successfully reject tumors *(140,141)*. However, the Th1/Th2 hypothesis is a model of cellular interactions still used to understand anticancer immune response *(142)*.

Critical cytokines produced by Th1 cells are IFN-γ, IL-12, and IL-2, whereas IL-4 and IL-10 are associated with Th2 cells. In agreement with this model of polarization, the presence of intratumoral T-cells, was found to correlate with improved outcome and increased expression of IFN-γ and IL-2 in human ovarian carcinoma *(4)*, whereas these cytokines were undetectable in tumors where T-cells were absent from tumor islets (but still present in surrounding stroma). In contrast, IL-10, the main function of which is to limit and eventually terminate inflammatory responses, has been reported overexpressed in different carcinomas, melanoma, and lymphoma/myeloma *(143)*. Immunosuppressive IL-10 is produced by both tumor cells and tumor-infiltrating leukocytes, e.g., CD14+CD16+CD54+ CD11a^{neg}CD11b^{neg} human leukocyte antigen-DR^{neg} monocytes in ovarian cancer *(144)*.

Chemokines cooperate with cytokines to establish polarity in the tumor microenvironment and by doing so, may directly contribute to tumor progression or rejection. For example, IFN-inducible protein (IP)-10 /CXCL10, IFN-inducible T-cell-α chemoattractant (I-TAC)/CXCL11, monokine-induced by IFN-γ (MIG)/CXCL9 and regulated on activation, normal T-cell-expressed and -secreted (RANTES)/CCL5 are upregulated by IFN-γ, an effect that is antagonized by IL-4 and IL-10 *(145)*. IFN-inducible chemokines play a central role in the orchestration of type 1 T-cell-mediated pathological responses, including transplant rejection, autoimmune inflammatory lesions, and atherosclerosis *(146– 149)*. MIG alone is capable of restoring rejection of allografts in IFN-γ knockout mice, whereas its neutralization abrogates the accumulation of T-cells and rejection of major histocompatibility mismatched skin allografts *(150)*. Th1 cells and CTLs with type 1 polarized cytokine production (Tc1) express receptors for type 1 chemokines including CXCR3 (receptor for IP-10, I-TAC, and MIG) and CCR5 (receptor for RANTES) at higher levels than Th2 and Tc2 cells *(25)*. In stage III ovarian carcinoma, MIG expression correlates significantly with the expression of IFN-γ and the presence of intratumoral T-cells (T-cells infiltrating tumor islets). Approximately 30% of CD8$^+$ T-cells isolated from peripheral blood of patients with expressed CXCR3 by flow cytometry. A marked upregulation of CXCR3 (and CD25) was noted following activation through CD3/CD28 co-stimulation ex vivo, suggesting that CXC3 ligands recruit effector CD8$^+$ T-cells to the tumor (our unpublished observations).

Two other chemokines that attract naïve or memory noneffector T-cells related to the presence of intratumoral T-cells in ovarian cancer are MDC/CCL22 and secondary lymphoid tissue chemokine/exodus 2/CCL21 *(4)*. Their expression may denote the organization of a secondary lymphoid organ-type inflammatory infiltrate, facilitating tumor antigen presentation through the interaction between mature APCs and naïve or memory T-cells in select tumors. Illustrating the relevance of chemokines in antigen presentation, a recent study demonstrated the induction of critical effector T-cells with mixtures of chemokines and tumor antigen or naked DNA plasmid vaccines *(151)*. However, MDC has also been implicated in the recruitment of Tregs, suggesting that chemokine networks cooperate with other factors in the tumor microenvironment to promote rejection or tolerance mechanisms.

Th2 cells express higher levels of CCR3, a low-specificity receptor for RANTES, eotaxins 1–3, and monocyte chemoattractant proteins (MCP)2–4; CCR4, a receptor for thymus and activation-regulated chemokine/CCL17 and MDC/CCL22; and CCR8, the receptor for I-309/CCL1. Peripheral blood CCR3$^+$ memory T-cells display a Th2 cytokine profile *(25)*, and T-cell clones derived from tissues with an ongoing allergic response express CCR3 *(152)*. Tc2 cells show a similar distribution of receptors for inflammatory chemokines, with markedly enhanced transcripts for CCR3, CCR4, and CCR8. Type 2 chemokines, such as IL-4 and IL-13, stimulate the production of eotaxin and MDC, which is counteracted by IFN-γ *(153)*.

In addition to being a key determinant of the polarity of TILs, chemokines regulate the trafficking of regulatory leukocytes. Tregs express known type 2 chemokine receptors, such as CCR3, CCR4, and CCR8, and respond to their cognate ligands *(154)*. For example, MDC/CCL22 recruits Tregs via CCR4 in ovarian cancer *(118)*. Notably, Tregs also respond to MIP-3/CCL20 *(121)*, which specifically interacts with CCR6. In human ovarian carcinoma, SDF-1α/CXCL12 produced by epithelial tumor cells recruits PDCs. This subtype of DCs expresses low levels of co-stimulatory molecules and induces tolerogenic IL-10-secreting T-cells *(27)*.

Finally, chemokines directly or indirectly regulate angiogenesis through the recruitment of cndothelial cell precursors or leukocytes that support angiogenesis. This topic has been reviewed extensively by others and is beyond the scope of the present chapter.

Suffice it to say, however, that type 1 chemokines, such as CXCR3 ligands MIG, IP-10, and I-TAC, exert antiangiogenic effects, whereas type 2 chemokines or chemokines involved in the recruitment of regulatory cell populations (e.g., SDF-1α) or monocytes and macrophages (e.g., MCP-1/CCL2) may promote angiogenesis, as the latter produce high levels of VEGF and metalloproteases *(155)*. Other angiogenic chemokines are the CXCL1 chemokines MIP-2 and cytokine-induced neutrophil chemoattractant, as well as neutrophil-activating peptide 2/CXCL7 and lipopolysaccharide-inducible CXC chemokine/CXCL5 (all through CXCR2) *(156)* and eotaxin/CCL11 (through CCR3) *(157)*. Microvascular endothelial cells also express CCR2 and respond chemotactically to MCP-1, thus providing a direct angiogenic mechanism. Thus, chemokines exert complex roles in the tumor microenvironment, which regulate immune cell trafficking, immune surveillance, and angiogenesis.

4. CONCLUDING REMARKS

After the disappointment of anticancer strategies paying attention solely to the tumor cell, during the last years the tumor microenvironment has been the subject of intensive research. It influences in a critical manner tumor growth and invasion, to the point that many primary tumor cells cannot grow in xenograft models in the absence of this favorable milieu. The tumor microenvironment determines many surprising immunological features associated with tumor immune evasion, allowing tumor cells to escape from cytotoxic effector cells. On the other hand, immune cells successfully recognize and attack select tumors. Understanding these mechanisms has evident implications for cancer immunotherapy and will help to tailor specific therapeutic strategies for each tumor. Unlike other anticancer strategies, manipulating the antitumor immune response offers two advantageous properties necessary for a definitive treatment: memory and specificity. However, there is a long way to go before we can effectively manipulate these remarkable features to fight tumors.

REFERENCES

1. Rosenberg SA. The identification of cancer antigens: impact on the development of cancer vaccines. *Cancer J* 2000; 6(Suppl 2):S142–149.
2. Zeng G. MHC class II-restricted tumor antigens recognized by CD4+ T cells: new strategies for cancer vaccine design. *J Immunother* 2001: 24:195–204.
3. Novellino L, Castelli C, Parmiani G. A listing of human tumor antigens recognized by T cells: March 2004 update. *Cancer Immunol Immunother* 2004: 54:187–207.
4. Zhang L, Conejo-Garcia JR, Katsaros D, et al. Intratumoral T cells, recurrence, and survival in epithelial ovarian cancer. *N Engl J Med* 2003, 348:203–213.
5. Schumacher K, Haensch W, Roefzaad C, Schlag PM. Prognostic significance of activated CD8(+) T cell infiltrations within esophageal carcinomas. *Cancer Res* 2001; 61:3932–3936.
6. Marrogi AJ, Munshi A, Merogi AJ, et al. Study of tumor infiltrating lymphocytes and transforming growth factor-beta as prognostic factors in breast carcinoma. *Int J Cancer* 1997; 74:492–501.
7. Vesalainen S, Lipponen P, Talja M, Syrjanen K. Histological grade, perineural infiltration, tumour-infiltrating lymphocytes and apoptosis as determinants of long-term prognosis in prostatic adenocarcinoma. *Eur J Cancer* 1994; 30A:1797–1803.
8. Halpern AC, Schuchter LM Prognostic models in melanoma. *Semin Oncol* 1997; 24:S2–S7.
9. Naito Y, Saito K, Shiiba K, et al. CD8+ T cells infiltrated within cancer cell nests as a prognostic factor in human colorectal cancer. *Cancer Res* 1998; 58:3491–3494.
10. Nakano O, Sato M, Naito Y, et al. Proliferative activity of intratumoral CD8(+) T-lymphocytes as a prognostic factor in human renal cell carcinoma: clinicopathologic demonstration of antitumor immunity. *Cancer Res* 2001; 61:5132–5136.

11. Conejo-Garcia JR, Benencia F, Courreges MC, et al. Ovarian carcinoma expresses the NKG2D ligand Letal and promotes the survival and expansion of CD28(−) antitumor T cells. *Cancer Res* 2004; 64: 2175–2182.

12. Dunn GP, Old LJ, Schreiber RD. The three Es of cancer immunoediting. *Annu Rev Immunol* 2004; 22: 329–360.

13. Iwai Y, Ishida M, Tanaka Y, Okazaki T, Honjo T, Minato N. Involvement of PD-L1 on tumor cells in the escape from host immune system and tumor immunotherapy by PD-L1 blockade. *Proc Natl Acad Sci USA* 2002; 99:12,293–12,297.

14. Streubel B, Chott A, Huber D, et al. Lymphoma-specific genetic aberrations in microvascular endothelial cells in B-cell lymphomas. *N Engl J Med* 2004; 351:250–259.

15. Kurose K, Hoshaw-Woodard S, Adeyinka A, Lemeshow S, Watson PH, Eng C. Genetic model of multi-step breast carcinogenesis involving the epithelium and stroma: clues to tumour-microenvironment interactions. *Hum Mol Genet* 2001; 10:1907–1913.

16. Lakhani SR, Jacquemier J, Sloane JP, et al. Multifactorial analysis of differences between sporadic breast cancers and cancers involving BRCA1 and BRCA2 mutations. *J Natl Cancer Inst* 1998; 90:1138–1145.

17. Moinfar F, Man YG, Arnould L, Bratthauer GL, Ratschek M, Tavassoli FA. Concurrent and independent genetic alterations in the stromal and epithelial cells of mammary carcinoma: implications for tumorigenesis. *Cancer Res* 2000; 60:2562–2566.

18. Banchereau J, Briere F, Caux C, et al. Immunobiology of dendritic cells. *Annu Rev Immunol* 2000; 18: 767–811.

19. Bhardwaj N. Processing and presentation of antigens by dendritic cells: implications for vaccines. *Trends Mol Med* 2001; 7:388–394.

20. Steinman RM, Turley S, Mellman I, Inaba K. The induction of tolerance by dendritic cells that have captured apoptotic cells. *J Exp Med* 2000; 191:411–416.

21. Yang L, Carbone DP. Tumor-host immune interactions and dendritic cell dysfunction. *Adv Cancer Res* 2004; 92:13–27.

22. Yang AS, Lattime EC. Tumor-induced interleukin 10 suppresses the ability of splenic dendritic cells to stimulate CD4 and CD8 T-cell responses. *Cancer Res* 2003; 63:2150–2157.

23. Tourkova IL, Yamabe K, Chatta G, Shurin GV, Shurin MR. NK cells mediate Flt3 ligand-induced protection of dendritic cell precursors in vivo from the inhibition by prostate carcinoma in the murine bone marrow metastasis model. *J Immunother* 2003; 26:468–472.

24. Furumoto K, Soares L, Engleman EG, Merad M. Induction of potent antitumor immunity by in situ targeting of intratumoral DCs. *J Clin Invest* 2004; 113:774–783.

25. Sallusto F, Lenig D, Mackay CR, Lanzavecchia A. Flexible programs of chemokine receptor expression on human polarized T helper 1 and 2 lymphocytes. *J Exp Med* 1998; 187:875–883.

26. Vicari AP, Treilleux I, Lebecque S. Regulation of the trafficking of tumour-infiltrating dendritic cells by chemokines. *Semin Cancer Biol* 2004; 14:161–169.

27. Zou W, Machelon V, Coulomb-L'Hermin A, et al. Stromal-derived factor-1 in human tumors recruits and alters the function of plasmacytoid precursor dendritic cells. *Nat Med* 2001; 7:1339–1346.

28. Bell D, Chomarat P, Broyles D, et al. In breast carcinoma tissue, immature dendritic cells reside within the tumor, whereas mature dendritic cells are located in peritumoral areas. *J Exp Med* 1999; 190:1417–1426.

29. Yang D, Chertov O, Bykovskaia SN, et al. Beta-defensins: linking innate and adaptive immunity through dendritic and T cell CCR6. *Science* 1999; 286:525–528.

30. Duits LA, Ravensbergen B, Rademaker M, Hiemstra PS, Nibbering PH. Expression of beta-defensin 1 and 2 mRNA by human monocytes, macrophages and dendritic cells. *Immunology* 2002; 106:517–525.

31. Conejo-Garcia JR, Benencia F, Courreges MC, et al. Tumor-infiltrating dendritic cell precursors recruited by a beta-defensin contribute to vasculogenesis under the influence of Vegf-A. *Nat Med* 2004; 10:950–958.

32. Sawaki K, Mizukawa N, Yamaai T, Yoshimoto T, Nakano M, Sugahara T. High concentration of beta-defensin-2 in oral squamous cell carcinoma. *Anticancer Res* 2002; 22:2103–2107.

33. Uehara N, Yagihashi A, Kondoh K, et al. Human beta-defensin-2 induction in Helicobacter pylori-infected gastric mucosal tissues: antimicrobial effect of overexpression. *J Med Microbiol* 2003; 52:41–45.

34. Hase K, Murakami M, Iimura M, et al. Expression of LL-37 by human gastric epithelial cells as a potential host defense mechanism against Helicobacter pylori. *Gastroenterology* 2003; 125:1613–1625.

35. Young AN, de Oliveira Salles PG, Lim SD, et al. Beta defensin-1, parvalbumin, and vimentin: a panel of diagnostic immunohistochemical markers for renal tumors derived from gene expression profiling studies using cDNA microarrays. *Am J Surg Pathol* 2003; 27:199–205.

36. Fujiwara K, Ochiai M, Ohta T, et al. Global gene expression analysis of rat colon cancers induced by a food-borne carcinogen, 2-amino-1-methyl-6-phenylimidazo[4,5-b]pyridine. *Carcinogenesis* 2004; 25:1495–1505.

37. Vlahou A, Schellhammer PF, Mendrinos S, et al. Development of a novel proteomic approach for the detection of transitional cell carcinoma of the bladder in urine. *Am J Pathol* 2001; 158:1491–1502.

38. Meyer JE, Harder J, Gorogh T, et al. Human beta-defensin-2 in oral cancer with opportunistic *Candida* infection. *Anticancer Res* 2004; 24:1025–1030.

39. Halder TM, Bluggel M, Heinzel S, Pawelec G, Meyer HE, Kalbacher H. Defensins are dominant HLA-DR-associated self-peptides from CD34(–) peripheral blood mononuclear cells of different tumor patients (plasmacytoma, chronic myeloid leukemia). *Blood* 2000; 95:2890–2896.

40. Vermi W, Bonecchi R, Facchetti F, et al. Recruitment of immature plasmacytoid dendritic cells (plasmacytoid monocytes) and myeloid dendritic cells in primary cutaneous melanomas. *J Pathol* 2003; 200: 255–268.

41. Steinman RM, Hawiger D, Liu K, et al. Dendritic cell function in vivo during the steady state: a role in peripheral tolerance. *Ann NY Acad Sci* 2003; 987:15–25.

42. Groux H, Fournier N, Cottrez F. Role of dendritic cells in the generation of regulatory T cells. *Semin Immunol* 2004; 16:99–106.

43. Rutella S, Lemoli RM. Regulatory T cells and tolerogenic dendritic cells: from basic biology to clinical applications. *Immunol Lett* 2004; 94:11–26.

44. Kalinski P, Hilkens CM, Wierenga EA, Kapsenberg ML. T-cell priming by type-1 and type-2 polarized dendritic cells: the concept of a third signal. *Immunol Today* 1999; 20:561–567.

45. Levings MK, Bacchetta R, Schulz U, Roncarolo MG. The role of IL-10 and TGF-beta in the differentiation and effector function of T regulatory cells. *Int Arch Allergy Immunol* 2002; 129:263–276.

46. Clement A, Pereboev A, Curiel DT, Dong SS, Hutchings A, Thomas JM. Converting nonhuman primate dendritic cells into potent antigen-specific cellular immunosuppressants by genetic modification. *Immunol Res* 2002; 26:297–302.

47. Gabrilovich D, Ishida T, Oyama T, et al. Vascular endothelial growth factor inhibits the development of dendritic cells and dramatically affects the differentiation of multiple hematopoietic lineages in vivo. *Blood* 1998; 92:4150–4166.

48. Gabrilovich DI, Chen HL, Girgis KR, et al. Production of vascular endothelial growth factor by human tumors inhibits the functional maturation of dendritic cells. *Nat Med* 1996; 2:1096–1103.

49. Oyama T, Ran S, Ishida T, et al. Vascular endothelial growth factor affects dendritic cell maturation through the inhibition of nuclear factor-kappa B activation in hemopoietic progenitor cells. *J Immunol* 1998; 160:1224–1232.

50. Almand B, Resser JR, Lindman B, et al. Clinical significance of defective dendritic cell differentiation in cancer. *Clin Cancer Res* 2000; 6:1755–1766.

51. Gabrilovich DI, Ishida T, Nadaf S, Ohm JE, Carbone DP. Antibodies to vascular endothelial growth factor enhance the efficacy of cancer immunotherapy by improving endogenous dendritic cell function. *Clin Cancer Res* 1999; 5:2963–2970.

52. Conejo-Garcia JR, Buckanovich RJ, Benencia F, et al. Vascular leukocytes contribute to tumor vascularization. *Blood* 2004; 105:679–681.

53. Curiel TJ, Cheng P, Mottram P, et al. Dendritic cell subsets differentially regulate angiogenesis in human ovarian cancer. *Cancer Res* 2004; 64:5535–5538.

54. Jonuleit H, Giesecke-Tuettenberg A, Tuting T, et al. A comparison of two types of dendritic cell as adjuvants for the induction of melanoma-specific T-cell responses in humans following intranodal injection. *Int J Cancer* 2001; 93:243–251.

55. McIlroy D, Gregoire M. Optimizing dendritic cell-based anticancer immunotherapy: maturation state does have clinical impact. *Cancer Immunol Immunother* 2003; 52:583–591.

56. Dhodapkar MV, Steinman RM, Krasovsky J, Munz C, Bhardwaj N. Antigen-specific inhibition of effector T cell function in humans after injection of immature dendritic cells. *J Exp Med* 2001; 193: 233–238.

57. Nair S, McLaughlin C, Weizer A, Su Z, et al. Injection of immature dendritic cells into adjuvant-treated skin obviates the need for ex vivo maturation. *J Immunol* 2003; 171:6275–6282.

58. Chomarat P, Banchereau J, Davoust J, Palucka AK. IL-6 switches the differentiation of monocytes from dendritic cells to macrophages. *Nat Immunol* 2000; 1:510–514.

59. Vicari AP, Chiodoni C, Vaure C, et al. Reversal of tumor-induced dendritic cell paralysis by CpG immunostimulatory oligonucleotide and anti-interleukin 10 receptor antibody. *J Exp Med* 2002; 196:541–549.

60. Whiteside TL, Stanson J, Shurin MR, Ferrone S. Antigen-processing machinery in human dendritic cells: up-regulation by maturation and down-regulation by tumor cells. *J Immunol* 2004; 173:1526–1534.

61. Chomarat P, Banchereau J. Interleukin-4 and interleukin-13: their similarities and discrepancies. *Int Rev Immunol* 1998; 17:1–52.

62. Nair S, Boczkowski D, Moeller B, Dewhirst M, Vieweg J, Gilboa E. Synergy between tumor immunotherapy and antiangiogenic therapy. *Blood* 2003; 102:964–971.

63. Bedrosian I, Mick R, Xu S, et al. Intranodal administration of peptide-pulsed mature dendritic cell vaccines results in superior CD8+ T-cell function in melanoma patients. *J Clin Oncol* 2003; 21:3826–3835.

64. La Montagne JR, Fauci AS. Intradermal influenza vaccination—can less be more? *N Engl J Med* 2004; 351:2330–2332.

65. Redfield RR, Innis BL, Scott RM, Cannon HG, Bancroft WH. Clinical evaluation of low-dose intradermally administered hepatitis B virus vaccine. A cost reduction strategy. *JAMA* 1985; 254:3203–3206.

66. Frech SA, Kenney RT, Spyr CA, et al. Improved immune responses to influenza vaccination in the elderly using an immunostimulant patch. *Vaccine* 2005; 23:946–950.

67. Saika T, Satoh T, Kusaka N, et al. Route of administration influences the antitumor effects of bone marrow-derived dendritic cells engineered to produce interleukin-12 in a metastatic mouse prostate cancer model. *Cancer Gene Ther* 2004; 11:317–324.

68. Schmidt T, Ziske C, Marten A, et al. Intratumoral immunization with tumor RNA-pulsed dendritic cells confers antitumor immunity in a C57BL/6 pancreatic murine tumor model. *Cancer Res* 2003; 63: 8962–8967.

69. Ehtesham M, Kabos P, Gutierrez MA, Samoto K, Black KL, Yu JS. Intratumoral dendritic cell vaccination elicits potent tumoricidal immunity against malignant glioma in rats. *J Immunother* 2003; 26: 107–116.

70. Candido KA, Shimizu K, McLaughlin JC, et al. Local administration of dendritic cells inhibits established breast tumor growth: implications for apoptosis-inducing agents. *Cancer Res* 2001; 61:228–236.

71. Triozzi PL, Khurram R, Aldrich WA, Walker MJ, Kim JA, Jaynes S. Intratumoral injection of dendritic cells derived in vitro in patients with metastatic cancer. *Cancer* 2000; 89:2646–2654.

72. Melero I, Vile RG, Colombo MP. Feeding dendritic cells with tumor antigens: self-service buffet or a la carte? *Gene Ther* 2000; 7:1167–1170

73. Melero I, Duarte M, Ruiz J, et al. Intratumoral injection of bone-marrow derived dendritic cells engineered to produce interleukin-12 induces complete regression of established murine transplantable colon adenocarcinomas. *Gene Ther* 1999; 6:1779–1784.

74. Miller PW, Sharma S, Stolina M, et al. Intratumoral administration of adenoviral interleukin 7 gene-modified dendritic cells augments specific antitumor immunity and achieves tumor eradication. *Hum Gene Ther* 2000; 11:53–65.

75. Kikuchi T, Moore MA, Crystal RG. Dendritic cells modified to express CD40 ligand elicit therapeutic immunity against preexisting murine tumors. *Blood* 2000; 96:91–99.

76. Mazzolini G, Alfaro C, Sangro B, et al. Intratumoral injection of dendritic cells engineered to secrete interleukin-12 by recombinant adenovirus in patients with metastatic gastrointestinal carcinomas. *J Clin Oncol* 2004; 23:999–1010.

77. Liu Y, Xia D, Li F, Zheng C, Xiang J. Intratumoral administration of immature dendritic cells following the adenovirus vector encoding CD40 ligand elicits significant regression of established myeloma. *Cancer Gene Ther* 2004; 12:122–132.

78. Tatsumi T, Huang J, Gooding WE, et al. Intratumoral delivery of dendritic cells engineered to secrete both interleukin (IL)-12 and IL-18 effectively treats local and distant disease in association with broadly reactive Tc1-type immunity. *Cancer Res* 2003; 63:6378–6386.

79. Ahmed SU, Okamoto M, Oshikawa T, et al. Anti-tumor effect of an intratumoral administration of dendritic cells in combination with TS-1, an oral fluoropyrimidine anti-cancer drug, and OK-432, a streptococcal immunopotentiator: involvement of toll-like receptor 4. *J Immunother* 2004; 27:432–441.

80. Chen Z, Xia D, Bi X, et al. Combined radiation therapy and dendritic cell vaccine for treating solid tumors with liver micro-metastasis. *J Gene Med* 2004; 7:506–517.

81. Teitz-Tennenbaum S, Li Q, Rynkiewicz S, et al. Radiotherapy potentiates the therapeutic efficacy of intratumoral dendritic cell administration. *Cancer Res* 2003; 63:8466–8475.

82. Tanaka F, Yamaguchi H, Ohta M, et al. Intratumoral injection of dendritic cells after treatment of anticancer drugs induces tumor-specific antitumor effect in vivo. *Int J Cancer* 2002; 101:265–269.

83. Tong Y, Song W, Crystal RG. Combined intratumoral injection of bone marrow-derived dendritic cells and systemic chemotherapy to treat pre-existing murine tumors. *Cancer Res* 2001; 61:7530–7535.

84. Mastrangelo MJ, Berd D, Maguire H Jr. The immunoaugmenting effects of cancer chemotherapeutic agents. *Semin Oncol* 1986; 13:186–194.

85. Machiels JP, Reilly RT, Emens LA, et al. Cyclophosphamide, doxorubicin, and paclitaxel enhance the antitumor immune response of granulocyte/macrophage-colony stimulating factor-secreting whole-cell vaccines in HER-2/*neu* tolerized mice. *Cancer Res* 2001; 61:3689–3697.

86. North RJ. Cyclophosphamide-facilitated adoptive immunotherapy of an established tumor depends on elimination of tumor-induced suppressor T cells. *J Exp Med* 1982; 155:1063–1074.

87. Juedes AE, Von Herrath MG. Using regulatory APCs to induce/maintain tolerance. *Ann NY Acad Sci* 2003; 1005:128–137.

88. Kalinski P, Hilkens CM, Snijders A, Snijdewint FG, Kapsenberg ML. IL-12-deficient dendritic cells, generated in the presence of prostaglandin E2, promote type 2 cytokine production in maturing human naive T helper cells. *J Immunol* 1997; 159:28–35.

89. Kalinski P, Vieira PL, Schuitemaker JH, de Jong EC, Kapsenberg ML. Prostaglandin E(2) is a selective inducer of interleukin-12 p40 (IL-12p40) production and an inhibitor of bioactive IL-12p70 heterodimer. *Blood* 2001; 97:3466–3469.

90. Waller EK, Rosenthal H, Sagar L. DC2 effect on survival following allogeneic bone marrow transplantation. *Oncology (Huntingt)* 2002; 16:19–26.

91. Akdis CA, Blaser K. Mechanisms of interleukin-10-mediated immune suppression. *Immunology* 2001; 103:131–136.

92. Lucas PJ, Kim SJ, Melby SJ, Gress RE. Disruption of T cell homeostasis in mice expressing a T cell-specific dominant negative transforming growth factor beta II receptor. *J Exp Med* 2000; 191:1187–1196.

93. Chen W, Wahl SM. Manipulation of TGF-beta to control autoimmune and chronic inflammatory diseases. *Microbes Infect* 1999; 1:1367–1380.

94. Krammer PH. CD95's deadly mission in the immune system. *Nature* 2000; 407:789–795.

95. Frauwirth KA, Riley JL, Harris MH, et al. The CD28 signaling pathway regulates glucose metabolism. *Immunity* 2002; 16:769–777.

96. Van Parijs L, Peterson DA, Abbas AK. The Fas/Fas ligand pathway and Bcl-2 regulate T cell responses to model self and foreign antigens. *Immunity* 1998; 8:265–274.

97. Whiteside TL, Rabinowich H. The role of Fas/FasL in immunosuppression induced by human tumors. *Cancer Immunol Immunother* 1998; 46:175–184.

98. Nagata S. Apoptosis by death factor. *Cell* 1997; 88:355–365.

99. Muzio M, Chinnaiyan AM, Kischkel FC, et al. FLICE, a novel FADD-homologous ICE/CED-3-like protease, is recruited to the CD95 (Fas/APO-1) death-inducing signaling complex. *Cell* 1996; 85: 817–827.

100. Griffith TS, Brunner T, Fletcher SM, Green DR, Ferguson TA. Fas ligand-induced apoptosis as a mechanism of immune privilege. *Science* 1995; 270:1189–1192.

101. Kauma SW, Huff TF, Hayes N, Nilkaeo A. Placental Fas ligand expression is a mechanism for maternal immune tolerance to the fetus. *J Clin Endocrinol Metab* 1999; 84:2188–2194.

102. Runic R, Lockwood CJ, Ma Y, Dipasquale B, Guller S. Expression of Fas ligand by human cytotrophoblasts: implications in placentation and fetal survival. *J Clin Endocrinol Metab* 1996; 81:3119–3122.

103. Rabinowich H, Reichert TE, Kashii Y, Gastman BR, Bell MC, Whiteside TL. Lymphocyte apoptosis induced by Fas ligand-expressing ovarian carcinoma cells. Implications for altered expression of T cell receptor in tumor-associated lymphocytes. *J Clin Invest* 1998; 101:2579–2588.

104. Restifo NP. Not so Fas: re-evaluating the mechanisms of immune privilege and tumor escape. *Nat Med* 2000; 6:493–495.

105. Abrahams VM, Straszewski SL, Kamsteeg M, et al. Epithelial ovarian cancer cells secrete functional Fas ligand. *Cancer Res* 2003; 63:5573–5581.

106. Dong H, Strome SE, Salomao DR, et al. Tumor-associated B7-H1 promotes T-cell apoptosis: a potential mechanism of immune evasion. *Nat Med* 2002; 8:793–800.

107. Latchman Y, Wood CR, Chernova T, et al. PD-L2 is a second ligand for PD-1 and inhibits T cell activation. *Nat Immunol* 2001; 2:261–268.

108. Brown JA, Dorfman DM, Ma FR, et al. Blockade of programmed death-1 ligands on dendritic cells enhances T cell activation and cytokine production. *J Immunol* 2003; 170:1257–1266.

109. Curiel TJ, Wei S, Dong H, et al. Blockade of B7-H1 improves myeloid dendritic cell-mediated anti-tumor immunity. *Nat Med* 2003; 9:562–567.
110. Munn DH, Sharma MD, Lee JR, et al. Potential regulatory function of human dendritic cells expressing indoleamine 2,3-dioxygenase. *Science* 2002; 297:1867–1870.
111. Munn DH, Sharma MD, Hou D, et al. Expression of indoleamine 2,3-dioxygenase by plasmacytoid dendritic cells in tumor-draining lymph nodes. *J Clin Invest* 2004; 114:280–290.
112. Lee GK, Park HJ, Macleod M, Chandler P, Munn DH, Mellor AL. Tryptophan deprivation sensitizes activated T cells to apoptosis prior to cell division. *Immunology* 2002; 107:452–460.
113. Munn DH, Mellor AL. IDO and tolerance to tumors. *Trends Mol Med* 2004; 10:15–18.
114. Fallarino F, Grohmann U, Vacca C, et al. T cell apoptosis by tryptophan catabolism. *Cell Death Differ* 2002; 9:1069–1077.
115. Hsieh CS, Liang Y, Tyznik AJ, Self SG, Liggitt D, Rudensky AY. Recognition of the peripheral self by naturally arising CD25+ CD4+ T cell receptors. *Immunity* 2004; 21:267–277.
116. Bluestone JA, Abbas AK. Natural versus adaptive regulatory T cells. *Nat Rev Immunol* 2003; 3:253–257.
117. Sakaguchi S. Naturally arising CD4+ regulatory t cells for immunologic self-tolerance and negative control of immune responses. *Annu Rev Immunol* 2004; 22:531–562.
118. Curiel TJ, Coukos G, Zou L, et al. Specific recruitment of regulatory T cells in ovarian carcinoma fosters immune privilege and predicts reduced survival. *Nat Med* 2004; 10:942–949.
119. O'Garra A, Vieira P. Regulatory T cells and mechanisms of immune system control. *Nat Med* 2004; 10:801–805.
120. Woo EY, Chu CS, Goletz TJ, et al. Regulatory CD4(+)CD25(+) T cells in tumors from patients with early-stage non-small cell lung cancer and late-stage ovarian cancer. *Cancer Res* 2001; 61:4766–4772.
121. Iellem A, Mariani M, Lang R, et al. Unique chemotactic response profile and specific expression of chemokine receptors CCR4 and CCR8 by CD4(+)CD25(+) regulatory T cells. *J Exp Med* 2001; 194:847–853.
122. Onizuka S, Tawara I, Shimizu J, Sakaguchi S, Fujita T, Nakayama E. Tumor rejection by in vivo administration of anti-CD25 (interleukin-2 receptor alpha) monoclonal antibody. *Cancer Res* 1999; 59:3128–3133.
123. Sutmuller RP, van Duivenvoorde LM, van Elsas A, et al. Synergism of cytotoxic T lymphocyte-associated antigen 4 blockade and depletion of CD25(+) regulatory T cells in antitumor therapy reveals alternative pathways for suppression of autoreactive cytotoxic T lymphocyte responses. *J Exp Med* 2001; 194:823–832.
124. Phan GQ, Yang JC, Sherry RM, et al. Cancer regression and autoimmunity induced by cytotoxic T lymphocyte-associated antigen 4 blockade in patients with metastatic melanoma. *Proc Natl Acad Sci USA* 2003; 100:8372–8377.
125. Hodi FS, Mihm MC, Soiffer RJ, et al. Biologic activity of cytotoxic T lymphocyte-associated antigen 4 antibody blockade in previously vaccinated metastatic melanoma and ovarian carcinoma patients. *Proc Natl Acad Sci USA* 2003; 100:4712–4717.
126. Frankel AE, Fleming DR, Hall PD, et al. A phase II study of DT fusion protein denileukin diftitox in patients with fludarabine-refractory chronic lymphocytic leukemia. *Clin Cancer Res* 2003; 9:3555–3561.
127. Dudley ME, Wunderlich JR, Robbins PF, et al. Cancer regression and autoimmunity in patients after clonal repopulation with antitumor lymphocytes. *Science* 2002; 298:850–854.
128. Bauer S, Groh V, Wu J, et al. Activation of NK cells and T cells by NKG2D, a receptor for stress-inducible MICA. *Science* 1999; 285:727–729.
129. Jamieson AM, Diefenbach A, McMahon CW, Xiong N, Carlyle JR, Raulet DH. The role of the NKG2D immunoreceptor in immune cell activation and natural killing. *Immunity* 2002; 17:19–29.
130. Wu J, Song Y, Bakker AB, et al. An activating immunoreceptor complex formed by NKG2D and DAP10. *Science* 1999; 285:730–732.
131. Diefenbach A, Jensen ER, Jamieson AM, Raulet DH. Rae1 and H60 ligands of the NKG2D receptor stimulate tumour immunity. *Nature* 2001; 413:165–171.
132. Girardi M, Oppenheim DE, Steele CR, et al. Regulation of cutaneous malignancy by gammadelta T cells. *Science* 2001; 294:605–609.
133. Roberts AI, Lee L, Schwarz E, et al. NKG2D receptors induced by IL-15 costimulate CD28-negative effector CTL in the tissue microenvironment. *J Immunol* 2001; 167:5527–5530.
134. Sutherland CL, Chalupny NJ, Schooley K, VandenBos T, Kubin M, Cosman D. UL16-binding proteins, novel MHC class I-related proteins, bind to NKG2D and activate multiple signaling pathways in primary NK cells. *J Immunol* 2002; 168:671–679.

135. Cosman D, Mullberg J, Sutherland CL, et al. ULBPs, novel MHC class I-related molecules, bind to CMV glycoprotein UL16 and stimulate NK cytotoxicity through the NKG2D receptor. *Immunity* 2001; 14:123–133.

136. Conejo-Garcia JR, Benencia F, Courreges C, et al. Letal, a tumor-associated NKG2D immunoreceptor ligand, induces activation and expansion of effector immune cells. *Cancer Biol Ther* 2003; 2:446–451.

137. Maus MV, Thomas AK, Leonard DG, et al. Ex vivo expansion of polyclonal and antigen-specific cytotoxic T lymphocytes by artificial APCs expressing ligands for the T-cell receptor, CD28 and 4-1BB. *Nat Biotechnol* 2002; 20:143–148.

138. Dudley ME, Wunderlich J, Nishimura MI, et al. Adoptive transfer of cloned melanoma-reactive T lymphocytes for the treatment of patients with metastatic melanoma. *J Immunother* 2001; 24:363–373.

139. Groh V, Wu J, Yee C, Spies T. Tumour-derived soluble MIC ligands impair expression of NKG2D and T-cell activation. *Nature* 2002; 419:734–738.

140. Wu CJ, Yang XF, McLaughlin S, et al. Detection of a potent humoral response associated with immune-induced remission of chronic myelogenous leukemia. *J Clin Invest* 2000; 106:705–714.

141. Dranoff G. Coordinated tumor immunity. *J Clin Invest* 2003; 111:1116–1118.

142. Kidd P. Th1/Th2 balance: the hypothesis, its limitations, and implications for health and disease. *Altern Med Rev* 2003; 8:223–246.

143. Moore KW, de Waal Malefyt R, Coffman RL, O'Garra A. Interleukin-10 and the interleukin-10 receptor. *Annu Rev Immunol* 2001; 19:683–765.

144. Loercher AE, Nash MA, Kavanagh JJ, Platsoucas CD, Freedman RS. Identification of an IL-10-producing HLA-DR-negative monocyte subset in the malignant ascites of patients with ovarian carcinoma that inhibits cytokine protein expression and proliferation of autologous T cells. *J Immunol* 1999; 163:6251–6260.

145. Gasperini S, Marchi M, Calzetti F, et al. Gene expression and production of the monokine induced by IFN-gamma (MIG), IFN-inducible T cell alpha chemoattractant (I-TAC), and IFN-gamma-inducible protein-10 (IP-10) chemokines by human neutrophils. *J Immunol* 1999; 162:4928–4937.

146. Mach F, Sauty A, Iarossi AS, et al. Differential expression of three T lymphocyte-activating CXC chemokines by human atheroma-associated cells. *J Clin Invest* 1999; 104:1041–1050.

147. Loetscher M, Loetscher P, Brass N, Meese E, Moser B. Lymphocyte-specific chemokine receptor CXCR3: regulation, chemokine binding and gene localization. *Eur J Immunol* 1998; 28:3696–3705.

148. Sorensen TL, Tani M, Jensen J, et al. Expression of specific chemokines and chemokine receptors in the central nervous system of multiple sclerosis patients. *J Clin Invest* 1999; 103:807–815.

149. Qin S, Rottman JB, Myers P, et al. The chemokine receptors CXCR3 and CCR5 mark subsets of T cells associated with certain inflammatory reactions. *J Clin Invest* 1998; 101:746–754.

150. Koga S, Auerbach MB, Engeman TM, Novick AC, Toma H, Fairchild RL. T cell infiltration into class II MHC-disparate allografts and acute rejection is dependent on the IFN-gamma-induced chemokine Mig. *J Immunol* 1999; 163:4878–4885.

151. Biragyn A, Tani K, Grimm MC, Weeks S, Kwak LW. Genetic fusion of chemokines to a self tumor antigen induces protective, T-cell dependent antitumor immunity. *Nat Biotechnol* 1999; 17:253–258.

152. Guironnet G, Dezutter-Dambuyant C, Vincent C, Bechetoille N, Schmitt D, Peguet-Navarro J. Antagonistic effects of IL-4 and TGF-beta1 on Langerhans cell-related antigen expression by human monocytes. *J Leukoc Biol* 2002; 71:845–853.

153. Romagnani S. Cytokines and chemoattractants in allergic inflammation. *Mol Immunol* 2002; 38:881–885.

154. Sebastiani S, Allavena P, Albanesi C, et al. Chemokine receptor expression and function in CD4+ T lymphocytes with regulatory activity. *J Immunol* 2001; 166:996–1002.

155. Conti I, Rollins BJ. CCL2 (monocyte chemoattractant protein-1) and cancer. *Semin Cancer Biol* 2004; 14:149–154.

156. Strieter RM, Polverini PJ, Arenberg DA, Kunkel SL. The role of CXC chemokines as regulators of angiogenesis. *Shock* 1995; 4:155–160.

157. Salcedo R, Young HA, Ponce ML, et al. Eotaxin (CCL11) induces in vivo angiogenic responses by human CCR3+ endothelial cells. *J Immunol* 2001; 166:7571–7578.

17 Manipulation of Lymphocyte Homeostasis for Enhancing Antitumor Immunity

Eduardo Davila and Esteban Celis

SUMMARY

Our appreciation of how the immune system recognizes and destroys cancer has led to the advancement of innovative approaches to be used for the treatment of cancer patients. The concept of immunotherapy is based on the body's immune system to combat potentially dangerous assaults to the host such as those occurring from infection, but also those from transformed malignant cells. T-lymphocytes are capable of eliminating transformed cells after recognizing specific tumor antigens expressed on their cell surface. Thus, one immediate goal of tumor immunology is the development of effective approaches to harness the immune system's natural tendency to eliminate cancer. However, the processes that govern the total size and diversity of the T-cell pool represent a major barrier for the induction of effective antitumor immune responses. We propose that cancer vaccines intended to generate effective antitumor responses have been unsuccessful to control disease because of inadequate T-cell activation, the fleeting duration of antitumor T-cell responses, and an active suppressor system that downplay immune responses.

Key Words: Immunotherapy; T-cells; homeostasis; immune tolerance; antitumor.

1. INTRODUCTION

During recent years, our understanding of how the immune system recognizes malignant tissue has lead to the development of novel approaches for the treatment against cancer. One such therapy uses the host's immune system to inhibit tumor cell growth. Immunotherapy seeks to generate T-lymphocytes that are capable of killing transformed cells after recognizing tumor antigens, which are preferentially expressed, by tumor cells. Effective T-cell-based immunotherapy leading to increased survival of cancer patients is dependent on the successful activation of sufficient numbers of tumor-reactive T-cells and the long-term persistence of such T-cell responses that will be necessary to prevent tumor recurrences. We believe that T-cell homeostasis, which governs the overall size and diversity of the T-cell pool by balancing lymphocyte generation, survival and death, poses a significant obstacle for the generation of effective antitumor immune responses. We hypothesize that

From: *Cancer Drug Discovery and Development: Immunotherapy of Cancer*
Edited by: M. L. Disis © Humana Press Inc., Totowa, NJ

cancer vaccines aimed at generating antitumor responses have failed to control disease due to suboptimal T-cell activation, in part resulting from low precursor frequencies against tumor antigens; the short-term duration of antitumor T-cell responses; and suppressor mechanisms that downregulate immune responses. In this chapter, we propose that we can achieve effective antitumor immune responses by manipulating some of the physiological mechanisms that control T-cell homeostasis. We present both theoretical and experimental arguments in support of this hypothesis.

2. ANTITUMOR IMMUNOTHERAPY

The most common approach to treat solid tumors is surgery, aimed at removing most of the malignant tissue. This is commonly followed by chemotherapy and/or radiotherapy, with the hope of eliminating any residual tumor cells. Unfortunately, these therapies all too often remain ineffective. For example, surgical procedures intended to remove the malignancy usually leave some tumor cells behind, yielding the possibility of continued tumor growth or metastases. Chemotherapy, on the other hand, involves the use of cytotoxic drugs to destroy rapidly dividing cancer cells. Sadly, as these drugs are carried in the bloodstream, they also destroy nonmalignant cells, routinely resulting in adverse side effects. Moreover, chemotherapeutic agents can often lead to the selection of tumors that are resistant to these forms of treatments, such as melanoma, nonsmall cell lung cancer, and breast cancer (1). Therefore, many of the current therapies intended to treat patients with cancer are not only poorly effective in eradicating disease, but they are also quite toxic and significantly hamper the patient's quality of life. Also, although a combination of these forms of therapies has proven effective in some cases, there is a need to consider alternate forms of therapy to treat cancer.

A novel, and perhaps more tolerable, form of cancer therapy is immunotherapy, which is based on the body's natural defense system to specifically recognize and destroy a variety of infectious pathogens, such as bacteria, viruses, parasites, and fungi. It has also become evident that the immune system can also react against endogenous assaults, such as those resulting from malignant transformation. Tumor immunotherapy includes a broad range of measures focused on eliciting effective immune responses against the malignant cells. Active immunotherapy seeks to elicit in vivo antitumor responses via vaccination. Passive, or adoptive, immunotherapy on the other hand, is based on the ex vivo generation of the immune-effector agents (i.e., cells, antibodies, lymphokines) that are administered to the patient with cancer. Actually, many of the currently explored immunotherapies for cancer are a combination of both strategies. For example, some recent therapeutic approaches that show great potential include the administration of vaccines composed of autologous antigen-pulsed dendritic cells (DCs) (3) or gene-modified tumor cells designed to produce immunostimulatory cytokines (2–4). Adoptive transfer of tumor-reactive T-lymphocytes (T-cell therapy) into some patients with cancer has also resulted in impressive antitumor responses (discussed in detail in this chapter). Although encouraging results using these therapeutic approaches have been observed in limited clinical trials, there are concerns as to whether these types of procedures will be effective against a broad spectrum of cancers and whether they can be applied to the general cancer patient population in a cost-effective manner.

A more appealing approach to stimulate specific tumor immunity revolves around the idea of using synthetic peptides or proteins as vaccines to induce antigen specific T-cell responses. In this model, the vaccines are composed of proteins or peptides that are derived from tumor-associated antigens (TAAs). The vaccines are administered with an immune adjuvant to enhance immunogenicity and facilitate antigen delivery to specialized antigen-presenting cells (APCs), such as DCs, which will stimulate the antitumor T-cell responses. Although the development of peptide or protein antitumor vaccines holds great promise for treating patients with cancer, there are still several challenges that must be overcome in order to generate potent and sustained antitumor responses. In our view, we consider three of the most significant hurdles that prevent the development of successful antitumor T cell-based therapy:

1. A low number of TAA-specific T-cell precursors.
2. The short-term duration of antitumor T-cell responses.
3. Inhibitory mechanisms that downregulate immune responses.

We propose that these obstacles may be overcome by altering lymphocyte homeostasis.

3. T-CELL HOMEOSTASIS AND TUMOR IMMUNITY

In most circumstances, lymphocyte responses are closely regulated following antigenic stimulation. Otherwise, uncontrolled proliferating clones of antigen-specific B- and T-cells, as well as their products, would overwhelm our bodies. As such, immune responses to foreign antigens are self-limiting and subside as the offending antigens are removed, leading to a return of the immune system to a state of natural equilibrium (i.e., lymphocyte homeostasis). Many regulatory processes ensure the maintenance of a constant and appropriate number of naïve, activated, and memory T-cells. The complex balance of T-lymphocyte generation, survival, proliferation, and death will ultimately determine the size and diversity of the T-cell pool throughout an individual's life. It is considered that because the "space" available to sustain these cells is limited, that T-cell expansion, because of antigen stimulation by an infection or an effective vaccine, will require altering the ongoing homeostatic control. In the case of infections, lymphocyte homeostasis is made evident by lymphocytosis, sometimes accompanied by splenomegaly and lymph node hypertrophy, reflecting the rapid generation of large numbers of pathogen-specific lymphocytes required for eliminating the offending agents, followed shortly by the return to a resting state. On the other hand, it is clear that the immune system reacts much more conservatively to immunological challenges represented by "inert" vaccines, such as those composed of peptides and proteins.

One of the ways that T-cell homeostasis attempts to maintain a constant number of T cells is through the availability of growth and survival factors (5). Various T-cell subsets, such as naïve, effector, and memory cells appear to compete for a limited amount of survival and proliferative signals. For example, naïve T-cell survival requires specific cytokines (interleukin [IL]-7 and perhaps IL-6 and IL-4) together with low-level T-cell receptor (TCR) stimulation (6,7). Similarly, memory CD8$^+$ T-cells depend on their access to specific cytokines (IL-15 and IL-7) in order to persist for long periods of time, whereas TCR–major histocompatibility complex–peptide interaction prompts quick effector actions, as well as rapid proliferative response (8–15).

Activation-induced cell death (AICD) is one important mechanism that ensures the waning of activated T-cell responses. Consequently, the use of such mechanisms ultimately leads to suboptimal antitumor effects. Additionally, unlike the maintenance of naïve or memory T-cells, which require growth factors and low-level TCR stimulation, the elimination of activated T-cells is mediated via the fatty acid synthase (Fas)/Fas ligand (FasL) death pathway *(16)*. This form of T-lymphocyte regulation plays not only a critical role in controlling the overall number of activated T-cells, but also establishes tolerance to self-antigens, such as TAAs *(17)*. In fact, procedures aimed at blocking FasL stimulation to prevent AICD represent an attractive way by which to maintain activated T-cell responses against tumors. In some circumstances, T-cells stimulated through their TCR may avoid AICD because the high expression of the antiapoptotic Fas-associated death domain-like IL-1β-converting enzyme-inhibitory protein (FLIP), which interferes with the formation of the death-inducing signaling complex. In a similar fashion, molecular approaches leading to the overexpression of other antiapoptotic proteins (i.e., B-cell leukemia [bcl]-2 and bcl-xl) disrupt the homeostatic process resulting in the buildup of lymphocytes *(18)*. An interesting similarity between the overexpression of antiapoptotic molecules in T-cells and T-cells induced to proliferate through homeostatic disruption, is their decreased susceptibility to various forms of cell death *(19–22)*. Therefore, strategies aimed at upregulating FLIP or other antiapoptotic proteins on antigen-activated antitumor T-cells could represent a useful approach to enhance the effectiveness of cancer vaccines.

Another mechanism involved in the downregulation of T-cell responses is via the stimulation of the cytotoxic-T-lymphocyte-associated antigen (CTLA)-4. Cell surface expression of CTLA-4 is a firmly ordered process, with the majority of the CTLA-4 protein located within intracellular vesicles and expressed on the cell surface following T-cell stimulation. On activation, cell surface expression of CTLA-4 competes with the activating receptor CD28 for ligation with CD80/B7-1 and CD86/B7-2 expressed on professional APCs. This interaction between CTLA-4 and B7 inhibits clonal T-cell expansion. The essential role of CTLA-4 as a negative modulator of T-cell homeostasis is clearly illustrated in CTLA-4-deficient mice that die within several weeks of birth because massive T-lymphocyte infiltration and destruction of organs *(23–28)*. In addition, CTLA-4 signaling mediates antigen-specific apoptosis of the activated T-cells and suppresses autoreactive responses *(29–31)*, demonstrating this pathway's importance in maintaining self-tolerance. For these reasons, an additional goal in the development of T-cell-based therapies is to be able to overcome or block CTLA-4 signals from occurring. In fact, CTLA-4 blockade utilizing nonagonistic anti-CTLA-4 antibodies has been among the most promising agents proposed for the use in the reversal of immune tolerance. Moreover, it is currently being explored for the enhancement of antitumor vaccines *(31–34)*. These findings demonstrate that by preventing normal physiological processes intended to downplay cell mediated immunity in cancer patients can result in the induction of T-cells that recognize normal self-sequences, such as TAA, that can be maintained for long periods.

T-regulatory (Tregs) lymphocytes represent another significant mechanism by which lymphocyte homeostasis is maintained. Studies conducted in numerous laboratories have demonstrated the existence of Treg subsets that prevent autoreactive T-cell responses *(35–38)* via the action of immunosuppressive soluble factors, such as IL-10 and tumor growth factor-β, as well as via other negative signals mediated by APCs (*[39]*; E. Davila, submitted manuscript). Whereas some studies have demonstrated that Treg cells can inhibit antigen-specific T-cell responses, other investigations have shown that Treg cells can modulate the expansion and preservation of the general T-cell population. Although this form of lymphocyte regulation is beneficial in controlling autoimmune disorders, the suppressive effects of Treg cells also tend to hinder the induction of T-cell mediated anti-tumor immunity *(34,37)*. In fact, the timely depletion of CD4+CD25+ Treg cells has been shown to enhance antitumor immunity, sometimes accompanied with autoimmunity, in both vaccinated and naïve animals *(34)*. Other studies have found that CD25+ cell depletion before vaccination or before the infusion of tumor-specific T-cells dramatically enhances antitumor immunity displaying prolonged responses *(40)*. In addition to impeding cell-mediated immunity, it has been suggested that Treg cells play a critical role in maintaining T-cell homeostasis. For example, the abrogation of the Treg-mediated suppression results in the transient increase of total T-cell numbers *(41)*. Consistent with this hypothesis is the recent work by Danke demonstrating that deletion of CD4+CD25+ Treg cells allows marked clonal expansion of human autoreactive T-cells *(42)*; studies by Curotto de Lafaille *(36)* showed that Treg cells also appear to maintain a balanced response to environmental antigens. The effect of Tregs on attenuating immune homeostasis is strikingly noted by severe and fatal lymphoproliferative syndrome observed in mice that are genetically deficient in genes required for the development and function of Treg cells *(43,44)*. Because Treg cells suppress cell-mediated immunity and help sustain T-cell homeostasis, these studies imply that in tumor-bearing patients, depletion of Treg cells before vaccination should improve vaccine efficacy.

In summary, the regulation of T-cell homeostasis affecting both naïve and antigen-experienced subsets relies on broad spectrum of signals provided by major histocompatibility complex/self-peptide complexes and soluble stimulatory and inhibitory factors, as well as direct effects mediated by Treg cells. We believe that by upsetting T-cell homeostasis in cancer patients through relatively simple procedures using therapies already in clinical practice, the effectiveness of antitumor vaccines will be significantly improved.

4. MODES OF T-CELL HOMEOSTASIS DISRUPTION

T-cell homeostasis is a tightly regulated process that ensures the survival of a constant number of activated and naïve lymphocytes, that is, except under infectious conditions. The signals that alert the immune system of the pending danger, represented by an infection that allows the disruption of homeostasis, are quite complex and probably derived from various sources. Moreover, because many of these signals function in the early phases of an infection, they are thought to act on the innate immune system. A major challenge that we encounter in the development of peptide-based cancer vaccines revolves around our understanding of the mechanisms that maintain T-cell homeostasis and the signals derived from acute infections that permit the disruption of this tightly regulated process.

The types of signals that promote lymphocyte homeostatic disruption are typically derived from a wide spectrum of pathogens whose effects are mediated by those cells responsible for innate immunity (e.g., DC, other APCs, and natural-killer [NK] cells). Among the diverse sorts of stimuli that induce DC and NK cells to promote T-cell expansion and alter transiently T-cell homeostasis are components derived from microorganisms, which are recognized by Toll-like receptors (TLRs) expressed on these cells. The foreign components that stimulate TLRs have been termed pathogen-associated molecular patterns and include bacterial DNA rich in cytosine–phosphate–guanine (CpG) motifs, lipopolysaccharide, flagellin, and single- and double-stranded RNA *(45,46)*. Initial work conducted in our laboratory using mice demonstrated that repeated administration of oligodeoxynucleotides (ODN) containing CpG motifs (CpG-ODN) dramatically augmented

Table 1
Cytosine–Phosphate–Guanine/Oligodeoxynucleotide Therapy
Increases the Number of Naïve and Activated T-Cells

| | Cell number per spleen (millions) | | |
	CpG-ODN	Neg-ODN	Fold increase
Total CD4$^+$	35.4 ± 2.2	9.44 ± 0.95	3.75
CD4$^+$ CD44^{low}	18.4 ± 2.4	5.74 ± 0.85	3.21
CD4$^+$ CD44^{high}	17.0 ± 2.6	3.70 ± 0.74	4.59
Total CD8$^+$	20.9 ± 3.1	5.50 ± 0.85	3.81
CD8$^+$ CD44^{low}	12.4 ± 3.0	3.30 ± 0.70	3.76
CD8$^+$ CD44^{high}	8.6 ± 0.5	2.20 ± 0.09	3.89

Repeated CpG-ODN administration induces an increase in CD4$^+$ and CD8$^+$ T-cell numbers. The number of CD44^{low} (naïve) and CD44^{high} (antigen-experienced) CD4$^+$/CD3$^+$ and CD8$^+$/CD3$^+$ T-cells in spleens for each treatment group was determined by triple-color flow cytometry. The total cell yield was calculated by multiplying the proportion of each cell subset by the total number of live cells obtained per organ. Values represent the means and standard deviations obtained from three animals. Results are representative of three separate experiments. (Reprinted with permission from ref. *48*.)
CpG, cytosine-phosphate-guanine; ODN, oligodeoxynucleotide.

T-cell responses to peptide and protein vaccines. Throughout the course of these studies, we observed that the repeated administration of CpG-ODNs (even in the absence of vaccine) resulted in a significant increase (three- to sevenfold) in the size of the local draining lymph nodes, as well as in the spleen *(47)*. These findings highlight two important points:

1. CpG adjuvant functions systemically as the both the proximal and distal lymph nodes and spleens were enlarged.
2. CpG stimulates the immune the system in an antigen-independent fashion.

The increase in the size of the peripheral tissue was, in general, because of the increased number of NK cells, B-cells, and DCs. However, on closer inspection we observed that the numbers of naïve and activated CD4$^+$ and CD8$^+$ T-cells were also amplified *(48)*. The results in Table 1 show that both CD4$^+$ and CD8$^+$ naïve (CD44^{low}) and activated/memory CD44^{high} T-cell subsets were increased by three- to fourfold. This finding is even more striking when we consider that the increase in T-cell numbers was obtained in the absence of exogenous antigen. Based on these results, we proposed that the administration of CpG-ODN likely stimulated the production of lymphokines that induced T-cell proliferation. Surprisingly, the increase in the number of T-lymphocytes was not because of the excessive T-cell proliferation, but instead because of an increase of antiapoptotic molecules in the T-cells, which prevented the natural demise of the cells *(48)*. The results presented in Fig. 1 show that CD4$^+$ and CD8$^+$ T-lymphocytes derived from CpG-treated mice (without antigen) expressed higher levels of several antiapoptotic molecules, including FLIP, bcl-2, and bcl-xl. Moreover, because this effect was not observed in CD28-deficient mice, and TLR-9 (the ligand for CpG-ODN) is not expressed on T-cells, we proposed that the administration of CpG-ODNs disrupted T-cell homeostasis through strong co-stimulatory signals provided by APCs. Similar reports by other groups demon-

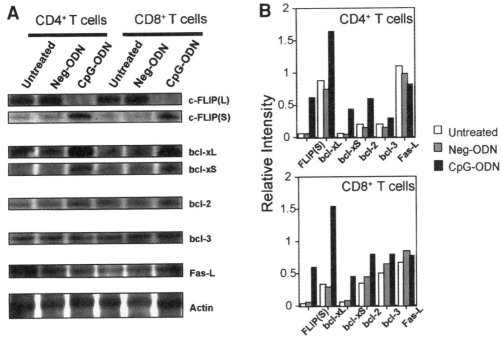

Fig. 1. Cytosine–phosphate–guanine (CpG)/oligodeoxynucleotide (ODN) therapy alters the protein expression of apoptotic-related genes in T-lymphocytes. **(A)** CD4+ and CD8+ T-cells were purified from untreated, CpG/ODN-treated, and Neg-ODN-treated mice 1 d after the final ODN injection. Total detergent cell lysates were used for Western blot analysis as described *(48)*. **(B)** Relative intensities were normalized to the corresponding actin intensity bands. (Reprinted with permission from ref. *48*.)

strated that molecular approaches that lead to the overt expression of antiapoptotic molecules or increased expression of T-cell co-stimulatory molecules, such as CD28, and OX40-L, in vivo also resulted in the expansion of the T-cell pool *(49–52)*, thus upsetting T-cell homeostasis. Noteworthy is whereas it is widely known that T-cell responses require both TCR and co-stimulation (usually in the form of anti-CD28 antibodies) to achieve optimal responses, T-cells induced to expand via homeostatic disruption bypass the need for co-stimulation and are less susceptible to various forms of death *(53,54)*.

Another major hurdle for inducing potent T-cell responses to peptide vaccines is the low precursor frequency of TAA-specific T-cells. Our published results looking at disrupting T-cell homeostasis with the administration of a peptide vaccine demonstrated a significant increase in the number of TAA-specific T-cells *(47)*. The results presented in Table 2 show an average 150-fold amplification in the number of TAA-specific T-cells above the administration of peptide vaccine alone and represented a dramatic increase in the percentage of TAA-specific cytotoxic T-lymphocytes (CTLs) from 0.0064 to 2.71%. Moreover, peptide immunization together with CpG-ODN routinely resulted in increased T-cell responses that provided protection against a subsequent tumor challenge. However, this vaccination protocol was not as effective against established tumors. To improve the effectiveness of peptide/protein-based vaccines, it was hypothesized that the presence of other immune regulatory mechanisms involved in maintaining T-cell homeostasis thwarted

Table 2
Cytosine-Phosphate-Guanine-1826 Increases the Number of Antigen-Specific Cytotoxic T-Lymphocyte Precursors Resulting From Peptide Vaccination

Treatment	CTL precursor frequency per 10^6 cells (per spleen)
Experiment 1	
PBS	8 (640)
CpG-1826 (single injection)	22 (3.3×10^3)
9X-CpG	71 (2.7×10^4)
Experiment 2	
PBS	3 (240)
CpG-1826 (single injection)	18 (3.6×10^3)
9X-CpG	185 (6.5×10^4)

Mice (three per group) were vaccinated with peptide simian virus (SV)40-IV mixed with Pan-DR T-helper cell epitopes in incomplete Freund's adjuvant in combination with a single CpG injection or 9X-CpG therapy. The number of CTL precursors was determined after pooling the spleens from each group by limiting dilution analysis using EL4 and peptide (SV40-IV)-pulsed EL-4 cells as targets. (Reprinted with permission from ref. *48*.)

CTL, cytotoxic T-lymphocyte; PBS, phosphate-buffered saline; CpG, cytosine-phosphate-guanine.

the generation and persistence of antitumor T-cell activity. Therefore, we examined the role of CpG-ODN plus CTLA-4 blockade in enhancing the effectiveness of peptide/protein vaccine to elicit therapeutic antitumor responses in mice. The results showed that the vaccination in combination with CpG-ODN and CTLA-4 blockade dramatically increased the antitumor effectiveness in the therapeutic setting *(55)*. What is even more surprising was that approx 20–30% of the lymph node CD8+ T-cell population from the vaccinated tumor-bearing mice recognized the peptide epitope used in the vaccine. Taken as a whole, these results imply that the effect of altering T-cell homeostasis during vaccination has the potential to skew the TCR repertoire toward one that contains more T-cells specific for the antigen vaccine formulation.

Alternative methods to disrupt T-cell homeostasis that could promote the induction and persistence of antitumor T-cell responses include common medical procedures that temporarily decrease lymphocyte numbers, such as irradiation, chemotherapy, and the administration of antibodies that induce specific in vivo T-cell depletion. In fact, early studies conducted by Hellstrom et al. demonstrated significant tumor growth regression specifically, if tumor-bearing mice underwent low-level, whole-body irradiation *(56,57)*. These authors proposed that tumor regression was likely because of the elimination of suppressor T-cells while leaving antitumor effector T-cells unaffected. In more-recent studies however, investigators administering sublethal doses of whole-body irradiation to mice, in order to alter T-cell homeostasis, revealed that adoptively transferred naive T-cells rapidly filled the T-cell compartment and acquired a semiactivated status that resembled memory T-cells, and underwent marked proliferation even in the absence of specific exogenous antigen *(58–64)*. More importantly, transferred T-cells that undergo this homeostatic proliferation also acquire memory and effector cell characteristics based on phenotypic analysis and by hypersensitivity to TCR stimulation. The significance of gaining an activation status becomes important, as these lymphocytes react to antigen stimulation at a quicker rate than do naïve T-cells, further potentiating antitumor effects. Therefore, based on our more recent understanding of homeostasis-driven proliferation of naïve and memory T-cells, specifically in irradiated hosts, an alternative explanation to the results of Hellstrom et al. is that the expanding T-cell population swelled in response to the "space" created by irradiation, and that antigenic stimulation, derived from the tumor cells, induced potent antitumor T-cell responses. This possible scenario is supported by the studies described herein.

Dummer et al. hypothesized that strong T-cell responses could be induced by homeostatic proliferation, and that these responses depended on the presentation of antigen by APCs during T-cell expansion. These studies demonstrated that tumor-bearing mice transfused with vast numbers of T-cells following homeostatic disruption (induced via low-level irradiation) elicited strong antitumor T-cell responses (7,8) resulting in dramatic tumor regressions. In another study, Hu et al. (65) showed that naïve T-cells reconstituted into lymphopenic hosts preferentially expanded the tumor-specific T-cell population, following a melanoma vaccine composed of melanoma cells genetically modified to secrete granulocyte-macrophage colony-stimulating factor (GM-CSF). In this model, tumor antigen was derived dying tumor cells, and the antitumor responses were augmented because of the DC-stimulating function of GM-CSF. Collectively, these results indicate that disrupting T-cell homeostasis elicits and augments vaccine-induced antigen-specific T-cell responses that generate potent antitumor effects.

Other approaches intended to disrupt T-cell homeostasis with the aim of inducing antitumor T-cell responses include the use of cytotoxic chemotherapeutic agents that modulate immune responses by temporarily depleting peripheral lymphocytes. Studies by Machiels et al. reported that the administration of low-dose chemotherapy (cyclophosphamide [Cy], doxyrubicin, or paclitaxel) (66), when given just before a GM-CSF secreting whole-cell vaccine, significantly delayed tumor growth and was associated with the generation of strong cytotoxic T-cell responses. These findings are also in agreement with numerous phase I and II clinical trials using similar anticancer drugs in cancer patients that also affect the human immune system (67 68). Ehrke et al. suggested that treatment of certain nonsolid malignancies with Cy correlated with tumor regression and sustained T-cell responses (69,70). Whereas in further studies, the combination of Cy and immunotherapies, typically consisting of ex vivo-activated T-cells, demonstrate belated tumor growth and eradication of metastatic tumors (71–73).

Interestingly, although the use of Cy in these previous studies was used for the induction of lymphopenia, Cy therapy has the added bonus of preferentially eliminating Treg cells. Early studies by North et al. found that low-dose Cy therapy induced immunological-mediated tumor regression by preferentially inhibiting Treg cells, thus facilitating the adoptive transfer of tumor-reactive T-cells (74,75). There are also other reports indicating that Cy can induce a polarized T-helper 1 cytokine phenotype (76), which is essential in inducing CTL responses, as well as supplementary data suggesting that Cy can overcome tolerance (77–80). Although the exact mechanism by which Cy enhances antitumor CTL responses is not known, there is ample evidence showing its therapeutic benefit. Therefore, it appears the use of Cy for inducing overall lymphodepletion has the further advantage of augmenting immune responses to "self" peptides, such as TAA, by removing Treg cells, which can inhibit T-cell responses against tumors and providing an optimal T-cell microenvironment.

In more recent clinical trials, Phan et al. reports that the co-administration of peptide vaccine plus α-CTLA blocking antibodies caused tumor shrinkage in most patients. What is more amazing, in 2 of the 14 patients in the study, all tumors (including lung and brain metastases) disappeared completely *(81)*. Studies conducted in our own laboratory demonstrated that TAA vaccination of tumor-bearing mice, given in combination with a strong adjuvant intended to disrupt lymphocyte homeostasis and CTLA-4 blockade, elicited long-lasting antitumor T-cell responses that extended mouse survival and delayed tumor growth kinetics *(55)*. In agreement with the idea that the disruption of T-cell homeostasis, administered with tumor antigens, can result in antitumor activity with clinical significance, Dudley et al. *(82)* recently found that the adoptive transfer of tumor-reactive T-cells into cancer patients exhibited a dramatic T-cell proliferation with sustained antitumor T-cell effector function following nonmyeloablative chemotherapy. Notably, 5 of 13 patients developed vitiligo, and tumor regression was observed in one or more metastases. Rosenberg et al. demonstrated that the autologous cell transfer of ex vivo expanded tumor-infiltrating lymphocytes proliferated in responses to the space created by lympho-depletion and caused significant tumor regression in patients with melanoma *(83)*. What is even more remarkable is that in some patients, tumor regression was accompanied by a dramatic increase of the tumor-reactive T-cells (up to 70% of CD8 T-cells in peripheral blood), which retained antitumor activity several months after transfer. Collectively, these results indicate that disruption of T-cell homeostasis before the administration of ex vivo expanded tumor-reactive T-cells can result in the induction of strong and long-lived antitumor immune responses with promising clinical benefit.

Although great success has been observed in clinical studies using adoptive cell transfer techniques to subdue certain cancers, for practical and economical reasons, we favor the use of peptide/protein-based vaccines that could be more widely used than cell-based therapies. However, we concede that current vaccination approaches are still far from attaining the impressive expansion of antitumor T-cells observed with adoptive immunotherapy. Currently, our laboratory is experimentally addressing what we consider several major obstacles in the in vivo generation of effective antitumor T-cell responses. First, we hope to generate sufficient numbers of tumor-reactive T-cells by utilizing a combination of optimized peptide T-cell epitopes, TLR ligand adjuvants, and co-stimulatory signals (via CD28, CD40 4-1BB, and OX40). The second obstacle—the short-term duration of antitumor immune activity—is being addressed by the timely induction of partial lympho-depletion before vaccination, to open space for homeostatic proliferation of tumor-reactive T-cells induced by the vaccine. Third, we intend to prevent some of the suppressor mechanisms that downregulate cellular immune responses. This challenge is being pursued by introducing CTLA-4 blockade postvaccination, and by depleting $CD4^+ CD25^+$ Treg cells using depleting antibodies or IL-2 toxin constructs, such as ONTAK. We theorize that by addressing these problems, we will be able to promote the preferential expansion and persistence of tumor-specific T-cells induced by vaccination, resulting in the prevention of tumor recurrences or metastatic diseases and perhaps even in the treatment of established bulky malignancies. This is certainly an attractive and more promising alternative to high dose chemotherapy and irradiation.

REFERENCES

1. Hsueh EC. Tumour cell-based vaccines for the treatment of melanoma. *BioDrugs* 2001; 15:713–720.
2. Toes RE, Offringa R, Blom RJ, Melief CJ, Kast WM. Peptide vaccination can lead to enhanced tumor growth through specific T-cell tolerance induction. *Proc Natl Acad Sci USA* 1996; 93:7855–7860.

3. Toes RE, Feltkamp MC, Ressing ME, et al. Cellular immunity against DNA tumour viruses: possibilities for peptide-based vaccines and immune escape. *Biochem Soc Trans* 1995; 23:692–696.

4. Siegel CT, Schreiber K, Meredith SC, et al. Enhanced growth of primary tumors in cancer-prone mice after immunization against the mutant region of an inherited oncoprotein. *J Exp Med* 2000; 191:1945–1956.

5. Schluns KS, Lefrançois L. Cytokine control of memory T-cell development and survival. *Nat Rev Immunol* 2003; 3:269–279.

6. Egerton M, Scollay R, Shortman K. Kinetics of mature T-cell development in the thymus. *Proc Natl Acad Sci USA* 1990; 87:2579–2582.

7. Dummer W, Ernst B, LeRoy E, Lee D, Surh C. Autologous regulation of naive T cell homeostasis within the T cell compartment. *J Immunol* 2001; 166:2460–2468.

8. Dummer W, Niethammer AG, Baccala R, et al. T cell homeostatic proliferation elicits effective antitumor autoimmunity. *J Clin Invest* 2002; 110:185–192.

9. Hassan J, Reen DJ. IL-7 promotes the survival and maturation but not differentiation of human post-thymic CD4+ T cells. *Eur J Immunol* 1998; 28:3057–3065.

10. Freitas AA, Rocha B. Lymphocyte survival: a red queen hypothesis [*see* comments]. *Science* 1997; 277:1950.

11. Freitas AA, Rocha B. Population biology of lymphocytes: the flight for survival. *Annu Rev Immunol* 2000; 18:83–111.

12. Freitas AA, Rocha BB. Lymphocyte lifespans: homeostasis, selection and competition [*see* comments]. *Immunol Today* 1993; 14:25–29.

13. Webb LM, Foxwell BM, Feldmann M. Interleukin-7 activates human naive CD4+ cells and primes for interleukin-4 production. *Eur J Immunol* 1997; 27:633–640.

14. Tough DF, Sprent J. Lifespan of lymphocytes. *Immunol Res* 1995; 14:1–12.

15. Tough DF, Sprent J. Life span of naive and memory T cells. *Stem Cells* 1995; 13:242–249.

16. Greil R, Anether G, Johrer K, Tinhofer I. Tracking death dealing by Fas and TRAIL in lymphatic neoplastic disorders: pathways, targets, and therapeutic tools. *J Leukoc Biol* 2003; 74:311–330.

17. Tschopp J, Irmler M, Thome M. Inhibition of fas death signals by FLIPs. *Curr Opin Immunol* 1998; 10:552–558.

18. Rathmell JC, Lindsten T, Zong WX, Cinalli RM, Thompson CB. Deficiency in Bak and Bax perturbs thymic selection and lymphoid homeostasis. *Nat Immunol* 2002; 3:932–939.

19. Colucci F, Bergman ML, Penha-Gonðcalves C, Cilio CM, Holmberg D. Apoptosis resistance of non-obese diabetic peripheral lymphocytes linked to the Idd5 diabetes susceptibility region. *Proc Natl Acad Sci USA* 1997; 94:8670–8674.

20. Colucci F, Cilio CM, Lejon K, Gonðcalves CP, Bergman ML, Holmberg D. Programmed cell death in the pathogenesis of murine IDDM: resistance to apoptosis induced in lymphocytes by cyclophosphamide. *J Autoimmun* 1996; 9:271–276.

21. Colucci F, Bergman ML, Lejon K, Holmberg D. Diabetes induction in C57BL/6 mice reconstituted with lymphocytes of nonobese diabetic ↔ C57BL/6 mouse embryo aggregation chimeras. *Scand J Immunol* 1998; 48:571–576.

22. Yang W, Hussain S, Mi QS, Santamaria P, Delovitch TL. Perturbed homeostasis of peripheral T cells elicits decreased susceptibility to anti-CD3-induced apoptosis in prediabetic nonobese diabetic mice. *J Immunol* 2004; 173:4407–4416.

23. Tivol EA, Borriello F, Schweitzer AN, Lynch WP, Bluestone JA, Sharpe AH. Loss of CTLA-4 leads to massive lymphoproliferation and fatal multiorgan tissue destruction, revealing a critical negative regulatory role of CTLA-4. *Immunity* 1995; 3:541–547.

24. Bachmann MF, Waterhouse P, Speiser DE, McKall-Faienza K, Mak TW, Ohashi PS. Normal responsiveness of CTLA-4-deficient anti-viral cytotoxic T cells. *J Immunol* 1998; 160:95–100.

25. Waterhouse P, Marengáere LE, Mittrèucker HW, Mak TW. CTLA-4, a negative regulator of T-lymphocyte activation. *Immunol Rev* 1996; 153:183–207.

26. Waterhouse P, Bachmann MF, Penninger JM, Ohashi PS, Mak TW. Normal thymic selection, normal viability and decreased lymphoproliferation in T cell receptor-transgenic CTLA-4-deficient mice. *Eur J Immunol* 1997; 27:1887–1892.

27. Waldmann TA, Dubois S, Tagaya Y. Contrasting roles of IL-2 and IL-15 in the life and death of lymphocytes: implications for immunotherapy. *Immunity* 2001; 14:105–110.

28. Waterhouse P, Penninger JM, Timms E, et al. Lymphoproliferative disorders with early lethality in mice deficient in Ctla-4. *Science* 1995; 270:985–988.

29. Greenwald RJ, Latchman YE, Sharpe AH. Negative co-receptors on lymphocytes. *Curr Opin Immunol* 2002; 14:391–396.

30. Greenwald RJ, Oosterwegel MA, van der Woude D, et al. CTLA-4 regulates cell cycle progression during a primary immune response. *Eur J Immunol* 2002; 32:366–373.

31. van Elsas A, Sutmuller RP, Hurwitz AA, et al. Elucidating the autoimmune and antitumor effector mechanisms of a treatment based on cytotoxic T lymphocyte antigen-4 blockade in combination with a B16 melanoma vaccine: comparison of prophylaxis and therapy. *J Exp Med* 2001; 194:481–489.

32. van Elsas A, Hurwitz AA, Allison JP. Combination immunotherapy of B16 melanoma using anti-cytotoxic T lymphocyte-associated antigen 4 (CTLA-4) and granulocyte/macrophage colony-stimulating factor (GM-CSF)-producing vaccines induces rejection of subcutaneous and metastatic tumors accompanied by autoimmune depigmentation. *J Exp Med* 1999; 190:355–366.

33. Gribben JG, Freeman GJ, Boussiotis VA, et al. CTLA4 mediates antigen-specific apoptosis of human T cells. *Proc Natl Acad Sci USA* 1995; 92:811–815.

34. Sutmuller RP, van Duivenvoorde LM, van Elsas A, et al. Synergism of cytotoxic T lymphocyte-associated antigen 4 blockade and depletion of CD25(+) regulatory T cells in antitumor therapy reveals alternative pathways for suppression of autoreactive cytotoxic T lymphocyte responses. *J Exp Med* 2001; 194:823–832.

35. Jonuleit H, Schmitt E. The regulatory T cell family: distinct subsets and their interrelations. *J Immunol* 2003; 171:6323–6327.

36. Curotto de Lafaille MA, Lafaille JJ. CD4(+) regulatory T cells in autoimmunity and allergy. *Curr Opin Immunol* 2002; 14:771–778.

37. Lanzavecchia A, Sallusto F. Regulation of T cell immunity by dendritic cells. *Cell* 2001; 106:263–266.

38. Lanzavecchia A, Sallusto F. The instructive role of dendritic cells on T cell responses: lineages, plasticity and kinetics. *Curr Opin Immunol* 2001; 13:291–298.

39. Tanchot C, Le Campion A, Lâeaument S, Dautigny N, Lucas B. Naive CD4(+) lymphocytes convert to anergic or memory-like cells in T cell-deprived recipients. *Eur J Immunol* 2001; 31:2256–2265.

40. Casares N, Arribillaga L, Sarobe P, et al. CD4+/CD25+ regulatory cells inhibit activation of tumor-primed CD4+ T cells with IFN-gamma-dependent antiangiogenic activity, as well as long-lasting tumor immunity elicited by peptide vaccination. *J Immunol* 2003; 171:5931–5399.

41. Read S, Malmstrèom V, Powrie F. Cytotoxic T lymphocyte-associated antigen 4 plays an essential role in the function of CD25(+)CD4(+) regulatory cells that control intestinal inflammation. *J Exp Med* 2000; 192:295–302.

42. Danke NA, Koelle DM, Yee C, Beheray S, Kwok WW. Autoreactive T cells in healthy individuals. *J Immunol* 2004; 172:5967–5972.

43. Furtado GC, Curotto de Lafaille MA, Kutchukhidze N, Lafaille JJ. Interleukin 2 signaling is required for CD4(+) regulatory T cell function. *J Exp Med* 2002; 196:851–857.

44. Fontenot JD, Rudensky AY. Molecular aspects of regulatory T cell development. *Semin Immunol* 2004; 16:73.

45. Akira S, Takeda K, Kaisho T. Toll-like receptors: critical proteins linking innate and acquired immunity. *Nat Immunol* 2001; 2:675–680.

46. Zuany-Amorim C, Hastewell J, Walker C. Toll-like receptors as potential therapeutic targets for multiple diseases. *Nat Rev Drug Discov* 2002; 1:797–807.

47. Davila E, Celis E. Repeated administration of cytosine-phosphorothiolated guanine-containing oligonucleotides together with peptide/protein immunization results in enhanced CTL responses with anti-tumor activity. *J Immunol* 2000; 165:539–547.

48. Davila E, Velez MG, Heppelmann CJ, Celis E. Creating space: an antigen-independent, CpG-induced peripheral expansion of naive and memory T-lymphocytes in a full T-cell compartment. *Blood* 2002; 100: 2537–2345.

49. Yu XZ, Bidwell SJ, Martin PJ, Anasetti C. CD28-specific antibody prevents graft-versus-host disease in mice. *J Immunol* 2000; 164:4564–4568.

50. Yu X, Fournier S, Allison JP, Sharpe AH, Hodes RJ. The role of B7 costimulation in CD4/CD8 T cell homeostasis. *J Immunol* 2000; 164:3543–3543.

51. Rogers PR, Song J, Gramaglia I, Killeen N, Croft M. OX40 promotes Bcl-xL and Bcl-2 expression and is essential for long-term survival of CD4 T cells. *Immunity* 2001; 15:445–455.

52. Dahl AM, Klein C, Andres PG, et al. Expression of bcl-X(L) restores cell survival, but not proliferation off effector differentiation, in CD28-deficient T lymphocytes. *J Exp Med* 2000; 191:2031–2038.

53. Jameson SC. Maintaining the norm: T-cell homeostasis. *Nat Rev Immunol* 2002; 2:547–556.
54. Prlic M, Blazar BR, Khoruts A, Zell T, Jameson SC. Homeostatic expansion occurs independently of costimulatory signals. *J Immunol* 2001; 167:5664–5668.
55. Davila E, Kennedy R, Celis E. Generation of antitumor immunity by cytotoxic T lymphocyte epitope peptide vaccination, CpG-oligodeoxynucleotide adjuvant, and CTLA-4 blockade. *Cancer Res* 2003; 63:3281–3288.
56. Hellstrèom KE, Hellstrèom I. Evidence that tumor antigens enhance tumor growth in vivo by interacting with a radiosensitive (suppressor?) cell population. *Proc Natl Acad Sci USA* 1978; 75:436–440.
57. Hellstrèom KE, Hellstrèom I, Kant JA, Tamerius JD. Regression and inhibition of sarcoma growth by interference with a radiosensitive T-cell population. *J Exp Med* 1978; 148:799–804.
58. Cho BK, Rao VP, Ge Q, Eisen HN, Chen J. Homeostasis-stimulated proliferation drives naive T cells to differentiate directly into memory T cells. *J Exp Med* 2000; 192:549–556.
59. Goldrath AW, Bevan MJ. Selecting and maintaining a diverse T-cell repertoire. *Nature* 1999; 402:255–262.
60. Goldrath AW, Bogatzki LY, Bevan MJ. Naive T cells transiently acquire a memory-like phenotype during homeostasis-driven proliferation. *J Exp Med* 2000; 192:557–564.
61. Bevan MJ, Goldrath AW. T-cell memory: you must remember this . . . *Curr Biol* 2000; 10:R338–R340.
62. Ge Q, Hu H, Eisen HN, Chen J. Naïve to memory T-cell differentiation during homeostasis-driven proliferation. *Microbes Infect* 2002; 4:555–558.
63. Ge Q, Palliser D, Eisen HN, Chen J. Homeostatic T cell proliferation in a T cell-dendritic cell coculture system. *Proc Natl Acad Sci USA* 2002; 99:2983–2988.
64. Tanchot C, Le Campion A, Martin B, Lêeaument S, Dautigny N, Lucas B. Conversion of naive T cells to a memory-like phenotype in lymphopenic hosts is not related to a homeostatic mechanism that fills the peripheral naive T cell pool. *J Immunol* 2002; 168:5042–5046.
65. Hu HM, Poehlein CH, Urba WJ, Fox BA. Development of antitumor immune responses in reconstituted lymphopenic hosts. *Cancer Res* 2002; 62:3914–3919.
66. Machiels JP, Reilly RT, Emens LA, et al. Cyclophosphamide, doxorubicin, and paclitaxel enhance the antitumor immune response of granulocyte/macrophage-colony stimulating factor-secreting whole-cell vaccines in HER-2/*neu* tolerized mice. *Cancer Res* 2001; 61:3689–3697.
67. Oehen S, Brduscha-Riem K. Naïve cytotoxic T lymphocytes spontaneously acquire effector function in lymphocytopenic recipients: A pitfall for T cell memory studies? *Eur J Immunol* 1999; 29:608–614.
68. Lu J, Higashimoto Y, Appella E, Celis E. Multiepitope Trojan antigen peptide vaccines for the induction of antitumor CTL and Th immune responses. *J Immunol* 2004; 172:4575–4582.
69. Ehrke MJ. Effect of cancer therapy on host response and immunobiology. *Curr Opin Oncol* 1991; 3: 1070–1077.
70. Ehrke MJ, Mihich E, Berd D, Mastrangelo MJ. Effects of anticancer drugs on the immune system in humans. *Semin Oncol* 1989; 16:230–253.
71. Gold JE, Malamud SC, LaRosa F, Osband ME. Adoptive chemoimmunotherapy using ex vivo activated memory T-cells and cyclophosphamide: tumor lysis syndrome of a metastatic soft tissue sarcoma. *Am J Hematol* 1993; 44:42.
72. Gold JE, Bleiweiss IJ, Goldfarb AB, et al. Adoptive cellular therapy of human breast and colorectal tumor targets using ex vivo activated memory T lymphocytes with potentiation by *cis*-diamminedichloroplatinum(II). *J Surg Oncol* 1994; 55:222–228.
73. Gold JE, Ross SD, Krellenstein DJ, LaRosa F, Malamud SC, Osband ME. Adoptive transfer of ex vivo activated memory T-cells with or without cyclophosphamide for advanced metastatic melanoma: results in 36 patients. *Eur J Cancer* 1995; 31A:698–708.
74. North RJ. Cyclophosphamide-facilitated adoptive immunotherapy of an established tumor depends on elimination of tumor-induced suppressor T cells. *J Exp Med* 1982; 155:1063–1074.
75. North RJ, Havell EA. Glucocorticoid-mediated inhibition of endotoxin-induced intratumor tumor necrosis factor production and tumor hemorrhagic necrosis and regression. *J Exp Med* 1989; 170:703–710.
76. Li L, Okino T, Sugie T, et al. Cyclophosphamide given after active specific immunization augments antitumor immunity by modulation of Th1 commitment of CD4+ T cells. *J Surg Oncol* 1998; 67:221–227.
77. Pâerez-Dâiez A, Butterfield LH, Li L, Chakraborty NG, Economou JS, Mukherji B. Generation of CD8+ and CD4+ T-cell response to dendritic cells genetically engineered to express the MART-1/Melan-A gene. *Cancer Res* 1998; 58:5305–5309.
78. Polak L, Geleick H, Turk JL. Reversal by cyclophosphamide of tolerance in contact sensitization. Tolerance induced by prior feeding with DNCB. *Immunology* 1975; 28:939–942.

79. Polak L, Turk JL. Reversal of immunological tolerance by cyclophosphamide through inhibition of suppressor cell activity. *Nature* 1974; 249:654–656.
80. Polak L, Frey JR, Turk JL. Antilymphocyte serum and cyclophosphamide in the induction of tolerance to skin allografts in guinea pigs. *Transplantation* 1972; 13:310–315.
81. Phan GQ, Yang JC, Sherry RM, et al. Cancer regression and autoimmunity induced by cytotoxic T lymphocyte-associated antigen 4 blockade in patients with metastatic melanoma. *Proc Natl Acad Sci USA* 2003; 100:8372–8377.
82. Dudley ME, Wunderlich JR, Robbins PF, et al. Cancer regression and autoimmunity in patients after clonal repopulation with antitumor lymphocytes. *Science* 2002; 298:850–854.
83. Rosenberg SA, Dudley ME. Cancer regression in patients with metastatic melanoma after the transfer of autologous antitumor lymphocytes. *Proc Natl Acad Sci USA* 2004; 101:14,639–14,645.

18 Fast-Lane Evolution in the Tumor Microenvironment

Gabriella Marincola
and Francesco M. Marincola

SUMMARY

Human tumor immunology is a compound biological discipline that combines complexities related to the evolutionary and epigenetic adaptation of the immune system to those related to the genetic instability of cancer cells. We have discussed elsewhere the relevance of immune polymorphism and immune adaptation to the study of tumor host interactions in the tumor microenvironment. In this chapter, we describe changes occurring during the natural history of cancer development. We discuss whether this process may be accelerated by immune editing or other conditions that could alter the natural biology of cancer cells in favor of their survival in the host. In particular, we address evidence of tumor escape through loss of antigen presentation or through secretion of factors that may influence the function of the arm of the innate or adaptive immune response. We describe novel technologies that could be applied for the study in real time of these phenomena directly in humans.

Key Words: Immunotherapy; melanoma; functional genomics; tumor escape; human polymorphism.

1. INTRODUCTION

Human tumor immunology is facing the fundamental question of why clearly recognizable adaptive immune responses against cancer cells cannot, in most cases, prevent or clear cancer development. Some suggested immune editing as a mechanism through which cancer cells can rapidly modify their biological characteristics to evade cognitive immune responses *(1)*. This point of view assumes that the immune system of the tumor-bearing host is capable of mounting an effective immune response that could efficiently induce tumor rejection, unless tumor cells could rapidly adapt though selection of immune-resistant mutants. We argue that, although animal models clearly demonstrate that this is a factual biological phenomenon, evidence that such modulation exists in humans is much more circumstantial and lacks definitive experimental evidence.

Others researchers hypothesize that, although cognitive immune responses against cancer can be identified in the tumor-bearing host, they do not reach either in quality or intensity the effector potential necessary to eliminate cancer cells. According to this model, cancer cells constitute a suitable target of immune recognition, but immune cells cannot

From: *Cancer Drug Discovery and Development: Immunotherapy of Cancer*
Edited by: M. L. Disis © Humana Press Inc., Totowa, NJ

effectively destroy them *(2–4)*. This hypothesis suggests that mechanism(s) other than the one-dimensional T-cell receptor/tumor antigen (TA) interaction is necessary for complete eradication of tumor masses. Obviously, a balance between the two points of view may be stricken by nature itself, as it is possible that immune responses against cancer in humans are not as strong as those observed in animal models and, therefore, these less effective immune responses lower the need for escape mechanisms. In that case, with increasing effectiveness of the immune responses induced by immunological manipulation, it could be expected that mechanisms promoted by immune selection may travel in a faster lane *(5)*. In this chapter, therefore, we discuss the evidence in humans that:

1. Cognitive immune responses against cancer naturally occur in the tumor-bearing host.
2. Such immune responses can be easily amplified by antigen-specific immunization.
3. They may localize to the tumor site.
4. They may not be intrinsically sufficient to induce tumor rejection.
5. Individual variation may be a factor influencing immune responses.
6. Heterogeneity of the tumor microenvironment may influence the effectiveness of the immune response (the mixed response phenomenon).
7. Such adaptation occurs rapidly in time in the tumor microenvironment and tools should be applied to study the kinetics of the immune responses to cancer in real time.

2. NATURALLY OCCURRING ANTICANCER IMMUNE RESPONSES

It has been long known that some human tumors harbor in their microenvironment T-cells capable of recognizing antigens expressed, processed, and presented by cancer cells in association with the major histocompatibility complex. Originally, Asano and Mandel *(6)* observed that cultures of tumor preparations from human breast cancer stimulated with phytohemagglutinin in soft agar yielded colonies of T-cells. In addition, Santer et al. *(7)* noted that mouse tumors harbored cytotoxic T-cells that could recognize and kill syngeneic cancer cells. These observations lead to the demonstration that lymphocytes cultured in vitro from human tumor preparations in the presence of interleukin (IL)-2 could be cytotoxic against tumor cells *(8–11)*, and that their recognition of target cells was human leukocyte antigen (HLA) class I-restricted *(12–14)*. Although the original identification of tumor-infiltrating lymphocytes in humans was done in breast cancer, most of the subsequent work was performed in the context of metastatic melanoma, perhaps because of the ease with which subcutaneous metastases could be accessed in this disease or because of the relative propensity of lymphocytes to grow in culture when expanded from melanoma lesions. Because most of the studies investigating the role of T-cells in human cancer were performed in melanoma, the discovery and molecular characterization of the first melanoma antigens recognized by T-cells occurred with this disease *(15)*. A large number of TAs recognized by T-cells have been subsequently identified in the context of melanoma and other solid tumors.

The observation of tumor-infiltrating lymphocytes that can be expanded from growing cancerous lesions and that could recognize tumor cells when activated in vivo suggested that the adaptive immune mechanisms are cognitive of tumor cells, but this recognition is not sufficient for the rejection of cancer. Two lines of thought could be envisioned to explain such phenomenon: there was either a discrepancy between the cytotoxic activity of T-cells expanded in vitro compared with their ability to destroy tumor cells in vivo, or the tumor cells could implement mechanisms in vivo that could protect them from immune recognition *(16)*.

The observation of the tumor-infiltrating lymphocyte phenomenon suggested that itinerant T-cells could reach and expand at tumor site. With the molecular identification of TAs recognized by tumor-infiltrating T-cells, it became possible to test whether the immune competence of the host was affected systemically by the presence of tumor burden by quantifying the immune responsiveness of antigen-specific circulating lymphocytes in tumor-bearing individuals and normal controls. Comparative analysis of TA-specific circulating T-cell responses in tumor-bearing vs normal individuals demonstrated that the tumor-bearing status primes in vivo the host immune system against cancer cells *(17)*. This observation validated further the concept that the adaptive immune system of humans is sensitized, at least in the context of metastatic melanoma, to the presence of tumor-specific antigens, but this level of immune competence is not sufficient for tumor rejection. In summary, therefore, it appears that the overall balance of tumor/immune system interactions scores, in the majority of cases, in favor of the tumor with a relatively peaceful coexistent of TA-specific T-cells and cancer cells within the tumor microenvironment.

3. ENHANCEMENT OF NATURAL OR NEWLY INDUCED IMMUNE RESPONSES AGAINST CANCER

Lack of tumor rejection by a cognitive immune system could be attributed to an insufficient intensity of the immune response. For this reason, the molecular characterization of TAs whose expression was shared by tumors from most individuals and the identification of individual epitopes associated with common HLA alleles lead to the development of active-specific immunization against cancer *(18)*. It became soon apparent that the in vivo administration of minimal epitopic determinants in adjuvant emulsions was sufficient to enhance greatly the frequency of circulating TA-specific T-cells *(19–24)*. Although promising results were achieved when active specific immunization was combined to the systemic administration of IL-2 *(25)*, in most cases, vaccination alone proved to consistently enhance pre-existing or induce *de novo* T-cell responses that, however, did not lead to tumor regression *(4,26–29)*. This observation corroborated the evidence that cognitive immune responses against antigens bore by cancer cells are not sufficient by themselves to induced cancer rejection.

Researchers have tried extensively to explain the reason for this paradoxical coexistence of cancer-specific T-cells and cancer cells in the same host, suggesting anergy, ignorance, or some other malfunctions of TA-specific T-cells that do not allow the exploitation of their full effector potential. We refer the reader to a recent review from our group on the subject *(4)*. We have concluded recently that the lack of tumor rejection by circulating cytotoxic T-cell induced by active specific immunization is a physiological behavior of T-cells intermittently exposed to antigen stimulation in the form of a vaccine. We postulated that T-cells need exposure to a co-stimulatory signal in addition to antigen-specific stimulation to be reactivated during the afferent phase of their life cycle *(30)*. The co-stimulation may be provided within the tumor microenvironment by proinflammatory stimuli constitutively produced by tumor or infiltrating normal cells, or could be induced by the coadministration of systemic immune enhancers, such as IL-2 *(31)*. Unfortunately, whereas extensive information about the requirements for T-cell activation is available in experimental systems, very little is known about the physiological requirements in vivo in humans because of the difficulty to extract this information directly from patients. In fact, the requirements for T-cell reactivation in the target organ (in our case, the tumor microenvironment) could be best analyzed by complementing the study of systemic immune responses with that of the direct interaction between tumor and immune cells within the tumor microenvironment where they are supposed to occur *(32)*. With this strategy, it is possible to verify whether immunization induced T-cells reach the tumors site, whether and how the heterogeneity of tumors may alter in different patients the effectiveness of T-cells, and, by serially analyzing the tumor microenvironment, it would be also possible to test whether dynamic changes of tumor cell phenotypes may balance the immunological wave induced by the immunization.

4. LOCALIZATION OF IMMUNE RESPONSES AT THE TUMOR SITE

It is intuitive and experimentally proven that localization at the tumor site is necessary for the fulfillment of the effector function of TA-specific cytotoxic T-cells. The adoptive administration of tumor-infiltrating lymphocytes labeled with [111]indium demonstrated that tumor regression occurs only when the adoptively transferred cells localize within the lesion *(33)*. This important observation underlines the relevance of the presence of antigen-specific T-cells at the tumor site as a mandatory contributor of tumor rejection. Although necessary, localization is not sufficient. In fact, in the same study, several cases where observed of localization without tumor regression. Similar observations could be made in the context of active-specific immunization. A comparative expansion of tumor-infiltrating lymphocytes from biopsies obtained before and after immunization suggested that it was easier to expand immunization-specific T-cells following immunization as compared with before immunization *(34)*. An even more important observation came from the analysis of interferon (IFN)-γ expression in melanoma metastases serially biopsied by fine needle aspiration (FNA). Material obtained from FNA performed during immunization had higher content of IFN-γ mRNA compared with those obtained before immunization *(35)*. The increase in IFN-γ mRNA levels could be attributed to the localization of vaccination-specific T-cells at the tumor site by identifying and enumerating them with tetrameric HLA/epitope complexes. Furthermore, the levels of IFN-γ correlated tightly with the expression by tumor cells of the antigen targeted by the vaccine. This suggests that not only the T-cells could localize at that tumor site, but also that they could also recognize tumor cells. Yet, this localization was not sufficient to induce tumor regression, because most of the lesions analyzed continued unaltered their growth.

These observations are very important because they confirm that TA-specific T-cells induced by vaccination are capable to reach the tumor site, but they are not able to expand in vivo and to exploit their potential anticancer activity in the tumor microenvironment. If this observation is correct, various explanations could be considered as discussed previously. We here focus on the possibility that circulating immunization-induced T-cells rest in a physiological quiescent status that allows them to leave the lymph nodes draining the immunization site where their locoregional exposure to the immunogen occurred *(30)*. This hypothesis suggests that after the primary stimulus, T-cells need to be reactivated in the target organ where they are reexposed to the cognate antigen, and that such reactivation requires a co-stimulatory stimulus, as well as antigen recall for the induction of successful effector T-cells. This is biologically intuitive in a teleological sense, because effector T-cells are most efficiently utilized if they are activated only in the presence of the relevant antigen and a danger signal that informs them of the necessity of their action *(36)*. In fact, in a recent analysis of vaccination-induced T-cells, we observed in an in vitro model that full activation of effector function, as well as massive proliferation, could be achieved only when T-cells were exposed to antigen recall plus IL-2 as a co-stimulating factor. In particular, we noted that both stimulations were required for the complete activation. If we are allowed to extrapolate the in vitro model to the in vivo situation, we can picture easily how, at the tumor site tumor, antigen-specific T-cells may be exposed to antigen recall, but seldom will sufficient co-stimulatory signals be present to induce their full activation *(2)*. This hypothesis raises the obvious question: what are the requirements within the tumor microenvironment for full T-cell activation that may influence the outcome of immunotherapy and switch a dormant recognition of cancer cells into an acute rejection of cancer, as observed in the context of acute rejection of solid transplant organs? This question points to the need of studying the tumor microenvironment and its complex biology.

5. HETEROGENEITY OF THE HOST AND IMMUNE POLYMORPHISM

Before addressing the question central to this chapter regarding the biology of the tumor microenvironment as a strong modulator of immune responses and its evolving nature, we address a factor independent of tumor biology that may also determine whether a patient is more likely to respond to therapy than another one. The influence that the genetic background of individual patients may have on the ability to respond to biological therapies remains largely unexplored. An oversimplification of the dynamics of the immune response may discriminate two distinct biological components that may influence immune responsiveness during biological therapy: the genetic background of the patient and the heterogeneous biology of individual tumors.

Although genetic background has often been proposed as a predictor of immune responsiveness, very little evidence exists that immune responsiveness is predetermined *(37)*. Specific markers that may affect immune responsiveness, such as the HLA complex genes responsible for coding molecules involved in antigen presentation, have not been conclusively linked to prognosis, response to therapy, and survival *(38–41)*. Associations between polymorphisms of cytokine genes and predisposition to develop melanoma or other cancers *(42,43)* suggest a genetic influence in the immune modulation of cancer growth. However, the relevance of immune polymorphism as a modulator of the immune response to biological therapy has never been addressed in the context of tumor immunology *(37,43)*. This factor should be considered in future studies as techniques are becoming available that are suitable for the screening at a genome wide level of polymorphisms in clinical settings *(37,44)*.

6. THE MIXED-RESPONSE PHENOMENON AND THE HETEROGENEITY OF TUMORS

Although genetic background may play a significant role in modulating immune responsiveness, it is possible that distinct phenotypes of tumor cells may play a key role in determining immune responsiveness. We have been particularly interested in this possibility because of the relatively frequent observation of mixed responses to identical treatment by synchronous metastatic lesions. Very little literature is available regarding this interesting biological phenomenon relatively well-known to clinicians treating with biological therapy metastatic cutaneous melanoma and patients with renal cell carcinoma. Multiple lesions in patients with advanced forms of these cancers have a propensity to respond differently to immunotherapy, with some regressing and others progressing in response to the same treatment. Considering the genetic background and immune status of the individual bearing such lesions as a constant at that point, the observation of the mixed responses suggests that different conditions in the microenvironment of distinct synchronous metastases present in the same individual may strongly affect the outcome. Because tumor immunology merges the intricacy of human immunology with the complex biology of cancer, the study of anticancer immune responses in humans should include, therefore, the analysis of the biology of individual tumors as, contrary to other immune phenomena, the immune systems confront in cancer a heterogeneous and potentially rapidly evolving target. This may also explain why experimental animal models created to bypass the complexity of humans through inbreeding and standardization of cancers cell clones rarely predict human response to therapy, although they have been extremely powerful tools for testing basic immunological concepts. The acceptance of complexity as an analytical tool, on the other hand, may provide useful insights if strategies could be applied to discern least-common denominators required for the existence of a biological process through the identification of required patterns comparable to those predictive of climatic changes that allow weather forecast using nonlinear mathematics approaches (45–47). Therefore, we gradually depart from hypothesis-driven, molecularly defined arguments as we progress in this story toward the part where the biology of human cancer is discussed as a movable target of immune recognition (31).

7. THE INTERACTIONS BETWEEN TUMOR CELLS AND TA-SPECIFIC T-CELLS

As discussed, it seems that the induction of IFN-γ in immunization-induced T-cells by tumor cells is not sufficient to induce tumor regression (35). For this reason, we hypothesized that TA-specific T-cells naturally or during therapy may reach the tumor microenvironment, but in most cases, they are not exposed to sufficient co-stimulation for their activation into full effector cells. Tumor cells may lack sufficient antigen presentation, or the tumor microenvironment may lack sufficient co-stimulatory properties (2). We favor the second hypothesis, because we have not been able to accumulate evidence that lack of antigen stimulation is a primary reason for tumor unresponsiveness. Indeed, transcriptional profiling of melanoma metastases assessed before therapy demonstrated that the level of expression of the target antigen is not predictive of immune responsiveness (48). These findings were also confirmed by immunohistochemical staining. Because this study was done in lesions that expressed the HLA antigen associated with the immunization (HLA-A*0201), HLA loss could also be excluded as responsible for the clinical outcome. In addition, lack of response was associated with a "silent" genetic profile characterized by no significant differences in global gene expression between treatment and pretreatment samples (49). Interestingly, whereas TA expression was not predictive of response, loss of TA expression was consistently observed during therapy in lesions destined to regress, whereas no changes were noted in lesions that did not respond (48). Loss of TA expression preceded clearance of tumor cell during response as the expression of other

TA irrelevant to the immunization remained stable and cytological analysis confirmed the presence of tumor cells. Thus, it is likely that TA-specific T-cells induced by immunization reach the tumor site, interact with tumor cells, and are exposed to antigen recall, but a secondary co-stimulation is lacking to expand further their number in vivo and activate their effector function (31).

8. THE TUMOR MICROENVIRONMENT

As observed previously, the microenvironment of human tumors is complex, heterogeneous, and ever-changing in adaptation to immune pressure, response to therapy, or simply as a consequence of the genetic instability of cancer cells (31). Although obvious, this concept has received little attention during the monitoring of anticancer immune responses, possibly because extensive analysis of the tumor microenvironment that requires repeated biopsies is technically challenging and ethically difficult to justify in humans. Thus, immune monitoring is mostly limited to the systemic immune response through analysis of circulating lymphocytes easy to access through venipuncture. Yet, tools are becoming available that allow the serial analysis of tumor lesions through FNA or similar strategies (32). In this fashion, it could be possible to predict immune responsiveness by sampling tumor lesions before the beginning of therapy, while directly linking experimental results to the clinical outcome (49). The same approach can be applied to the study of the mechanism of actions of therapeutic agents, as we demonstrated for systemically administered IL-2 (50). Advancements in mRNA amplification technology allow the utilization of material from a limited source for extensive genetic profiling of metastatic lesions (51–53). These analyses have shown that the tumor microenvironment of a relatively homogenous sample of tumors, such as a collection of subcutaneous melanoma metastases, can vary greatly in expression of potent immune modulatory genes including cytokines, chemokines, metalloproteinases, angioregulatory factors, and growth factors (31). In addition, it is becoming apparent that metastatic melanoma harbors a genetic profile quite different from other solid tumors, and that such differences are in part related to the frequency of expression of immune regulatory genes mostly belonging to the effector arm of the innate immune response (54). Obviously, much more needs to be learned through discovery-driven descriptions of human tumors before relevant theories can be framed about the interactions between immune and tumor cells in humans.

9. FAST-LANE EVOLUTION
IN THE TUMOR MICROENVIRONMENT

Cancer is a disease characterized by extreme genetic instability (55). Individual differences in telomere size (56), different patterns of methylation (57), and other factors may influence the patterns of growth and adaptation to the surrounding environment of cancer cells. The question arises of whether environmental pressure mediated by immune selection or other biologically relevant conditions may alter the rate of this natural dedifferentiation process. Animal models strongly support the possibility that the immune system plays a major role in regulating and modifying tumor growth. This concept has been recently termed "immune editing" (1,58), and it differs from the old idea of immune surveillance (59,60), because not only does it suggest that the immune system may control tumor growth, but that also by sculpting the immunogenic phenotype of tumor cells it might facilitate tumor progression (1). Most recently, Dunn et al. (58) suggested that immune editing proceeds through three stages: elimination (of target cells by immune cells), equilibrium (a balance is stricken between the host and the tumor), and escape (tumor cells acquire a phenotype that allows them to avoid immune recognition).

Although intuitive, evidence in humans of immune editing is less easy to demonstrate for the simple reason that the type of experimentation necessary to confirm that the dedifferentiation occurring naturally during the neoplastic process is influenced by the surrounding environment is often impractical and in some circumstances, unethical. A few observations support the concept that neoplastic phenotype evolution is accelerated by immune selection:

1. The neoplastic process is by nature unstable *(55)*; gene expression profiling has shown that the transcriptional program of cancer cells evolves early in the determination of the disease. Subsequently, alteration in the behavior of tumors occurs because the most dedifferentiated and aggressive cellular phenotypes take over the other milder ones *(61,62)*.
2. Immune suppression, whether related to immune deficient pathology or to pharmaceutical manipulation for the control of transplant rejection, is associated with an increased rate of several cancers *(63–69)*.
3. Anecdotal examples have described phenotype changes of tumor cells that promote their escape specifically to relevant to the immune therapies received by the patients *(70–75)*.

The evolution of cancer cell phenotypes can be altered by treatment other than immune manipulation, and some have argued that gene expression analysis should be applied to study the dynamic profile of cancers undergoing various forms of therapy *(76)*. Similarly, we have proposed that tools are now available to dissect in real-time changes related and specific to a given therapy through serial FNA *(32)*. With this strategy, we observed that the pretreatment level of expression of the gene targeted by active-specific immunization (in this case, the melanoma differentiation antigen gp100/PMel17) did not predict the immune responsiveness of melanoma metastases *(48)*. However, the short-term kinetics of TA expression during therapy was very informative and demonstrated a rapid loss of gp100/PMel17 in lesions undergoing clinical regression, whereas no changes were observed in progressing lesions. TA loss was partially specific because other tumor-specific antigens belonging to the cancer/testis family and expressed selectively by tumor cells did not change their level of expression. Interestingly, the expression of melanoma antigen recognized by T-cells 1/MelanA decreased in association with the expression of gp100/PMel17, although the former was not targeted by vaccination. Indeed, we had observed previously by immunohistochemical analysis that the expression of the two melanoma differentiation antigens is relatively, although not absolutely, coordinated in the majority of melanoma metastases *(77–79)*.

Recently, we compared the genetic profile of melanoma metastases and noted that the expression of melanoma differentiation antigens including gp100/PMle17, melanoma antigen recognized by T-cells 1/MelanA, tyrosinase, tyrosinase-related protein 1 and preferentially expressed antigen in melanoma was tightly coordinated, suggesting that their downregulation or loss of expression during melanoma progression may be related to a central regulatory pathway not yet identified *(54)*. This finding may have important repercussions in the design of antigen-specific immunization protocols and at the same time, may complicate the interpretation of TA loss variant analysis by broadening loss of expression to antigens other than those targeted by a given therapy. More broadly, this example underlines the importance of studying the genetic evolution of cancer using high-throughput technologies that allow a global understanding of biological processes framing individual gene expression alterations in the context of the whole transcriptional profile relevant to a given situation. Genetic profiling has been quite useful in analyzing cancer progression in natural conditions and during therapy. Global transcript analysis can differentiate tumors into subclasses beyond the discriminatory power of histopathological observation, and such distinction may have diagnostic and prognostic value *(49,52, 80–86)*. However, we have recently argued that, whereas, in some cases, molecular subclasses may represent distinct disease taxonomies associated to specific biological behaviors, temporal changes associated with the dedifferentiation of cancer may contribute to the segregation of taxonomically identical entities into separate groups. For instance, although we noticed originally that melanoma metastases can be segregated into two molecular subclasses believed to represent distinct disease entities *(82)*, serial sampling of identical metastases by FNA suggested that the two subclasses most likely represented temporal phenotypic changes, because material from the same lesions could cluster within either subgroup with a unilateral shift of the later samples toward a less differentiated phenotype. This observation questions rigid classifications of morphologically identical diseases based on single time-point observations *(31,49)*.

Most recently, to estimate exactly the influence of ontogeny on the transcriptional profile of cancer, we analyzed a series of primary renal cell cancer (RCC) tissues accompanied by normal renal tissue, subjected to identical surgical manipulation and experimental preparation. The transcriptional analysis of the paired specimens was compared with archival frozen samples of melanoma metastases representing a putative extreme of diversity with regard to ontogenesis and neoplastic progression, as well as with various primary epithelial cancers, to frame the origin of similarities and discrepancies in the transcriptional program. This study demonstrated that primary RCC tissues do segregate into at least two molecular subgroups, one of which contained only RCC samples, whereas the other contained a mixture of RCC and normal renal specimens. The genes responsible for the differences noted between the two subclasses of RCC belonged predominantly to the renal lineage and were mostly coexpressed by the group including RCC and normal renal tissues, suggesting that global transcript separated RCC tissues based on their level of differentiation. Thus, we concluded that, if no information was available about the transcriptional profile of paired normal tissues, it would have been difficult to explain the separation of the two major classes of RCC, and it might have been tempting to attribute such differences to separate taxonomies of disease, as previously done in the context of metastatic melanoma *(49,82)*. Comparison of the genetic profile of RCC and other primary tumors suggested that only a minority of genes related to oncogenesis was renal-specific, whereas in a large majority, the oncogenic process was similar among all primary tumors but quite different from the metastatic ones. The implication of this observation is critical, because it stresses the necessity of studying immune editing and cancer cell evolution in a dynamic fashion, while respecting the time lines that might be most relevant to a particular therapy.

10. CONCLUSIONS

In conclusion, there is overwhelming evidence that the tumor microenvironment changes rapidly during cancer progression. In addition, animal models suggest that tumor cell phenotype changes could be, at least in part, accelerated by immune surveillance or immune editing. There is, however, only circumstantial evidence immune editing occurs in humans. Nevertheless, whatever the cause, the ever-changing cancer phenotypes, whether in response to environmental pressure or the result of the natural evolution of neoplasia, may affect significantly the ability of immune cells to recognize and destroy cancer cells. Therefore, future studies should take into account tumor heterogeneity and its dynamic essence when monitoring the response to immunotherapy. Tools are now available that allow such analyses, at least in the translational medicine settings, and we believe that this opportunity should not be missed by clinical researchers.

REFERENCES

1. Dunn GP, Bruce AT, Ikeda H, Old LJ, Schreiber RD. Cancer immunoediting: from immunosurveillance to tumor escape. *Nat Immunol* 2002; 3:991–998.
2. Fuchs EJ, Matzinger P. Is cancer dangerous to the immune system? *Semin Immunol* 1996; 8:271–280.
3. Ochsenbein AF, Klenerman P, Karrer U, et al. Immune surveillance against a solid tumor fails because of immunological ignorance. *Proc Natl Acad Sci USA* 1999; 96:2233–2238.
4. Monsurro' V, Wang E, Panelli MC, Nagorsen D, Jin P, Smith K, et al. Active-specific immunization against cancer: is the problem at the receiving end? *Sem Cancer Biol* 2003; 13:473–480.
5. Khong HT, Restifo NP. Natural selection of tumor variants in the generation of "tumor escape" phenotypes. *Nat Immunol* 2002; 3:999–1005.
6. Asano S, Mandel TE. Colonies formed in agar from human breast cancer and their identification as T-lymphocytes. *J Natl Cancer Inst* 1981; 67:25–32.
7. Santer V, Mastromarino JH, Lala PK. Characterization of lymphocyte subsets in spontaneous mouse mammary tumors and host lymphoid organs. *Int J Cancer* 1980; 25:159–168.
8. Kimura H, Yamaguchi Y, Fujisawa T. Cytotoxicity of autologous and allogeneic lymphocytes against cultured human lung cancer cells: optimal conditions for the production of cytotoxic lymphocytes. *Gann* 1984; 75:1006–1016.
9. Vose BM, Moore M. Human tumor-infiltrating lymphocytes: a marker of host response. *Semin Hematol* 1985; 22:27–40.
10. Itoh K, Tilden AB, Balch CM. Interleukin 2 activation of cytotoxic T-lymphocytes infiltrating into human metastatic melanomas. *Cancer Res* 1986; 46:3011–3017.
11. Rabinowich H, Cohen R, Bruderman I, Steiner Z, Klajman A. Functional analysis of mononuclear cells infiltrating into tumors: lysis of autologous human tumor cells by cultured infiltrating lymphocytes. *Cancer Res* 1987; 47:173–177.
12. Wolfel T, Klehmann E, Muller C, Schutt KH, Meyer zum Buschenfelde KH, Knuth A. Lysis of human melanoma cells by autologous cytolytic T cell clones. Identification of human histocompatibility leukocyte antigen A2 as a restriction element for three different antigens. *J Exp Med* 1989; 170:797–810.
13. Kawakami Y, Zakut R, Topalian SL, Stotter H, Rosenberg SA. Shared human melanoma antigens. Recognition by tumor-infiltrating lymphocytes in HLA-A2.1-transfected melanomas. *J Immunol* 1992; 148:638–643.
14. Anichini A, Maccalli C, Mortarini R, et al. Melanoma cells and normal melanocytes share antigens recognized by HLA-A2-restricted cytotoxic T cell clones from melanoma patients. *J Exp Med* 1993; 177: 989–998.
15. van der Bruggen P, Traversari C, Chomez P, et al. A gene encoding an antigen recognized by cytolytic T lymphocytes on a human melanoma. *Science* 1991; 254:1643–1647.
16. Marincola FM, Jaffe EM, Hicklin DJ, Ferrone S. Escape of human solid tumors from T cell recognition: molecular mechanisms and functional significance. *Adv Immunol* 2000; 74:181–273.
17. Marincola FM, Rivoltini L, Salgaller ML, Player M, Rosenberg SA. Differential anti-MART-1/MelanA CTL activity in peripheral blood of HLA-A2 melanoma patients in comparison to healthy donors: evidence for in vivo priming by tumor cells. *J Immunother* 1996; 19:266–277.
18. Boon T, Gajewski TF, Coulie PG. From defined human tumor antigens to effective immunization? *Immunol Today* 1995; 16:334–336.
19. Cormier JN, Salgaller ML, Prevette T, et al. Enhancement of cellular immunity in melanoma patients immunized with a peptide from MART-1/Melan A [*see* comments]. *Cancer J Sci Am* 1997; 3:37–44.
20. Salgaller ML, Marincola FM, Cormier JN, Rosenberg SA. Immunization against epitopes in the human melanoma antigen gp100 following patient immunization with synthetic peptides. *Cancer Res* 1996; 56:4749–4757.

21. Parmiani G, Castelli C, Dalerba P, et al. Cancer immunotherapy with peptide-based vaccines: what have we achieved? Where are we going? *J Natl Cancer Inst* 2002; 94:805–818.

22. Marchand M, van Baren N, Weynants P, et al. Tumor regressions observed in patients with metastatic melanoma treated with an antigenic peptide encoded by gene MAGE-3 and presented by HLA-A1. *Int J Cancer* 1999; 80:219–230.

23. Marshall JL, Hoyer RJ, Toomey MA, et al. Phase I study in advanced cancer patients of a diversified prime-and-boost vaccination protocol using recombinant vaccinia virus and recombinant nonreplicating avipox virus to elicit anti-carcinoembryonic antigen immune responses. *J Clin Oncol* 2000; 18:3964–3973.

24. Jaeger E, Bernhard H, Romero P, et al. Generation of cytotoxic T-cell responses with synthetic melanoma-associated peptides in vivo: implications for tumor vaccines with melanoma-associated antigens. *Int J Cancer* 1996; 66:162–169.

25. Rosenberg SA, Yang JC, Schwartzentruber D, et al. Immunologic and therapeutic evaluation of a synthetic tumor associated peptide vaccine for the treatment of patients with metastatic melanoma. *Nat Med* 1998; 4:321–327.

26. Parmiani G, Castelli C, Rivoltini L, et al. Immunotherapy of melanoma. *Sem Cancer Biol* 2003; 13:391–400.

27. Talebi T, Weber JS. Peptide vaccine trials for melanoma: preclinical background and clinical results. *Sem Cancer Biol* 2003; 13:431–438.

28. Andersen MH, Gehl J, Reker S, et al. Dynamic changes of specific T cell responses to melanoma correlate with IL-2 administration. *Semin Cancer Biol* 2003; 13:449–459.

29. Paczesny S, Ueno H, Fay J, Banchereau J, Palucka AK. Dendritic cells as vectors for immunotherapy of cancer. *Semin Cancer Biol* 2003; 13:439–447.

30. Monsurro' V, Wang E, Yamano Y, et al. Quiescent phenotype of tumor-specific CD8+ T cells following immunization. *Blood* 2004; 104:1970–1978.

31. Marincola FM, Wang E, Herlyn M, Seliger B, Ferrone S. Tumors as elusive targets of T cell-directed immunotherapy. *Trends Immunol* 2003; 24:334–341.

32. Wang E, Marincola FM. A natural history of melanoma: serial gene expression analysis. *Immunol Today* 2000; 21:619–623.

33. Pockaj BA, Sherry RM, Wei JP, et al. Localization of [111]indium-labeled tumor infiltrating lymphocytes to tumor in patients receiving adoptive immunotherapy. Augmentation with cyclophosphamide and correlation with response. *Cancer* 1994; 73:1731–1737.

34. Panelli MC, Riker A, Kammula US, et al. Expansion of tumor/T cell pairs from fine needle aspirates (FNA) of melanoma metastases. *J Immunol* 2000; 164:495–504.

35 Kammula US, Lee K-H, Riker A, et al. Functional analysis of antigen-specific T lymphocytes by serial measurement of gene expression in peripheral blood mononuclear cells and tumor specimens. *J Immunol* 1999; 163:6867–6879.

36 Matzinger P. Danger model of immunity. *Scand J Immunol* 2001; 54:2–3.

37 Jin P, Wang E. Polymorphism in clinical immunology. From HLA typing to immunogenetic profiling. *J Transl Med* 2003; 1:8.

38. Wang E, Marincola FM, Stroncek D. Human leukocyte antigen (HLA) and human neutrophil antigen (HNA) systems. In: Hoffman R, Benz EJ, Shattil SJ, Furie B, Cohen HJ, Silberstein LE et al., eds. *Hematology: Basic Principles and Practice*. Philadelphia: Elsevier Science. 2003.

39. Rubin JT, Adams SD, Simonis T, Lotze MT. HLA polymorphism and response to IL-2 bases therapy in patients with melanoma. *Proc Soc Biol Ther Annu Meet* 1991; 1:18.

40. Marincola FM, Shamamian P, Rivoltini L, et al. HLA associations in the anti-tumor response against malignant melanoma. *J Immunother* 1996; 18:242–252.

41. Lee JE, Reveille JD, Ross MI, Platsoucas CD. HLA-DQB1*0301 association with increased cutaneous melanoma risk. *Int J Cancer* 1994; 59:510–513.

42. Howell WM, Bateman AC, Turner SJ, Collins A, Theaker JM. Influence of vascular endothelial growth factor single nucleotide polymorphisms on tumour development in cutaneous malignant melanoma. *Genes Immun* 2002; 3:229–232.

43. Howell WM, Calder PC, Grimble RF. Gene polymorphisms, inflammatory diseases and cancer. *Proc Nutr Soc* 2002; 61:447–456.

44. Wang E, Adams S, Zhao Y, et al. A strategy for detection of known and unknown SNP using a minimum number of oligonucleotides. *J Transl Med* 2003; 1:4.

45. Schwab ED, Pienta KJ. Cancer as a complex adaptive system. *Med Hypotheses* 1996; 47:235–241.

46. Cucuianu A. Chaos in cancer? *Nat Med* 1998; 4:1342–1343.

47. Dalgleish A. The relevance of non-linear mathematics (chaos theory) to the treatment of cancer, the role of the immune response and the potential for vaccines. *QJM* 1999; 92:347–359.
48. Ohnmacht GA, Wang E, Mocellin S, et al. Short term kinetics of tumor antigen expression in response to vaccination. *J Immunol* 2001; 167:1809–1820.
49. Wang E, Miller LD, Ohnmacht GA, et al. Prospective molecular profiling of subcutaneous melanoma metastases suggests classifiers of immune responsiveness. *Cancer Res* 2002; 62:3581–3586.
50. Panelli MC, Wang E, Phan G, et al. Genetic profiling of peripheral mononuclear cells and melanoma metastases in response to systemic interleukin-2 administration. *Genome Biol* 2002; 3:RESEARCH0035.
51. Wang E, Miller L, Ohnmacht GA, Liu E, Marincola FM. High-fidelity mRNA amplification for gene profiling using cDNA microarrays. *Nat Biotech* 2000; 17:457–459.
52. Wang E, Panelli MC, Marincola FM. Genomic analysis of cancer. *Princ Pract Oncol* 2003; 17:1–16.
53. Wang E, Panelli MC, Monsurro' V, Marincola FM. Gene expression profiling of anti-cancer immune responses. *Curr Opin Mol Ther* 2004; 6:288–295.
54. Wang E, Panelli MC, Zavaglia K, et al. Melanoma-restricted genes. *J Transl Med* 2004; 2:34.
55. Lengauer C, Kinzler KW, Vogelstein B. Genetic instabilities in human cancers. *Nature* 1998; 396:643–649.
56. Londono-Vallejo JA. Telomere length heterogeneity and chromosome instability. *Cancer Lett* 2004; 212: 135–144.
57. Szyf M, Pakneshan P, Rabbani SA. DNA methylation and breast cancer. *Biochem Pharmacol* 2004; 68: 1187–1197.
58. Dunn GP, Old LJ, Schreiber RD. The three Es of cancer immunoediting. *Annu Rev Immunol* 2004; 22: 329–360.
59. Burnet FM. The concept of immunological surveillance. *Prog Exp Tumor Res* 1970; 13:1–27.
60. Smyth MJ, Godfrey DI, Trapani JA. A fresh look at tumor immunosurveillance and immunotherapy. *Nat Immunol* 2001; 2:293–299.
61. Klein CA. The systemic progression of human cancer: a focus on the individual disseminated cancer cell —the unit of selection. *Adv Cancer Res* 2003; 89:35–67.
62. Klein CA. Gene expression signatures, cancer cell evolution and metastatic progression. *Cell Cycle* 2004; 3:29–31.
63. Cottrill CP, Bottomley DM, Phillips RH. Cancer and HIV infection. *Clin Oncol (R Coll Radiol)* 1997; 9:365–380.
64. Grulich AE. Update: cancer risk in persons with HIV/AIDS in the era of combination antiretroviral therapy. *AIDS Read* 2000; 10:341–346.
65. Robertson P, Scadden DT. Immune reconstitution in HIV infection and its relationship to cancer. *Hematol Oncol Clin North Am* 2003; 17:703–716, vi.
66. Abgrall S, Orbach D, Bonhomme-Faivre L, Orbach-Arbouys S. Tumors in organ transplant recipients may give clues to their control by immunity. *Anticancer Res* 2002; 22:3597–3604.
67. Lutz J, Heemann U. Tumours after kidney transplantation. *Curr Opin Urol* 2003; 13:105–109.
68. Ulrich C, Schmook T, Sachse MM, Sterry W, Stockfleth E. Comparative epidemiology and pathogenic factors for nonmelanoma skin cancer in organ transplant patients. *Dermatol Surg* 2004; 30(Pt 2):622–627.
69. Euvrard S, Ulrich C, Lefrancois N. Immunosuppressants and skin cancer in transplant patients: focus on rapamycin. *Dermatol Surg* 2004; 30(Pt 2):628–633.
70. Marincola FM, Shamamian P, Alexander RB, et al. Loss of HLA haplotype and B locus down-regulation in melanoma cell lines. *J Immunol* 1994; 153:1225–1237.
71. Jager E, Ringhoffer M, Karbach J, Arand M, Oesch F, Knuth A. Inverse relationship of melanocyte differentiation antigen expression in melanoma tissues and CD8+ cytotoxic-T-cell responses: evidence for immunoselection of antigen-loss variants in vivo. *Int J Cancer* 1996; 66:470–476.
72. Restifo NP, Marincola FM, Kawakami Y, Taubenberger J, Yannelli JR, Rosenberg SA. Loss of functional beta 2-microglobulin in metastatic melanomas from five patients receiving immunotherapy. *J Natl Cancer Inst* 1996; 88:100–108.
73. Jager E, Ringhoffer M, Altmannsberger M, et al. Immunoselection in vivo: independent loss of MHC class I and melanocyte differentiation antigen expression in metastatic melanoma. *Int J Cancer* 1997; 71:142–147.
74. Lee K-H, Panelli MC, Kim CJ, et al. Functional dissociation between local and systemic immune response following peptide vaccination. *J Immunol* 1998; 161:4183–4194.
75. Hicklin DJ, Marincola FM, Ferrone S. HLA class I antigen downregulation in human cancers: T-cell immunotherapy revives an old story. *Mol Med Today* 1999; 5:178–186.

76. Ellis MJ. Breast cancer gene expression analysis—the case for dynamic profiling. *Adv Exp Med Biol* 2003; 532:223–234.
77. Marincola FM, Hijazi YM, Fetsch P, et al. Analysis of expression of the melanoma associated antigens MART-1 and gp100 in metastatic melanoma cell lines and in in situ lesions. *J Immunother* 1996; 19: 192–205.
78. Cormier JN, Hijazi YM, Abati A, et al. Heterogeneous expression of melanoma-associated antigens (MAA) and HLA-A2 in metastatic melanoma in vivo. *Int J Cancer* 1998; 75:517–524.
79. Cormier JN, Abati A, Fetsch P, et al. Comparative analysis of the in vivo expression of tyrosinase, MART-1/Melan-A, and gp100 in metastatic melanoma lesions: implications for immunotherapy. *J Immunother* 1998; 21:27–31.
80. Alizadeh AA, Eisen MB, Davis RE, et al. Distinct types of diffuse large B-cell lymphoma identified by gene expression profiling. *Nature* 2000; 403:467–578.
81. Perou CM, Sertle T, Eisen MB, et al. Molecular portraits of human breast tumorurs. *Nature* 2000; 406: 747–752.
82. Bittner M, Meltzer P, Chen Y, et al. Molecular classification of cutaneous malignant melanoma by gene expression: shifting from a continuous spectrum to distinct biologic entities. *Nature* 2000; 406:536–840.
83. van't Veer LJ, Dai H, van de Vijver MJ, et al. Gene expression profiling predicts clinical outcome of breast cancer. *Nature* 2002; 415:530–536.
84. Boer JM, Huber WK, Sultmann H, et al. Identification and classification of differentially expressed genes in renal cell carcinoma by expression profiling on a global human 31,500-element cDNA array. *Genome Res* 2001; 11:1861–1870.
85. Young AN, Amin MB, Moreno CS, et al. Expression profiling of renal epithelial neoplasms: a method for tumor classification and discovery of diagnostic molecular markers. *Am J Pathol* 2001; 158:1639–1651.
86. Takahashi M, Yang XJ, Sugimura J, et al. Molecular subclassification of kidney tumors and the discovery of new diagnostic markers. *Oncogene* 2003; 22:6810–6818.

Leisha A. Emens, R. Todd Reilly, and Elizabeth M. Jaffee

SUMMARY

Initial clinical trials have demonstrated the safety and bioactivity of cancer vaccines, but vaccine-induced immune responses have seldom translated into clinically meaningful tumor regressions, particularly in advanced disease. It is increasingly clear that tumor-specific immune tolerance represents a layered system of controls that keep the immune system turned off. Immunoregulatory checkpoints map locoregionally to the tumor microenvironment and draining lymph nodes, and arise from the dynamic interactions between the tumor and the immune system. It is now apparent that cancer vaccines will have to be combined with other therapeutics that abrogate immune tolerance, further amplify vaccine-induced T-cell responses, or modify the tumor microenvironment to make it more conducive to the concerted action of innate and antigen-specific immune effector mechanisms. Here, we review the host–tumor dynamic from the perspective of immune tolerance and review current data supporting the integration of cancer vaccines with standard and novel therapeutic agents that can maximize their activity.

Key Words: Cancer vaccines; immune tolerance; tumor microenvironment; costimulation; regulatory T-cells; myeloid suppressor cells; combinatorial vaccination; chemotherapy; monoclonal antibodies.

1. INTRODUCTION

Efforts to optimize the use of surgery, radiation therapy, and chemotherapy for cancer treatment have produced a minimal improvement in survival for most solid tumors. The intrinsic therapeutic resistance of tumor cells is a major limitation to traditional cancer treatments. Their use is further dose-limited by the narrow therapeutic window defined by their efficacy and the magnitude of collateral damage to normal tissues resulting from the imprecise specificity of radiation and chemotherapy. These problems have generated great interest in applying advances in basic scientific research to develop highly targeted therapies that specifically disable regulatory pathways critical for transformation and metastasis. Harnessing the power of the patient's own immune system to reject breast

From: *Cancer Drug Discovery and Development: Immunotherapy of Cancer*
Edited by: M. L. Disis © Humana Press Inc., Totowa, NJ

cancer in a targeted, antigen-specific fashion expands this strategy beyond passive drug therapy to establish a durable process of cancer control through the phenomenon of immunologic memory. Several clinical trials testing distinct immunization strategies for cancer treatment support the safety and promise of cancer vaccines *(1)*. Despite the clear advantages of vaccine therapy, applying immunization to the problem of cancer treatment poses significant challenges. First, the potency of cancer vaccines is limited by strongly entrenched systemic mechanisms of immune tolerance *(2)*. Second, their therapeutic efficacy is frequently abrogated within the tumor microenvironment by local mechanisms of immune tolerance *(3)*. Third, dysregulated signaling pathways intrinsic to the transformed mammary epithelial cell itself represent a significant barrier to successful vaccine-induced tumor regression *(4)*. Fourth, in advanced cancers, vaccination is limited the simple mismatch between the sheer physical burden of metastatic tumor cells and the magnitude of vaccine-induced antitumor immune response *(5)*. Finally, many established cancer therapies are known to have an inhibitory effect on the immune system *(6)*. In this chapter, we consider strategies for combining breast cancer vaccines with a variety of standard and novel breast cancer treatment modalities and/or specifically targeted immune modulators. These combinatorial vaccination strategies are designed to break through established regulatory checkpoints to maximize the activity of the individual therapeutic components.

2. IMMUNE TOLERANCE:
A FORMIDABLE BARRIER TO CANCER IMMUNOTHERAPY

A complex system of checks and balances for controlling antigen-specific immune responses has evolved to protect the host from immunologic self-destruction, yet maintain the capacity for responding to and eliminating exogenous infectious threats. Whereas immune tolerance is essential for self- /nonself-discrimination and the prevention of autoimmunity, it represents a seemingly intractable barrier to the efficacy of tumor immunotherapy. Understanding the multilayered control of immune responses to tumor antigens, and complementary mechanisms of immune evasion, is essential for developing effective vaccination strategies for cancer treatment that can overcome immune tolerance.

2.1. Systemic Mechanisms of Immune Tolerance

Systemic mechanisms of immune tolerance can be broadly divided into those that occur centrally in the thymus, and those that occur peripherally in extrathymic tissues *(2)*. Specific tolerance can be achieved through central or peripheral deletional mechanisms, whereby a particular antigen-specific T-cell clone is physically eliminated from the repertoire. Because tumor cells arise endogenously and are recognized as self, elements of the tumor antigen-specific T-cell repertoire with the highest affinity for tumor antigens are most frequently deleted centrally in the thymus. Those that survive thymic deletion may be deleted peripherally by activation-induced cell death in the setting of widely disseminated tumor. These deletional processes result in the establishment of an alternate, lower affinity T-cell repertoire specific for the tumor that may be inherently less functional. However, high-affinity autoreactive T-cells can escape thymic and peripheral deletion, adding a very small population of highly reactive antigen-specific T-cells to the broader repertoire of low affinity T-cells. Complementary mechanisms exist that keep the activity of both high- and low-affinity T-cells in check once they reach the periphery. They may be rendered anergic (nonreactive) by suboptimal activation stimuli, or they may be directly suppressed by a variety of immunoregulatory cells.

2.2. Co-Stimulation and Counterstimulation: An Immunological Rheostat

Primary T-cell activation occurs as the result of two signals. One is provided by engagement of the antigen-specific T-cell receptor with the antigen/major histocompatibility complex (MHC), and the second is provided by the interactions of accessory molecules present on the surface of the T-cell with their ligands on antigen presenting cells (APCs). Importantly, although they express antigens on their surface, neither normal nor transformed somatic cells normally express positive co-stimulatory molecules. Thus, a potent mechanism of immune evasion by tumor cells is the presentation of tumor-associated antigens in the absence of appropriate accessory molecules for co-stimulation. In this case, tumor antigen-specific signaling without co-stimulation turns the T-cell off, resulting in anergy *(2)*. In contrast, professional APCs are programmed to provide effective co-stimulation, thereby activating antitumor immunity. This second signal provides a mechanism for fine-tuning the antigen-specific immune response by delivering positive and negative signals for T-cell activation that are integrated to determine the final magnitude of immune activation *(7)*. These second signals can be provided by a number of molecules in the B7 (Tables 1 and 2) or tumor necrosis factor receptor (TNFR) (Fig. 1) protein families.

2.2.1. THE B7 FAMILY

The B7 family is a system of receptor–ligand pairs characterized by a pair that transmits a positive signal and a counterregulatory pair that transmits a negative signal *(8)*. The prototype set of pairs is represented by the positive interactions of B7-1 (CD80)/B7-2 (CD86) with CD28, and the negative interactions of B7-1 (CD80)/B7-2 (CD86) with cytotoxic T-lymphocyte-associated antigen (CTLA)-4. Whereas CTLA-4-derived negative signals can be integrated with positive T-cell activation signals to raise the threshold for T-cell activation, it appears to preferentially attenuate stronger signals delivered by the T-cell receptor in order to limit T-cell expansion *(9)*. Interestingly, the preferential recruitment of CD28 by B7-2 and CTLA-4 by B7-1 to the immune response creates a mechanism whereby the activating potential of the APC is determined by its relative expression of B7-1 and B7-2 *(10)*. Importantly, newer members of the B7 family can not only regulate immune responses in lymphoid tissues, but also in nonlymphoid tissues (*see* Tables 1 and 2) *(11)*. Accordingly, these newer B7 family members collaborate with CD28/CTLA-4 signaling to orchestrate later stages of T-cell activation.

2.2.2. THE TNFR FAMILY

The TNFR family is essential for the initiation, expansion, and durability of the effector T-cell response (Fig. 2) *(25)*. Six receptor–ligand pairs positively regulate T-cell activation: CD40/CD40L, OX40/OX40L, 4-1BB/4-1BBL, CD27/CD70, CD30/CD30L, and herpes virus entry mediator (HVEM)/LIGHT (homologous to lymphotoxins, shows inducible expression, and competes with herpes simplex virus glycoprotein D for HVEM). CD40 is constitutively expressed on highly proliferative cell types, including hematopoietic progenitor cells, epithelial, and endothelial cells, and on all APCs *(26)*. Activated immune cells express CD40L. This pathway is critical for T-cell-dependent humoral immunity, and can substitute for T-cell help in priming CD4$^+$ and CD8$^+$ T-cell responses.

Table 1
Fine Control of T-Cell Activation by B7 Family Members

APC	T-cell	Signal	Function	Reagents	Reference
B7-1 (CD-80) B7-2 (CD-86)	CD28	+	Naïve T-cell activation IL-2 production T-cell proliferation and survival	No	8–10
B7-1 (CD-80) B7-2 (CD-86)	CTLA-4	–	Attenuation of T-cell responses	Yes[a]	8–10
ICOS ligand	ICOS	+ and –	Increases T-cell proliferation Increases T-helper type 2 responses Promotes T-cell-dependent humoral immunity Negative effects remain undefined	No	11–13[b]
B7-H3	?	+ and –	Increases T-cell proliferation Increases IFN-γ secretion Decreases T-helper type 1 responses	No	11,14–17[c]
B7-DC (PD-L2)	PD-1/?[d]	– and +	Inhibits T-cell proliferation (low Ag) Inhibits cytokine production (high Ag) Augments T-cell proliferation Promotes T-helper type 1 responses	No	11,18–21[d]
B7-H1 (PD-L1)	PD-1/?	– and +	Inhibits T-cell activation Increases T-cell proliferation Increases IL-10 production	No	11,22
B7-H4	BTLA-4	–	Inhibits T-cell proliferation Inhibits cytokine production	No	23

IL, interleukin; ICOS, inducible costimulator; IFN, interferon; PD, programmed death receptor; Ag, antigen; BTLA, B- and T-lymphocyte attenuator.

[a]Reagents available to modulate cytotoxic T-lymphocyte-associated antigen 4 signaling are the monoclonal antibodies CP-675206 and MDX010.

[b]Expression of ICOS ligand in tumor cells facilitates tumor rejection.

[c]Expression of B7-H3 in plasmacytoma or EL-4 lymphoma cells results in CD8+ T-cell-mediated tumor regression.

[d]PD-1 is the negative coreceptor for B7-DC; its positive coreceptor remains undefined.

[e]B7-DC expression on tumor cells promotes CD8+ T-cell-mediated tumor rejection.

In general, OX40, 4-1BB, and CD30 are induced by T-cell activation, with B7/CD28 signaling augmenting the level and kinetics of expression of these downstream molecules. CD27 and HVEM are constitutively expressed, with downregulation of HVEM on T-cell activation and reexpression on return to the resting state. OX40L, 4-1BBL, CD70, and CD30L are induced with APC activation. In contrast, LIGHT is expressed by immature dendritic cells (DCs) and is downregulated with maturation. Interestingly, forced expression of LIGHT within the tumor microenvironment incites a vigorous tumor rejection response (27). Together, these molecules determine the quality of the T-cell response.

2.3. Peripheral and Intratumoral Regulatory Cells Keep Tumor-Specific Immune Responses at Bay

Three types of regulatory cells keep immune responses in check: immature DCs, myeloid suppressor cells (MSCs), and regulatory T-cells (Tregs). In the absence of inflamma-

Table 2
B7 Family Members Expressed in the Tumor
Microenvironment Control Local Immune Responses

Tumor cell	T-cell	Signal	Function	Reagents	Reference
B7-DC	PD-1	+	Augments T-cell activity Promotes tumor rejection	No	*21*
B7-H1	PD-1	−	Causes apoptosis of effector CD8$^+$ T-cells	No	*11,24*
B7-H4	BTLA-4	−	Inhibits T-cell proliferation Inhibits effector CD8$^+$ T-cell function	No	*11,23*

PD, programmed death receptor; Ag, antigen, BTLA, B. and T-lymphocyte attenuator.

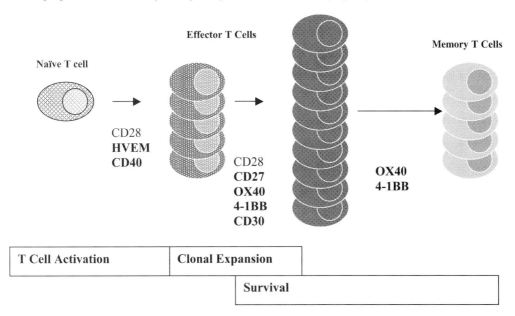

Fig. 1. The tumor necrosis factor receptor (TNFR) family regulates T-cell activation, expansion, and survival. B7-CD28 signaling provides the initial stimulus for the costimulation of naïve T-cells at the time of immune priming. Superimposed on the integrated signals of the B7 family, members of the TNFR family are activated in a timed sequential fashion to complement B7-CD28 signaling, and promote T-cell expansion and survival. This sequence of events culminates in established effector and memory T-cell populations.

tion, immature DCs enforce peripheral tolerance to tissue-specific antigens, thereby maintaining immunological homeostasis *(2)*. Improper antigen presentation by these cells results in a tepid antigen-specific T-cell response. Immature DCs express Toll-like receptors (TLRs) in the resting state, which bind the pathogen-associated molecular patterns highly characteristic of invading microbes during acute infections. The TLR–pathogen-associated molecular pattern interaction induces the maturation and migration of DCs from peripheral tissues to the draining lymph node. The primed DC has activated the costimulatory pathways critical for effective T-cell activation, and is thus positioned to activate efficiently a potent, antigen-specific immune response. Under such proinflammatory conditions, MSCs are recruited to contain the immune response *(28)*. In mice, MSCs

Immunologic Checkpoints

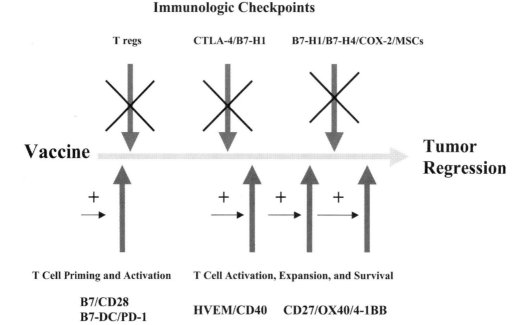

Fig. 2. Combinatorial vaccination regimens are critical to the success of cancer vaccines. Multiple combinatorial immunization strategies to maximize vaccine-induced tumor immunity can be designed based on current knowledge of molecular events underlying immune activation. One approach is to abrogate immunological checkpoints, releasing the antitumor immune response. Another strategy is to amplify the co-stimulatory pathways that support T-cell activation, expansion, and survival. A third is to manipulate the tumor microenvironment to render it receptive to the activity of immune effector cells. It is likely that exacting combinations of novel therapeutics will be required to optimize the antitumor response for distinct tumor types.

represent a mixed population of immature and mature myeloid cells that express Gr-1 and CD11b, and inhibit the activation and expansion of cytotoxic T-lymphocytes (CTLs); a CD34$^+$ population in humans with similar properties has been identified (29). MSCs develop from bone marrow-derived hematopoietic precursors on exposure to interleukin (IL)-3, granulocyte-macrophage colony-stimulating factor (GM-CSF), and vascular endothelial growth factor (VEGF). Activated T-cells trigger MSCs to block reversibly the development of CTLs by expressing inducible nitric oxide synthase or arginase 1. These enzymes generate nitric oxide or deplete the environment of arginine, respectively. Importantly, simultaneous induction of both enzymes causes CTL apoptosis. Tregs represent a third important suppressive arm of the immune system (30). Naturally occurring CD4$^+$CD25$^+$ Tregs constitute 5 to 10% of CD4$^+$ lymphocytes in mice and humans. They express CTLA-4 and glucocorticoid-induced tumor necrosis factor receptor, secrete IL-10 and transforming growth factor (TGF)-β, and are specifically characterized by the expression of the fork head/winged helix transcription factor. A similarly active population of inducible Tregs producing IL-10 and TGF-β has also been described. Tregs inhibit CD8$^+$ T-cell responses in an IL-2-dependent fashion through direct cell contact or through inhibition mediated by IL-10 and TGF-β. These cells prevent autoimmunity, but also profoundly inhibit the antitumor immune response. In vivo, the abrogation of Treg-mediated suppression requires the secretion of IL-6 by TLR-activated DCs (31).

2.4. Tumor Cells Create a Hostile Environment for the Immune Response

The negative influence of immunoregulatory cells is further amplified by close proximity to, and interactions with, the tumor cells themselves. Tumors produce a variety of factors that either promote Treg (cyclo-oxygenase (COX)-2 /prostaglandin E2) or MSC (GM-CSF/VEGF) activity, or inhibit DC activity (IL-10, TGF-β, VEGF). These tumor-derived factors can upregulate the signal transducer and activator of transcription 3 pathway, which prevents DC maturation (28,32,33). Thus, the lack of inflammatory stimuli is compounded by the presence of multiple suppressive factors that prevent immune activity where it is most needed. The depletion of the nutrients arginine and tryptophan within the tumor microenvironment by arginase 1 and indoleamine 2,3'dioxygenase (IDO) creates an even harsher environment for immune effector cells. Tumor cells both express IDO and recruit IDO-expressing APCs. It has been suggested further that IDO-arrested T-cells acquire a Treg phenotype, thereby further short-circuiting the immune response (34). If a local immune response does develop, tumors also frequently downregulate the expression of proteins critical for the effector T-cell response, including pivotal tumor antigens and components of the antigen processing pathways (MHC class I and II molecules, proteasome subunits, and the transporter associated with antigen processing transporter) (35). Thus, antitumor immunity can fail locally at multiple levels. Importantly, these regulatory mechanisms offer many opportunities for targeted manipulation of the immune system to enhance the activity of cancer vaccines by combining immunization rationally with other therapeutics.

3. COMBINATORIAL VACCINATION REGIMENS CAN OVERCOME DIVERSE MECHANISMS OF IMMUNE TOLERANCE

The multifaceted system of immune tolerance and evasion offers multiple opportunities for combining cancer vaccines with drugs that promote immune responses by amplifying co-stimulatory pathways, abrogating suppressive immune cells, capitalizing on immunoregulatory mechanisms for maintaining immunological homeostasis, modifying the tumor microenvironment, or altering the biology of the tumor cells themselves. Therapeutic interventions that can be added to cancer vaccines to potentiate their activity include therapeutic monoclonal antibodies (MAbs), chemotherapeutic agents, radiation therapy, and small biologically targeted molecules. Their immunomodulatory activity is summarized in Table 3.

3.1. Therapeutic MAbs and Tumor Immunity

Therapeutic MAbs can be broadly divided into those that target costimulatory pathways of the immune response itself and those that directly target the biology of tumor cells. Thus far, MAbs that block CTLA-4 have been tested clinically, but other immunoregulatory therapeutic MAbs are under preclinical development. MAbs already in routine clinical use that modify tumor cell biology, and have immunomodulatory activity include Trastuzumab, Cetuximab, Rituximab, and Bevacizumab. We consider each group in turn.

3.1.1. MAbs That Modulate B7 or TNFR Co-Stimulation

The B7 family offers multiple opportunities for amplifying co-stimulatory signaling or abrogating counterregulatory mechanisms during immune priming, or potentiating immune effector activity within the tumor microenvironment. The TNFR family expands

Table 3
Modulation of Tumor Immunity by Chemotherapy,
Radiation, Therapeutic Monoclonal Antibodies, and Small Biologicals

Mechanism	Chemotherapy	Radiation	Therapeutic MAbs/ small biologicals
Immune tolerance			
T-cell co-stimulation	Bleomycin Melphalan	Yes	
Regulatory T-cells	Cyclophosphamide		Denileukin Difitox
Myeloid suppressor cells			Retinoic acid
			Bevacizumab?
DC migration and maturation	Paclitaxel		Celecoxib
	Docetaxel		Celecoxib
			STI-571
			Bryostatin
			Retinoic acid
			Bevacizumab
Cytokine deviation	Cyclophosphamide		Celecoxib
			Paclitaxel
			Melphalan
Tumor microenvironment			
Innate immune effectors			Trastuzumab
			Rituximab
Cytokine secretion	Cyclophosphamide	Yes	Celecoxib
	Bleomycin		
	Melphalan		
Antigen presentation	5-Aza'-2'-deoxycytidine	Yes	STI-571
	5-Fluorouracil		Bryostatin
	Paclitaxel		Retinoic acid
			Trastuzumab
Angiogenesis	Cyclophosphamide	Yes	Celecoxib
	Paclitaxel		
	Doxorubicin		
	Vinblastine		
Host environment	Cyclophosphamide +Fludarabine	Yes	Bevacizumab
	BMT/ASCT		

MAbs, monocolonal antibodies; DC, dendritic cell; BMT, bone marrow transplant; ASCT, autologous stem cell transplant.

therapeutic opportunities to later phases of the T-cell immune response, including effector T-cell expansion, survival, and memory cell differentiation.

3.1.2. αCTLA-4 MAB

MAb-blocking CTLA-4 have already entered clinical development. Preclinical studies established that αCTLA-4 MAbs induced a CD8+ T-cell-dependent regression of established tumors, even in the absence of vaccination (9). Combining CTLA-4 blockade with GM-CSF-secreting vaccines exerts synergistic antitumor activity compared with either antibody or vaccine alone *(36,37)*. Two clinical trials testing a humanized MAb specific for CTLA-4 have been reported. The first included nine previously vaccinated patients with metastatic melanoma or ovarian carcinoma; five had been immunized with GM-CSF-secreting autologous tumor cells, and four with gp100 or melanoma-associated antigen 1-targeted vaccines for melanoma *(38)*. Three patients with melanoma previously vaccinated with GM-CSF-secreting vaccines developed extensive tumor necrosis with associated immune infiltrates, and two ovarian patients with cancer displayed stable or declining CA-125 levels. In the second study, 14 patients with metastatic melanoma were immunized with gp100-specific peptide vaccination in the setting of weekly infusions of αCTLA-4 MAbs *(39)*. Six research subjects (43%) developed grade III autoimmunity (dermatitis, enterocolitis, hepatitis, hypophysitis), and three (21%) developed evidence of tumor regression.

3.1.3. αB7-DC MAb

Few preclinical studies have been reported with MAbs specific for B7-DC. Pease and colleagues identified a naturally occurring immunoglobulin M antibody specific for B7-DC that augments DC survival, antigen processing, and IL-12 production *(40)*. This MAb also augments naïve T-cell activation. Notably, administration of this antibody to mice induced a CD4$^+$ and CD8$^+$ T-cell-dependent immune response capable of mediating the rejection of established B16 melanomas *(41)*. The development of additional B7-DC-specific immunomodulators is currently the focus of intense investigation.

3.1.4. αB7-H1, αB7-H4, AND α-INDUCIBLE CO-STIMULATOR MABS

MAbs that abrogate B7-H1 signaling augment tumor immunity by multiple mechanisms. Myeloid DCs present in the blood, draining lymph nodes, and tumor nodules of ovarian cancer patients express B7-H1, and a blocking MAb specific for B7-H1 augmented myeloid DC-mediated T-cell activation in one report *(42)*. The role of B7-H1 in promoting T-cell apoptosis within the tumor microenvironment suggests that blocking B7-H1 MAbs could further exert immune-enhancing effects not only during immune priming, but also at the level of T-cell effector function. The ability of B7-H1 blockade to augment adoptive T-cell immunotherapy for squamous cell carcinoma lends credence to this hypothesis *(43)*. Neither B7-H4- nor inducible co-stimulator-directed immunomodulation has been reported.

3.1.5. αCD40 MAb

CD40-mediated co-stimulation is crucial for effective CD4$^+$ T-helper responses and T-cell dependent humoral immunity *(26)*. It also plays a key role in the activation of memory but not naïve T-cell precursors. αCD40 MAbs are particularly effective against B-cell malignancies, because they promote tumor cell lysis by direct binding, increase antigen presentation by the transformed B-cells, and augment tumor-specific CTL activity. The expression of CD40 by epithelial and mesenchymal tumors suggests that this activity could extend to those tumor types as well. The effect of CD40 modulation is maximized when αCD40 MAbs are combined with antigen-specific vaccines. This combination therapy is thought to both promote the maturation of endogenous DC and augment the crosspresentation of tumor-associated antigens to break immune tolerance *(44, 45)*. αCD40 MAbs are just entering human clinical trials.

3.1.6. αOX40 MAb

OX40 co-stimulation promotes the activation and survival of effector CD4⁺ T-cells after antigen priming, thereby augmenting humoral immune responses and enlarging the CD4⁺ memory T-cell pool *(46)*. It also likely augments the function of OX40⁺ CD8⁺ effector T-cells directly, and facilitates T-cell trafficking through the tumor microvasculature into tissues through engaging OX40L expressed on endothelial cells. Importantly, MAbs that augment OX40 signaling in vivo circumvent CD4⁺ T-cell tolerance *(47)*, in part by inhibiting peripheral deletion *(48)* and abrogating the suppressive influence of CD4⁺CD25⁺ Treg cells *(49)*. Treatment of tumor-bearing mice with αOX40 MAbs alone results in prolonged CD4⁺ and CD8⁺ T-cell-dependent tumor-free survival in models of melanoma, sarcoma, colon cancer, breast cancer, and glioma *(46)*. Moreover, CD4⁺ memory T-cells derived from these OX40-specific MAb-treated mice protect naïve mice from homologous tumor challenge. Importantly, the impact of OX40 ligation is potentiated by concomitant 41BB ligation (in the presence of IL-12) *(50)* or GM-CSF exposure *(51)*, with combinatorial therapy resulting in a marked antitumor response. A human OX40-specific mouse MAb will enter phase I clinical trials in advanced-stage cancer patients in 2006 *(46)*.

3.1.7. α41BB MAb

The administration of MAbs specific for 41BB causes the regression of even poorly immunogenic tumors in a CD4⁺ and CD8⁺ T-cell- and natural-killer cell-dependent fashion *(52)*. MAbs specific for 41BB also potentiate the activity of preactivated CD8⁺ T-cells in part by prolonging their survival *(53)*. When α41BB MAbs are combined with vaccines, they abrogate immunological ignorance, promote the CD4⁺ T-helper response, and potentiate pre-existing (albeit ineffective) tumor-specific immune responses to synergistically effect tumor rejection *(54)*. A humanized 41BB MAb has minimal toxicity and inhibits T-cell-dependent antibody responses in nonhuman primates, but has not yet been tested in phase I clinical trials *(55)*.

3.1.7.1. MAbs That Modulate CD4⁺CD25⁺ Treg Cells. MAbs specific for CD25 or glucocorticoid-induced tumor necrosis factor receptor can deplete or (in the latter case) abrogate the function of Tregs in vivo to overcome immune tolerance and effect tumor rejection even in the absence of tumor-specific vaccination *(56,57)*. Importantly, the depletion of CD4⁺CD25⁺ Tregs with MAbs specific for CD25 in the setting of concomitant CTLA-4 blockade and GM-CSF-secreting tumor cell vaccination resulted in synergistic antitumor effects in a poorly immunogenic melanoma model *(58)*. The two Treg-depleting drugs currently available for clinical development include a MAb specific for CD25, and Denileukin difitox (ONTAK®), a diphtheria toxin-based therapeutic that targets CD25 (the IL-2R α-chain). Although initial clinical studies testing the depletion of Tregs in the context of vaccination have already begun *(59)*, current drugs have significant limitations. First, because CD25 is expressed by both Tregs and activated effector T-cells, repetitive dosing of drugs that inhibit the activity of CD25⁺ T-cells could abrogate the vaccine-induced antitumor immune response. Second, Denileukin difitox is associated with significant infusion-related reactions that can be life threatening. Drugs that more specifically target Tregs and have a more favorable side effect profile are clearly needed.

3.1.7.2. MAbs That Modulate Tumor Cell Biology. Emerging data suggests that humoral immunity is likely to play a greater role in antitumor immune responses that previously appreciated, cooperating with the cellular arm of the response to maximize tumor immunity *(60–65)*. Therapeutic MAbs already in clinical use thus have great potential to synergize with active immunotherapy by passively recapitulating the humoral immune response, modifying the biology of the tumor cells, modulating the antitumor immune response induced by vaccination, and/or by modulating the host tumor microenvironment in which the immune response takes place. Trastuzumab, Rituximab, Cetuximab, and Bevacizumab all have the potential to affect at least one of these features of the therapeutic response.

3.1.7.2.1. Trastuzumab: αHER-2/neu MAb. Trastuzumab is a MAb specific for HER-2/*neu*, a protooncogene overexpressed by about 30% of breast cancers. Trastuzumab is widely used for the treatment of stage IV breast cancer alone and in combination with chemotherapy, and is under active investigation in combination or in sequence with adjuvant chemotherapy for early breast cancer as well *(66)*. The MAb can potentiate antitumor immune responses in a variety of ways. Trastuzumab recruits innate immune effectors to the tumor microenvironment to effect antibody-dependent cellular cytotoxicity (ADCC) *(67,68)*. It also enhances the lytic activity of MHC class I-restricted HER-2/*neu*-specific CTLs against HER-2/*neu*-overexpressing breast and ovarian carcinoma tumor cells *(69)*. It has been shown to augment the ubiquitination and degradation of internalized HER-2/*neu* molecules, thus increasing proteasome-dependent antigen presentation *(70,71)*. Trastuzumab also exerts a direct antitumor effect by both disrupting growth-promoting signaling pathways and by rendering tumor cells more susceptible to apoptosis. Supporting the notion that antigen-specific humoral and cellular immune effectors act in concert, we have shown that the adoptive transfer of HER-2/*neu*-specific antibody with HER-2/*neu*-specific CTLs results in a greater antitumor response than the passive administration of either alone in severe combined immunodeficient mice *(61)*. Extending these observations to tolerized HER-2/*neu* transgenic mice, we further showed that the combination of HER-2/*neu*-specific MAbs and a HER-2/*neu*-directed GM-CSF-secreting cellular vaccine exerts a more robust antitumor effect than either exerts alone, curing about 40% of tumor-bearing mice *(72)*. The addition of HER-2/*neu*-specific MAbs to vaccination augmented the number of vaccine-induced, TNF-secreting HER-2/*neu*-specific CD8+ T-cells as measured by enzyme-linked immunospot assay (ELISPOT). Interestingly, the MAbs themselves induced new CD8+ T-cell immunity specific for HER-2/*neu*. Others have shown that HER-2/*neu*-specific antibody induced by peptide vaccination can inhibit tumor cell growth and mediate ADCC *(73)*. These observations together provide a compelling argument for testing HER-2/*neu*-targeted vaccines in combination with Trastuzumab in patients with HER-2/*neu*-overexpressing high-risk primary or metastatic breast cancer. M. L. Disis and colleagues are currently conducting a clinical trial testing this concept.

3.1.7.2.2. Rituximab: aCD20 MAb. Rituximab is a MAb specific for CD20, a surface molecule expressed by more than 95% of B-cell lymphomas and leukemias *(74)*. CD20 modulates *src* tyrosine kinase signaling during B-cell activation, and is a Ca^{2+} channel that may further modulate activation by regulating Ca^{2+} influx. Rituximab modulates tumor immunity by effecting ADCC and complement-mediated lysis, and by directly inhibiting progrowth signaling pathways and triggering apoptosis. By modulating *src* tyrosine kinase signaling, Rituximab decreases the production of IL-10 by B-cell lymphocyte 2-expressing follicular lymphoma cells *(75)*. Notably, IL-10 normally supports the constitutive expression of signal transducer and activator of transcription 3, resulting in sustained B-cell lymphocyte 2 expression. Thus, Rituximab can abrogate the intrinsic resistance to apoptosis that is characteristic of follicular lymphoma. This mechanism underlies the synergistic activity of Rituximab in combination with chemotherapy. Clinical trials combining Rituximab with GM-CSF-secreting cancer vaccines are in the planning stages.

3.1.7.2.3. Other Therapeutic MAbs. Cetuximab is a MAb specific for epidermal growth factor receptor. Epidermal growth factor receptor is a transmembrane tyrosine kinase receptor overexpressed by a variety of epithelial tumors, including breast, prostate, ovarian, and those of aerodigestive origin. Cetuximab also inhibits progrowth signaling pathways, and promotes apoptosis. Its ability to facilitate ADCC has not yet been reported. Cetuximab is Food and Drug Administration-approved for the treatment of refractory metastatic colorectal cancer in combination with the chemotherapeutic Irinotecan (76), but it has not been evaluated in combination with other immune-based therapy. Bevacizumab is a MAb specific for VEGF. It is Food and Drug Administration-approved for the first-line treatment of metastatic colorectal cancer in combination with 5-fluorouracil. As discussed, VEGF is immunosuppressive. At levels found in advanced cancer patients, it causes thymic atrophy, inhibits the development of T-cells, and disrupts DC function (77). Gabrilovich and colleagues have demonstrated that MAbs specific for VEGF can significantly improve the number and function of DCs in tumor-bearing mice, potentiating the antitumor effect of DC-based immunotherapy (78). These studies suggest that combining Bevacizumab with cancer vaccines may potentiate their therapeutic efficacy in advanced cancer.

4. CHEMOTHERAPEUTIC AGENTS, BIOLOGICALLY TARGETED DRUGS, RADIATION, AND TUMOR IMMUNITY

Chemotherapy is widely used for cancer treatment, directly cytoreducing both established and micrometastatic tumors. Standard chemotherapy is widely considered immunosuppressive, and is used commonly to treat severe autoimmune disease. This inhibitory effect extends to the antitumor immune response. One study demonstrated a reduced number of carcinoembryonic antigen (CEA)-specific T-cell precursors in research subjects receiving a greater number of prior chemotherapy regimens in close proximity to vaccination with the CEA-specific attenuated canary pox vaccine ALVAC-CEA (79). Jaffee and colleagues conducted a phase I clinical trial of a GM-CSF-secreting, mesothelin-expressing pancreatic cancer vaccine incorporated in the adjuvant treatment of high-risk stage II and III pancreatic cancer (80). Research subjects received the first vaccine immediately after surgery and just before 6 mo of adjuvant chemoradiation; those that continued to have no evidence of disease received three additional vaccinations after standard therapy. In this study, the number of vaccine-induced mesothelin-specific CD8[+] T-cells enumerated by serial ELISPOT became undetectable after aggressive adjuvant chemoradiation, and recovered only with multiple subsequent vaccinations after adjuvant chemoradiation was complete.

Despite the clear immunosuppressive effects of standard chemotherapy, a large body of data supports the immunomodulatory activity of a variety of cytotoxic drugs (6). Chemotherapy can both modulate mechanisms of immune tolerance to activate latent immunity and render the tumor microenvironment more vulnerable to the lytic activity of tumor-specific CD8[+] effector T-cells. Bleomycin and Melphalan modulate cytokine secretion by tumor cells, promoting the activity of CTLs *(81–83)*. Melphalan and Bleomycin can upregulate co-stimulatory molecules of the B7 family, thereby promoting crosspriming directly within the tumor mass itself *(84)*. Chemotherapeutics also enhance antigen presentation. 5-Aza-2'-deoxycytidine and 5-fluorouracil can restore MHC class I and/or tumor antigen expression and reenable CTL-mediated lysis *(85–87)*. Many cytotoxics, including Paclitaxel (PTX), augment antigen presentation by inducing apoptosis *(84,88–90)*. Marked apoptosis itself stimulates DC maturation, thereby further promoting antigen presentation and immune priming *(91)*. One report has demonstrated a correlation between the extent of apoptosis and mitotic arrest after one cycle of neoadjuvant PTX for breast cancer with overall therapeutic response and the development of tumor-infiltrating lymphocytes *(91)*. Furthering its potential to promote antigen crosspresentation, PTX has lipopolysaccharide-mimetic activity, binding to TLR-4 and inducing the secretion of proinflammatory cytokines in rodents *(92,93)*. These effects are independent of TLR-4 but dependent on MyD88 in humans, suggesting the involvement of an alternative TLR *(94)*.

The alternative effects of chemotherapy are complex, and dependent not only on the drug, but also on its dose and schedule. For example, many cytotoxics have dose- and sequence-specific antiangiogenic activity. The repeated administration of very low dose cyclophosphamide (CY), PTX, Doxorubicin (DOX), or Vinblastine at frequent intervals (metronomic scheduling) preferentially targets the tumor vasculature over the tumor cells themselves *(95,96)*. This may augment tumor immunity by increasing tumor cell apoptosis and vascular access early on, but ultimately, inhibit antitumor immunity by destroying tumor access. Furthermore, low doses of chemotherapy can either potentiate or antagonize immunity, depending on the drug and the timing of its administration in relation to antigen exposure *(6)*. CY augments antigen-specific immunity if given before antigen exposure, but induces tolerance and/or abrogates immune induction if given concomitant with or subsequent to the antigen exposure. DOX augments immunity if given 3–5 d prior or 7 d after antigen exposure. Gemcitabine given every 3 d for five doses inhibits antigen-specific humoral immunity without affecting cellular immunity *(97)*. We found that Gemcitabine profoundly inhibits vaccine-induced antitumor immunity in HER-2/*neu* transgenic mice (unpublished data).

Importantly, low, immunomodulatory doses of chemotherapy can modify active mechanisms of tumor-specific immune tolerance. CY, PTX, and Melphalan promote the T-helper type I phenotype critical for antitumor activity *(82,98)*, and CY further upregulates type I interferon production, thus promoting the outgrowth of CD44[hi] memory T-cells in treated mice *(99)*. Based on its ability to abrogate the influence of suppressor T-cells, low-dose CY pretreatment has been used to augment the activity of tumor vaccines in a variety of preclinical and clinical studies during the last decade *(6)*. Although this activity was attributed to CY before the characterization of Tregs as they are currently defined, recent studies have shown that low-dose CY does modulate CD4[+]CD25[+] Tregs to augment antitumor immunity *(100)*. Conversely, high-dose chemotherapy can facilitate the development of antitumor immunity because of homeostatic proliferation *(101)*. Thus, whereas standard dose chemotherapy typically inhibits adaptive immunity by inducing lymphopenia (without homeostatic proliferation), low- or high-dose chemotherapy can idiosyncratically promote the antitumor immune response.

4.1. Combining Chemotherapy With Tumor Vaccines

Tumor vaccines can be directly combined with chemotherapy utilizing two therapeutic strategies: incorporating low-dose chemotherapeutic agents into the immunization protocol as a vaccine adjuvant, and conditioning the vaccine recipient with high-dose chemotherapy followed by autologous or allogeneic stem cell support to produce an altered host environment for vaccination. DOX or PTX have been reported to augment the antitumor effect of RNA-based vaccines *(102)*, and PTX was found to augment the efficacy of DC-based vaccines *(103)*; both of these studies were in breast cancer models. The use of low-to standard-dose chemotherapy with GM-CSF-secreting vaccines has been systematically examined using two preclinical model systems *(98,104)*. In a BALB/c model of CT26 colon carcinoma, a variety of cytotoxics was administered in sequence with a GM-CSF-secreting CT26 cellular vaccine *(104)*. Whereas most drugs reduced vaccine efficacy, low-dose DOX given with or subsequent to vaccination augmented CT26-specific T-cell immunity. Mice treated with vaccine followed by DOX were fully protected from a subsequent tumor challenge, and 40% of tumor-bearing mice were cured of pre-established tumors with combined therapy. Tumor-bearing mice treated with vaccine or DOX alone had cure rates of 30 and 10%, respectively. DOX given 1 wk before vaccine abrogated vaccine activity. Pretreatment with CY in this system did not augment vaccine activity, and abrogated it if given simultaneously with or subsequent to immunization.

We extended these studies to the tolerogenic HER-2/*neu* transgenic mouse model of spontaneous breast cancer *(98)*. Parental FVB/N mice vigorously reject large HER-2/*neu*-expressing tumors after vaccination with a HER-2/*neu*-targeted, GM-CSF-secreting vaccine *(105)*. Reflective of pre-existing immune tolerance, HER-2/*neu* transgenic mice mount a tepid HER-2/*neu*-specific immune response to vaccination that is completely ineffective against established tumors, and only modestly protective against a subsequent tumor challenge *(105)*. Characterization of the HER-2/*neu*-specific immune responses at the molecular level revealed that the CD8+ effector T-cells activated in nontolerized parental mice are exclusively specific for a single immunodominant peptide epitope derived from rat HER-2/*neu*, $RNEU_{420-429}$ *(106)*. T-cells specific for this epitope are almost undetectable in vaccinated HER-2/*neu* transgenic mice, which develop a more heterogeneous T-cell population that recognizes cryptic, subdominant HER-2/*neu* epitopes.

Timed, sequential therapy with defined doses of some chemotherapeutics and the vaccine can partially overcome some mechanisms of immune tolerance in HER-2/*neu* transgenic mice *(98)*. Both parental and HER-2/*neu* transgenic mice develop a more vigorous tumor rejection response to a HER-2/*neu*-targeted, GM-CSF-secreting cellular vaccine combined with either CY or PTX 1 d before vaccination compared with either treatment alone. Sequencing the vaccine with DOX 7 d later also enhanced vaccine-induced antitumor responses, but only in HER-2/*neu* transgenic mice. The productive interaction between the drugs and the vaccine diminished with nadiring T-cell counts (produced with increasing drug doses), and was completely abrogated by reversing the order of administration of each drug with vaccine. That the drugs were functioning as immunological adjuvants was confirmed by their ability to recapitulate this result in tumor protection experiments, and confirmed by the measurement of increased numbers of HER-2/*neu*-specific T-helper type 1 responses by ELISPOT (CY and PTX only). Thus, these two drugs circumvented immune tolerance in part by reversing immunological skew. The multiagent regimen incorporating CY 1 d before vaccination and DOX 1 wk later was most potent, curing up to 30% of tolerized HER-2/*neu* transgenic mice of pre-existing tumor burdens. The analysis of immune responses in these cured mice demonstrated the development of robust, high-avidity T-cell responses specific for RNEU$_{420-429}$, suggesting that chemotherapy-modulated vaccination resulted in the recruitment of latent populations of high-avidity T-cells to the antitumor immune response *(106a)*. We are currently conducting a phase I clinical trial testing time sequential therapy with CY, DOX, and an allogeneic GM-CSF-secreting cellular breast cancer vaccine, which explores the safety and bioactivity of this combined modality immunization regimen in patients with metastatic breast cancer *(107)*. Additional clinical trials testing GM-CSF-secreting vaccines preceded by CY alone in patients with metastatic pancreatic cancer and metastatic nonsmall cell lung cancer have recently completed accrual.

High-dose chemotherapy can potentially promote a favorable balance between the sheer physical burden of tumor cells and the kinetics and magnitude of the antigen-specific antitumor immune response by providing an environment for lymphophenia-induced homeostatic T-cell proliferation after optimal tumor debulking *(108,109)*. Manipulating the T-cell repertoire with cancer vaccines during immunological reconstitution after lymphoablative treatments can potentially reprogram the immune system to recognize tumor antigens that more efficiently result in tumor rejection *(101)*. Consistent with this idea, the selective induction and expansion of functional melanoma-specific T-cells by treating lymphopenic, tumor-bearing mice with GM-CSF-secreting vaccination resulted in significant tumor regression *(110)*. Multiple preclinical studies have also shown that vaccinating tumor-bearing mice with GM-CSF-secreting tumor vaccines during early engraftment after syngeneic or allogeneic T-cell-depleted bone marrow transplantation augments the effectiveness of vaccine-induced immunity *(111,112)*. Other preclinical studies have demonstrated that altering the host environment before immunization can promote the development of an effective tumor-specific immune response *(113,114)*. Although the phenomenon of homeostatic proliferation has not yet been rigorously demonstrated in patients, the adoptive transfer of melanoma-specific tumor-infiltrating lymphocytes to patients with metastatic melanoma after nonmyeloablative conditioning with CY and fludarabine suggests that it might be clinically relevant *(115)*. Because many traditional cancer therapies result in lymphopenia, thoroughly characterizing the influence of chemotherapy on the kinetics, durability, and functional quality of antigen-specific immune reconstitution will be required in order to incorporate effectively cancer vaccines into clinical practice. Clinical trials testing the bioactivity of GM-CSF-secreting cell-based vaccines during immune reconstitution after autologous stem cell transplantation in acute myelogenous leukemia and multiple myeloma have recently completed accrual.

4.2. Combining Radiation Therapy With Tumor Vaccines

Radiation therapy is also known to modulate the immunobiology of the tumor microenvironment. Radiation can upregulate the expression of B7 molecules within the tumor microenvironment *(84)*. Sublethal doses of radiation were more recently shown to upregulate the expression of the death receptor fatty acid synthase (Fas) in CEA-expressing murine colon cancer cells, making them more sensitive to CTL-mediated lysis in vitro and in vivo *(116)*. Combining local tumor irradiation with CEA-TRICOM® vaccination in human CEA transgenic mice resulted in a dramatic Fas-dependent tumor rejection associated with a massive infiltration of T-cells not seen with either therapy alone. Mice treated with combinatorial therapy developed CD4[+] and CD8[+] T-cell responses specific for CEA, with broadening of the tumor antigen-specific response to include epitopes derived from other antigens (gp70 and p53). Extension of this work to human cancer cell lines (prostate, lung, and colon) demonstrated upregulation of Fas, MHC class I, intercellular adhesion molecule 1, and the tumor antigens mucin 1 and CEA *(117)*. This upregulation was associated with the enhanced CTL-mediated tumor cell lysis of HLA-A2[+] tumor cell lines expressing CEA.

4.3. Biologically Targeted Cancer Drugs and Tumor Immunity

Biologically targeted cancer drugs are relatively new, but there are already significant data that support their potential immunomodulatory activity. Celecoxib is a selective COX-2 inhibitor that decreases prostaglandin E2 production by tumor cells *(118)*. Tumor-associated COX-2 expression is associated with resistance to apoptosis, increased angiogeneis, and immunosuppression. COX-2 overexpression results in T-helper type 1 to T-helper type 2 skew, DC dysfunction, and a preponderance of IL-10 compared with IL-12 within the tumor microenvironment *(119–121)*. Celecoxib therapy restores the IL-10/IL-12 balance, reverses immunological skew, and restores DC function *(120– 122)*. Combining Celecoxib therapy with CEA-TRICOM vaccination in the CEA transgenic/multiple intestinal neoplasia mouse model of spontaneous colon cancer reduced tumor formation by 95% compared with Celecoxib therapy (65%) or vaccination alone (54%) *(123)*. Imatinib mesylate (STI-571) is a tyrosine kinase inhibitor selective for the *bcr/abl* tyrosine kinase activity underlying chronic myelogenous leukemia (CML). Recent data suggest that it can enhance the antigen presentation potential of DCs, restoring the responsiveness of tolerized CD4[+] T-cells from tumor-bearing hosts *(124)*. In this study, STI-571 prevented the tolerization of adoptively transferred tumor-specific CD4[+] T-cells, and augmented the efficacy of antigen-specific vaccination in tumor-bearing mice. Similar to chemotherapy, the effect may be dose-dependent, with higher doses of STI-571 inhibiting antitumor immune responses. Two clinical studies have tested STI-571 with peptide vaccination for CML, and have found that combination therapy is more effective in generating cytogenetic and molecular responses in the setting of ongoing CML-specific CD8[+] T-cell responses *(125,126)*. Bryostatin, a small-molecule protein kinase C inhibitor, can similarly augment the maturation and antigen-presentation potential of DCs *(127)*. This activity, together with its ability to induce tumor cell apoptosis, suggests that it might synergistically augment antigen presentation. It can also enhance T-cell activation, expansion, and the acquisition of antigen-specific effector function, particularly in the presence of IL-2 *(128)*. Although it has not been combined with therapeutic vaccines, Bryostatin exposure can augment the therapeutic effect of adoptively transferred, vaccine-activated T-lymphocytes against established mammary cancers in mice *(129)*. Similarly, selective retinoic acid analogs trigger the maturation of DCs, increasing the expression of MHC class II molecules and co-stimulatory molecules to prime more effectively the antigen-specific T-cell response *(130)*. Retinoids also augment antigen presentation in tumor cell lines by upregulating various subunits of the immunoproteasome, enhancing the sensitivity of neuroblastoma cells to MHC class I-restricted and unrestricted CTL lysis *(131)*. Complementing these activities, all-transretinoic acid can eliminate MSCs from tumor-bearing mice to augment the efficacy of CD4[+] and CD8[+] antitumor responses in response to vaccination *(132)*. Further studies have demonstrated that liposomal all-transretinoic acid collaborates with adaptive tumor-specific immune responses to effect long-term molecular remissions in mice with acute promyelocytic leukemia *(133)*. An emerging area of drug development is the development of agents that directly target TLRs, thereby conditioning DCs to respond maximally to an antigenic challenge by priming the most effective immune response *(134)*. These data together provide a compelling argument for the careful preclinical modeling of cancer vaccines not only in combination with standard cancer therapies, but also with highly specific biologically targeted cancer therapies as well.

5. SUMMARY AND CONCLUSIONS

Rapid advances in our understanding of the molecular and cellular underpinnings of the antitumor immune response have resulted in substantial progress in the preclinical development of cancer vaccines. Initial clinical trials have provided data supporting their safety and bioactivity, but have been largely disappointing with regard to clinical efficacy. This argues for the development of immunization strategies that potentiate vaccine bioactivity by directly manipulating immunoregulatory pathways or removing barriers to immune effector function within the tumor microenvironment. Indeed, combinatorial vaccination regimens that incorporate vaccines with novel targeted immunotherapeutics to abrogate immunological checkpoints or positively manipulate distinct phases of immune priming and T-cell activation are already in clinical testing (*see* Fig. 2). In addition, clinical studies to elucidate further the pharmacodynamic interactions between cancer vaccines and standard or novel therapies directed at the tumor cell itself are underway. Such innovative combination regimens should push cancer vaccines past the tipping point of weak to modest bioactivity to release the full power of the immune system to effect tumor regression. Coordinated research efforts that seamlessly link the laboratory and the clinic should realize the potential of engaging the immune system in the fight against malignancy, ultimately establishing cancer vaccines as part of standard cancer therapy.

ACKNOWLEDGMENTS

Supported in part by K23 CA098498-01, DAMD 17-01-1-0281, the Maryland Cigarette Restitution Fund; NIH P50 CA88843, RO1 CA 93714-1, the National Cooperative Drug Discovery Group Grant U10CA72108; and the AVON Foundation. Dr. Jaffee is the Dana and Albert "Cubby" Broccoli Professor of Oncology at the Sidney Kimmel Cancer Center at Johns Hopkins.

REFERENCES

1. Emens LA, Jaffee EM. Cancer vaccines: an old idea comes of age. *Cancer Biol Ther* 2003; 2(Suppl 1): S161–S168.
2. Walker LS, Abbas AK. The enemy within: keeping self-reactive T cells at bay in the periphery. *Nat Rev Immunol* 2001; 21:11–19.
3. Marincola FM, Jaffee EM, Hicklin DJ, Ferrone S. Escape of human solid tumors from T-cell recognition: molecular mechanisms and functional significance. *Adv Immunol* 2000; 74:181–273.
4. Spaner DE. Amplifying cancer vaccine responses by modifying pathogenic gene programs in tumor cells. *J Leukoc Biol* 2004; 76:338–351.
5. Perez-Diaz A, Spiess PJ, Restifo NP, Matzinger P, Marincola FM. Intensity of the vaccine-elicited immune response determines tumor clearance. *J Immunol* 2002; 168:338–347.
6. Emens LA, Machiels J-PH, Reilly RT, Jaffee EM. Chemotherapy: friend or foe to cancer vaccines? *Curr Opin Mol Ther* 2001; 3:77–82.

7. Pardoll DM. Spinning molecular immunology into successful immunotherapy. *Nat Rev Immunol* 2002; 2:227–238.

8. Carreno BM, Collins M. The B7 family of ligands and its receptors: new pathways for costimulation and inhibition of immune responses. *Annu Rev Immunol* 2002; 20:29–53.

9. Egen JG, Kuhns MS, Allison JP. CTLA-4: new insights into its biological function and use in tumor immunotherapy. *Nat Immunol* 2002; 3:611–618.

10. Pentcheva-Hoang T, Egen JG, Wojnoonski K, Allison JP. B7-1 and B7-2 selectively recruit CTLA-4 and CD28 to the immunological synapse. *Immunity* 2004; 21:401–413.

11. Khoury SJ, Sayegh MH. The roles of the new negative T cell costimulatory pathways in regulating auto-immunity. *Immunity* 2004; 20:529–538.

12. McAdam AJ, Greenwald RJ, Levin MA, et al. ICOS is critical for CD40-mediated antibody class-switching. *Nature* 2001; 409:102–105.

13. Wallin JJ, Liang L, Bakardjiev A, Sha W. New regulatory co-receptors: inducible co-stimulator and PD-1. *Curr Opin Immunol* 2002; 14:779–782.

14. Chapoval AI, Ni J, Lau JS, et al. B7-H3: a costimulatory molecule for T cell activation and IFN-γ production. *Nat Immunol* 2001; 2:269–274.

15. Luo L, Chapoval AI, Flies DB, et al. B7-H3 enhances tumor immunity in vivo by costimulating rapid clonal expansion of antigen-specific CD8+ cytolytic T cells. *J Immunol* 2004; 173:5445–5450.

16. Sun X, Vale M, Leung E, Kanwar JR, Gupta R, Krissansen GW. Mouse B7-H3 induces antitumor immunity. *Gene Ther* 2003; 10:1728–1734.

17. Suh WK, Gajewska BU, Okada H, et al. The B7 family member B7-H3 preferentially down-regulates T helper type 1-mediated immune responses. *Nat Immunol* 2003; 4:899–906.

18. Latchman Y, Wood CR, Chernova T, et al. PD-L2 is a second ligand for PD-1 and inhibits T cell activation. *Nat Immunol* 2001; 2:261–268.

19. Tseng SY, Otsuji M, Gorski K, et al. B7-DC, a new dendritic cell molecule with potent costimulatory properties for T cells. *J Exp Med* 2001; 193:839–845.

20. Shin T, Kennedy G, Gorski K, et al. Cooperative B7-1/2 (CD80/86) and B7-DC costimulation of CD4+ T cells independent of the PD-1 receptor. *J Exp Med* 2003; 198:31–38.

21. Liu X, Gao JX, Wen J, et al. B7-DC/PD-L2 promotes tumor immunity by a PD-1-independent mechanism. *J Exp Med* 2003; 197:1721–1730.

22. Freeman GJ, Long AJ, Iwai Y, et al. Engagement of the PD-1 immunoinhibitory receptor by a novel B7 family member leads to negative regulation of lymphocyte activation. *J Exp Med* 2000; 192:1027–1034.

23. Sica GL, Choi IH, Zhu G, et al. B7-H4, a molecule of the B7 family, negatively regulates T cell immunity. *Immunity* 2003; 18:849–861.

24. Dong H, Strome SE, Salomao DR, et al. Tumor-associated B7-H1 promotes T-cell apoptosis: a potential mechanism of immune evasion. *Nat Med* 2002; 8:793–800.

25. Croft M. Co-stimulatory members of the TNFR family: keys to effective T-cell immunity? *Nat Rev Immunol* 2003; 3:609–620.

26. Tong AW, Stone MJ. Prospects for CD-40-directed experimental therapy of human cancer. *Cancer Gene Ther* 2002; 10:1–13.

27. Yu P, Lee Y, Liu W, et al. Priming of naive T cells inside tumors leads to eradication of established tumors. *Nat Immunol* 2004; 5:141–149.

28. Bronte V, Serafini P, Mazzoni A, Segal D, Zanovello P. L-Arginine metabolism in myeloid cells controls T-lymphocyte functions. *Trends Immunol* 2003; 24:301–305.

29. Young MR, Lathers DM. Myeloid progenitor cells mediate immune suppression in patients with head and neck cancers. *Int J Immunopharmacol* 1999; 21:241–252.

30. O'Garra A, Vierira P. Regulatory T cells and mechanisms of immune system control. *Nat Med* 2004; 10:801–805.

31. Pasare C, Medzhitov R. Toll pathway-dependent blockade of CD4+CD25+ T cell-mediated suppression by dendritic cells. *Science* 2004; 299:1033–1036.

32. Wang T, Niu G, Kortylewski M, et al. Regulation of the innate and adaptive immune responses by Stat-3-signaling in tumor cells. *Nat Med* 2004; 10:48–54.

33. Munn DH, Mellor AL. IDO and tolerance to tumors. *Trends Mol Med* 2004; 10:15–18.

34. Mellor AL, Munn DH. Tryptophan catabolism and regulation of adaptive immunity. *J Immunol* 2003; 170:5809–5813.

35. Ferrone S, Finerty JF, Jaffee EM, Nabel GJ. How much longer will tumour cells fool the immune system? *Immunol Today* 2000; 21:70–72.

36. Hurwitz AA, Yu TF, Leach DR, Allison JP. CTLA-4 blockade synergizes with tumor-derived granu-locyte-macrophage colony-stimulating factor for treatment of an experimental mammary carcinoma. *Proc Natl Acad Sci USA* 1998; 18:10,067–10,071.

37. van Elsas A, Hurwitz AA, Allison JP. Combination immunotherapy of B16 melanoma using anti-cytotoxic T lymphocyte-associated antigen-4 (CTLA-4) and granulocyte-macrophage colony-stimu-lating factor (GM-CSF)-producing vaccines induces rejection of subcutaneous and metastatic tumors accompanied by autoimmune depigmentation. *J Exp Med* 1999; 190:355–366.

38. Hodi FS, Mihm MC, Soiffer RJ, et al. Biologic activity of cytotoxic T lymphocyte-associated antigen 4 antibody blockade in previously vaccinated metastatic melanoma and ovarian carcinoma patients. *Proc Natl Acad Sci USA* 2003; 100:4712–4717.

39. Phan GQ, Yang JC, Sherry RM, et al. Cancer regression and autoimmunity induced by cytotoxic T lymphocyte-associated antigen 4 blockade in patients with metastatic melanoma. *Proc Natl Acad Sci USA* 2003; 100:8372–8377.

40. Radhakrishnan S, Nguyen LT, Ciric B, et al. Naturally occurring human IgM antibody that binds B7-DC and potentiates T cell stimulation by dendritic cells. *J Immunol* 2003; 170:1830–1838.

41. Radhakrishnan S, Nguyen LT, Ciric B, et al. Immunotherapeutic potential of B7-DC (PD-L2) cross-linking antibody in conferring antitumor immunity. *Cancer Res* 2004; 64:4965–4972.

42. Curiel TJ, Wei S, Dong H, et al. Blockade of B7-H1 improves myeloid dendritic cell-mediated anti-tumor immunity. *Nat Med* 2003; 9:562–567.

43. Strome SE, Dong H, Tamura H, et al. B7-H1 blockade augments adoptive T-cell immunotherapy for squamous cell carcinoma. *Cancer Res* 2003; 63:6501–6505.

44. Diehl L, den Boer AT, van der Voort EI, Melief CJ, Offringa R, Toes RE. The role of CD40 in peripheral T cell tolerance and immunity. *J Mol Med* 2000; 78:363–371.

45. Sotomayor EM, Borrello I, Tubb E, et al. Conversion of tumor-specific CD4$^+$ T-cell tolerance to T-cell priming through in vivo ligation of CD40. *Nat Med* 1999; 5:780–787.

46. Sugamura K, Ishii N, Weinberg AD. Therapeutic targeting of the effector T-cell co-stimulatory mole-cule OX40. *Nat Rev Immunol* 2004; 4:420–431.

47. Bansal-Pakala P, Jember A-H, Croft M. Signaling through OX40 (CD134) breaks peripheral T-cell tolerance. *Nat Med* 2001; 7:907–902.

48. Maxwell JR, Weinberg A, Prell RA, Vella AT. Danger and OX40 receptor signaling synergize to enhance memory T cell survival by inhibiting peripheral deletion. *J Immunol* 2000; 164:107–112.

49. Takeda I, Ine S, Killeen N, et al. Distinct roles for the OX40-OX40 ligand interaction in regulatory and nonregulatory T cells. *J Immunol* 2004; 172:3580–3589.

50. Pan PY, Zang Y, Weber K, Meseck ML, Chen SH. OX40 ligation enhances primary and memory cytotoxic T lymphocyte responses in an immunotherapy for hepatic colon metastases. *Mol Ther* 2002; 6:528–536.

51. Gri G, Gallo E, Di Carlo E, Musiani P, Colombo MP. OX40 ligand-transduced tumor cell vaccine syn-ergizes with GM-CSF and requires CD40-APC signaling to boost the host T cell antitumor response. *J Immunol* 2003; 170:99–106.

52. Melero I, Shuford WW, Newby SA, et al. Monoclonal antibodies against the 4-1BB T-cell activation molecule eradicate established tumors. *Nat Med* 1997; 3:682–685.

53. May KJ, Chen L, Zheng P, Liu Y. Anti-4-1BB monoclonal antibody enhances rejection of large tumor burden by promoting survival but not clonal expansion of tumor-specific CD8$^+$ T cells. *Cancer Res* 2002; 62:3459–465.

54. Wilcox RA, Flies DB, Zhu G, et al. Provision of antigen and CD137 signaling breaks immunological ignorance, promoting regression of poorly immunogenic tumors. *J Clin Invest* 2002; 109:651–659.

55. Hong HJ, Lee JW, Park SS, et al. A humanized anti-4-1BB monoclonal antibody suppresses antigen-induced humoral immune responses in nonhuman primates. *J Immunother* 2000; 23:613–621.

56. Onizuka S, Tawara I, Shimizu J, Sakaguchi S, Fujita T, Nakayama E. Tumor rejection by in vivo administration of anti-CD25 (interleukin-2 receptor alpha) monoclonal antibody. *Cancer Res* 1999; 59:3128–3133.

57. Shimizu J, Yamazaki S, Takahashi T, Ishida Y, Sakaguchi S. Stimulation of CD25$^+$CD4$^+$ regulatory T cells through GITR breaks immunological self-tolerance. *Nat Immunol* 2002; 3:135–142.

58. Sutmuller RP, van Duivenvoorde LM, van Elsas A, et al. Synergism of cytotoxic T lymphocyte-associated antigen-4 blockade and depletion of CD25$^+$ regulatory T cells in antitumor therapy reveals alternative pathways for suppression of autoreactive cytotoxic T lymphocyte responses. *J Exp Med* 2001; 194:824–832.

59. Vieweg J, Su Z, Dannull J. Enhancement of antitumor immunity following depletion of CD4⁺CD25⁺ regulatory T cells. *Proc Am Soc Clin Oncol* 2004; Abstract no. 23:164.

60. Dyall R, Vasovic LV, Clynes RA, Nikolic-Zugic J. Cellular requirements for the monoclonal antibody-mediated eradication of an established solid tumor. *Eur J Immunol* 1999; 29:30–37.

61. Reilly RT, Machiels J-PH, Emens LA, et al. The collaboration of both humoral and cellular HER-2-targeted immune responses is required for the complete eradication of HER-2/*neu*-expressing tumors. *Cancer Res* 2001; 61:880–883.

62. Reilly RT, Emens LA, Jaffee EM. Humoral and cellular immune responses: independent forces or collaborators in the fight against cancer? *Curr Opin Invest Drugs* 2001; 2:133–135.

63. Vasovic LV, Dyall R, Clynes RA, Ravetch JV, Nicolic-Zugic J. Synergy between an antibody and CD8⁺ cells in eliminating an established tumor. *Eur J Immunol* 1997; 27:374–382.

64. Wu CJ, Yang XF, McLaughlin S, et al. Detection of a potent humoral response associated with immune-induced remission of chronic myelogenous leukemia. *J Clin Invest* 2000; 106:705–714.

65. Yang XF, Wu CJ, McLaughlin S, et al. CML66, a broadly immunogenic tumor antigen, elicits a humoral immune response associated with remission of chronic myelogenous leukemia. *Proc Natl Acad Sci USA* 2001; 98:7492–7497.

66. Emens LA, Davidson NE. Trastuzumab in breast cancer. *Oncology* 2004; 18:1117–1128.

67. Clynes RA, Towers TL, Presta LG, Ravetch JV. Inhibitory Fc receptors modulate in vivo cytoxicity against tumor targets. *Nat Med* 2000; 6:443–446.

68. Gennari R, Menard S, Fagnoni F, et al. Pilot study of the mechanism of action of preoperative Trastuzumab in patients with primary operable breast tumors overexpressing HER2. *Clin Cancer Res* 2004; 10:5650–5645.

69. zum Buschenfelde CM, Hermann C, Schmidt B, Peschel C, Bernhard H. Antihuman epidermal growth factor receptor 2 (HER2) monoclonal antibody Trastuzumab enhances cytolytic activity of Class I-restricted HER2-specific T lymphocytes against HER2-overexpressing tumor cells. *Cancer Res* 2002; 62:2244–2247.

70. Castilleja A, Ward NE, O'Brian CA, et al. Accelerated HER-2 degradation enhances ovarian tumor recognition by CTL. Implications for tumor immunogenicity. *Mol Cell Biochem* 2001; 217:21–33.

71. Klapper LN, Waterman H, Sela M, Yarden Y. Tumor-inhibitory antibodies to HER-2/ErbB-2 may act by recruiting c-Cbl and enhancing ubiquitination of HER-2. *Cancer Res* 2000; 60:3384–3348.

72. Wolpoe ME, Lutz ER, Ercolini AM, et al. HER-2/*neu*-specific monoclonal antibodies collaborate with HER-2-targeted granulocyte macrophage colony-stimulating factor secreting whole cell vaccination to augment CD8⁺ T cell effector function and tumor-free survival in HER-2/*neu* transgenic mice. *J Immunol* 2003; 15:2161–2169.

73. Jasinska J, Wagner S, Radauer C, et al. Inhibition of tumor cell growth by antibodies induced after vaccination with peptides derived from the extracellular domain of HER-2/*neu*. *Int J Cancer* 2003; 107:976–983.

74. Olszewski AJ, Grossbard ML. Empowering targeted therapy: lessons from Rituximab. *Science STKE* 2004; 241:pe30.

75. Vega MI, Huerta-Yepaz S, Garban H, Jazirehi C, Emmanouilides C, Bonavida B. Rituximab inhibits p38 MAPK activity in 2F7 B NHL and decreases IL-10 transcription: pivotal role of p38 MAPK in drug resistance. *Oncogene* 2004; 23:3530–3540.

76. Cunningham D, Humblet Y, Siena S, et al. Cetuximab monotherapy and cetuximab plus irinotecan in irinotecan-refractory metastatic colorectal cancer. *N Engl J Med* 2004; 351:337–345.

77. Almand B, Resser JR, Lindman B, et al. Clinical significance of defective dendritic cell differentiation in cancer. *Clin Cancer Res* 2000; 6:1755–1766.

78. Gabrilovich DI, Ishida T, Nadaf S, Ohm JE, Carbone DP. Antibodies to vascular endothelial growth factor enhance the efficacy of cancer immunotherapy by improving dendritic cell function. *Clin Cancer Res* 1999; 5:2963–2970.

79. von Mehren M, Arlen P, Gulley J, et al. The influence of granulocyte macrophage colony-stimulating factor and prior chemotherapy on the immunological response to a vaccine (ALVAC-CEA B7.1) in patients with metastatic carcinoma. *Clin Cancer Res* 2001; 7:1181–1191.

80. Thomas AM, Santarsiero LM, Lutz ER, et al. Mesothelin-specific CD8⁺ T cell responses provide evidence of in vivo cross-priming by antigen-presenting cells in vaccinated pancreatic cancer patients. *J Exp Med* 2004; 200:297–306.

81. Yuan L, Kuramitsu Y, Li Y, Kobayashi M, Hosokawa M. Restoration of interleukin-2 production in tumor-bearing rats through reduction of tumor-derived transforming growth factor β by treatment with Bleomycin. *Cancer Immunol Immunother* 1995; 41:355–341.

82. Gorelik L, Prokhorova A, and Mokyr MB. Low-dose melphalan-induced shift in the production of a Th2-type cytokine to a Th1-type cytokine in mice bearing a large MOPC-315 tumor. *Cancer Immunol Immunother* 1994; 39:117–125.

83. Jovasevic VM, Mokyr MB. Melphalan-induced expression of IFN-β in MOPC-315 tumor-bearing mice and its importance for the up-regulation of TNF-α expression. *J Immunol* 2001; 167:4895–4901.

84. Sojka DK, Donepudi M, Bluestone JA, Mokyr MB. Melphalan and other anticancer modalities up-regulate B7-1 gene expression in tumor cells. *J Immunol* 2000; 164:6230–5236.

85. Serrano A, Tanzarella S, Lionello I, et al. Expression of HLA class I antigens and restoration of antigen-specific CTL response in melanoma cells following 5-aza-2'-deoxycytidine treatment. *Int J Cancer* 2001; 94:243–251.

86. Coral S, Sigalotti L, Altomonte M, et al. 5-Aza-2'-deoxycytidine-induced expression of functional cancer testis antigens in human renal cell carcinoma: immunotherapeutic implications. *Clin Cancer Res* 2002; 8:2690–2695.

87. Correale P, Aquino A, Giuliani A, et al. Treatment of colon and breast carcinoma cells with 5-fluorouracil enhances expression of carcinoembryonic antigen and susceptibility to HLA-A*02.01 restricted, CEA-peptide-specific cytotoxic T cells in vitro. *Int J Cancer* 2003; 104:437–445.

88. Keane MM, Ettenberg SA, Nau MM, Russell EK, Lipkowitz S. Chemotherapy augments TRAIL-induced apoptosis in breast cell lines. *Cancer Res* 1999; 59:734–741.

89. Zisman A, Ng CP, Pantuck AJ, Bonavida B, Belldegrun AS. Actinomycin D and Gemcitabine synergistically sensitize androgen-independent prostate cancer cells to Apo2/TRAIL-mediated apoptosis. *J Immunother* 2001; 24:459–471.

90. Nimmanapalli R, Perkins CL, Orlando M, O'Bryan E, Nguyen D, Bhalla KN. Pretreatment with Paclitaxel enhances Apo-2 ligand/tumor necrosis factor-related apoptosis ligand-induced apoptosis of prostate cancer cells by inducing death receptors 4 and 5 protein levels. *Cancer Res* 2001; 61:759–763.

91. Demaria S, Volm MD, Shapiro RL, et al. Development of tumor-infiltrating lymphocytes in breast cancer after neoadjuvant paclitaxel chemotherapy. *Clin Cancer Res* 2001; 7:3025–3303.

92. Kawasaki K, Akashi S, Shimazu R, Yoshida T, Miyake K, Nishijima M. Mouse toll-like receptor 4.MD-2 complex mediates lipopolysaccharide-mimetic signal transduction by Taxol. *J Biol Chem* 2000; 275:2251–2254.

93. Bryd-Leifer CA, Block EF, Takeda K, Akira S, Ding A. The role of MyD88 and TLR4 in the LPS-mimetic activity of Taxol. *Eur J Immunol* 2001; 31:2448–2457.

94. Wang J, Kobayashi M, Han M, et al. MyD88 is involved in the signaling pathway for Taxol-induced apoptosis and TNF-alpha expression in human myelomonocytic cells. *Br J Haematol* 2002; 118:638–645.

95. Hanahan D, Bergers G, Bergsland E. Less is more, regularly: metronomic dosing of cytotoxic drugs can target tumor angiogenesis in mice. *J Clin Invest* 2000; 105:1045–1047.

96. Bocci G, Nicolaou KC, Kerbel RS. Protracted low-dose effects on human endothelial cell proliferation and survival *in vitro* reveal a selective antiangiogenic window for various chemotherapeutic agents. *Cancer Res* 2002; 62:6938–6943.

97. Nowak AK, Robinson BW, Lake RA. Gemcitabine exerts a selective effect on the humoral immune response: implications for combination chemo-immunotherapy. *Cancer Res* 2002; 62:2353–2358.

98. Machiels J-PH, Reilly RT, Emens LA, et al. Cyclophosphamide, Doxorubicin, and Paclitaxel enhance the anti-tumor immune response of GM-CSF secreting whole-cell vaccines in HER-2/*neu* tolerized mice. *Cancer Res* 2001; 61:3689–3697.

99. Schiavoni G, Mattei F, Di Pucchio T, Santini SM, Bracci L, Belardelli FE. Cyclophosphamide induced type I interferon and augments the number of CD44[hi] T lymphocytes in mice: implications for strategies of chemoimmunotherapy for cancer. *Blood* 2000; 95:20,224–20,230.

100. Ghiringhelli F, Larmonier N, Schmitt E, et al. CD4+CD25+ regulatory T cells suppress tumor immunity but are sensitive to Cyclophosphamide which allows immunotherapy of established tumors to be curative. *Eur J Immunol* 2004; 34:336–344.

101. Mackall CL, Bare CV, Granger LA, Sharrow SO, Titus JA, Gress RE. Thymic-independent T cell regeneration occurs via antigen-driven expansion of peripheral T cells resulting in a repertoire that is limited in diversity and prone to skewing. *J Immunol* 1996; 156:4609–416.

102. Eralp Y, Wang X, Wang JP, Maughan MF, Polo JM, Lachman LB. Doxorubicin and Paclitaxel enhance the antitumor efficacy of vaccines directed against HER-2/*neu* in a murine mammary carcinoma model. *Breast Cancer Res* 2004; 6:R275–R283.

103. Yu B, Kusmartsev S, Cheng F, et al. Effective combination of chemotherapy and dendritic cell administration for the treatment of advanced-stage experimental cancer. *Clin Cancer Res* 2003; 9:285–294.

104. Nigam A, Yacavone RF, Zahurak ML, et al. Immunomodulatory properties of antineoplastic drugs administered in conjunction with GM-CSF-secreting cancer cell vaccines. *Int J Cancer* 1998; 12:161–170.

105. Reilly RT, Gottlieb MBC, Ercolini AM, et al. HER-2/*neu* is a tumor rejection target in tolerized HER-2/*neu* transgenic mice. *Cancer Res* 2000; 60:3569–3576.

106. Ercolini AM, Machiels J-PH, Chen Y, et al. Identification and characterization of the immunodominant rat HER-2/*neu* MHC Class I epitope presented by spontaneous mammary tumors from HER-2/*neu* transgenic mice. *J Immunol* 2003; 170:4273–4280.

106a. Ercolini AM, Ladle BH, Manning EA, et al. Recruitment of latent pools of high avidity CD8+ T-cells to the antitumor immune response. *J Exp Med* 2005; 201:1591–1602.

107. Emens LA, Armstrong DK, Biedrzycki B, et al. A phase I vaccine safety and chemotherapy dose-finding trial of an allogeneic GM-CSF-secreting breast cancer vaccine given in a specifically timed sequence with immunomodulatory doses of Cyclophosphamide and Doxorubicin. *Human Gene Ther* 2004; 15: 313–337.

108. Goldrath AW, Bogatzki LY, Bevan MJ. Naïve T cells transiently acquire a memory-like phenotype during homeostasis-driven proliferation. *J Exp Med* 2000; 192:557–564.

109. Cho BK, Rao VP, Ge Q, Eisen HN, Chen J. Homeostasis-stimulated proliferation drives naive T cells to differentiate directly into memory T cells. *J Exp Med* 2000; 192:549–556.

110. Hu HM, Poehlein CH, Urba WJ, Fox BA. Development of antitumor immune responses in reconstituted lymphopenic hosts. *Cancer Res* 2002; 62:3914–3919.

111. Borrello I, Sotomayor EM, Rattis FM, Cooke SK, Gu L, Levitsky HI. Sustaining the graft-versus-tumor effect through posttransplant immunization with granulocyte-macrophage colony-stimulating factor (GM-CSF)-producing tumor vaccines. *Blood* 2000; 95:3011–3019.

112. Teshima T, Mach N, Hill GR, et al. Tumor cell vaccine elicits potent antitumor immunity after allogeneic T-cell-depleted bone marrow transplantation. *Cancer Res* 2001; 61:162–171.

113. Dummer W, Niethammer AG, Baccala R, et al. T cell homeostatic proliferation elicits effective antitumor autoimmunity. *J Clin Invest* 2002; 110:185–192.

114. Luznik L, Slansky JE, Jalla S, et al. Successful therapy of metastatic cancer using tumor vaccines in mixed allogeneic bone marrow chimeras. *Blood* 2003; 101:1645–1652.

115. Dudley ME, Wunderlich JR, Robbins PF, et al. Cancer regression and autoimmunity in patients after clonal repopulation with antitumor lymphocytes. *Science* 2002; 298:850–854.

116. Chakarborty M, Abrams SI, Coleman CN, Camphausen K, Schlom J, Hodge JW. External beam radiation of tumors alters phenotype of tumor cells to render them susceptible to vaccine-mediated T-cell killing. *Cancer Res* 2004; 64:4328–4337.

117. Garnett CT, Palena C, Chakarborty M, Tsang KY, Schlom J, Hodge JW. Sublethal irradiation of human tumor cells modulates phenotype resulting in enhanced killing by cytotoxic T lymphocytes. *Cancer Res* 2004; 64:7985–7994.

118. Gasparini G, Longo R, Sarmiento R, Morabito A. Inhibitors of cyclooxygenase 2: a new class of anticancer agents? *Lancet Oncol* 2003; 4:605–615.

119. Huang M, Stolina M, Sharma S, et al. Non-small cell lung cancer cyclooxygenase-2-dependent regulation of cytokine balance in lymphocytes and macrophages: up-regulation of interleukin 10 and down-regulation of interleukin 12 production. *Cancer Res* 1998; 58:1208–1216.

120. Sharma S, Stolina M, Yang SC, et al. Tumor cyclooxygenase 2-dependent suppression of dendritic cell function. *Clin Cancer Res* 2003; 9:961–968.

121. Pockaj BA, Basu GD, Pathangey LB, et al. Reduced T-cell and dendritic cell function is related to cyclooxygenase-2 overexpression and prostaglandin E2 secretion in patients with breast cancer. *Ann Surg Oncol* 2004; 11:328–339.

122. Stolina M, Sharma S, Lin Y, et al. Specific inhibition of cyclooxygenase 2 restores antitumor reactivity by altering the balance of IL-10 and IL-12 synthesis. *J Immunol* 2000; 164:361–370.

123. Zeytin HE, Patel AC, Rogers CJ, et al. Combination of a poxvirus-based vaccine with a cyclooxygenase-2 inhibitor (Celecoxib) elicits antitumor immunity and long-term survival in CEA.Tg/MIN mice. *Cancer Res* 2004; 64:3668–3678.

124. Wang H, Cheng F, Cuenca A, et al. Imatinib mesylate (STI-571) enhances antigen presenting cell function and overcomes tumor-induced CD4+ T-cell tolerance. *Blood* 2004; 105:1135–1143.

125. Gentilli S, Abruzzese E, Fanelli A, et al. Imatinib plus CMLVAX100 (p210-derived multipeptide vaccine): Induction of complete molecular responses in patients with CML showing persistent residual disease during treatment with Imatinib Mesylate. *Blood* 2003; 102:30a.

126. Li Z, Qiao Y, Laska E, et al. Autologous leukocyte-derived heat shock protein 70-peptide complex as a vaccine for chronic myelogenous leukemia in chronic phase: an updated phase I study. *Blood* 2003; 102:911a.

127. Do Y, Hegde VL, Nagarkatti PS, Nagarkatti M. Bryostatin-1 enhances the maturation and antigen-presenting ability of murine and human dendritic cells. *Cancer Res* 2004; 64:6756–6765.

128. Kos FJ, Cornell DL, Lipke AB, Graham LJ, Bear HD. Protective role of IL-2 during activation of T cells with bryostatin 1. *Int J Immunopharm* 2000; 22:645–652.

129. Parviz M, Chin CS, Graham LJ, et al. Successful adoptive immunotherapy with vaccine-sensitized T cells, despite no effect with vaccination alone in a weakly immunogenic tumor model. *Cancer Immunol Immunother* 2003; 52:739–750.

130. Geissmann F, Revy P, Brousse N, et al. Retinoids regulate survival and antigen presentation by immature dendritic cells. *J Exp Med* 2003; 198:623–634.

131. Vertuani S, De Geer A, Levitsky V, Kogner P, Kiessling R, Levitskaya J. Retinoids act as multistep modulators of the major histocompatibility class I presentation pathway and sensitize neuroblastomas to cytotoxic lymphocytes. *Cancer Res* 2003; 63:8006–8013.

132. Kusmartsev S, Cheng F, Yu B, et al. All-trans-retinoic acid eliminates immature myeloid cells from tumor-bearing mice and improves the effect of vaccination. *Cancer Res* 2003; 63:4441–4449.

133. Westervelt P, Pollock JL, Oldfather KM, et al. Adaptive immunity cooperates with liposomal all-trans-retinoic acid (ATRA) to facilitate long-term molecular remissions in mice with acute promyelocytic leukemia. *Proc Natl Acad Sci USA* 2002; 99:9468–9473.

134. Zuany-Amorim C, Hastewell J, Walker C. Toll-like receptors as potential therapeutic targets for multiple diseases. *Nat Rev Drug Discov* 2002; 1:797–807.

20

Interleukin-2 as Cancer Therapy

Joseph I. Clark and Kim A. Margolin

SUMMARY

Interleukin (IL)-2 is the only interleukin that has fully evolved from a partially puri-fied product of activated T-cells to a commercially approved, bacterially produced recom-binant human protein. Since 1992, IL-2 has been marketed for the treatment of advanced renal cancer, and its approval for advanced melanoma followed several years later. Whereas early efforts to characterize the mechanisms of action of IL-2 led to heightened understanding of cellular and cytokine interactions in malignancy and nonmalignant states, more recent efforts have focused on improving the therapeutic index of IL-2-based therapy. Optimal combinations of IL-2 with other agents such as antibodies, chemo-therapeutics, and other cytokines for use in solid tumors, hematological malignancies, and nonmalignant diseases remain under active investigation. Other strategies that have emerged from the relative success of IL-2-based therapies include the development of immunocytokines and other structures containing an active IL-2 molecule covalently bound to a second molecule that redirects effector cells, prolongs the half-life, or alters the pharmacology of the IL-2 molecule. The use of IL-2 in immunization strategies is another area of active investigation, particularly for vaccine approaches that include ex vivo sensitization of T-cells to tumor antigens by antigen-presenting cells. Comple-menting the rapid advances in IL-2-based therapeutic manipulations of immune effec-tor subsets is the recent discovery of IL-2-receptor-bearing regulatory T-cells and other counterregulatory mechanisms of control or "escape" that will require careful study as more effective immunotherapy regimens are designed.

Key Words: Interleukin 2; cancer therapy, immunotherapy; malignancy; immuno-cytokines.

1. INTRODUCTION AND HISTORY:
THE PROMISE OF INTERLEUKIN-2 AS A T-CELL GROWTH FACTOR

Interleukin (IL)-2 was originally isolated as a soluble factor with the property of enhanc-ing T-lymphocyte proliferation in studies of the human immunodeficiency virus (1). The earliest studies of its activity in the cellular therapy of cancer used partially purified IL-2 from the Jurkat human T-cell line, and subsequent studies used recombinant IL-2 produced in *Escherichia coli*, an unlimited source of this valuable cytokine that has been used more than any other immunological agent for laboratory and clinical investigations of immuno-therapy for malignant and nonmalignant disease. Proof of concept for the potent activity

From: *Cancer Drug Discovery and Development: Immunotherapy of Cancer*
Edited by: M. L. Disis © Humana Press Inc., Totowa, NJ

of IL-2-activated killer cells (lymphokine-activated killer [LAK] cells) against established malignancy in animal models was provided in the extensive series of reports from Rosenberg and the Surgery Branch of the National Cancer Institute (NCI) beginning in the mid-1980s (2–4). The earliest human studies used Jurkat-derived IL-2 and ex vivo-activated autologous LAK cells derived from leukapheresis of patients with advanced cancer who received intravenous IL-2 before mononuclear cell collections, and additional IL-2 following the reinfusion of autologous lymphocytes that had undergone further exposure to IL-2 ex vivo for several days. The encouraging level of activity against renal cancer and melanoma, including a 5–7% rate of durable complete remission, was particularly gratifying in light of the marked resistance of these two malignancies to chemotherapy and other biological agents, such as interferon (IFN). Subsequent clinical trials demonstrated that ex vivo exposure of patient cells to IL-2 was not necessary, as the in vivo exposure appeared to be associated with a comparable likelihood of antitumor response (5). At the same time, the success of this approach at centers outside of the NCI was confirmed with a series of studies by the Cytokine Working Group and other institutions (6–9).

2. TOXICITIES OF IL-2
AND ATTEMPTS TO MITIGATE IT WITH SELECTIVE AGENTS

The animal models of IL-2 in the treatment of cancer suggested a close relationship between the amount of IL-2 exposure, the number of LAK cells reinfused, and the overall clinical benefit of this approach. Phase I clinical studies confirmed these dose-limiting toxicities and demonstrated the potential of IL-2 to cause severe, dose-related multiorgan toxicities, with nearly all toxicities resolving completely within hours to days following the last exposure to IL-2. The common mechanism appeared to be a "capillary leak syndrome" that allowed for the movement of plasma and activated lymphocytes into the interstitial spaces of nearly all organs examined. A common pattern of initial profound vasodilatation, resulting in hypotension, followed by fluid retention and evidence of "third-space" accumulation of the excess volume resulting from support of the intravascular volume using intravenous crystalloid was experienced by all patients. Individual toxicities that limited the cumulative exposure to IL-2 included hypotension with hypoperfusion of end organs exacerbated by the use of vasopressors to support the arterial blood pressure, acidosis and renal insufficiency, pulmonary insufficiency, cardiac arrhythmias or myocarditis, dermatitis and occasional mucositis, and central nervous system dysfunction. After randomized and nonrandomized trials in patients with various malignancies suggested the equivalence of high-dose IL-2 alone and IL-2 plus LAK cells, the subsequent elimination of the ex vivo LAK cell component, increasing experience with high-dose IL-2, and a trend to decreasing total IL-2 administration, resulted in an improved overall safety profile, particularly with regard to pulmonary, acid–base, and hemodynamic toxicities (10).

Whereas the vast majority of high-dose IL-2 toxicities are completely reversible, occasional patients in the early investigations developed evidence of myocardial damage manifested by myocardial dysfunction, electrocardiogram changes, chemical evidence of myocarditis, and in the rare fatal cases, pathological evidence of a lymphocytic myocardial infiltrate believed to be responsible for the damage (10–17). The incidence of this type of toxicity is now rare, presumably because of continued use of rigorous screening to exclude patients at risk for cardiovascular complications, as well as the general trend to reduced IL-2 exposure in recent series. The other irreversible toxicity, although nonlife-threatening, is the common development of thyroid dysfunction, usually hypothyroidism, in patients who survive for prolonged intervals following IL-2 therapy. The etiology of thyroid dysfunction is presumed to be an autoimmune thyroiditis resulting from IL-2-mediated dysregulation of a thyroid-reactive T-cell clone or some form of crossreactivity between thyroid and tumor antigens stimulated by IL-2 *(18–23)*. All of the other toxicities of IL-2, although challenging to patients undergoing therapy and the physicians who manage them, are reversible within a few hours to several days, and represent varying degrees of sensitivity to capillary leakage or direct infiltration by IL-2-activated lymphocytes or the secondary effects of other cytokines induced by lymphocytes in response to IL-2. These include dermatitis, usually a diffuse, maculopapular erythema resembling a drug eruption and sometimes intensely pruritic; gastrointestinal toxicities ranging from nausea, emesis, diarrhea, and occasional stomatitis to mild to moderate hepatobiliary dysfunction (variable enzyme and bilirubin elevation, synthetic dysfunction, as well as hepatomegaly, sometimes tender); and flu-like symptoms including the "first-dose" occurrence of chills and fever followed variably by fatigue, malaise, and occasional arthralgias and myalgias. Most patients experience some degree of alteration of mental status, ranging from mild confusion to the rare development of visual hallucinations, severe depression, and delirium or combative behavior. Asymptomatic but occasionally dose-limiting hematological alterations include lymphopenia, eosinophilia, anemia, and thrombocytopenia sometimes requiring transfusion support, and a "rebound" lymphocytosis following discontinuation of IL-2 (reviewed in refs. *24* and *25)*. Paradoxical increases in the susceptibility to bacterial infection during and after IL-2 therapy result from a cytokine-induced neutrophil chemotactic dysfunction and the susceptibility of tissues lacking their usual barriers to infection, such as the skin and gastrointestinal tract *(26,27)*.

3. CURRENT STATUS OF HIGH-DOSE IL-2 IN RENAL CANCER

The original experience using high-dose IL-2 in patients with cancer was reviewed by Dr. Steven Rosenberg, who pioneered this approach with colleagues at the NCI Surgery Branch *(4)*. This pooled series of 652 patients contained 155 patients who received high-dose IL-2 alone, 214 with LAK cells, 66 with tumor-infiltrating lymphocytes cultured from patient tumors and reinfused with high-dose IL-2, and 128 with IFN-α A smaller number of patients received IL-2 with chemotherapy or other cytokines. Two hundred seven patients in this series had renal cancer, and the response rate, which varied from 22 to 35%, appeared to favor the inclusion of LAK cells. However, subsequent randomized trials and sequential comparative trials in which patients were rigorously screened using the same eligibility criteria did not suggest a benefit for this component *(5,28)*. The use of other cell types, such as tumor-infiltrating lymphocytes *(29)*, and the use of other cytokines, such as IFN-α *(30–34)* added to the complexities and toxicities of the regimens without apparent benefit, so the regimen approved in 1992 by the Food and Drug Administration and used as the "gold standard" for achieving durable complete responses and long-term survivals in renal cancer is high-dose IL-2 alone. Subsequent series and pooled databases have demonstrated the reproducible level of activity and provided a basis for the design of regimens with reduced toxicity or improved therapeutic efficacy *(35,36)*.

A series of such studies was carried out by the Cytokine Working Group (previously known as the Extramural NCI-LAK Working Group), based on an initial contract to six cancer centers to reproduce the clinical results of Rosenberg and colleagues at the Surgery

Branch *(4,37)*. In summary, the Cytokine Working Group confirmed the activity, including durable complete remissions in a small fraction of patients, of high-dose IL-2 in advanced renal cancer. This group also demonstrated the lack of benefit associated with alternative schedules such as continuous intravenous infusion (less activity *[38]*) and the use of chemotherapy-containing combinations (more unfavorable therapeutic index *[39]*). Using novel methods to assess the impact of potential modulators of IL-2 toxicity, this group also showed that inhibitors of tumor necrosis factor, IL-1, lipid-mediators of inflammatory signal transduction, and cytokine-inducible nitric oxide synthase did not provide significant toxicity reduction *(40–45)*.

The results of this group's most recent study, a large phase III randomized trial of inpatient high-dose IL-2 vs a popular, fairly well-tolerated outpatient combination of lower-dose IL-2 and IFN-α, have been analyzed and are the basis for several correlative analyses of pathology, immunological, and metabolic parameters in predicting the benefit of high-dose IL-2 *(46–48)*. Overall, responses were more than twice as frequent in the group receiving high-dose inpatient IL-2 (23 vs 9%), but the primary end points of overall and progression-free survival were not significantly affected by the treatment arm. At the time of trial design, prestratifications were limited to performance status, sites of disease, and presence of the primary renal cancer. At the conclusion of the study, the groups were analyzed by separating the patients in each treatment arm into additional categories based on more recently identified factors. The unanticipated finding was that patients with the most unfavorable characteristics (primary tumor in place, hepatic and/or osseous metastases) benefited significantly from treatment with high-dose, inpatient IL-2, whereas those with the more favorable characteristics did equally well with either regimen. The outcomes from this study have also been analyzed with respect to new information regarding pathological prognostic and predictive features for patients with advanced renal cancer undergoing IL-2-based therapy, and the results are currently undergoing validation testing in phase III trials of IL-2-based therapy with other biological agents.

The need for high-dose IL-2, with its associated toxicities, expense, and the need for experienced physicians in specialized centers, has also been investigated in a novel phase III trial design by Yang and colleagues at the NCI Surgery Branch. In the first part of this randomized trial, patients were assigned to receive high-dose IL-2 on the standard regimen or one-tenth of the standard dose, using the same schedule and route of administration. After initial analysis of the data suggested the lack of a significant benefit of high-dose IL-2 over the low-dose regimen *(49)*, a third treatment arm was added, consisting of outpatient subcutaneous IL-2 using a regimen that had been reported in European multicenter studies to be effective and tolerable when self-administered. The results of this trial, reported in 2003, confirmed that the response rate to high-dose IL-2 at the Surgery Branch was now predictably in the same range reported outside of the NCI. Patients randomized to receive low-dose intravenous IL-2 or the outpatient subcutaneous regimen had a lower response rate, but their survival that did not differ significantly from that of the patients assigned to high-dose therapy *(50)*. Although the overall activity of high-dose IL-2 remains disappointing, the results of this trial also confirmed that durable complete remissions were achieved more frequently with high-dose therapy.

In addition to the need for better identification of patients who will benefit from IL-2 for advanced renal cancer, there is a desperate need for effective adjuvant therapy for patients with resected disease who are at a high risk of recurrence. The Cytokine Working Group recently reported the results of a small phase III trial to assess the benefit of a single course (two 5-d cycles) of high-dose IL-2 for patients with renal cancer at risk of recurrence following nephrectomy. In view of the toxicities of high-dose IL-2, the trial was designed to detect a large benefit that would justify further manipulations of the regimen in larger, more definitive trials; further, the end point of progression-free, rather than overall survival, was chosen because of the high likelihood that patients would receive IL-2-based therapy at the time of relapse, thus potentially negating the survival impact of adjuvant IL-2. The results of this study, which accrued 44 primary nephrectomy patients and another 25 who were randomized following surgical excision of a single or limited number of metastases, did not demonstrate a benefit in progression-free interval for patients assigned to IL-2 *(51)*. It is likely that with the emergence of new therapies for renal cancer, IL-2 will become a component of combination regimens containing agents with complementary mechanisms of antitumor activity and minimally overlapping toxicities.

4. CURRENT STATUS OF HIGH-DOSE IL-2 IN MELANOMA

Like renal cancer, melanoma is a tumor with minimal responsiveness to chemotherapies or other cytokines that has been the focus of extensive study using IL-2-based approaches. Initial studies in melanoma were designed exactly like those used for renal cancer, which are summarized in the preceding paragraphs. In the 1989 Rosenberg/NCI Surgery Branch review, 270 of the 652 pooled patients had advanced melanoma. The results of their treatment with high-dose IL-2 and LAK cells (66 patients), IL-2 alone (60 patients), or one of the other combinations (with IFN-α, tumor necrosis factor, antibody, cyclophosphamide, or tumor-infiltrating lymphocytes) mirrored those of the patients with advanced renal cancer receiving IL-2 alone, again suggesting that there is a maximum achievable response rate in the range of 20% (about one-third of which are durable complete responses) for IL-2 alone that is not enhanced by the addition of other agents *(4)*.

Investigators working in the field of IL-2-based immunotherapy of malignancy have taken advantage of important differences in the biology of renal cancer and melanoma. The two most important features of melanoma that lend themselves to the development of innovations in IL-2-based therapy include the availability of chemotherapeutic agents with activity against melanoma that possess only partially overlapping toxicities with those of IL-2, and the availability of well-characterized tumor antigens in melanoma that have been studied in combination with IL-2 and other immunostimulatory agents in both the advanced disease and the adjuvant setting. Although many chemotherapy combinations with IL-2 with or without other cytokines (often called "biochemotherapy") appeared promising when first reported, recent data from randomized studies have nearly all shown disappointing results, suggesting the lack of benefit for using complex, multiagent regimens containing one or more chemotherapies and IL-2 with or without IFN-α *(52)*. Although these results were not surprising, in view of the more empiric than rational design of the regimens used, there has continued to be a dedicated group of investigators who have applied cutting-edge principles from the explosive growth in cancer immunology to design regimens more likely to succeed in human advanced cancer. One example involves the combination of high-dose IL-2 with melanoma-specific peptides *(53,54)*. In addition, in a complex but promising recent report, patients with advanced melanoma underwent high-dose, nonmyeloablative chemotherapy followed by the reinfusion of highly selected T-cell "clones" with reactivity against known melanoma peptide antigens *(55)*. The chemotherapy in this case was designed to reduce the number of regulatory T-cells that are believed to quench the activity of the cytolytic CD8 cells with peptide-specific, human leukocyte antigen-restricted antitumor activity. Confirmatory trials of this approach are ongoing, and further studies of the mechanisms of resistance and escape from immune control will be an important correlate of these investigations.

5. IL-2-BASED THERAPY OF HEMATOLOGICAL MALIGNANCIES

During the time that IL-2-based therapies for solid tumors were under intense investigation, the potential of IL-2 for the treatment of hematological malignancies was also explored. In the case of leukemias and lymphomas, additional opportunities included the study of effector T-cells and natural-killer (NK) cells in the marrow and stem cell compartment, as well as the differentiation of hematopoietic precursor cells into dendritic cells, yielding a population of cells that could present its own antigens and be a target for immunotherapeutic eradication. Based on this extensive body of preclinical data, clinical trials were carried out at several centers to assess the feasibility of IL-2 with or without ex vivo IL-2-activated cells in the primary and adjunctive treatment of leukemia and lymphoma *(56–60)*; there was at that time also a renewed interest in the potential role of IL-2-activated hematopoietic cells as a component of regimens using high-dose chemotherapy with stem cell support for solid tumors *(61,62)*. The latter approach has largely been abandoned because of the lack of sufficient evidence for efficacy of the cytoreductive "conditioning" regimen against solid tumors, although other approaches to cellular immunotherapy for these diseases remain under active investigation. However, the results of ongoing or recently completed randomized controlled trials are eagerly awaited: the first was a Children's Oncology Group trial assessing IL-2 consolidation for acute myelogenous leukemia in remission *(63)*; the second is a recently completed Southwest Oncology Group trial assessing IL-2 following autologous stem cell transplant for intermediate-grade B-cell non-Hodgkin's lymphoma in second remission (J. A. Thompson/SWOG 9438, manuscript in preparation). IL-2 has also been evaluated for its ability to enhance antibody-dependent cellular cytotoxicity, specifically in combination with rituximab, a chimeric monoclonal antibody widely used in the treatment of indolent and aggressive B-cell lymphomas; a randomized trial of rituximab with or without IL-2 is expected to begin accrual in 2004 (D. Hurst, personal communication), and its potential for combination with other antibodies to produce additive or synergistic benefit will likely follow.

6. IL-2 IN OTHER MALIGNANCIES

The value of IL-2 or IL-2-containing combinations in other tumor types has been little studied, because:

1. Most other tumors are more responsive to cytotoxic therapies than melanoma and renal cancer.
2. Most of these cytotoxic therapies have predictable toxicities that are better tolerated by a higher fraction of patients than IL-2 in patients with these malignancies.
3. There has been inadequate study of the potential important interactions between IL-2 and other agents like cytotoxic agents, other cytokines, or other biological molecules with potentially complementary mechanisms.

It may well turn out that the most important activity of IL-2 is as an adjuvant to other types of immunotherapy. These may be antigen-specific (as with the rituximab combination, as well as in combination with tumor-derived peptides that elicit an antigen-specific T-cell response). Alternatively, they may occur via stimulation of the "innate" branch of the immune system (i.e., NK cell-mediated cytotoxicity, which is governed by very different intercellular interactions than T-cell responses) and may be based on IL-2 alone or in synergistic combinations with agents that possess different mechanisms, such as inhibitors of angiogenesis or cell signaling pathways.

7. ALTERNATIVE IL-2 MOLECULES

Many investigators and biotechnology corporations have endeavored to design a "better" IL-2, particularly because the disappointing results of several modulator trials were published *(40–45)*. Efforts have included single-amino acid substitutions, resulting in preferential binding to the IL-2 receptor of T-cells over that of NK cells *(64)*, or chemical modification of IL-2 to produce a molecule with markedly prolonged half-life that enhances overall exposure while minimizing the episodes of high peak concentrations that might be associate more with toxicity than benefit *(65,66)*. IL-2 has also been covalently linked to an antibody molecule that targets or traffics the IL-2 to the site where effector cells can be concentrated for both sensitization to tumor antigen and for optimal cytotoxic activity following activation by IL-2 *(67)*.

8. IL-2 AND OTHER BIOLOGICAL AGENTS

Except for the extensive experience with IFN combinations, primarily -α but also -γ, the use of IL-2 in combination with other cytokines has been limited. With the interferons, the successful development of a combination based on agents with non- or only partially overlapping toxicities has not been realized. Furthermore, the antitumor activity of such combinations has not been superior to that of either agent alone, and the only IL-2-containing combination that has achieved even moderate appeal in the community setting is in the outpatient, subcutaneously administered regimen presented in this chapter. The role of other combinations, such as with IL-6, IL-10, IL-12, and probably many others, remains to be further elucidated by carefully designed protocols with a solid preclinical and clinical rationale, a proven record of safety and tolerability, and appropriate correlative laboratory studies.

9. CONCLUSIONS

In the nearly two decades since the discovery of IL-2, the expansion of its role in various approaches to the biological therapy of malignant disease has taken several promising directions. Whereas the original application of IL-2 in supraphysiological doses continues to provide remissions, sometimes durable, in a small fraction of patients with advanced renal cancer and melanoma, its mechanisms of action remain speculative, ranging from antigen-driven T-cell-based effects to nonspecific activation of NK cells against tumor. IL-2 continues to be an essential element of more precisely defined strategies, such as vaccines that involve dendritic cells and other methods of optimized antigen presentation, to induce cytolytic T-cell responses in an antigen-specific, human leukocyte antigen-restricted fashion. Promising combinations of IL-2 with other cytokines, chemotherapeutic agents, angiogenesis inhibitors, and small molecules with defined molecular targets are likely to find a niche in the near future. More innovative approaches, such as bispecific IL-2-containing molecules that retarget effector lymphocytes and derivative molecules that provide enhanced activity and/or reduced toxicity, are also in development. Experience with the design of translational studies of IL-2 over the past 20 yr has provided the framework for the study of other immunotherapies, which will continue to evolve as the field expands into the 21st century.

REFERENCES

1. Smith KA. Interleukin-2: inception, impact, and implications. *Science* 1988; 240:1169–1176.
2. Rosenberg SA, Lotze MT, Muul LM, et al. Observations on the systemic administration of autologous lymphokine-activated killer cells and recombinant interleukin-2 to patients with metastatic cancer. *N Engl J Med* 1985; 313:1485–1492.
3. Rosenberg SA, Lotze MT, Muul LM, et al. A progress report on the treatment of 157 patients with advanced cancer using lymphokine-activated killer cells and interleukin-2 or high-dose interleukin-2 alone. *N Engl J Med* 1987; 316:889–897.
4. Rosenberg SA, Lotze MT, Yang JC, et al. Experience with the use of high-dose interleukin-2 in the treatment of 652 cancer patients. *Ann Surg* 1989; 210:474–484; discussion 484–485.
5. Law TM, Motzer RJ, Mazumdar M, et al. Phase III randomized trial of interleukin-2 with or without lymphokine-activated killer cells in the treatment of patients with advanced renal cell carcinoma. *Cancer* 1995; 76:824–832.
6. Dutcher JP, Creekmore S, Weiss GR, et al. A phase II study of interleukin-2 and lymphokine-activated killer cells in patients with metastatic malignant melanoma. *J Clin Oncol* 1989; 7:477–485.
7. Weiss GR, Margolin KA, Aronson FR, et al. A randomized phase II trial of continuous infusion interleukin-2 or bolus injection interleukin-2 plus lymphokine-activated killer cells for advanced renal cell carcinoma. *J Clin Oncol* 1992; 10:275–281.
8. Hawkins MJ, Atkins MB, Dutcher JP, et al. A phase II clinical trial of interleukin-2 and lymphokine-activated killer cells in advanced colorectal carcinoma. *J Immunother* 1994; 15:74–78.
9. Sparano JA, Fisher RI, Weiss GR, et al. Phase II trials of high-dose interleukin-2 and lymphokine-activated killer cells in advanced breast carcinoma and carcinoma of the lung, ovary, and pancreas and other tumors. *J Immunother Emphasis Tumor Immunol* 1994; 16:216–223.
10. Kammula US, White DE, Rosenberg SA, et al. Trends in the safety of high dose bolus interleukin-2 administration in patients with metastatic cancer. *Cancer* 1998; 83:797–805.
11. Du Bois JS, Udelson JE, Atkins MB, et al. Severe reversible global and regional ventricular dysfunction associated with high-dose interleukin-2 immunotherapy. *J Immunother Emphasis Tumor Immunol* 1995; 18:119–123.
12. White RL Jr, Schwartzentruber DJ, Guleria A, et al. Cardiopulmonary toxicity of treatment with high dose interleukin-2 in 199 consecutive patients with metastatic melanoma or renal cell carcinoma. *Cancer* 1994; 74:3212–3222.
13. Zhang J, Yu ZX, Hilbert SL, et al. Cardiotoxicity of human recombinant interleukin-2 in rats. A morphological study. *Circulation* 1993; 87:1340–1353.
14. Marshall ME, Cibull ML, Pearson T, et al. Human recombinant interleukin-2 provokes infiltration of lymphocytes into myocardium and liver in rabbits. *J Biol Response Mod* 1990; 9:279–287.
15. Samlowski WE, Ward JH, Craven CM, et al. Severe myocarditis following high-dose interleukin-2 administration. *Arch Pathol Lab Med* 1989; 113:838–841.
16. Kragel AH, Travis WD, Feinberg L, et al. Pathologic findings associated with interleukin-2-based immunotherapy for cancer: a postmortem study of 19 patients. *Hum Pathol* 1990; 21:493–502.
17. Eisner RM, Husain A, Clark JI. Case report and brief review: IL-2 induced myocarditis. *Cancer Invest* 2004; 22:401–404.
18. Krouse RS, Royal RE, Heywood G, et al. Thyroid dysfunction in 281 patients with metastatic melanoma or renal carcinoma treated with interleukin-2 alone. *J Immunother Emphasis Tumor Immunol* 1995; 18:272–278.
19. Vialettes B, Guillerand MA, Viens P, et al. Incidence rate and risk factors for thyroid dysfunction during recombinant interleukin-2 therapy in advanced malignancies. *Acta Endocrinol (Copenh)* 1993; 129:31–38.
20. Kruit WH, Bolhuis RL, Goey SH. Interleukin-2-induced thyroid dysfunction is correlated with treatment duration but not with tumor response. *J Clin Oncol* 1993; 11:921–924.

21. Schwartzentruber DJ, White DE, Zweig MH, et al. Thyroid dysfunction associated with immunotherapy for patients with cancer. *Cancer* 1991; 68:2384–2390.
22. Pichert G, Jost LM, Zobeli L. Thyroiditis after treatment with interleukin-2 and interferon alpha-2a. *Br J Cancer* 1990; 62:100–104.
23. Atkins MB, Mier JW, Parkinson DR, et al. Hypothyroidism after treatment with interleukin-2 and lymphokine-activated killer cells. *N Engl J Med* 1988; 318:1557–1563.
24. Margolin K. The clinical toxicities of high-dose interleukin-2. In: Atkins MB, Mier JW, eds. *Therapeutic Applications of Interleukin-2*. New York: Marcel Dekker. 1993: pp. 331–362.
25. Siegel JP, Puri RK. Interleukin-2 toxicity. *J Clin Oncol* 1991; 9:694–704.
26. Klempner MS, Noring R, Mier JW, et al. An acquired chemotactic defect in neutrophils from patients receiving interleukin-2 immunotherapy. *N Engl J Med* 1990; 322:959–965.
27. Pockaj BA, Topalian SL, Steinberg SM, et al. Infectious complications associated with interleukin-2 administration: a retrospective review of 935 treatment courses. *J Clin Oncol* 1993; 11:136–147.
28. Fyfe G, Fisher RI, Rosenberg SA, et al. Results of treatment of 255 patients with metastatic renal cell carcinoma who received high-dose recombinant interleukin-2 therapy. *J Clin Oncol* 1995; 3:688–696.
29. Yannelli JR, Hyatt C, McConnell S, et al. Growth of tumor-infiltrating lymphocytes from human solid cancers: summary of a 5-year experience. *Int J Cancer* 1996; 65:413–421.
30. Ilson DH, Motzer RJ, Kradin RL, et al. A phase II trial of interleukin-2 and interferon alfa-2a in patients with advanced renal cell carcinoma. *J Clin Oncol* 1992; 10:1124–1130.
31. Atkins MB, Sparano J, Fisher RI, et al. Randomized phase II trial of high-dose interleukin-2 either alone or in combination with interferon alfa-2b in advanced renal cell carcinoma. *J Clin Oncol* 1993;11:661–670.
32. Vogelzang NJ, Lipton A, Figlin RA, et al. Subcutaneous interleukin-2 plus interferon alfa-2a in metastatic renal cancer: an outpatient multicenter trial. *J Clin Oncol* 1993; 11:1809–1816.
33. Marincola FM, White DE, Wise AP, et al. Combination therapy with interferon alfa-2a and interleukin-2 for the treatment of metastatic cancer. *J Clin Oncol* 1995; 13:1110–1122.
34. Negrier S, Escudier B, Lasset C, et al. Recombinant human interleukin-2, recombinant human interferon alfa-2a, or both in metastatic renal-cell carcinoma. *N Engl J Med* 1998; 338:1272–1278.
35. Dutcher JP, Atkins M, Fisher R, et al. Interleukin-2-based therapy for metastatic renal cell cancer: the Cytokine Working Group Experience, 1989–1997. *Cancer J Sci Am* 1997; 3(Suppl 1):S73–S78.
36. Atkins MB, Dutcher J, Weiss G, et al. Kidney cancer: the Cytokine Working Group experience (1986–2001): part I. IL-2-based clinical trials. *Med Oncol* 2001; 18:197–207.
37. Fisher RI, Coltman CA, Doroshow JH, et al. Metastatic renal cancer treated with interleukin-2 and lymphokine-activated killer cells. *Ann Intern Med* 1988; 108:518–523.
38. Weiss GR, Margolin KA, Aronson FR, et al. A randomized phase II trial of continuous infusion interleukin-2 or bolus injection interleukin-2 plus lymphokine-activated killer cells for advanced renal cell carcinoma. *J Clin Oncol* 1992; 10:275–281.
39. Dutcher JP, Logan T, Gordon M, et al. Phase II trial of interleukin 2, interferon alpha, and 5-fluorouracil in metastatic renal cell cancer: a Cytokine Working Group study. *Clin Cancer Res* 2000; 6:3442–3250.
40. Sosman, JA, Weiss GR, Margolin KA, et al. Phase IB clinical trial of anti-CD3 followed by high-dose bolus interleukin-2 in patients with metastatic melanoma and advanced renal cell carcinoma: clinical and immunologic effects. *J Clin Oncol* 1993; 11:1496–1505.
41. Margolin KM, Atkins M, Sparano J, et al. Prospective randomized trial of lisofylline for the prevention of toxicities of high-dose interleukin 2 therapy in advanced renal cancer and malignant melanoma. *Clin Cancer Res* 1997; 3:565–572.
42. Trehu EG, Mier JW, Dubois JS, et al. Phase I trial of interleukin 2 in combination with the soluble tumor necrosis factor receptor p75 IgG chimera. *Clin Cancer Res* 1996; 2:1341–1351.
43. Du Bois JS, Trehu EG, Mier JW, et al. Randomized placebo-controlled clinical trial of high-dose interleukin-2 in combination with a soluble p75 tumor necrosis factor receptor immunoglobulin g chimera in patients with advanced melanoma and renal cell carcinoma. *J Clin Oncol* 1997; 15:1052–1062.
44. McDermott DF, Trehu EG, Mier JW, et al. A two-part phase I trial of high-dose interleukin 2 in combination with soluble (Chinese hamster ovary) interleukin 1 receptor. *Clin Cancer Res* 1998; 5:1203–1213.
45. Atkins MB, Redman B, Mier J, et al. A phase I study of CNI-1493, an inhibitor of cytokine release, in combination with high-dose interleukin-2 in patients with renal cancer and melanoma. *Clin Cancer Res* 2001; 7:486–492.
46. McDermott DF, Parker RA, Youmans AL. The effect of recent nephrectomy on treatment with high-dose interleukin-2 (HD IL-2) or subcutaneous (SC) IL-2/interferon alfa-2b (IFN) in patients with metastatic renal cell carcinoma (RCC). *Proc Am Soc Clin Oncol* 2003; 22:1547 (abstract no. 385).

47. Zea AH, Atkins MB, McDermont D, et al. Role of CD35 expression and arginase activity in predicting response and survival in metastatic renal cell carcinoma (mRCC) patients receiving IL-2. *Proc Am Soc Clin Oncol* 2004; 22:2535.

48. Upton MP, Parker RA, Youmans A, et al. Histologic predictors of renal cell carcinoma (RCC) response to interleukin-2-based therapy. *Proc ASCO* 2003; 22:851 (abstract no. 3420).

49. Yang JC, Topalian SL, Parkinson D, et al. Randomized comparison of high-dose and low-dose intravenous interleukin-2 for the therapy of metastatic renal cell carcinoma: an interim report. *J Clin Oncol* 1994; 12:1572–1576.

50. Yang JC, Sherry RM, Steinberg SM, et al. Randomized study of high-dose and low-dose interleukin-2 in patients with metastatic renal cancer. *J Clin Oncol* 2003; 21:3127–3132.

51. Clark JI, Atkins MB, Urba WJ, et al. Adjuvant high-dose bolus interleukin-2 for patients with high-risk renal cell carcinoma: a cytokine working group randomized trial. *J Clin Oncol* 2003; 21:3133–3140.

52. Margolin K. Biochemotherapy of melanoma—rational therapeutics in the search for weapons of melanoma destruction (editorial). *Cancer* 2004; 101:435–438.

53. Rosenberg SA, Yang JC, Schwartzentruber DJ, et al. Immunologic and therapeutic evaluation of a synthetic peptide vaccine for the treatment of patients with metastatic melanoma. *Nat Med* 1998; 4:321–327.

54. Gollob J, Flaherty L, Smith J, et al. A Cytokine Working Group (CWG) phase II trial of a modified gp100 melanoma peptide (gp100 [209M]) and high dose interleukin-2 (HD IL-2) administered q3 weeks in patients with stage IV melanoma: limited anti-tumor activity. *Proc Am Soc Clin Oncol* 2001; 20:357a (abstract no. 1423).

55. Dudley ME, Wunderlich JR, Robbins PF, et al. Cancer regression and autoimmunity in patients after clonal repopulation with antitumor lymphocytes. *Science* 2002; 298:850–854.

56. Stein AS, O'Donnell MR, Slovak ML, et al. Interleukin-2 after autologous stem-cell transplantation for adult patients with acute myeloid leukemia in first complete remission. *J Clin Oncol* 2003; 21:615–623.

57. Blaise D, Attal M, Reiffers J, et al. Randomized study of recombinant interleukin-2 after autologous bone marrow transplantation for acute leukemia in first complete remission. *Eur Cytokine Netw* 2000; 11:91–98.

58. Margolin KA, Negrin RS, Wong KK, et al. Cellular immunotherapy and autologous transplantation for hematologic malignancy. *Immunol Rev* 1997; 157:231–240.

59. Margolin KA, Forman SJ. Immunotherapy with interleukin-2 after hematopoietic cell transplantation for hematologic malignancy. *Cancer J Sci Am* 2000; 6(Suppl 1):S33–S38.

60. Van Besien K, Mehra R, Wadehra N, et al. Phase II study of autologous transplantation with interleukin-2-incubated peripheral blood stem cells and posttransplantation interleukin-2 in relapsed or refractory non-Hodgkin lymphoma. *Biol Bone Marrow Transplant* 2004; 10:386–394.

61. Sosman JA, Stiff P, Moss SM, et al. Pilot trial of interleukin-2 with granulocyte colony-stimulating factor for the mobilization of progenitor cells in advanced breast cancer patients undergoing high-dose chemotherapy: expansion of immune effectors within the stem-cell graft and post-stem-cell infusion. *J Clin Oncol* 2001; 19:634–644.

62. Meehan KR, Verma UN, Cahill R, et al. Interleukin-2-activated hematopoietic stem cell transplantation for breast cancer: investigation of dose level with clinical correlates. *Bone Marrow Transplant* 1997; 20:643–651.

63. Sievers EL, Lange BJ, Sondel PM, et al. Children's Cancer Group trials of Interleukin-2 therapy to prevent relapse of acute myelogenous leukemia. *Cancer J Sci Am* 2000; 6(Suppl 1):S39–S44.

64. Hartmann G. Technology evaluation: BAY-50-4798, Bayer. *Curr Opin Mol Ther* 2004; 6:221–227.

65. Meyers FJ, Paradise C, Scudder SA, et al. A phase I study including pharmacokinetics of polyethylene glycol conjugated interleukin-2. *Clin Pharmacol Ther* 1991; 49:307–313.

66. Yao Z, Dai W, Perry J, et al. Effect of albumin fusion on the biodistribution of interleukin-2. *Cancer Immunol Immunother* 2003; 53:404–410.

67. Lode HN, Reisfeld RA. Targeted cytokines for cancer immunotherapy. *Immunol Res* 2000; 21:279–288.

21

Biological and Clinical Properties of the Type 1 Interferons

Douglas W. Leaman,
Shaun Rosebeck, and Ernest C. Borden

SUMMARY

Interferons (IFNs) are class 2 cytokines that carry out important physiological functions in higher vertebrates, particularly in the regulation of host adaptive and innate immune responses. The complex type 1 IFN family, which includes IFN-α and IFN-β, will be the focus of this chapter. Virus and other innate immune stimuli induce expression of type 1 IFNs, which then act on responsive cells to establish an antiviral state. Type 1 IFN effects are mediated by the protein products of IFN-responsive genes, the identities and functions of which are only now starting to emerge fully. In a clinical setting, type 1 IFNs, IFN-α in particular, have shown effectiveness against a variety of malignancies. Current efforts aimed at improving pharmacokinetic and pharmacodynamic profiles of IFNs, identifying subtypes with novel biological activities and/or establishment of combined treatment modalities involving type 1 IFNs should lead to future improvements in therapeutic effectiveness.

Key Words: Interferon subtypes; interferon signaling; interferon-stimulated genes; melanoma; myeloma.

1. INTRODUCTION: INTERFERONS

Interferons (IFNs) *(1)* are class 2 cytokines that carry out important physiological functions in higher vertebrates, particularly in the regulation of host adaptive and innate immune responses *(2,3)*. Known IFNs are currently subclassified as either type 1 or type 2 based on common biochemical features including receptor crossreactivities and/or amino acid sequence similarities, although recently discovered "IFN-like" molecules may soon lead to expansion of the current classification system to include a third IFN type. The only type 2 member, IFN-γ, is structurally unrelated to the type 1 IFNs, but shares some overlap in signaling mechanisms and biological responses. IFN-γ regulates immune cell function, including aspects of T-cell maturation and stimulation of cytokine production. This chapter will focus only on type 1 IFNs, because several recent reviews have provided a thorough analysis of IFN-γ regulation, function, and therapeutic application *(4–8)*. It should be appreciated, however, that type 1 and 2 IFNs have convergent and often synergistic effects on responsive cells, and that in the course of viral or bacterial infections both IFN types are important.

From: *Cancer Drug Discovery and Development: Immunotherapy of Cancer*
Edited by: M. L. Disis © Humana Press Inc., Totowa, NJ

1.1. Type 1 IFN Classification

All type 1 IFNs share a common cell surface receptor and most, if not all, are evolutionarily related. The complex type 1 IFN family is divided into distinct subtypes based on nucleotide and amino acid sequence identities, unique biological functions, or species-restricted distributions *(9–13)*. Depending on the species in question, six to eight unique type 1 IFN subtypes may be expressed, each designated by a distinct Greek symbol: α, β, δ, ϵ, κ, τ, and ω. The recently discovered murine limitin and limitin-like mole-cules are also considered type 1 IFNs, but have not yet received Greek letter designations *(14)*. Multiple functional genes exist for many of the individual IFN subtypes and most mammalian species possess a total of 30 or more type 1 IFN genes and/or pseudogenes, all clustered on a single chromosomal arm (reviewed in ref. *15*). The type 1 IFN gene clusters reside on chromosome 9 in humans, chromosome 4 in mice, and chromosome 8 in cattle, although within these loci the relative spatial orientations, gene copy numbers, and intervening non-IFN genes differ between species.

The best-characterized type 1 IFNs are the IFN-αs and IFN-βs, which are also the two most ancient subtypes and thus the most broadly distributed among mammals *(15)*. *IFN-α* genes have been highly amplified in all species examined to date. *IFN-β*, on the other hand, has remained as a single-copy gene in most species, including humans and mice, but has amplified to high copy number in others, such as cattle and sheep *(16,17)*. *IFN-ω* and the related *IFN-τ* emerged sequentially from *IFN-α* more recently, and, in the case of the *IFN-τ*, have evolved interesting and unique biological functions, which will be discussed in Subheading 1.1.4. Evolutionary relationships among the other family members (*IFN-ϵ, -δ, -κ*, and *limitin*) have not yet been determined precisely. The following sections will address some of the unique aspects of the various type 1 IFNs, focusing on their species distributions, tissues of origin, biological effects, and therapeutic applications.

1.1.1. INTERFERON-α

As implied earlier, the most complex IFN subtype is the IFN-α family of proteins *(18)*. Between 14 and 28 *IFN-α* genes and pseudogenes may be present, depending on the species in question, and in humans, at least 13 distinct IFN molecules are expressed, not counting allelic variants *(19)*. The IFN-α members studied to date are produced predominantly by a subset of CD4$^+$CD3$^-$CD11c$^-$ plasmacytoid precursor type 2 dendritic cells, the so-called "professional" IFN-α-producing cells *(20)*. IFN-α expression is also detected in many other cell types, but typically in quantities that are orders of magnitude lower than those observed in precursor type 2 dendritic cells.

Underlying reasons for *IFN-α* gene amplification in mammals remain obscure, but may reflect the need for diverse *IFN-α* gene inducibilities to allow the host to respond effectively to a variety of different virus types *(21)*. Evidence for a hierarchical induction of different IFN-α subtypes to amplify the overall IFN response is discussed in Subheading 1.4. The various IFN-α subtypes also exhibit different relative biological potencies in vitro and in vivo *(22,23)*. Of the 13 functional IFN-α proteins expressed in humans, IFN-α preparations currently used in clinical settings are derived almost exclusively from allelic variations of a single subtype, IFN-α2. These allelic variants, designated IFN-α2a, -α2b, and -α2c, differ by single-amino acid substitutions and have virtually indistinguishable biological activities *(24)*. Each of the IFN-α2 allelic variants exhibits slightly higher specific activities as compared with IFN-α1 or IFN-α4. Although IFN-α1 had lower specific activity and receptor-binding properties in vitro as compared with IFN-α2, in vivo studies have suggested that IFN-α1 exhibited fewer side effects *(25)* and thus may permit higher dosing in a clinical setting. A few in vitro studies have suggested that IFN-α8 may be even more potent than IFN-α2 *(26)*, but surprisingly little attention has been paid to this and the other IFN-α subtypes, which remain a relatively untapped resource for therapeutic development.

Attempts have been made to improve on the activities of the naturally occurring IFN-αs, including production of a "consensus IFN-α" that incorporates the most conserved amino acid residues of the known human IFN-α *(27,28)*. Consensus IFN-α was slightly more active than naturally occurring IFNs in cell-based antiviral and cell proliferation assays and was thus hypothesized to exhibit improved effectiveness in patients that failed to respond to wild-type IFN-α *(29,30)*. However, pharmacological stabilizing modifications to IFN-α, pegylation in particular, have proved more effective in enhancing IFN clinical responses. In vitro, pegylated IFN-α was as effective as unconjugated IFN-α in promoting cellular growth arrest or apoptosis and in establishing an antiviral state when applied at equivalent activity units *(31,32)*. Enhanced in vivo stability of the pegylated molecules has resulted in improved clinical responsiveness while reducing frequency of administration, features that are likely to enhance the therapeutic potential of IFN-α (*see* Subheading 4.4.).

1.1.2. INTERFERON-β

IFN-β evolved from IFN-α approx 400 million yr ago, and since that time, the two subtypes have retained approx 35% amino acid sequence identity and similar, but not identical, receptor-binding properties. Originally called "fibroblast IFN," IFN-β is produced by nearly all cell types following treatment with virus or viral mimetics, such as double stranded RNA (dsRNA) or imiquimod *(33,34)*. Mechanisms underlying the transcriptional regulation of the *IFN-β* gene following treatment of cells with these stimuli have been the focus of extensive research, and the *IFN-β* gene promoter has served as an important experimental model for studying the details of inducible gene expression in mammals *(35)*. These studies have identified a variety of virus-induced chromatin-remodeling events and transcription factor modifications that culminate in IFN-β transcription, work that has been elegantly reviewed in several recent articles *(36–39)* and will be touched on briefly in Subheading 1.4.

In vitro, IFN-β protein is more effective at regulating cellular antiproliferative or apoptotic responses in nonhematopoietic cell types as compared with IFN-α *(40)*. Enhanced receptor binding affinity and slightly extended activation kinetics may contribute to these effects, but the exact molecular details underlying these differences are still unknown. A critical role for IFN-β in antiviral responses in vivo was demonstrated by disrupting the single IFN-β locus in mice *(41)*. These knockout animals were profoundly more sensitive to vaccinia virus *(41)* or Coxsackievirus *(42)* infection, indicating that the specific sites of production or biological consequences of IFN-β expression cannot be replaced by the remaining IFN-α or other type 1 IFN genes. Despite the apparent superior in vitro biological activity of IFN-β as compared with IFN-α *(43)*, IFN-β is currently used only for treatment of multiple sclerosis in humans. Future stabilizing modifications (*see* Subheading 4.4.) or improved delivery methods may lead to more widespread application in malignant disease.

1.1.3. INTERFERON-ω

The IFN-ω subtype was first identified more than 20 yr ago, but comparatively little is known about IFN-ω's physiological function. Multiple genes, including pseudogenes, are found in humans and ruminants *(15)*, and IFN-ω expression patterns mirror those of IFN-α, with strong induction in peripheral blood mononuclear cells following treatment with virus, dsRNA, or imiquimod *(44)*. The IFN-ω proteins share, on average, 65 and 35% amino acid sequence identity with IFN-α and IFN-β, respectively. However, the relative contribution of IFN-ω to a full antiviral response in vivo is currently unknown, and the absence of this specific subtype in mice *(44)* has excluded experimental perturbation of IFN-ω in this important model organism. Therapeutic applications of IFN-ω have not been pursued in humans, although a feline IFN-ω has been used in trials to treat diseases as diverse as feline leukemia *(45)*, canine parvovirus *(46)*, and akoya-virus infection in Japanese pearl oysters *(47)*. Successes in these animal systems could one day lead to use of IFN-ω as a second line of treatment of malignant or viral diseases in humans because neutralizing antibodies occasionally limit long-term effectiveness of IFN-α or IFN-β.

1.1.4. INTERFERON-τ

The IFN-τ proteins are closely related to IFN-ω, and in fact may have been classified as such if not for several critical biological distinctions. Firstly, IFN-τ is restricted to animals within the *Ruminantia* suborder of the order *Artiodactyla (16)*. Whereas sheep, cattle, goats, and related ungulates contain multiple IFN-τ genes and pseudogenes, IFN-τ genes are absent from mice, humans, and all other nonruminant species assessed to date. IFN-τ evolved from IFN-ω less than 35–40 million yr ago, and thus may represent one of the "youngest" members of the type 1 IFN family *(16,48)*. Unlike other known type 1 IFNs, the IFN-τ function primarily not as antiviral agents but as critical mediators of pregnancy recognition in ruminant species *(48)*. Expression is observed in trophoblast cells of the periimplantation conceptus, where production is massive for several days in early pregnancy, then subsides. Transcription is regulated in a manner that is distinct from the other type 1 IFNs, possibly involving a developmentally regulated signal *(49)*. Despite their restriction to ruminants, therapeutic applications outside of the animal husbandry realm have been proposed. Treatment of a murine model of autoimmune disease (experimental allergic encephalomyelitis) with IFN-τ led to effective reversal of the disease with few associated side effects *(50)*. Oral or gastric delivery also led to amelioration of experimental allergic encephalomyelitis symptoms, albeit at higher doses than effective with injection *(51)*. Because humans do not possess IFN-τ, oral administration for the treatment of multiple sclerosis has been proposed, to avoid immune response to the recombinant ovine or bovine proteins *(52)*. Whereas such studies have the potential to provide insight into the cross-species application of IFNs, it should be appreciated that the use of low-dose oral IFN remains controversial and will require extensive validation before becoming more widely accepted.

1.2. Novel Type 1 IFNs

Genome data mining studies, expressed sequence tag (EST) analyses, and biological activity screens have led to the recent identification of four new IFN subtypes: IFN-δ, -ε, -κ, and limitin (plus limitin-like molecules). These have been classified tentatively as type 1 based on primary amino acid sequence similarities and/or crossreactivity with the type 1 receptor, and all are clustered with or near the prototypical type 1 IFN genes in their respective species. Although completion of the human genome sequencing project has presumably ruled out identification of additional human type 1 IFN genes (beyond those that follow), novel family members in other species are certain to continue to emerge in the coming years.

1.2.1. Interferon-δ and Interferon-ε

IFN-δ was identified as a trophectodermal protein secreted during early pregnancy in pigs *(53)*. Unlike IFN-τ, IFN-δ does not appear to play a role in early pregnancy recognition in this species, and its transcriptional regulation in the conceptus appears to mirror IFN-γ more closely than type 1 IFNs *(53)*. Whereas IFN-δ cross-reacts with the type 1 IFN receptor complex and has potent antiviral and antiproliferative properties *(3)*, little is known about its physiological function in pigs or other species. Similarly ambiguous, IFN-ε has been described only as a novel IFN-like gene sequence embedded within the type 1 IFN gene cluster in mice and humans *(54)*. Although initially incorrectly classified as IFN-τ variants, the human and murine IFN-ε orthologs are clearly more ancient and may even predate IFN-α/β divergence (M. Roberts, personal communication). IFN-ε mRNA is reportedly expressed in ovaries and the uterus *(54)*, but the putative protein product has not yet been characterized in the scientific literature. As with IFN-δ, additional information on IFN-ε expression patterns and biological functions are needed before therapeutic potential can be ascertained.

1.2.2. Interferon-κ

First identified in keratinocytes, IFN-κ has biological properties similar to those associated with other type 1 IFNs, including upregulation by virus or dsRNA *(55)*, transcriptional induction of prototypical IFN-stimulated genes (ISGs) in responsive cells, and the ability to induce cytokine gene expression in monocytes or dendritic cells *(56)*. The IFN-κ gene is located on syntenic regions of chromosomes 4 and 9 in mice and human, respectively, separated from the other clustered type 1 IFN genes by approx 6 Mb. Human IFN-κ shares about 35% amino acid identity with IFN-α, -β, and -ω, and antibodies that blocked binding to the type 1 IFN receptor neutralized IFN-κ activity in vitro. Forced expression of IFN-κ in the pancreas led to diabetes in transgenic mice *(57)*, mirroring the effects of other IFNs, but few other animal-based studies have been reported, and little is known about the normal physiological function of IFN-κ.

1.2.3. Limitin

Limitin is the final putative member of the type 1 IFN gene family. Like IFN-κ, murine limitin shares 30–35% sequence identity with other murine type 1 IFNs and appears to signal via the prototypical type 1 IFN receptor complex *(58,59)*. A recent murine study suggested that the antiviral and antiproliferative effects of limitin were as potent as those observed with IFN-α, but that toxic side effects were significantly lower as compared with traditional type 1 IFNs *(60)*. Although these features would be desirable in novel human therapeutics, to date, human limitin orthologs have not been identified and may not exist. Thus, it is currently unclear whether limitin will ever be applicable to human disease, unless humanizing modifications to the murine molecules can be developed in the future.

1.3. Interferon-λ

Before discussing examples of the biological and clinical impacts of type 1 IFNs, it is important to note that a family of novel IFN-related molecules was recently identified in peripheral blood mononuclear cells *(61,62)*. At least three related genes have been cloned, and these have been termed either IFN-λa, -λb and -λc, or interleukin (IL)-28, IL-28a, and IL-29, respectively *(63)*. These antiviral cytokines bind to a unique receptor-binding chain called either IFN-λR1 or IL-28R, and utilize the shared IL-10R2 chain for full signaling *(14,64)*. Genes for IFN-λ/IL28/29 reside on chromosome 19 in humans, and are thus well removed from the type 1 IFN gene cluster *(65)*. Low-sequence identities and distinct receptor-binding characteristics clearly precludes classifying IFN-λ/IL-28/IL-29 proteins as type 1 IFNs, and they may instead qualify as the first members of a "type III" IFN family, although they have not yet been officially sanctioned as such.

1.4. Type 1 IFN Gene Induction

The primary regulators of type 1 IFN expression under normal physiological conditions are microbial pathogens, particularly viruses, whose presence must be detected before the body can mount an immune response. The mammalian innate immune system recognizes invading pathogens, in part, by using a family of cell surface and endosomal receptors known as the Toll-like receptors (TLRs) *(66)*. Components of the viral genome or replicative intermediates, such as single-stranded RNA or dsRNA, can serve as ligands for TLRs, which then trigger cytoplasmic signaling cascades that culminate in the induction of target genes, including the type 1 IFNs and other stress cytokines *(66)*. TLR3 recognizes dsRNA *(67)*, whereas TLR7 in mice and TLR8 in humans recognize single-stranded RNA *(68)*. The TLR7/8 pathway is also activated in response to imiquimod, a well-known in vivo IFN stimulant *(69)*. TLR-activated signaling cascades eventually lead to activation of transcription factors, such as nuclear factor-κB, ATF/c-jun, and members of the IFN regulatory factor (IRF) family of proteins *(70–72)*. These and other cellular virus-detection mechanisms do not regulate all IFN genes identically. IFN-β and IFN-α1 (IFN-α4 in the mouse) are induced early in infection through viral-dependent activation of the constitutively expressed IRF-3 *(73,74)*. However, the enhancer elements of other IFN-α subtypes cannot bind IRF-3 and these "late" responder IFNs, IFN-α2, -α4, and -α14 (-α2, -α5, -α6, and -α8 in the mouse *[75]*) are expressed only after secondary transcriptional induction of IRF-7 by the earlier IFNs *(76,77)*. The result is a sustained and potent IFN response that affects cellular function well beyond the cells that were initially infected with virus.

2. BIOLOGICAL ACTIVITIES OF TYPE 1 IFNs

Cells treated with IFNs in vitro exhibit a variety of responses, including acquisition of a viral resistant phenotype, reduced proliferation, growth arrest or apoptosis (depending on the dose and cell type under investigation), and induced expression of cell surface antigens. In vivo, additional effects include immune cell modulation and inhibition of angiogenesis. Work over the past 25–30 yr has led to a better understanding of the molecular details behind these therapeutically relevant biological responses, and the following sections will emphasize some of the intracellular changes that contribute to IFN-dependent influences on cell function as they pertain to cancer.

2.1. Type 1 IFN Receptors and Signaling

Biological activities associated with IFNs result from receptor-mediated changes in gene expression patterns in target cells. Type 1 IFN receptors are high-affinity, low-copy number, heterodimeric cell surface molecules found on nearly every cell type in the body *(78)*. Engagement of the monomeric IFN protein to the type 1 receptor, composed of IFNAR1 and IFNAR2C chains, leads to activation of the receptor-associated protein tyrosine kinases, Tyk2 and Janus kinase (Jak)1 *(79)*. Tyk2 and Jak1 are activated through transmolecular phosphorylation events, resulting in phosphorylation of tyrosine-466 on the cytoplasmic tail of IFNAR1 *(78,80)*. This phosphotyrosine moiety serves as a binding site for the Src homology 2 domain of the latent transcription factor signal transducer and activator of transcription (Stat)2. Stat2 is phosphorylated on tyrosine-690, which then serves to recruit Stat1 to the receptor complex *(11)*. Stat1 is in turn phosphorylated on tyrosine-701, and Stat1/2 heterodimers formed via reciprocal phosphotyrosine/Src homology 2 domain interactions leave the receptor and associate with a third cytoplasmic factor, IRF-9 (p48), to form IFN-stimulated gene factor 3 *(80)*. IFN-stimulated gene factor 3 translocates to the nucleus, where it activates transcription by binding to the IFN-stimulated response element found in the regulatory regions of most type 1 IFN-regulated genes *(11,12,80)*. Stat1 homodimer is also formed in response to type 1 or type 2 IFNs, and can activate a distinct subset of responsive genes by binding to a different DNA element called the γ activated sequence *(81)*. Involvement of transcriptional coactivators, such as CBP/p300, and synergistic association with adjacent transcription factors provides additional specificity to the transcriptional responses to type 1 IFNs *(39)*.

Additional signaling cascades are activated in response to type 1 IFNs. For example, Stat1 phosphorylation on serine-727 is required for maximum gene induction *(82,83)*, and several serine kinases have been implicated in this process, including p38 mitogen-activated protein kinase and calcium/calmodulin dependent kinase II *(84,85)*. Methylation of Stat1 on arginine-31 by type 1 IFN receptor-associated protein arginine methyl-transferase 1 has been proposed to enhance DNA-binding activity *(86)*, although recent data have raised some concerns about those observations and the overall significance of Stat1 methylation *(87)*. A variety of other signaling molecules have been implicated in IFN responses *(3,11,77,79,84)*, but the Jak–Stat proteins are clearly the components most integral to biological effects of IFNs.

2.2. IFN Signal Termination

Following initial upregulation, IFN responses must be suppressed to prevent long-term deleterious effects on cell viability. Negative regulators of type 1 IFN signaling include the suppressors of cytokine signaling (SOCS) and the protein inhibitor of activated STAT molecules. SOCS members affect IFN signaling pathways through direct interactions with phosphorylated Jaks or the activated receptor complexes, leading to an inhibition of Jak–Stat activity *(88–91)*. SOCS proteins also bind to elongins B and C, components of an E3 ubiquitin ligase complex, to target activated Jaks and Stats for proteasomal degradation *(92,93)*. Constitutive SOCS1 and/or SOCS3 expression leads to IFN-α insensitivity in melanoma *(94)*, chronic myelogenous leukemia *(95,96)* and tumor cells, and may contribute to IFN-resistance in cells infected with hepatitis C virus *(97)*. The protein inhibitor of activated Stat family of proteins also modulate Stat transcriptional activity by blocking Stat/DNA interaction *(98)* or by modifying Stat half-life through attachment of small ubiquitin-related modifier moieties to lysine residues on Stat1, a process that is less well understood *(99)*. Cytoplasmic and nuclear tyrosine phosphatases also appear to downmodulate Jak and Stat activities *(100,101)*. Although these factors combine to terminate an active IFN signaling cascade, details underlying the transcriptional suppression of IFN responsive genes under basal conditions have not been fully defined.

3. IFN-STIMULATED GENES

As mentioned, IFNs do not possess inherent biological activities, but instead regulate physiological effects via the transcriptional regulation of target genes, the ISGs *(11)*. ISGs are early response genes that are typically induced within 2 h of stimulation, most commonly peaking in expression 8–16 h after receptor activation. Gene induction is transient, with most ISG mRNA returning to baseline levels within hours, even in the continued presence of IFN *(11,102)*. Whereas the underlying events that regulate ISG expression have been well established, the identities and individual functions of many ISG protein products are only now becoming clear. This section will emphasize several of the IFN-regulated genes and proteins that contribute to IFN biological effects.

3.1. ISG Assessment

The advent of gene array technologies has allowed identification of the full repertoire of IFN-regulated transcripts, and numerous published studies have used a variety of IFN subtypes, treatment durations, doses, and array formats to assess ISG expression in cells of differing histologies *(103–111)*. At least several hundred genes are upregulated following treatment with IFN-α or IFN-β. Of these, about 50 represent "traditional" ISGs that were identified previously by functional assays or differential expression approaches, many of which are highly upregulated (10- to 500-fold induction) in response to IFN treatment. The rest are composed of a variety of novel (including ESTs) and known genes not previously associated with IFN biology. Potent ISGs, such as *ISG12, ISG15,* and *ISG6-16,* are typically induced by IFN-α or IFN-β in all responsive cell types, although the magnitude of induction varies between cell types *(103,108,111)*. Induction of some genes, however, is tissue type or cell line-specific. For example, potent IFN-dependent induction of K12 (a transmembrane protein) and galectin 9 (a galactosidase-binding lectin) was observed only in subsets of the cells examined by gene array *(108)*. Other cell types, although fully responsive to IFNs, did not exhibit induction of these transcripts. This diversity observed in cells treated in vitro suggests that gene expression changes are likely to be complex when evaluated in different cells and tissue types following in vivo treatment. Use of gene array to identify transcriptional changes indicative of clinical responsiveness to IFNs may one day assist in identifying patients that are strong candidates for IFN therapy and/or to monitor cytotoxicity *(106,112)*, although much larger profiling studies are needed to control for sample variability. Nevertheless, this approach may one day identify a handful of regulated genes whose expression provides important evaluative data in a clinical setting.

3.2. Categorization of ISG Function

Because of the pleiotropic nature of type 1 IFNs, not all induced genes will contribute to all biological responses. Some are easily assigned to a particular effect, such as the signaling molecules Stat1, Stat2, and IRF-9, whose induction by IFN provides a positive feedback to amplify subsequent responses *(11)*. Others, such as ribonuclease L (RNase L), have multiple biological functions, including viral inhibition and tumor suppression, as outlined in the following two subheadings. What follows is a brief synopsis of a few ISGs whose protein products have been implicated in specific biological effects, although it must be appreciated that the majority of IFN regulated genes have not yet been functionally characterized with respect to their roles in mediating IFN responses.

3.2.1. ANTIVIRAL ENZYMES

Several ISGs encode enzymes that are critical components of the cellular antiviral response. One of these is protein kinase R (PKR), a latent cytoplasmic serine–threonine kinase that is activated on binding dsRNA *(113,114)*. Once activated, PKR phosphorylates specific cellular target proteins including the α-subunit of the translation initiation factor eIF-2, thereby inhibiting its activity and blocking protein synthesis *(115)*. Several viral types, including encephalomyocarditis virus (EMCV), herpes simplex virus (HSV)-1, and vaccinia virus are sensitive to the antiviral actions of PKR *(116)*. Replication of other viruses, such as vesicular stomatitis virus (VSV), was unaffected, suggesting that the contribution of PKR to antiviral responses depends on the particular virus–host cell system in question.

Like PKR, the 2',5'-oligoadenylate (2-5A) synthetases are a family of IFN-inducible enzymes whose activities are regulated by dsRNA binding. Once activated, 2-5A synthetases polymerize adenosine triphosphate into 2',5'-linked oligoadenylates, which serve to activate latent cellular RNase L, which then targets mRNA and rRNA for degradation *(117)*. Although RNase L is indiscriminant in its activity, 2-5 A oligomers are relatively unstable, and so their synthesis in close proximity of viral RNA may target RNase L activity preferentially toward viral RNA *(118)*. Inactivation of the 2-5A/RNase L system by targeted ablation of the *RNase L* gene in mice attenuated IFN-β efficacy against HSV-1 replication in a trigeminal ganglion cell culture model system *(119)*. RNase L-null mice with ocular HSV-1 infection showed significantly more severe herpetic keratitis and higher mortality *(120)*. Interestingly, mice triply deficient in PKR, RNase L, and Mx (another IFN-regulated antiviral protein) were able to mount an antiviral response against infection with EMCV or VSV after IFN-α treatment *(121,122)*, suggesting the existence of additional innate antiviral pathways *(123)*. RNase L has also been implicated in the apoptotic response to virus and other cellular stresses. Thymocytes from RNase L-null mice were resistant to various apoptotic stimuli such as Fas ligand and engagement of the T-cell co-stimulatory receptor CD3 *(122)*. Dominant-negative RNase L reduced apoptotic responsiveness to IFN/dsRNA combined treatment or poliovirus infection, whereas forced activation of RNase L was sufficient to induce apoptosis in 3T3 cells *(124,125)*. Reduced levels of functional RNase L have also been implicated in prostate tumorigenesis, and several recent studies have linked the hereditary prostate cancer 1 allele to the *RNase L* gene *(126–131)*. These data highlight the importance of RNase L in various physiological processes involved in limiting viral and malignant disease progression.

Other ISG-encoded antiviral enzymes include guanylate binding protein 1, a small cellular guanosine triphosphatase that has been shown to inhibit replication of both VSV and EMCV when overexpressed in HeLa cells *(132)*. The RNA-specific adenosine deaminase is another IFN-regulated dsRNA-binding protein that can inhibit efficient replication of adenovirus *(133)*. ISG20 (HEM45) is a newly described RNase that can confer resistance to VSV when overexpressed in HeLa cells *(134)*.

3.2.2. OTHER ANTIVIRAL ISGs

A variety of additional, less characterized ISGs have been implicated in antiviral responses, although their exact mechanisms of action may require further verification. P56, encoded by the *ISG56* gene, is a potently induced protein regulated directly by IFNs, virus infection, or dsRNA stimulation *(135)*. It is part of a gene cluster that includes other IFN-induced genes, such as *ISG54*, *ISG60*, and *ISG58 (136)*. P56 appears to play a role in blocking protein synthesis through binding to and inhibiting the eIF-3 complex *(137)*. The *ISG9-27* gene product has been shown to block replication of VSV, although not as effectively as MxA *(138)*. Finally, the *cig5* gene product, viperin, has been implicated in blocking human cytomegalovirus replication by disrupting human cytomegalovirus protein processing through the Golgi apparatus *(139)*. Thus, a significant number of ISGs have important antiviral functions, but only a small fraction have been characterized as such relative to the total number of ISGs identified.

3.2.3. ANTIGROWTH/APOPTOTIC

Because type 1 IFNs possess antigrowth activities in vitro, it has been assumed that these activities contribute, at least in part, to their antitumor effectiveness. Over the past few years, it has become apparent that IFNs also possess proapoptotic effects, and a few genes involved in this response have been identified. Some ISGs, such as those in the p200 family *(140)*, promyelocytic leukemia gene product (Pml) *(141)*, Fas ligand *(142)*, and XAF1 *(143)*, among others, appear to have profound effects on cell proliferation or viability. Apoptosis induction by IFNs is indirect, requiring intervening gene transcription and protein synthesis. Numerous studies have now demonstrated an obligatory role for tumor necrosis factor-related apoptosis-inducing ligand (TRAIL) in IFN-induced apoptosis in myeloma *(144)*, melanoma *(40,145,146)*, T-cells *(147)*, B-cells *(148)*, hepatoma *(149)*, and lymphoma cells *(150)*. Coculture of cells with IFN and neutralizing TRAIL antibody or TRAIL decoy receptor is sufficient to block IFN-induced apoptosis *(40,144)*. However, other ISG protein products are clearly also needed to sensitize cells to the effects of TRAIL, because direct administration of recombinant TRAIL or TRAIL receptor agonists, in the absence of IFN pretreatment, is frequently ineffective at inducing apoptosis *(146,151)*. Recent studies have suggested that the nuclear protein Pml may be involved in IFN-induced TRAIL expression in myeloma cells *(152)*. Pml is a tumor suppressor involved in a variety of cellular apoptotic responses *(153)*. Pml expression is induced by IFN treatment, and mice deficient in Pml are largely resistant to IFN-induced apoptosis *(153)*. Expression of XAF1, a newly discovered ISG, was also correlated with the ability of cells to respond to the proapoptotic effects of TRAIL *(143)*. As a potential regulator of the inhibitor of apoptosis molecule XIAP *(154)*, XAF1 induction may allow TRAIL to fully activate downstream caspase cleavage events, but additional studies are needed to confirm this hypothesis. Several recent reviews have addressed other aspects of IFN-regulated apoptosis that are beyond the scope of this chapter *(34,145)*.

3.2.4. ANTIANGIOGENIC

IFNs can inhibit tumor vascularization at doses that are well within therapeutically achievable ranges *(155,156)*. A few IFN-regulated genes have been implicated in this effect, including genes that are downregulated in endothelial cells following IFN treatment. Basic fibroblast growth factor has been shown in numerous in vivo studies to decrease in expression following type 1 IFN treatment *(156,157)*. Downregulation of other angiogenic factors, including collagenase type IV, IL-8, matrix metalloproteinase (MMP)-2, and MMP-9 has also been reported *(155,158,159)*. The timing of the antiangiogenic response suggests that secondary effectors are required, and recent studies have implicated a role for a member of the IFN-inducible p200 gene family, *p202*, in these effects. P202 is a transcriptional repressor strongly upregulated by IFN treatment *(160)*, and ectopic expression of P202 in tumor cells lead to decreased production of IL-8, vascular endothelial growth factor, and MMP-2, resulting in reduced vascularity and tumor regression in vivo *(160)*. Additional IFN-stimulated proteins, such as IP-10 (CXCL10) and tryptophanyl-tRNA synthetase, exhibit angiostatic activities *(161,162)*. Thus, direct induction of angiostatic factors, coupled with secondary downregulation of angiogenic factors, may contribute to the overall IFN-dependent inhibition of angiogenesis.

3.2.5. Immunomodulatory

Direct effects of IFNs on tumor cell growth and viability has been demonstrated using orthologous murine tumor model systems. Treatment of nude mice implanted with human tumor cells with human type 1 IFN effectively controlled tumor growth and in some cases, promoted tumor cell apoptosis *(163,164)*. Because murine cells cannot respond to the human IFN, these antitumor effects were clearly direct. However, several recent studies have also highlighted the importance of immune cell regulation by type 1 IFNs in their antitumor effects. Stat1 knockout mice implanted with IFN-responsive tumors did not exhibit enhanced survival in response to IFN-α therapy *(165)*, whereas wild-type (Stat1$^{+/+}$) animals implanted with Stat1-null tumor cells were able to mount an effective antitumor response following IFN treatment *(166)*, suggesting that the antitumor response to IFN relies more on the effects on host tissues than the tumor itself. Cell depletion studies were performed to assess the types of immune cells involved, and these highlighted the critical importance of natural-killer (NK) cells in the antitumor effects of IFN treatment *(165)*. Identities of the IFN-regulated factors that contribute to these responses remain uncertain. IFN-α, along with IL-12, can induce NK cell production of IFN-γ and maturation of T-helper 1 cells and cytotoxic T-lymphocytes *(167)*. IFNs also augment presentation of certain antigens in a wide variety of cell types. Foreign protein antigens must be broken down within endosomes or lysosomes to generate suitable peptides that will form complexes with class II major histocompatibility complex molecules for presentation to T-cells. Type 1 IFNs potently upregulate class I (but not class II) major histocompatibility complex expression, and regulate expression of specific proteins involved in antigen processing, such as the lysosomal protease legumain *(108)*. However, specific requirements for these proteins in IFN-regulated antitumor effects will have to await future studies.

3.2.6. Protein Stability

IFNs can influence steady-state levels of proteins not only by influencing gene transcription and protein translation, but also by regulating protein stability. *ISG15* encodes a low-molecular-weight protein that is structurally related to ubiquitin. Like ubiquitin, the ISG15 protein is covalently conjugated to target proteins, including Stat1 and Jak1 proteins, that are required for type 1 IFN signaling *(168)*. Unlike ubiquitination, however, ISG15 conjugation (also called ISGylation) appears to stabilize proteins. In the case of Jak and Stat conjugation, the result appears to be augmentation of IFN responsiveness *(169)*. Interestingly, three of the proteins associated with ISGylation, UBP43, UBE1L, and Ubc8, are also transcriptionally upregulated by type 1 IFNs. UBE1L is the E1 enzyme *(170)* and Ubc8 is the E2 ligase *(171)* involved in conjugating ISG15 to proteins, whereas UBP43 (USP18) is an isopeptidase that specifically cleaves ISG15 from conjugated proteins *(172,173)*. The physiological significance of ISGylation is only now becoming known,

Table 1
Effectiveness of Interferon-α in Phase II and Phase III Clinical Trials

Chronic leukemias	Malignant melanoma[a]
Myeloid[a,b]	Mid-gut carcinoids
Hairy cell[a,b]	Renal carcinomas[a]
Myeloproliferative syndromes[a]	Kaposi's sarcomas[c]
Lymphomas	Ovarian carcinomas[c]
Follicular[a,b]	Basal cell carcinomas[c]
T-cell[b]	Bladder carcinoma
Large cell	Breast carcinomas
Multiple myeloma	

[a]Improved survival in Phase III trials.
[b]Response rates more than 40%.
[c]Intralesional or regional administration.
For more complete references, see http://www.ncbi.nlm.nih.gov/entrez/query.
fcgi?cmd=Search&db=books&doptcmdl=GenBookHL&term=borden+++
interferon++AND+352336%5Buid%5D&rid=cmed6.table.13992.
Nonmalignant proliferative processes of papilloma virus origin (laryngeal warts, genital warts) are also approved by regulatory authorities in many countries.

but early work suggests that this system contributes to the regulation of IFN responses. Mice lacking the UBP43 isopeptidase exhibited increased ISG15 conjugation to proteins, shortened lifespan, hypersensitivity to IFNs *(169)*, and enhanced antiviral responses *(174)*. Interest in the effects of IFNs on stability of other proteins is likely to increase as these studies provide new insight into the influence of IFNs on posttranslational modifications.

4. CLINICAL ANTITUMOR EFFECTS

IFNs have achieved a significant role in clinical medicine and were the first human proteins to be effective as a cancer treatment modality. They have improved therapeutic outcomes for viral diseases and malignancies, and increased quality and quantity of life for patients with hematological malignancies and solid tumors. Findings have led to regulatory approvals around the world. The clinical roles of IFNs go well beyond that of the selective antiviral envisioned at discovery.

Clinically beneficial therapeutic activity of IFN-α2 as a single agent has been demonstrated in more than a dozen malignancies (Table 1). The molecular and cellular effects of IFNs (summarized herein) complement the mechanisms of actions of other effective anticancer therapies. When combined with these other therapies in cell and animal tumor preclinical studies, IFNs have augmented, often-synergistic effectiveness for tumor types of diverse histologies. Combinations of IFNs with other modalities thus seem likely to result in new and more effective clinical applications that will be further enhanced by the continued development of second generation IFNs *(175)*.

IFNs have faced the same challenges in clinical development as any new therapy: definition of optimal dose and schedule, understanding side effects, and demonstration of reproducible activity in a defined clinical stage. It is important to understand that a single clinical trial is essentially equivalent to a single laboratory experiment, compounded in complexity by uncontrolled genetic and environmental variables. To provide a basis for understanding clinical development and impact of IFN-α, clinical findings in a solid tumor (melanoma) and a hematologic malignancy (myeloma) will be detailed here. For melanoma, marketing approval has been achieved. For myeloma, single-agent antitumor activity has resulted, but findings have yet to be substantial enough to warrant regulatory approval. Clinical results for both may improve with second generation IFNs now being introduced (*see* Subheading 4.4).

4.1. Solid Tumors: Melanoma

For renal carcinoma and melanoma, IFN-α2 has resulted in response rates in metastatic disease equivalent to the best chemotherapeutic approaches. Response rates from 4 to 26% have been reported in trials of recombinant IFN-α2 in metastatic renal carcinoma with a mean response of 15% (*176*). When compared with other modalities in phase III trials, IFN-α2 has demonstrated significant survival benefit (*177–179*). Two randomized trials suggest survival may be prolonged in patients who have nephrectomies, despite the presence of metastases, and then receive IFN-α2 (*180,181*).

IFNs for metastatic melanoma, when administered systemically, result in disease regression in 15–20% of patients (*182,183*). These findings, with other preclinical and clinical actions of IFNs in melanoma and in other malignancies, have resulted in continuing multi-institutional trials with IFNs in both the United States and Europe. For patients with metastatic disease, IFNs are more effective against smaller tumor masses than for larger tumor masses. As described in Subheading 3.2., IFNs modulate expression of a number of critical genes influencing immune effector cell recognition. These finding have led to combinations of IFNs with IL-2 and chemotherapy for metastatic disease.

Positive clinical results in the initial trials with buffy-coat IFN-α administered intramuscularly in cooperative trials of the American Cancer Society (*184*), and in a separate trial with patients receiving lymphoblastoid IFN-α (*185*), led to clinical assessment of IFN-α2, produced by recombinant technology, in patients with metastatic melanoma. As predicted by the experience with nonrecombinant IFNs, IFN-α2 had therapeutic activity. In one trial of 31 patients treated with IFN-α2, seven had regression of their disease, including four partial and three complete responses (CR) that lasted from 3 to 11.2 mo (*186*). Because the high dose used resulted in the development of fatigue in more than 80% of patients, a lower dose was used in a subsequent trial of 40 patients with metastatic melanoma (*187*). Although fewer complete responses occurred, the results were statistically significant. In another trial, 10 patients with lung, skin, or lymph node metastases had objective responses, four of which were complete (*188*). IFN-α2 produced four responses (two CR) in 23 evaluable patients treated intravenously or intramuscularly 5 d per week for 4 wk at daily doses of 10, 20, 50, or 100×10^6 U (*189*). Intramuscular injection was used in a trial of escalating doses that yielded two CR in 20 patients (*190*), and in another study using IFN-α2 on a daily dose schedule escalating to 36×10^6 U daily or on a fixed schedule of 18×10^6 U three times weekly, 5 of 62 patients treated responded (*191*). In a trial using IFN-α2 as an induction regimen of high dose daily, followed by a 50% decreased dose three times per week, 3 of 26 patients with good performance status responded (2 CR) (*192*). IFN-γ has been evaluated in phase I and II trials and has little activity against melanoma (between 6 and 11% response rate) (*193–197*). Overall, the trials of recombinant IFN-α2 on various doses and schedules summarized above have resulted in an overall objective response rate of 15% (39 of 249 patients). All trials have reported CRs, and the durable nature of some complete responses has been emphasized. For metastatic melanoma, overall level of activity of IFN-α2 has been equivalent to the best single-agent chemotherapy.

Trials combining IFN-α2 with surgery for patients with high-risk primary melanoma have been conducted in the United States and Europe. The rationale for these trials is the postulated greater effectiveness of IFN-α against minimal (microscopic) disease than against bulky tumor, a rationale supported by murine studies *(198)*. Multi-institutional North American trials (EST 1684, EST 1690, and EST 1694) have involved sufficient numbers of patients to allow statistical powering for defined stage groups. These trials have focused on patients with deeply invasive primary melanomas or those with node metastasis but no clinical evidence of metastatic disease. The two initial studies randomized patients to the standard of care at the time (careful observation) or IFN-α2. EST 1684 enrolled 287 patients from 1985 until 1990 *(199)*. Patients were randomized to either observation or 1 yr of IFN-α2. The median follow-up of patients when the study was reported was 6.9 yr, with a range of 0.6–9.6 yr. A highly significant affect on disease-free survival with IFN-α2 was demonstrated: 1.72 vs 0.98 yr, ($p < 0.01$). This translated to a 42% improvement in relapse-free survival for patients treated with IFN-α2 compared to those observed. Overall survival was positively affected, though less substantially on a statistical basis ($p = 0.04$). Benefit of IFN appeared in the first year of treatment, the period during which the patients were receiving therapy. Ten-year follow-up data has now confirmed affect on disease-free survival but not overall survival in this trial *(200)*.

To evaluate and extend the initial results of EST 1684, another trial, EST 1690, was initiated. With a median follow-up of 4.9 yr (of 642 patients entered), an almost identical survival curve for patients receiving high-dose IFN-α2 was obtained when compared with the earlier trial. However, statistical comparison of the two studies identified a highly significant difference in the results for patients randomized to observation *(201)*. Median overall survival for the observation patients in EST 1684 was 2.8 yr, with a 5-yr survival of 37%, compared with a median overall survival of the observation patients in EST 1690 of 5.9 yr, with a 5-yr survival of 55%. Thus, patients randomized to observation on EST 1690 had a 3.1-yr improvement in median survival compared with EST 1684, begun 6 yr earlier *(185)*. With recurrence, a significant number of the patients on the observation arm received IFN-α2, which may have further confounded analysis of outcomes. No other major difference in study eligibility or patient management could be identified that would account for this marked improvement in survival on the observation arm. In the most recent of these trials, a comparison to a ganglioside vaccine resulted in a 48% decrease in risk of death for those patients receiving IFN-α2 ($p < 0.01$) *(202)*. The greatest benefit appeared to have occurred in patients without histopathological evidence of node involvement *(202)*.

Other large trials have randomized patients to IFN-α2 treatment or careful observation for high-risk, primary melanoma. One that was similar in dose to the trials described above involved 262 patients with stage IIA or stage III disease who received 3 mo of treatment *(203)*. This contrasted with the 52 wk utilized in EST 1684 and EST 1690. A trend toward a delay in recurrence, particularly in the node-positive patients ($p = 0.04$) was identified, but no affect on survival was apparent. Both EST 1684 and EST 1690 included patients on a high-dose program of 10×10^6 U IFN-α2/m^2 three times weekly after a month of even higher-dose intravenous induction. EST 1690 also evaluated a low dose of IFN-α2 given at 3×10^6 U. This latter regimen resulted in no significant impact on therapeutic outcome.

Thus, the weight of evidence in the adjuvant setting points to greater effectiveness of higher doses. Although other trials have been negative, as summarized in recent meta-analyses, the overall results from these trials confirm a strong statistical affect on progression-free survival but, at best, only a marginal affect on overall survival *(204,205)*. The potential benefit of a short, high-dose treatment in patients who only have molecular evidence of nodal involvement is currently being assessed *(206)*. Prolonged treatment is being assessed in a trial involving pegylated IFN-α2 (*see* Subheading 4.4.) administered for 5 yr at doses adjusted to maintain patient quality of life. Outcomes will be compared with a control group receiving no systemic therapy *(207)*. Although further improvement is clearly needed, IFNs remain the most active adjuvant therapy for melanoma for patients staged as at highest risk for recurrence.

The data for patients with metastatic disease are less clear. Combinations of IFNs with other active modalities, such as chemotherapy and/or IL-2, might increase response rates and potentially survival in metastatic melanoma *(208, 209)*. These encouraging phase II findings, particularly the high response rates with combination chemotherapy, led to prospectively randomized phase III trials. Although the higher response rate could sometimes be confirmed when a regimen containing IFN-α2 and IL-2 was compared with the chemotherapy alone, the critical parameters of progression-free survival and overall survival were not prolonged (*[210]*; M. Atkins, personal communication). Thus, IFN-α2 in combination with chemotherapy can increase tumor regression frequency but with a significant increase in toxicity and without impact on eventual outcome. However, in phase I trials of pegylated IFN-α2 (*see* Subheading 4.4.), two out of six patients with metastatic melanoma responded *(211)*. Thus, pegylated IFN-α2 is active in melanoma and should be evaluated critically in phase II and phase III trials.

Progress has been made in identifying genes that when mutated or lost result in melanoma. One such chromosomal locus, at 9p21, codes for at least two protein products that influence cell cycle progression *(212,213)*. The genes for the IFN-αs lie at 9p22, another locus commonly lost in melanoma *(214)*. In melanoma patients, a loss of IFNs may lead to a lessened host response to the transformed cells. Acting in concert with the loss of the cell cycle regulatory proteins at 9p21, the IFN system may be a critical element in controlling progression of transformed melanocytes to malignant tumor masses.

4.2. Hematological Malignancies: Myeloma

Like melanoma, myeloma was evaluated in American Cancer Society trials with buffy-coat IFNs *(215)*. Beneficial clinical effects resulted in initiation of clinical trials with the first introduction of recombinant IFN-α2 *(216,217)*. However, it was the degree of activity and improvement in quality of life of patients with hairy cell leukemia (a leukemia refractory to other anticancer drugs) that resulted in the first licensed approval for an IFN in the United States. Following IFN treatment, a gradual decrease resulted in bone marrow infiltration with hairy cells, as well as a reversal of anemia, leukopenia, and thrombocytopenia *(218)*. This reduced morbidity from the disease process, an effect that increased with continuous treatment *(219)*. IFN's role in hairy cell leukemia has now been supplanted in clinical use by other even more effective drugs. However, Food and Drug Administration approval in hairy cell leukemia opened the way for expanded clinical trials of IFN-α2 in other disease states *(220)*.

In another chronic leukemia, chronic myeloid leukemia (CML), IFN-α2 resulted in sustained therapeutic response in more than 75% of newly diagnosed patients *(221,222)*. In addition to reduction in leukemic cell mass, a reduction occurred in frequency of cells bearing the pathogenic 9–22 chromosomal translocation *(222)*. Median and 10-yr survival data demonstrated significant advantage for IFN-α2 when compared with chemotherapy *(223)*. An increase in cytogenetic response frequency and clinical survival occurred with addition of cytosine arabinoside to IFN-α2, although this was accompanied by increased toxicity (224,225). Whether IFN-α2 will be used to clinical advantage in CML to augment the therapeutic advances that have resulted from imatinib mesylate is just beginning to be assessed. However, IFN-α2 and imatinib in vitro have synergistic effectiveness in inhibiting CML precursor proliferation (226,227).

Cytotoxic drugs result in disease response in more than 70% of patients with myeloma. However, complete remissions are unusual and the median survival in most reported series is 24–36 mo (228–230). Melphalan and glucocorticoids remain widely used but a recent meta-analysis has shown no survival advantage for other combination chemotherapies (231,232). More recently, stem cell transplantation has been introduced with possibly improved outcomes, but is limited in application for younger patients because of the associated increased morbidity and eventual relapse. With a desire to improve outcomes, various biological approaches, such as IFNs, have been investigated.

Human buffy-coat leukocyte IFN-α was administered to four patients in the first study in which IFN-α was utilized as a single agent for therapy of previously untreated myeloma patients (233). All patients achieved a response lasting from 3 to 19 mo, results that lead to further evaluation of recombinant IFN-α2. The early clinical studies on IFN-α2 showed response rates ranging from 20 to 100%, with an overall response rate of about 30% (234–236). Subsequently, the Myeloma Group of Central Sweden reported results of a randomized trial comparing the administration of human leukocyte IFN-α with oral melphalan and prednisone (MP) (237). Of patients treated with MP, 44% achieved responses, whereas only 14% of the patients treated with IFN-α responded. However, in the immunoglobulin A and Bence-Jones myeloma subgroups, the response rate was similar in both treatment groups. In another initial trial, IFN-α2 was associated with normalization of suppressed immunoglobulins, a characteristic infrequently altered by chemotherapy (216).

Several studies have since been undertaken using IFN-α2 in combination with chemotherapy to exploit synergistic antitumor effects. The Eastern Cooperative Oncology Group designed a study to evaluate the effect of adding alternating 6-wk cycles of IFN-α2 or early intensification with high-dose cyclophosphamide (for patients <70 yr old) to a combination chemotherapy regimen for previously untreated patients (238). Treatment was continued for 2 yr. Of the 653 patients entered, 628 were eligible for the study. With median follow-up for surviving patients of 54 mo, the median survival duration was 42 mo, 1 yr longer than usually reported for MP. A comparison of the three regimens revealed no significant difference in the rates of survival or objective response. However, more CR occurred among patients receiving chemotherapy and IFN-α2 when compared to chemotherapy alone (18 vs 10%, $p = 0.03$). Patients treated with chemotherapy and IFN-α2 also had a longer response duration (30 vs 25 mo, $p = 0.035$). There was a greater response rate with the IFN-α2 regimen among elderly patients (objective response and CR = 67 and 31%, respectively). Thus, combination chemotherapy plus IFN-α2 yielded a higher rate of CR and longer response duration than chemotherapy alone, but made no difference in the rates of overall response or survival (238). The superior ability of chemotherapy and IFN-α2 in this trial to produce CR and more-durable responses, as well as its activity in older patients and in those with immunoglobulin A myeloma, suggest that this therapy has important biological activity meriting further clinical investigation.

IFN-α2 has more frequently been studied as a maintenance treatment aimed at prolonging chemotherapy-induced disease control. An Italian group compared IFN-α2 maintenance with no treatment, and the relapse rate after 33 mo of follow-up was reduced from

56 to 24% *(239)*. However, a subsequent UK study found no survival benefit of IFN-α2 *(240)*. Although opinion is divided on this issue, a recent meta-analysis of 24 randomized trials involving 4000 patients showed that IFN-α2 produced a moderate improvement in relapse-free survival and a minor improvement in overall survival *(241)*. Survival was somewhat better at 3 yr with IFNs (3-yr survival: 53 vs 49%, $p = 0.01$). An effect of similar magnitude was observed in both primary treatment and maintenance use with increases in median survival of about 2 and 7 mo, respectively. CR were both significantly better with IFNs in both induction ($p < 0.0003$) and maintenance ($p < 0.00001$) trials: median relapse-free survival increased by about 6 mo in both, and 3-yr relapse-free survival were improved by 7 and 12%, respectively, with some suggestion of prolonged stability in disease beyond 4 yr for IFN treated patients.

When initial results of maintenance IFN-α2 were reported, greatest benefit was in patients with the lowest tumor burden at the start of therapy *(239)*. Thus, an ideal group of patients for investigation of the role of IFN-α2 would be those who have undergone high-dose chemotherapy and achieved substantial disease regression. This hypothesis was the basis for 84 patients entered on a trial where induction treatment consisted of intensive combination chemotherapy given until maximum response was achieved *(242)*. Autologous marrow stem cell support 6 wk after the last chemotherapy cycle was planned, and randomization to the IFN group was carried out at hematological recovery following autologous bone marrow transplant. Follow-up has failed to demonstrate the benefits of IFN-α2 and may be the result of 17 of 33 patients in the control group who, on relapse, subsequently received IFN-α2. Only 4 of 31 patients who relapsed after IFN-α2 maintenance were further treated with IFN-α2 for possible disease suppression *(242)*. Thus, the trial was really a "crossover" of treatment potentially negating survival benefit.

Several other studies have examined use of IFN-α2 following high-dose treatment, but all these studies were nonrandomized. A 28% event-free survival and 52% overall survival at 5 yr was reported in one trial, and a retrospective analysis suggested a similar favorable trend for patients with CR (37% CR rate) on maintenance posthigh-dose chemotherapy *(243,244)*. IFN-α2 has been used to increase CR rates in patients not in CR when evaluated 4 mo after allogeneic stem cell transplant. No increased toxicity occurred from graft-vs-host disease when compared with those patients not receiving IFN-α2, and durable CRs were achieved in 4 of 13 patients *(245)*.

The beneficial effects in the meta-analyses and individual trials must be balanced against possible toxicity and financial costs of IFN-α2. No specific disease or patient characteristics have been defined that would allow us to identify patients who are most likely to benefit from IFN-α2. However, in analogy to other cancers, low tumor load, excellent performance status, young age, and remission from high-dose chemotherapy seem to be factors associated with beneficial effects of IFN. A randomized, multicenter study was designed to compare two schedules of a maintenance therapy in order to assess the difference in effectiveness and tolerance *(246)*. Patients with low-risk myeloma (i.e., with serum β2 microglobulin <6.0 mg/L and serum albumin >3.0 g/L) were enrolled; 27 patients were randomly assigned to receive IFN-α2 three times weekly, and 25 patients received daily treatments. Progression-free survival was 11.9 mo in the three-times-weekly group and 38.3 mo in the other *(246)*. Thus, dose and schedule might play a role in the quality of response and require further exploration. Second-generation IFNs may resolve the issue of toxicity limiting dose intensity and/or may resolve the inconveniences of daily dosing.

Table 2
Clinical Side Effects of Interferons

Acute fever	Chronic fatigue
Chills	Anorexia
Malaise	Weight loss
Myalgias	Granulocytopenia
Headaches	Hepatic transaminase increases
Nausea	Depression, mental slowing
	Less common: thrombocytopenia,
	diarrhea, nausea, and vomiting

4.3. Side Effects

Like other potent physiological mediators, such as glucocorticoids, IFNs have toxicities when administered on pharmacological doses or schedules (Table 2). Side effects with initial dose are predominantly constitutional dominated by malaise, fever, and chills, which begin a few hours after a dose and last for 2–8 h *(247–250)*. These influenza-like symptoms, whereas dose-related but individually variable in severity, occur uniformly following the initial injection. However, even after an initial low dose, these symptoms do not recur with subsequent daily injections. Flu-like symptoms can be partially controlled with acetaminophen.

Fatigue and anorexia are dose-limiting toxicities associated with chronic administration; weight loss occurs and can be more than 10% *(247–250)*. Chronic fatigue may necessitate dose reduction; tolerance can be improved with lower doses. Although individual variability can be marked, older patients generally have greater difficulty with these side effects than do younger patients. Neither the cause nor effective treatment for this syndrome has been identified *(249,251–254)*. Thus, it has been difficult not only for patients, but also for nurses and physicians involved in their management, particularly because these patients, in contrast to many of those with metastatic disease, are otherwise well. The most frequent neurological side effects (other than the possible relationship of the fatigue) are somnolence, confusion, and depression. A small, randomized trial has suggested that paroxetine may partially ameliorate the depression *(255)*.

Despite side effects, 80% of protocol-defined doses were received by patients treated for melanoma on EST 1684 *(199)*. Despite the fatigue and anorexia associated with 1 yr of IFN administration, quality-of-life analysis identified a significant advantage in favor of treatment *(256)*. This quality-adjusted time without symptoms and toxicity analysis identified more quality-adjusted survival time for patients receiving treatment even considering side effects. Also, because a survival advantage accrued to patients treated on this study, results could be demonstrated to have a magnitude of economic benefit associated with advantageous medical interventions *(257)*.

Hematological effects include moderate granulocytopenia with a reduction in counts by 40–60%, followed by normalization several days after discontinuation. Granulocytopenia is rarely dose limiting. Anemia occurs with chronic therapy but is rarely severe. This may reflect an influence on the erythropoiesis because return to normal hematocrit has often required weeks or months. Mild thrombocytopenia has been reported in 5–50% of patients and can be accentuated by marrow infiltration with tumor. Elevation of transaminases, usually mild, has occurred more commonly in the presence of pretreatment hepatic abnormalities and is also dose-related. The most common renal toxicity described has been mild proteinuria. Although little or no IFN can be identified in urine, renal failure reduces but does not eliminate clearance, suggesting catabolism by renal tubular cells is one degradation pathway *(258)*.

With chronic administration, a minority of patients develop neutralizing antibody to the administered IFN-α2 and IFN-β *(259–262)*. Antibody development is a function of dose, schedule, route, and possibly underlying disease. Antibodies have rarely been identified with less than 4 mo of IFN administration. Particularly when present in high titer, neutralizing antibodies may be correlated with disease progression *(263)*.

4.4. Second-Generation IFNs

Clinical effectiveness may be further enhanced by the introduction of second generation IFNs with different biological effects and/or pharmacokinetic/pharmacodynamic profiles. As mentioned earlier, quantitative difference in the in vitro activities of the various eukaryotic cell produced IFN-αs have been reported *(264)*, yet only IFN-α2 has been broadly assessed clinically. Limited phase I trials of IFN-α1 have been conducted in the United States. Significantly fewer side effects resulted *(265)*. For example, maximum peak temperature was significantly less from IFN-α1 than resulting from IFN-α2 in this randomized clinical comparison. Nevertheless, IFN-α1 was as effective in inducing 2-5A synthetase and NK cell cytotoxicity as was IFN-α2 *(265,266)*. IFN-α1 has been more widely assessed in China, where it has been used mostly for chronic hepatitis B and hepatitis C infections, with good effectiveness. Reported side effects have been fewer and less severe. IFN-α1 has had only limited trial in malignancies in China, although it has clinical activity in CML and hairy cell leukemia.

Pegylated IFN-αs have polyethylene glycol (PEG) linked with a single covalent bond. PEG is an uncharged polymer of various lengths that reduces immunogenicity, reduces sensitivity to proteolysis, and lengthens serum half-life. PEG has been utilized effectively for therapeutic proteins such as erythropoietin, thrombopoietin, and adenosine deaminase. Pharmacokinetics have been characterized by a dose-related increase in serum concentrations and delayed elimination of PEG-IFN-α2 compared to IFN-α2 *(211)*. Mean elimination half-life (50+ h) was approximately sevenfold greater with PEG-IFN-α2 when compared with IFN-α2. The volume of distribution was the same for either preparation (1 L/kg). PEG-IFN-α2 has proven to be safe and allows once or twice weekly dosing. Tumor regressions have resulted in renal carcinomas, melanoma, and CML *(211,267,268)*.

Although IFN-β binds to the same receptor on the cell surface as IFN-α, it does so with higher affinity *(269)*. IFN-β has effects on gene induction and cell differentiation, proliferation and apoptosis, which contrast with IFN-α *(40,108,270–276)*. In the nude mouse, human IFN-β inhibited growth of three different melanoma xenografts and resulted in greater antitumor effects than IFN-α2 *(276,277)*. In humans, a deficiency in IFN-β production has been identified in the epidermis overlying melanomas, with a concomitant increase in angiogenesis *(278)*. Because IFN-β has antiangiogenic effects in the nude mouse, these antitumor effects may result from vascular inhibition in addition to direct effects on tumor. A high-dose daily infusion of IFN-β $(60 \times 10^6$ U) for 4 d resulted in partial responses in 3 of 15 patients with metastatic melanoma *(279)*. A lower dose (up to 20×10^6 U intravenously) two times weekly was ineffective *(280)*. In studies in both cancer and multiple sclerosis, IFN-β has proven better tolerated than anticipated based on side effects of IFN-α2. For example, in studies in cancer, little or no weight loss has resulted *(281,282)*.

Table 3
Unanswered Clinical Questions in Melanoma and Myeloma

Roles of different IFN types	Dose intensity
Induced genes	Cause of side effects
Mechanism of antitumor action	Optimal clinical stage for therapy
Prediction of therapeutic response	Duration of therapy
	Effectiveness of combinations

IFN, interferon.

In multiple sclerosis, frequency of cumulative side effects over the first 3 mo between placebo and control have been difficult to discern (283).

IFN-inducers, functioning through stimulation of toll-like receptors on dendritic cells, include low-molecular-weight compounds (such as imiquimod) and modified single-strand cytosine–phosphate–guanine (CpG)-oligodeoxynucleotides (ODNs) with a phophoro-thioate backbone. The former, whereas active orally and potent inducers, cause dose-limiting fatigue when given systemically (284). Although requiring injection, the synthetic CpG-ODNs have been better tolerated, with only mild fatigue and injection-site sore-ness. In addition to IFN induction, the CpG-ODNs are also potent immunomodulators and have demonstrated antitumor effects in preclinical murine models (285–289). Although an optimal dose and schedule are still being defined, based on immunological and clinical data, phase II/III trials are being initiated assessing different doses and in combination with chemotherapy.

5. UNANSWERED QUESTIONS

Despite these advances in IFN application to malignant disease for the past 20+ yr, a number of important questions remain unanswered. What are the physiological roles of the various members of the type 1 IFN family? Will pharmacologically and therapeutically important differences in cancer responses be identified after utilization of IFN inducers or pegylated IFNs? Will identified differences in genes induced by individual IFNs enable better understanding of antitumor mechanisms? Our working hypotheses are that these differences will be clinically realized and that, as additional members of the IFN family or IFN inducers are introduced, additional clinical effectiveness and/or lesser side effects will result. These will enable the full therapeutic potential of the IFN system for cancer to be realized (Table 3).

REFERENCES

1. Isaacs A, Lindenmann J. Virus interference. 1. The interferon. *Proc R Soc Lond Ser B: Biol Sci* 1957; 147:258–267.
2. Pfeffer LM, Dinarello CA, Herberman RB, et al. Biological properties of recombinant alpha-interferons: 40th anniversary of the discovery of interferons. *Cancer Res* 1998; 58:2489–2499.
3. Pestka S, Krause CD, Walter MR. Interferons, interferon-like cytokines, and their receptors. *Immunol Rev* 2004; 202:8–32.
4. Young HA, Hardy KJ. Role of interferon-gamma in immune cell regulation. *J Leukoc Biol* 1995; 58: 373–381.
5. Boehm U, Klamp T, Groot M, Howard JC. Cellular responses to interferon-gamma. *Annu Rev Immunol* 1997; 15:749–795.
6. Pestka S, Kotenko SV, Muthukumaran G, Izotova LS, Cook JR, Garotta G. The interferon gamma (IFN-gamma) receptor: a paradigm for the multichain cytokine receptor. *Cytokine Growth Factor Rev* 1997; 8:189–206.

7. Dorman SE, Holland SM. Interferon-gamma and interleukin-12 pathway defects and human disease. *Cytokine Growth Factor Rev* 2000; 11:321–333.

8. Schroder K, Hertzog PJ, Ravasi T, Hume DA. Interferon-gamma: an overview of signals, mechanisms and functions. *J Leukoc Biol* 2004; 75:163–189.

9. Kontsek P. Human type 1 interferons: structure and function. *Acta Virol* 1994; 38:345–360.

10. De Maeyer E, De Maeyer-Guignard J. Type 1 interferons. *Int Rev Immunol* 1998; 17:53–73.

11. Stark GR, Kerr IM, Williams BRG, Silverman RH, Schreiber RD. How cells respond to interferons. *Annu Rev Biochem* 1998; 67:227–264.

12. Leaman DW. Mechanisms of interferon action. *Prog Mol Subcell Biol* 1998; 120:101–142.

13. Samuel C. Antiviral actions of interferons. *Clin Microbiol Rev* 2001; 14:778–809.

14. Pestka S, Krause CD, Sarkar D, Walter MR, Shi Y, Fisher PB. Interleukin-10 and related cytokines and receptors. *Annu Rev Immunol* 2004; 22:929–979.

15. Roberts RM, Lui L, Guo Q, Leaman D, Bixby J. The evolution of the Type 1 interferons. *J Interferon Cytokine Res* 1998; 18:805–816.

16. Leaman DW, Cross JC, Roberts RM. The genes for the trophoblast interferons and their distribution among mammals. *Mol Reprod Fert* 1992; 4:349–353.

17. Ryan AM, Womack JE. Type 1 interferon genes in cattle: restriction fragment length polymorphisms, gene numbers and physical organization on bovine chromosome 8. *Anim Genet* 1993; 24:9–16.

18. Weissmann C, Nagata S, Boll W, et al. Structure and expression of human IFN-alpha genes. *Philos Trans R Soc Lond* 1982; 299:7–28.

19. Allen G, Diaz MO. Nomenclature of the human interferon proteins. *J Interferon Cytokine Res* 1996; 16:181–184.

20. Siegal FP, Kadowski N, Shodell M, et al. The nature of the principal type 1 interferon-producing cells in human blood. *Science* 1999; 284:1835–1837.

21. Hiscott J, Cantell K, Weissman C. Differential expression of human interferon genes. *Nucleic Acids Res* 1984; 12:3727–3749.

22. Fish EN, Banerjee K, Stebbing N. Human leukocyte interferon subtypes have different antiproliferative and antiviral activities on human cells. *Biochem Biophys Res Commun* 1983; 112: 537–546.

23. Foster GR, Rodrigues O, Ghouze F, et al. Interferon-alpha 2 variants in the human genome. *J Interferon Cytokine Res* 1995; 15:341–349.

24. Lee N, Ni D, Brissette R, Chou M, et al. Interferon-alpha 2 variants in the human genome. *J Interferon Cytokine Res* 1995; 15:341–349.

25. Edwards BS, Hawkins MJ, Borden EC. Comparative in vivo and in vitro activation of human natural killer cells by two recombinant alpha-interferons differing in antiviral activity. *Cancer Res* 1984; 44: 3135–3139.

26. Foster GR, Rodriques O, Ghouze F, et al. Different relative activities of human cell-derived interferon-a subtype: IFN-a8 has very high antiviral potency. *J Interferon Cytokine Res* 1996; 16:1027–1033.

27. Koyama AH, Arakawa T, Adachi A. Comparison of an antiviral activity of recombinant consensus interferon with recombinant interferon-alpha-2b. *Microbes Infect* 1999; 1:1073–1077.

28. Mecchia M, Matarrese P, Malorni W, et al. Type 1 consensus interferon (CIFN) gene transfer into human melanoma cells up-regulates p53 and enhances cisplatin-induced apoptosis: implications for new therapeutic strategies with IFN-alpha. *Gene Ther* 2000; 7:167–179.

29. Pockros PJ, Reindollar R, McHutchinson J, et al. The safety and tolerability of daily infergen plus ribavirin in the treatment of naive chronic hepatitis C patients. *J Viral Hepat* 2003; 10:55–60.

30. Miglioresi L, Bacosi M, Russo F, et al. Consensus interferon versus interferon-alpha 2b plus ribavirin in patients with relapsing HCV infection. *Hepatol Res* 2003; 27:253–259.

31. Bailon P, Palleroni A, Schaffer CA, et al. Rational design of a potent, long-lasting form of interferon: a 40 kDa branched polyethylene glycol-conjugated interferon alpha-2a for the treatment of hepatitis C. *Bioconjug Chem* 2001; 12:195–202.

32. Vyas K, Brassard DL, DeLorenzo MM, et al. Biologic activity of polyethylene glycol12000-interferon-alpha2b compared with interferon-alpha2b: gene modulatory and antigrowth effects in tumor cells. *J Immunother* 2003; 26:202–211.

33. Megyeri K, Au WC, Rosztoczy I, et al. Stimulation of interferon and cytokine gene expression by imiquimod and stimulation by Sendai virus utilize similar signal transduction pathways. *Mol Cell Biol* 1995; 15:2207–2218.

34. Barber GN. Host defense, viruses and apoptosis. *Cell Death Differ* 2001; 8:113–126.

35. Ohno S, Taniguchi T. Inducer-responsive expression of the cloned human interferon beta 1 gene introduced into cultured mouse cells. *Nucleic Acids Res* 1982; 10:967–977.
36. Agalioti T, Lomvardas S, Parekh B, Yie J, Maniatis T, Thanos D. Ordered recruitment of chromatin modifying and general transcription factors to the IFN-beta promoter. *Cell* 2000; 103:667–678.
37. Lomvardas S, Thanos D. Modifying gene expression programs by altering core promoter chromatin architecture. *Cell* 2002; 110:261–271.
38. Smale ST, Fisher AG. Chromatin structure and gene regulation in the immune system. *Annu Rev Immunol* 2002; 20:427–462.
39. Yang H, Ma G, Lin CH, Orr M, Wathelet MG. Mechanism for transcriptional synergy between interferon regulatory factor (IRF)-3 and IRF-7 in activation of the interferon-beta gene promoter. *Eur J Biochem* 2004; 271:3693–3703.
40. Chawla-Sarkar M, Leaman DW, Borden EC. Preferential induction of apoptosis by interferon-β compared to interferon-α: correlation with TRAIL/Apo2L induction in melanoma cell lines. *Clin Cancer Res* 2001; 7:1821–1831.
41. Deonarain R, Alcami A, Alexiou M, Dallman MJ, Gewert DR, Porter AC. Impaired antiviral response and alpha/beta interferon induction in mice lacking beta interferon. *J Virol* 2000; 74:3404–3409.
42. Deonarain R, Cerullo D, Fuse K, Liu PP, Fish EN. Protective role for interferon-beta in coxsackievirus B3 infection. *Circulation* 2004; 110:3540–3543.
43. Leadbeater L, Thomas HC. Different relative activities of human cell-derived interferon-alpha subtypes: IFN-alpha 8 has very high antiviral potency. *J Interferon Cytokine Res* 1996; 16:1027–1033.
44. Adolf GR. Human interferon omega—a review. *Mult Scler* 1995; 1(Suppl 1):S44–47.
45. de Mari K, Maynard L, Sanquer A, Lebreux B, Eun HM. Therapeutic effects of recombinant feline interferon-omega on feline leukemia virus (FeLV)-infected and FeLV/feline immunodeficiency virus (FIV)-coinfected symptomatic cats. *J Vet Intern Med* 2004; 18:477–482.
46. Minagawa T, Ishiwata K, Kajimoto T. Feline interferon-omega treatment on canine parvovirus infection. *Vet Microbiol* 1999; 69:51–53.
47. Miyazaki T, Nozawa N, Kobayashi T. Clinical trial results on the use of a recombinant feline interferon-omega to protect Japanese pearl oysters, *Pinctada fucata martensii*, from akoya-virus infection. *Dis Aquat Organ* 2000; 43:15–26.
48. Roberts RM, Cross JC, Leaman DW. Interferons as hormones of pregnancy. *Endocrine Rev* 1992; 13: 432–452.
49. Roberts RM, Ezashi T, Rosenfeld CS, Ealy AD, Kubisch HM. Evolution of the interferon *tau* genes and their promoters, and maternal-trophoblast interaction in control of their expression. *Reprod Suppl* 2003; 61:239–251.
50. Soos JM, Subramaniam PS, Hobeika AC, Schiffenbauer J, Johnson HM. The IFN pregnancy recognition horomone, IFN-tau, blocks both development and superantigen reactivation of experimental allergic encephalomyelitis without associated toxicity. *J Immunol* 1995; 155:2747–2753.
51. Soos JM, Mujtaba MG, Subramaniam PS, Streit WJ, Johnson HM. Oral feeding of interferon tau can prevent the acute and chronic relapsing forms of experimental allergic encephalomyelitis. *J Neuroimmunol* 1997; 75:43–50.
52. Soos JM, Stüve O, Youssef S, et al. Cutting edge: oral type 1 IFN-τ promotes a th2 bias and enhances suppression of autoimmune encephalomyelitis by oral glatiramer acetate. *J Immunol* 2002; 169:2231–2235.
53. Lefevre F, Guillomot M, D'Andrea S, Battegay S, La Bonnardiere C. Interferon-delta: the first member of a novel type 1 interferon family. *Biochimie* 1998; 80:779–788.
54. Hardy MP, Owczarek CM, Jermiin LS, Ejdeback M, Hertzog PJ. Characterization of the type 1 interferon locus and identification of novel genes. *Genomics* 2004; 84:331–345.
55. LaFleur DW, Nardelli B, Tsareva T, et al. Interferon-kappa, a novel type 1 interferon expressed in human keratinocytes. *J Biol Chem* 2001; 276:39,765–39,771.
56. Nardelli B, Zaritskaya L, Semenuk M, et al. Regulatory effect of IFN-kappa, a novel type 1 IFN, on cytokine production by cells of the innate immune system. *J Immunol* 2002; 169:4822–4830.
57. Vassileva G, Chen SC, Zeng M, et al. Expression of a novel murine type 1 IFN in the pancreatic islets induces diabetes in mice. *J Immunol* 2003; 170:5748–5755.
58. Oritani K, Kincade PW, Zhang C, Tomiyama Y, Matsuzawa Y. Type 1 interferons and limitin: a comparison of structures, receptors, and functions. *Cytokine Growth Factor Rev* 2001; 12:337–348.
59. Kawamoto S, Oritani K, Asakura E, et al. A new interferon, limitin, displays equivalent immunomodulatory and antitumor activities without myelosuppressive properties as compared with interferon-alpha. *Exp Hematol* 2004; 32:797–805.

60. Kawamoto S, Oritani K, Asada H, et al. Antiviral activity of limitin against encephalomyocarditis virus, herpes simplex virus, and mouse hepatitis virus: diverse requirements by limitin and alpha inter-feron for interferon regulatory factor 1. *J Virol* 2003; 77:9622–9631.

61. Kotenko SV, Gallagher G, Baurin VV, et al. IFN-lambdas mediate antiviral protection through a distinct class II cytokine receptor complex. *Nat Immunol* 2003; 4:69–77.

62. Dumoutier L, Tounsi A, Michiels T, Sommereyns C, Kotenko SV, Renauld JC. Role of the interleukin (IL)-28 receptor tyrosine residues for antiviral and antiproliferative activity of IL-29/interferon-lambda 1: similarities with type 1 interferon signaling. *J Biol Chem* 2004; 279:32,269–32,274.

63. Kontsek P, Karayianni-Vasconcelos G, Kontsekova E. The human interferon system: characterization and classification after discovery of novel members. *Acta Virol* 2003; 47:201–215.

64. Sheppard P, Kindsvogel W, Xu W, et al. IL-28, IL-29 and their class II cytokine receptor IL-28R. *Nat Immunol* 2003; 4:63–68.

65. Donnelly RP, Sheikh F, Kotenko SV, Dickensheets H. The expanded family of class II cytokines that share the IL-10 receptor-2 (IL-10R2) chain. *J Leukoc Biol* 2004; 76:314–321.

66. Iwasaki A, Medzhitov R. Toll-like receptor control of the adaptive immune responses. *Nat Immunol* 2004; 5:987–995.

67. Alexopoulou L, Holt AC, Medzhitov R, Flavell RA. Recognition of double-stranded RNA and activation of NF-kappaB by Toll-like receptor 3. *Nature* 2001; 413:732–738.

68. Heil F, Hemmi H, Hochrein H, et al. Species-specific recognition of single-stranded RNA via toll-like receptor 7 and 8. *Science* 2004; 303:1526–1529.

69. Syed TA. A review of the applications of imiquimod: a novel immune response modifier. *Expert Opin Pharmacother* 2001; 2:877–882.

70. Fitzgerald KA, McWhirter SM, Faia KL, et al. IKKepsilon and TBK1 are essential components of the IRF3 signaling pathway. *Nat Immunol* 2003; 4:491–496.

71. Sharma S, tenOever BR, Grandvaux N, Zhou G, Lin R, Hiscott J. Triggering the interferon antiviral response through an IKK-related pathway. *Science* 2003; 300:1148–1151.

72. Kim TK, Maniatis T. The mechanism of transcriptional synergy of an in vitro assembled interferon-beta enhanceosome. *Mol Cell* 1997; 1:119–129.

73. Lin R, Genin P, Mamane Y, Hiscott J. Selective DNA binding and association with the CREB binding protein coactivator contribute to differential activation of alpha/beta interferon genes by interferon regulatory factors 3 and 7. *Mol Cell Biol* 2000; 20:6342–6353.

74. Levy DE, Marie I, Smith E, Prakash A. Enhancement and diversification of IFN induction by IRF-7-mediated positive feedback. *J Interferon Cytokine Res* 2002; 22:87–93.

75. Marie I, Durbin JE, Levy DE. Differential viral induction of distinct interferon-alpha genes by positive feedback through interferon regulatory factor-7. *EMBO J* 1998; 17:6660–6669.

76. Yeow W-S, Au W-C, Juang Y-T, et al. Reconstitution of virus-mediated expression of interferon α genes in human fibroblast cells by ectopic interferon regulatory factor-7. *J Biol Chem* 2000; 275:6313–6320.

77. Decker T, Stockinger S, Karaghiosoff, Muller M, Kovarik P. IFNs and STATs in innate immunity to microorganisms. *J Clin Invest* 2002; 109:1271–1277.

78. Uzé G, Lutfalla G, Mogensen KE. α and β interferons and their receptor and their friends and relations. *J Interferon Cytokine Res* 1995; 15:3–26.

79. Schindler C, Darnell JE Jr. Transcriptional responses to polypeptide ligands: the JAK-STAT pathway. *Annu Rev Biochem* 1995; 64:621–651.

80. Darnell Jr JE, Kerr IM, Stark GR. Jak STAT pathways and transcriptional activation in response to IFNs and other extracellular signaling proteins. *Science* 1994; 264:1415–1421.

81. Decker T, Kovarik P, Meinke A. GAS elements: a few nucleotides with a major impact on cytokine-induced gene expression. *J Interferon Cytokine Res* 1997; 17:121–134.

82. Wen Z, Darnell JE Jr. Mapping of Stat3 serine phosphorylation to a single residue (727) and evidence that serine phosphorylation has no influence on DNA binding of Stat1 and Stat3. *Nucleic Acids Res* 1997; 25:2062–2067.

83. Wen Z, Zhong Z, Darnell JE Jr. Maximal activation of transcription by Stat1 and Stat3 requires both tyrosine and serine phosphorylation. *Cell* 1995; 82:241–250.

84. Platanias LC. The p38 mitogen-activated protein kinase pathway and its role in interferon signaling. *Pharmacol Ther* 2003; 98:129–142.

85. Nair JS, DaFonseca CJ, Tjernberg A, et al. Requirement of Ca^{2+} and CaMKII for Stat1 Ser-727 phosphorylation in response to IFN-gamma. *Proc Natl Acad Sci USA* 2002; 99:5971–5976.

86. Mowen KA, Tang J, Zhu W, et al. Arginine methylation of STAT1 modulates IFNalpha/beta-induced transcription. *Cell* 2001; 104:731–734.
87. Meissner T, Krause E, Lodige I, Vinkemeier U. Arginine methylation of STAT1: a reassessment. *Cell* 2004; 119:587–590.
88. Starr R, Willson TA, Viney EM, et al. A family of cytokine-inducible inhibitors of signalling. *Nature* 1997; 387:917–921.
89. Endo TA, Masuhara M, Yokouchi M, et al. A new protein containing an SH2 domain that inhibits JAK kinases. *Nature* 1997; 387:921–924.
90. Naka T, Narazaki M, Hirata M, et al. Structure and function of a new STAT-induced STAT inhibitor. *Nature* 1997; 387:924–929.
91. Kile BT, Alexander WS. The suppressors of cytokine signalling (SOCS). *Cell Mol Life Sci* 2001; 58: 1627–1635.
92. Kamura T, Sato S, Haque D, et al. The Elongin BC complex interacts with the conserved SOCS-box motif present in members of the SOCS, ras, WD-40 repeat, and ankyrin repeat families. *Genes Dev* 1998; 12:3872–3881.
93. Zhang JG, Farley A, Nicholson SE, et al. The conserved SOCS box motif in suppressors of cytokine signaling binds to elongins B and C and may couple bound proteins to proteasomal degradation. *Proc Natl Acad Sci USA* 1999; 96:2071–2076.
94. Li Z, Metze D, Nashan D, et al. Expression of SOCS-1, suppressor of cytokine signalling-1, in human melanoma. *J Invest Dermatol* 2004; 123:737–745.
95. Roman-Gomez J, Jimenez-Velasco A, Castillejo JA, et al. The suppressor of cytokine signaling-1 is constitutively expressed in chronic myeloid leukemia and correlates with poor cytogenetic response to interferon-alpha. *Haematologica* 2004; 89:42–48.
96. Sakai I, Takeuchi K, Yamauchi H, Narumi H, Fujita S. Constitutive expression of SOCS3 confers resistance to IFN-alpha in chronic myelogenous leukemia cells. *Blood* 2002; 100:2926–2931.
97. Vlotides G, Sorensen AS, Kopp F, et al. SOCS-1 and SOCS-3 inhibit IFN-alpha-induced expression of the antiviral proteins 2,5-OAS and MxA. *Biochem Biophys Res Commun* 2004; 320:1007–1014.
98. Liu B, Liao J, Rao X, et al. Inhibition of Stat1-mediated gene activation by PIAS1. *Proc Natl Acad Sci USA* 1998; 95:10626–10631.
99. Rogers RS, Horvath CM, Matunis MJ. SUMO modification of STAT1 and its role in PIAS-mediated inhibition of gene activation. *J Biol Chem* 2003; 278:30,091–30,097.
100. Neel BG. Structure and function of SH2-domain containing tyrosine phosphatases. *Semin Cell Biol* 1993; 4:419–432.
101. Neel BG, Tonks NK. Protein tyrosine phosphatases in signal transduction. *Curr Opin Cell Biol* 1997; 9:193–204.
102. Larner A, Reich NC. Interferon signal transduction. *Biotherapy* 1996; 8:175–181.
103. Der SD, Zhou A, Williams BRG, Silverman RH. Identification of genes differentially regulated by interferon α, β or γ using oligonucleotide arrays. *Proc Natl Acad Sci USA* 1998; 95:15,623–15,628.
104. Baechler EC, Batliwalla FM, Karypis G, et al. Interferon-inducible gene expression signature in peripheral blood cells of patients with severe lupus. *Proc Natl Acad Sci USA* 2003; 100:2610–2615.
105. Crow MK, Kirou KA, Wohlgemuth J. Microarray analysis of interferon-regulated genes in SLE. *Autoimmunity* 2003; 36:481–490.
106. Ji X, Cheung R, Cooper S, Li Q, Greenberg HB, He XS. Interferon alpha regulated gene expression in patients initiating interferon treatment for chronic hepatitis C. *Hepatology* 2003; 37:610–621.
107. Koike F, Satoh J, Miyake S, et al. Microarray analysis identifies interferon beta-regulated genes in multiple sclerosis. *J Neuroimmunol* 2003; 139:109–118.
108. Leaman DW, Chawla-Sarkar M, Jacobs B, et al. Novel growth and death related interferon (IFN) stimulated genes (ISGs) in melanoma: GREATER POTENCY of IFN-beta compared to IFN-alpha. *J Interferon Cytokine Res* 2003; 23:745–756.
109. Brassard DL, Delorenzo MM, Cox S, et al. Regulation of gene expression by pegylated IFN-alpha2b and IFN-alpha2b in human peripheral blood mononuclear cells. *J Interferon Cytokine Res* 2004; 24: 455–469.
110. Taylor MW, Grosse WM, Schaley JE, et al. Global effect of PEG-IFN-alpha and ribavirin on gene expression in PBMC in vitro. *J Interferon Cytokine Res* 2004; 24:107–118.
111. Tracey L, Spiteri I, Ortiz P, Lawler M, Piris MA, Villuendas R. Transcriptional response of T cells to IFN-alpha: changes induced in IFN-alpha-sensitive and resistant cutaneous T cell lymphoma. *J Interferon Cytokine Res* 2004; 24:185–195.

112. Stürzebecher S, Wandinger KP, Rosenwald A, et al. Expression profiling identifies responder and non-responder phenotypes to interferon-§ in multiple sclerosis. *Brain* 2003; 126:1419–1429.

113. Clemens MJ, Elia A. The double-stranded RNA-dependent protein kinase PKR: structure and function. *J Interferon Cytokine Res* 1997; 17:503–524.

114. Williams BR. PKR; a sentinel kinase for cellular stress. *Oncogene* 1999; 18:6112-6120.

115. Samuel CE. The eIF-2 alpha protein kinases, regulators of translation in eukaryotes from yeasts to humans. *J Biol Chem* 1993; 268:7603–7606.

116. Stewart MJ, Blum MA, Sherry B. PKR's protective role in viral myocarditis. *Virology* 2003; 314:92–100.

117. Silverman RH. Fascination with 2-5A-dependent RNase: a unique enzyme that functions in interferon action. *J Interferon Res* 1994;1 4:101–104.

118. Staeheli P. Interferon-induced proteins and the antiviral state. *Adv Virus Res* 1990; 38:147–200.

119. Al-khatib K, Williams BR, Silverman RH, Halford W, Carr DJ. The murine double-stranded RNA-dependent protein kinase PKR and the murine 2',5'-oligoadenylate synthetase-dependent RNase L are required for IFN-beta-mediated resistance against herpes simplex virus type 1 in primary trigeminal ganglion culture. *Virology* 2003; 313:126–135.

120. Zheng X, Silverman RH, Zhou A, et al. Increased severity of HSV-1 keratitis and mortality in mice lacking the 2-5A-dependent RNase L gene. *Invest Ophthalmol Vis Sci* 2001; 42:120–126.

121. Zhou AJ, Paranjape TL, Brown TL, et al. Interferon action and apoptosis are defective in mice devoid of 2',5'-oligoadenylate-dependent RNase L. *EMBO J* 1997; 16:6355–6363.

122. Zhou A, Paranjape JM, Der SD, Williams BR, Silverman RH. Interferon action in triply deficient mice reveals the existence of alternative antiviral pathways. *Virology* 1999; 258:435–440.

123. Choudhary S, Gao J, Leaman DW, De BP. Interferon action against human parainfluenza virus type 3: involvement of a novel antiviral pathway in the inhibition of transcription. *J Virol* 2001; 75:4823–4831.

124. Castelli JC, Hassel BA, Wood KA, et al. A study of the interferon antiviral mechanism: apoptosis activation by the 2-5A system. *J Exp Med* 1997; 186:967–972.

125. Castelli JC, Hassel BA, Maran A, et al. The role of 2'-5' oligoadenylate-activated ribonuclease L in apoptosis. *Cell Death Differ* 1998; 5:313–320.

126. Carpten J, Nupponen N, Isaacs S, et al. Germline mutations in the ribonuclease L gene in families showing linkage with HPC1. *Nat Genet* 2002; 30:181–184.

127. Rokman A, Ikonen T, Seppala EH, et al. Germline alterations of the RNASEL gene, a candidate HPC1 gene at 1q25, in patients and families with prostate cancer. *Am J Hum Genet* 2002; 70:1299–1304.

128. Casey G, Neville PJ, Plummer SJ, et al. RNASEL Arg462Gln variant is implicated in up to 13% of prostate cancer cases. *Nat Genet* 2002; 32:581–583.

129. Xiang Y, Wang Z, Murakami J, et al. Effects of RNase L mutations associated with prostate cancer on apoptosis induced by 2',5'-oligoadenylates. *Cancer Res* 2003; 63:6795–6801.

130. Downing SR, Hennessy KT, Abe M, Manola J, George DJ, Kantoff PW. Mutations in ribonuclease L gene do not occur at a greater frequency in patients with familial prostate cancer compared with patients with sporadic prostate cancer. *Clin Prostate Cancer* 2003; 2:177–180.

131. Nupponen NN, Wallen MJ, Ponciano D, et al. Mutational analysis of susceptibility genes RNASEL/HPC1, ELAC2/HPC2, and MSR1 in sporadic prostate cancer. *Genes Chromosomes Cancer* 2004; 39:119–125.

132. Anderson SL, Carton JM, Lou J, Xing L, Rubin BY. Interferon-induced guanylate binding protein-1 (GBP-1) mediates an antiviral effect against vesicular stomatitis virus and encephalomyocarditis virus. *Virology* 1999; 256:8–14.

133. Lei M, Liu Y, Samuel CE. Adenovirus VAI RNA antagonizes the RNA-editing activity of the ADAR adenosine deaminase. *Virology* 1998; 245:188–196.

134. Espert L, Degols G, Gongora C, et al. ISG20, a new interferon-induced RNase specific for single-stranded RNA, defines an alternative antiviral pathway against RNA genomic viruses. *J Biol Chem* 2003; 278:16,151–16,158.

135. Guo J, Peters KL, Sen GC. Induction of the human protein P56 by interferon, double-stranded RNA, or virus infection. *Virology* 2000; 267:209–219.

136. Sen GC. Viruses and interferons. *Annu Rev Microbiol* 2001; 55:255–281.

137. Guo J, Hui D, Merrick WC, Sen GC. A new pathway of translational regulation mediated by eukaryotic initiation factor 3. *EMBO J* 2001; 19:6891–6899.

138. Alber D, Staeheli P. Partial inhibition of vesicular stomatitis virus by the interferon-induced human 9-27 protein. *J Interferon Cytokine Res* 1996; 16:375–380.

139. Chin KC, Cresswell P. Viperin (cig5), an IFN-inducible antiviral protein directly induced by human cytomegalovirus. *Proc Natl Acad Sci USA* 2001; 98:15,125–15,130.

140. Lengyel P, Choubey D, Li S, Datta B. The interferon-activatable gene 200 cluster: from structure toward function. *Sem Virol* 1995; 6:202–213.

141. Wu WS, Xu ZX, Hittelman WN, Salomoni P, Pandolfi PP, Chang KS. Promyelocytic leukemia protein sensitizes tumor necrosis factor alpha-induced apoptosis by inhibiting the NF-kappaB survival pathway. *J Biol Chem* 2003; 278:12,294–12,304.

142. Kirou KA, Vakkalanka RK, Butler MJ, Crow MK. Induction of Fas ligand-mediated apoptosis by interferon-alpha. *Clin Immunol* 2000; 95:218–226.

143. Leaman DW, Chawla-Sarkar M, Vyas K, et al. Identification of X-linked inhibitor of apoptosis-associated factor-1 (XAF1) as an interferon-stimulated gene that augments TRAIL/Apo2L-induced apoptosis. *J Biol Chem* 2002; 277:28,504–28,511.

144. Chen Q, Gong B, Mahmoud-Ahmed AS, et al. Apo2L/TRAIL and Bcl-2-related proteins regulate type 1 interferon-induced apoptosis in multiple myeloma. *Blood* 2001; 98:2183–2192.

145. Chawla-Sarkar M, Lindner DJ, Liu YF, et al. Apoptosis and interferons: role of interferon-stimulated genes as mediators of apoptosis. *Apoptosis* 2003; 8:237–249.

146. Chawla-Sarkar M, Leaman DW, Jacobs BS, Borden EC. IFN-β pretreatment sensitizes human melanoma cells to tumor necrosis factor-related apoptosis-inducing ligand (TRAIL/Apo2L) induced apoptosis. *J Immunol* 2003; 169:847–855.

147. Ballestrero A, Nencioni A, Boy D, et al. Tumor necrosis factor-related apoptosis-inducing ligand cooperates with anticancer drugs to overcome chemoresistance in antiapoptotic Bcl-2 family members expressing Jurkat cells. *Clin Cancer Res* 2004; 10:1463–1470.

148. Ucur E, Mattern J, Wenger T, Okouoyo S, Schroth A, Debatin KM, Herr I. Induction of apoptosis in experimental human B cell lymphomas by conditional TRAIL-expressing T cells. *Br J Cancer* 2003; 89:2155–2162.

149. Shigeno M, Nakao K, Ichikawa T, et al. Interferon-alpha sensitizes human hepatoma cells to TRAIL-induced apoptosis through DR5 upregulation and NF-kappa B inactivation. *Oncogene* 2003; 22:1653–1662.

149. Oshima K, Yanase N, Ibukiyama C, et al. Involvement of TRAIL/TRAIL-R interaction in IFN-alpha-induced apoptosis of Daudi B lymphoma cells. *Cytokine* 2001; 22:1653–1662.

149. Yagita H, Takeda K, Hayakawa Y, Smyth MJ, Okumura K. TRAIL and its receptors as targets for cancer therapy. *Cancer Sci* 2004; 95:777–783.

150. Crowder C, Dahle O, Davis RE, Gabrielsen OS, Rudikoff S. PML mediates IFN-α induced apoptosis in myeloma by regulating TRAIL induction. *Blood* 2004; 105:1280–1287.

153. Wang ZG, Ruggero D, Ronchetti S, et al. PML is essential for multiple apoptotic pathways. *Nat Genet* 1998; 20:220–222.

154. Holcik M, Gibson H, Korneluk RG. XIAP: apoptotic brake and promising therapeutic target. *Apoptosis* 2001; 6:253–261.

155. Fidler IJ. Angiogenesis and cancer metastasis. *Cancer J* 2000; 6:S134–S141.

156. Lindner DJ. Interferons as antiangiogenic agents. *Curr Oncol Rep* 2002; 4:510–514.

157. Riedel F, Gotte K, Bergler W, Rojas W, Hormann K. Expression of basic fibroblast growth factor protein and its down-regulation by interferons in head and neck cancer. *Head Neck* 2000; 22:183–189.

158. Ma Z, Qin H, Benveniste EN. Transcriptional suppression of matrix metalloproteinase-9 gene expression by IFN-gamma and IFN-beta: critical role of STAT-1alpha. *J Immunol* 2001; 167:5150–5159.

159. Huang S, Bucana CD, Van Arsdall M, Fidler IJ. Stat1 negatively regulates angiogenesis, tumorigenicity and metastasis of tumor cells. *Oncogene* 2002; 21:2504–2512.

160. Wen Y, Yan DH, Wang B, et al. p202, an interferon-inducible protein, mediates multiple antitumor activities in human pancreatic cancer xenograft models. *Cancer Res* 2001; 61:7142–7147.

161. Yang J, Richmond A. The angiostatic activity of interferon-inducible protein-10/CXCL10 in human melanoma depends on binding to CXCR3 but not to glycosaminoglycan. *Mol Ther* 2004; 9:846–855.

162. Wakasugi K, Slike BM, Hood J, et al. A human aminoacyl-tRNA synthetase as a regulator of angiogenesis. *Proc Natl Acad Sci USA* 2002; 99:173–177.

163. Sanceau J, Poupon MF, Delattre O, Sastre-Garau X, Wietzerbin J. Strong inhibition of Ewing tumor xenograft growth by combination of human interferon-alpha or interferon-beta with ifosfamide. *Oncogene* 2002; 21:7700–7709.

164. Qin XQ, Tao N, Dergay A, et al. Interferon-beta gene therapy inhibits tumor formation and causes regression of established tumors in immune-deficient mice. *Proc Natl Acad Sci USA* 1998; 95:14,411–14,416.

165. Lesinski GB, Anghelina M, Zimmerer J, et al. The antitumor effects of IFN-alpha are abrogated in a STAT1-deficient mouse. *J Clin Invest* 2003; 112:170–180.

166. Badgwell B, Lesinski GB, Magro C, Abood G, Skaf A, Carson W III. The antitumor effects of interferon-alpha are maintained in mice challenged with a STAT1-deficient murine melanoma cell line. *J Surg Res* 2004; 116:129–136.

167. Malmgaard L. Induction and regulation of IFNs during viral infections. *J Interferon Cytokine Res* 2004; 24:439–454.

168. Malakhov MP, Kim KI, Malakhova OA, Jacobs BS, Borden EC, Zhang DE. High-throughput immuno-blotting. Ubiquitin-like protein ISG15 modifies key regulators of signal transduction. *J Biol Chem* 2003; 278:16,608–16,613.

169. Malakhova OA, Yan M, Malakhov MP, et al. Protein ISGylation modulates the JAK-STAT signaling pathway. *Genes Dev* 2003; 17:455–460.

170. Yuan W, Krug RM. Influenza B virus NS1 protein inhibits conjugation of the interferon (IFN)-induced ubiquitin-like ISG15 protein. *EMBO J* 2001; 20:362–371.

171. Kim KI, Giannakopoulos NV, Virgin HW, Zhang DE. Interferon-inducible ubiquitin E2, Ubc8, is a conjugating enzyme for protein ISGylation. *Mol Cell Biol* 2004; 24:9592–9600.

172. Malakhov MP, Malakhova OA, Kim KI, Ritchie KJ, Zhang DE. UBP43 (USP18) specifically removes ISG15 from conjugated proteins. *J Biol Chem* 2002; 277:9976–9981.

173. Tokarz S, Berset C, La Rue J, et al. The ISG15 isopeptidase UBP43 is regulated by proteolysis via the SCFSkp2 ubiquitin ligase. *J Biol Chem* 2004; 279:46,424–46,430.

174. Ritchie KJ, Hahn CS, Kim KI, et al. Role of ISG15 protease UBP43 (USP18) in innate immunity to viral infection. *Nat Med* 2004; 10:1374–1380.

175. Masci P, Bukowski RM, Patten PA, Osborn BL, Borden EC. New and modified interferon alfas: pre-clinical and clinical data. *Curr Oncol Rep* 2003; 5:108–113.

176. Nelson BE, Borden EC. Interferons: biological and clinical effects. *Semin Surg Oncol* 1989; 5:391–401.

177. Collaborators MRCRC. Interferon-α and survival in metastatic renal carcinoma: early results of a randomized controlled trial. *Lancet* 1999:14–17.

178. Pyrhonen S, Salminen E, Ruutu M, et al. Prospective randomized trial of interferon alfa-2a plus vinblastine versus vinblastine alone in patients with advanced renal cell carcinoma. *J Clin Oncol* 1999; 17:2859–2867.

179. Hernberg M, Pyrhonen S, Muhonen T. Regimens with or without interferon-alpha as treatment for metastatic melanoma and renal cell carcinoma: an overview of randomized trials. *J Immunother* 1999; 22:145–154.

180. Mickisch GH, Garin A, van Poppel H, de Prijck L, Sylvester R. European Organisation for Research and Treatment of Cancer (EORTC) Genitourinary Group. Radical nephrectomy plus interferon-alpha-based immunotherapy compared with interferon alpha alone in metastatic renal-cell carcinoma: a randomized trial. *Lancet* 2001; 358:966–970.

181. Flanigan RC, Salmon SE, Blumenstein BA, et al. Nephrectomy followed by interferon alpha-2b compared with interferon alpha-2b alone for metastatic renal-cell cancer. *N Engl J Med* 2001; 345:1655–1659.

182. Creagan E, Ahmann DL, Green SJ. Phase II study of recombinant leukocyte interferon (rIFN-Alpha-A) in disseminated malignant melanoma. *Cancer* 1984; 54:2844–2849.

183. Robinson W, Mughal TI, Thomas MR, Johnson M, Spiegel RJ. Treatment of metastatic melanoma with recombinant interferon alpha 2. *Immunobiology* 1986; 172:275–282.

184. Krown SE, Burk MW, Kirkwood JM, Kerr D, Morton DL, Oettgen HF. Human leukocyte (alpha) interferon in metastatic malignant melanoma: The American Cancer Society phase II trial. *Cancer Treat Rep* 1984; 68:723–726.

185. Retsas S, Priestman TJ, Newton KA, Westbury G. Evaluation of human lymphoblastoid interferon in advanced malignant melanoma. *Cancer* 1983; 51:273–276.

186. Creagan ET, Ahmann DL, Green SJ. Phase II study of recombinant leukocyte A interferon (rIFN-alpha A) in disseminated malignant melanoma. *Cancer* 1984; 54:2844–2849.

187. Creagan ET, Ahmann DL, Long HJ, Frytak S, Sherwin SA, Chang MN. Phase II study of recombinant interferon-gamma in patients with disseminated malignant melanoma. *Cancer Treat Rep* 1987; 71:843–844.

188. Robinson WA, Mughal TI, Thomas MR, Johnson M, Spiegel RJ. Treatment of metastatic malignant melanoma with recombinant interferon alpha-2. *Immunobiology* 1986; 172:275–282.

189. Kirkwood JM, Ernstoff MS, Davis CA, Reiss M, Ferraresi R, Rudnick SA. Comparison of intramuscular and intravenous recombinant interferon in melanoma and other cancers. *Ann Intern Med* 1985; 103: 32–36.

190. Hersey P, Hasic E, MacDonald M, Edward A, Spurling A, Coates AS. Effects of recombinant leukocyte interferon (rIFN-alpha A) on tumour grow and immune responses in patients with metastatic melanoma. *Br J Cancer* 1985; 51:815–826.

191. Legha SS, Papadopoulos NE, Plager C, et al. Clinical evaluation of recombinant interferon alfa-2A (Roferon-A) in metastatic melanoma using two different schedules. *J Clin Oncol* 1987; 5:1240–1246.

192. Miller RL, Steis RG, Clark JW, et al. Randomized trial of recombinant alpha 2B-interferon with or without indomethacin in patients with metastatic malignant melanoma. *Cancer Res* 1989; 49:1871–1876.

193. Ernstoff MS, Trautman T, Davis CA, et al. A randomized phase I/II study of cutaneous versus intermittent intravenous interferon gamma in patients with metastatic malignant melanoma. *J Clin Oncol* 1987; 5:1804–1810.

194. Kurzrock R, Quesada JR, Talpaz M, et al. Phase I study of multiple dose intramuscularly administered recombinant gamma interferon. *J Clin Oncol* 1986; 4:1101–1109.

195. Kirkwood JM, Ernstoff MS, Trautman T, et al. In vivo biological response to recombinant interferon-gamma during a phase I done-response trial in patients with metastatic melanoma. *J Clin Oncol* 1990; 8:1070–1082.

196. Meyskens FL Jr, Kopecky KJ, Taylor CW, et al. Randomized trial of adjuvant human interferon gamma versus observation in high-risk cutaneous melanoma: a Southwest Oncology Group study. *J Natl Cancer Inst* 1995; 87:1710–1713.

197. Schiller JH, Pugh M, Kirkwood JM, Karp D, Larson M, Borden E. Eastern cooperative group trial of interferon gamma in metastatic melanoma: an innovative study design. *Clin Cancer Res* 1996; 2:29–36.

198. Gresser I. How does interferon inhibit tumour growth? *Philos Trans R Soc Lond B Biol Sci* 1982; 299: 69–76.

199. Kirkwood JM, Strawderman MH, Ernstoff MS, Smith TJ, Borden EC, Blum RH. Interferon alfa-2b adjuvant therapy of high-risk resected cutaneous melanoma: the Eastern Cooperative Oncology Group trial EST 1684. *J Clin Oncol* 1996; 14:7–17.

200. Kirkwood JM, Manola J, Ibrahim J, Sondak V, Ernstoff MS, Rao U, Eastern Cooperative Oncology Group. A pooled analysis of eastern cooperative oncology group and intergroup trials of adjuvant high-dose interferon for melanoma. *Clin Cancer Res* 2004; 10:1670–1677.

201. Kirkwood JM, Ibrahim JG, Sondak VK, et al. High- and low-dose interferon alfa-2b in high-risk melanoma: first analysis intergroup trial E1690/S9111/C9190. *J Clin Oncol* 2000; 18:2444–2458.

202. Kirkwood JM, Ibrahim JG, Sosman JA, et al. High-dose interferon alfa-2b significantly prolongs relapse-free and overall survival compared with the GM2-KLH/QS-21 vaccine in patients with resected stage IIB-III melanoma: results of intergroup trial. *J Clin Oncol* 2001; 19:2370–2380.

203. Creagan ET, Dalton RJ, Ahmann DL, et al. Randomized, surgical adjuvant clinical trial of recombinant interferon alfa-2a in selected patients with malignant melanoma. *J Clin Oncol* 1995; 13:2776–2783.

204. Pirard D, Heenen M, Melot C, Vereeken P. Interferon alpha as adjuvant postsurgical treatment of melanoma: a meta-analysis. *Dermatology* 2004; 208:43–48.

205. Wheatley K, Ives N, Hancock B, Gore M, Eggermont A, Suciu S. Does adjuvant interferon-alpha for high-risk melanoma provide a worthwhile benefit? A meta-analysis of the randomised trials. *Cancer Treat Res* 2003; 29:241–252.

206. McMasters KM, Noyes RD, Reintgen DS, et al. Lessons learned from the Sunbelt Melanoma Trial. *J Surg Oncol* 2004; 86:212–223.

207. Eggermont AM, Punt CJ. Does adjuvant systemic therapy with interferon-alpha for stage II-III melanoma prolong survival? *Am J Clin Dermatol* 2003; 4:531-536.

208. Legha SS RS, Eton O, Bedikian A, Buzaid AC, Plager C, Papadopoulos N. Development of a biochemotherapy regimen with concurrent administration of cisplatin, vinblastine, dacarbazine, interferon alfa, and interleukin-2 for patients with metastatic melanoma. *J Clin Oncol* 1998; 16:1752–1759.

209. Richards J, Gale D, Mehta N, Lestingi T. Combination of chemotherapy with interleukin-2 and interferon alfa for the treatment of metastatic melanoma. *J Clin Oncol* 1999; 17:651–657.

210. Eton O, Legha SS, Bedikian AY, et al. Sequential biochemotherapy versus chemotherapy for metastatic melanoma: results from a phase III randomized trial. *J Clin Oncol* 2002; 20:2045–2052.

211. Bukowski R, Ernstoff MS, Gore ME, et al. Pegylated interferon alfa-2b treatment for patients with solid tumors: a phase I/II study. *J Clin Oncol* 2002; 20:3841–3849.

212. Chin L, Merlino G, DePinho RA. Malignant melanoma: modern black plague and genetic black box. *Genes Den* 1998; 12:3467–3481.
213. Castellano M, Pollock PM, Walters MK, et al. CDKN2A/p16 is inactivated in most melanoma cell lines. *Cancer Res* 1998; 57:4868–4875.
214. Bastian BC, LeBoit PE, Hamm H, Brocker EB, Pinkel D. Chromosomal gains and losses in primary cutaneous melanomas detected by comparative genomic hybridization. *Cancer Res* 1998; 58:2170–2121.
215. Borden EC. Progress toward therapeutic application of interferons, 1979–1983. *Cancer* 1984; 54:2770–2776.
216. Quesada JR, Hawkins M, Horning S, et al. Collaborative phase I-II study of recombinant DNA-produced leukocyte interferon (clone A) in metastatic breast cancer, malignant lymphoma, and multiple myeloma. *Am J Med* 1984; 77:427–432.
217. Ludwig H, Cortelezzi A, Van Camp BG, et al. Treatment with recombinant interferon-alpha-2C: multiple myeloma and thrombocythaemia in myeloproliferative diseases. *Oncology* 1985; 42:19–25.
218. Quesada J, Hersh EM, Manning J, et al. Treatment of hairy cell leukemia with recombinant alpha interferon. *Blood* 1985; 1986:493–497.
219. Golomb HM, Jacobs A, Fefer A, et al. Alpha-2 interferon therapy of hairy-cell leukemia: a multicenter study of 64 patients. *J Clin Oncol* 1986; 4:900–905.
220. Ratain MJ, Golomb HM, Bardawil RG, et al. Durability of responses to interferon alpha-2b in advanced hairy cell leukemia. *Blood* 1987; 69:872–877.
221. Kantarjian HM, Deisseroth A, Kurzrock R, Estrov Z, Talpaz M. Chronic myelogenous leukemia: a concise update. *Blood* 1993; 82:691–703.
222. Talpaz M. Use of interferon in the treatment of chronic myelogenous leukemia. *Semin Oncol* 1994; 21:3–7.
223. The Italian Cooperative Study Group on Chronic Myeloid Leukemia. Long-term follow-up of the Italian trial of interferon-alpha versus conventional chemotherapy in chronic myeloid leukemia. *Blood* 1998; 92:1541–1548.
224. Guilhot F, Chastang C, Michallet M, et al. Interferon alfa-2b combined with cytarabine versus interferon alone in chronic myelogenous leukemia. French Chronic Myeloid Leukemia Study Group [*see* comments]. *N Engl J Med* 1997; 337:223–229.
225. Hughes TP, Kaeda J, Branford S, et al. Frequency of major molecular responses to imatinib or interferon alfa plus cytarabine in newly diagnosed chronic myeloid leukemia. *N Engl J Med* 2003; 349:1423–1432.
226. Thiesing JT, Ohno-Jones S, Kolibaba KS, Druker BJ. Efficacy of STI571, an abl tyrosine kinase inhibitor, in conjunction with other antileukemic agents against bcr–abl-positive cells. *Blood* 2000; 96:3195–3199.
227. Kano Y, Akutsu M, Tsunoda S, et al. In vitro cytotoxic effects of a tyrosine kinase inhibitor STI571 in combination with commonly used antileukemic agents. *Blood* 2001; 97:1999–2007.
228. Osterborg A, Ahre A, Bjorkholm M, et al. Alternating combination chemotherapy (VCMP/VBAP) is not superior to melphalan/prednisolone in the treatment of multiple myeloma stage III: a randomized study from MGCS. *Eur J Haematol* 1989; 43:54–62.
229. MacLennan ICM, Chapman C, Dunn J, Kelly K. Combined chemotherapy with ABCM versus melphalan for treatment of myelomatosis. *Lancet* 1991; 339:200–205.
230. Conde J, Moro MJ, Alonso C, et al. Alternating combination VCMP/VBAP chemotherapy versus melphalan/prednisolone in the treatment of multiple myeloma: a randomized multicentric study of 487 patients. *J Clin Oncol* 1993; 11:1165–1171.
231. Alexanian R, Haut A, Khan AU, et al. Treatment for multiple myeloma: combination chemotherapy with different melphalan dose regimens. *JAMA* 1969; 208:1680–1685.
232. Gregory WM, Richards MA, Malpas JS. Combination chemotherapy versus melphalan and prednisolone in the treatment of multiple myeloma: an overview of published trials. *J Clin Oncol* 1992; 10:334–342.
233. Mellstedt H, Ahre A, Bjorkholm M, Holm G, Johansson B, Strander H. Interferon therapy in myelomatosis. *Lancet* 1979; 1:245–247.
234. Costanzi JJ, Pollard RB. The use of interferon in the treatment of multiple myeloma. *Semin Oncol* 1987; 14:24–28.
235. Ludwig H, Cortelezzi A, Scheithauer W, et al. Recombinant interferon alpha-2c versus polychemotherapy (VMCP) for treatment of multiple myeloma: a prospective randomized trial. *Eur J Cancer Clin Oncol* 1986; 22:1111–1116.

236. Ahre A, Bjorkholm M, Osterborg A, et al. High doses of natural α-interferon (α-IFN) in the treatment of multiple myeloma. A pilot study from the myeloma group of central Sweden (MCCS). *Eur J Haematol* 1988; 41:123–130.

237. Ahre A, Bjorkholm M, Mellstedt H, et al. Human leukocyte interferon and intermittent high-dose melphalan-prednisone administration in the treatment of multiple myeloma: a randomized clinical trial from the myeloma group of central Sweden (MCCS). *Cancer Treat Rep* 1984; 68:1331–1338.

238. Oken MM, Leong T, Lenhard RE Jr, et al. The addition of interferon or high dose cyclophosphamide to standard chemotherapy in the treatment of patients with multiple myeloma: phase III eastern cooperative oncology group clinical trial EST 9846. *Cancer* 1999; 86:957–988.

239. Mandelli F, Avvisati G, Amadori S, et al. Maintenance treatment with recombinant interferon alfa-2b in patients with multiple myeloma responding to conventional induction chemotherapy. *N Engl J Med* 1990; 322:1430–1434.

240. Drayson MT, Chapman CE, Dunn JA, Olujohungbe AB, MacLennan IC. MRC trial of interferon-alfa 2b maintenance therapy in first plateau phase of multiple myeloma. *Br J Haem* 1998; 101:195–202.

241. Wheatley J. Which myeloma patients benefit from interferon therapy? An overview of 24 randomized trials with 4000 patients. *Br J Haem* 1998; 102:140.

242. Cunningham D, Powles R, Malpas J, et al. A randomized trial of maintenance interferon following high-dose chemotherapy in multiple myeloma: long-term follow-up results. *Br J Haem* 1998; 102:495–502.

243. Attal M, Harousseau JL, Stoppa AM, et al. A prospective randomized trial of autologous bone marrow transplantation and chemotherapy in multiple myeloma. *N Eng J Med* 1996; 335:91–97.

244. Harousseau JL, Attal M, Divine M, et al. Autologous stem cell transplantation after first remission induction treatment in multiple myeloma: a report of the French registry on autologous transplantation in multiple myeloma. *Blood* 1995; 85:3077–3085.

245. Byrne JL, Carter GI, Bienz N, Haynes AP, Russell NH. Adjuvant alpha-interferon improves complete remission rates following allogeneic transplantation for multiple myeloma. *Bone Marrow Transplant* 1998; 22:639–643.

246. Offidani M, Olivieri A, Montillo M, et al. Two dosage interferon-alpha 2b maintenance therapy in patients affected by two low risk multiple myeloma in plateau phase: a randomized trial. *Haematologica* 1998; 83:40–477.

247. Weiss K. Safety profile of interferon-alpha therapy. *Semin Oncol* 1998; 25:9–13.

248. Quesada JR, Talpaz M, Rios A, Kurzrock R, Gutterman JU. Clinical toxicity of interferons in cancer patients: a review. *J Clin Oncol* 1986; 4:234–243.

249. Borden EC, Parkinson D. A perspective on the clinical effectiveness and tolerance of interferon-alpha. *Semin Oncol* 1998; 25:3–8.

250. Kirkwood JM, Bender C, Agarwala S, et al. Mechanism and management of toxicities associated with high-dose interferon alfa-2b therapy. *J Clin Oncol* 2002; 20:3703–3718.

251. Licinio J, Kling MA, Hauser P. Cytokines and brain function: relevance to interferon-alpha-induced mood and cognitive changes. *Semin Oncol* 1998; 25:30–38.

252. Valentine AD, Meyers CA, Kling MA, Richelson E, Hauser P. Mood and cognitive side effects of interferon-alpha therapy. *Semin Oncol* 1998; 25:39–47.

253. Jones TH, Wadler S, Hupart KH. Endocrine-mediated mechanisms of fatigue during treatment with interferon-alpha. *Semin Oncol* 1998; 25:54–63.

254. Plata-Salaman CR. Cytokines and anorexia: a brief overview. *Semin Oncol* 1998; 25:64–72.

255. Musselman DL, Lawson DH, Gumnick JF, et al. Paroxetine for the prevention of depression induced by high-dose interferon alfa. *N Engl J Med* 2001; 344:961–966.

256. Cole BF, Gelber RD, Kirkwood JM, Goldhirsch A, Barylak E, Borden E. Quality-of-life-adjusted survival analysis of interferon alfa-2b adjuvant treatment for high-risk resected cutaneous melanoma: an Eastern Cooperative Oncology Group study (E1684). *J Clin Oncol* 1996; 14:2666–2673.

257. Hillner BE, Kirkwood JM, Atkins MB, Johnson ER, Smith TJ. Economic analysis of adjuvant interferon alfa-2b in high-risk melanoma based on projections from Eastern Cooperative Oncology Group 1684. *J Clin Oncol* 1997; 15:2351–2358.

258. Gotoh A, Hara I, Fujiwawa M, et al. Pharmacokinetics of natural human IFN-α in hemodialysis patients. *J Interferon Cytokine Res* 1999;19:1117–1123.

259. Freund M, von Wussow P, Diedrich H, et al. Recombinant human interferon (IFN) alpha-2b in chronic myelogenous leukaemia: dose dependence of response and frequency of neutralizing anti-interferon antibodies. *Brit J Haem* 1989; 72:350–356.

260. Itri LM, Sherman MI, Palleroni AV, et al. Incidence and clinical significance of neutralizing antibodies in patients receiving recombinant IFN-alpha-2a. *J Interferon Res* 1989; 9:S9–S15.

261. Larocca AP, Leung S, Marcus SG, Coby CB, Borden EC. Evaluation of neutralizing antibodies in patients treated with recombinant interferon-betaser. *J Interferon Res* 1989; 9:S.

262. Bertolotto A, Gilli F, Sala A, et al. Persistent neutralizing antibodies abolish the interferon beta bioavailability in MS patients. *Neurology* 2003; 60:634–639.

263. von Wussow P, Pralle H, Hochkeppel HK, et al. Effective natural interferon-alpha therapy in recombinant interferon-alpha-resistant patients with hairy cell leukemia. *Blood* 1991; 78:38–43.

264. Pestka S. The human interferon-alpha species and hybrid proteins. *Semin Oncol* 1997; 24:S9–4, S9–17.

265. Hawkins MJ, Borden EC, Merritt JA, et al. Comparison of the biologic effects of two recombinant human interferon alpha (rA and rD) in humans. *J Clin Oncol* 1984; 2:221–226.

266. Edwards BS, Hawskins MJ, Borden EC. Comparative in vivo and in vitro activation of human natural killers cells by two recombinant alpha interferons differing in antiviral activity. *Cancer Res* 1984; 44: 3135–3139.

267. Michallet M, Maloisel F, Delain M, et al. Pegylated recombinant interferon alpha-2b vs recombinant interferon alpha-2b for the initial treatment of chronic-phase chronic myelogenous leukemia: a phase III study. *Leukemia* 2004; 18:309–315.

268. Bukowski RM, Tendler C, Cutler D, Rose E, Laughlin MM, Statkevich P. Treating cancer with PEG Intron: pharmacokinetic profile and dosing guidelines for an improved interferon-alpha-2b formulation. *Cancer* 2002; 95:389–396.

269. Ruzicka FJ, Jach ME, Borden EC. Binding of recombinant-produced interferon beta_{ser} to human lymphoblastoid cells: evidence for two binding domains. *J Biol Chem* 1987; 262:16,142–16,149.

270. Hamburger A, White CP, Siebenlist RE, Sedmak JJ. Grossberg SE. Cytotoxicity of human beta interferon for differentiating leukemic HL-60 cells. *Cancer Res* 1985; 45:5369–5373.

271. Borden EC, Hogan TF, Voelkel J. The comparative antiproliferative activity in vitro of natural interferons α and β for diploid and transformed human cells. *Cancer Res* 1982; 42:4948–4953.

272. Schiller JH, Willson JKV, Bittner G, Wolberg WH, Hawkins MJ, Borden EC. Antiproliferative effects of interferons on human melanoma cells in the human tumor colony forming assay. *J Interferon Cytokine Res* 1986; 6:612–625.

273. Kopf J, Hanson C, Delle U, Weimarck A, Stierner U. Action of interferon alpha and beta on four human melanoma cell lines in vitro. *Anticancer Res* 1996; 2:791–798.

274. Nagatani T, Okazawa H, Kambara T, et al. Effect of natural interferon-beta on the growth of melanoma cell lines. *Melanoma Res* 1998; 8:295–299.

275. Chawla-Sarkar M, Bae SI, Reu FJ, Jacobs BS, Lindner DJ, Borden EC. Downregulation of Bcl-2, FLIP or IAPs (XIAP and survivin) by siRNAs sensitizes resistant melanoma cells to Apo2L/TRAIL-induced apoptosis. *Cell Death Differ* 2004; 1:915–923.

276. Johns TG, Mackay IR, Callister KA, Hertzog PJ, Devenish RJ, Linnane AW. Antiproliferative potencies of interferons on melanoma cell lines with xenografts: higher efficacy of interferon beta. *J Natl Cancer Inst* 1991; 84:1185–1190.

277. Gomi K, Morimoto M, Nakamizo N. Antitumor effect of recombinant interferon-beta against human melanomas transplanted into nude mice. *J Pharmacobiodyn* 1984; 12:951–961.

278. McCarthy MG, Bucan CD, Fidler IJ. Melanoma-induced epidermal hyperplasia and increased angiogenesis is mediated by TGF-α through down-regulation of IFN-β. *Cancer Res* 2000; 41:5155–5161.

279. Abdi EA, Tan YH, McPherson TA. Natural human interferon-beta in metastatic melanoma. A phase II study. *Acta Oncol* 1988; 6:815–817.

280. Sarna G, Figlin RA, Percheck M. Phase II study of betaseron (beta ser 17-interferon) as treatment of advanced malignant melanoma. *J Biol Response Mod* 1987; 4:375–378.

281. Borden EC, Rinehart J, Storer BM, Trump DL, Paulnock DM, Teitelbaum AP. Biological and clinical effects of interferon beta_{ser} at two doses. *J Interferon Cytokine Res* 1990; 10:559–570.

282. Hawkins M, Horning S, Konrad M, et al. Phase I evaluation of a synthetic mutant of interferon β. *Cancer Res* 1985; 45:5914–5920.

283. PRISMS Study Group. Randomised double-blind placebo-controlled study of interferon beta-la in relapsing/remitting multiple sclerosis. *Lancet* 1998; 352:1498–1504.

284. Litton G, Hong R, Grossberg SE, Echlekar D, Goodavish CN, Borden EC. Biological and clinical effects of the oral immunomodulator 3,6-bis (2-piperidinoethoxy) acridine trihydrochloride in patients with advance malignancy. *J Biol Resp Mod* 1990; 9:61–70.

285. Cooper CL, Davis HL, Morris ML, et al. Safety and immunogenicity of CPG 7909 injection as an adjuvant to Fluarix influenza vaccine. *Vaccine* 2004; 22:3136–3143.
286. Wooldridge JE, Weiner GJ. CpG DNA and cancer immunotherapy: orchestrating the antitumor immune response. *Curr Opin Oncol* 2003; 15:440–445.
287. Whitmore MM, DeVeer MJ, Edling A, et al. Synergistic activation of innate immunity by double-stranded RNA and CpG DNA promotes enhanced antitumor activity. *Cancer Res* 2004; 64:5850–5860.
288. Lonsdorf AS, Kuekrek H, Stern BV, Boehm BO, Lehmann PV, Tary-Lehmann M. Intratumor CpG-oligodeoxynucleotide injection induces protective antitumor T cell immunity. *J Immunol* 2003; 171: 3941–3946.
289. Krieg AM. CpG motifs in bacterial DNA and their immune effects. *Annu Rev Immunol* 2002; 20:709–760.

22 Promising γ-Chain Cytokines for Cancer Immunotherapy

Interleukins-7, -15, and -21 as Vaccine Adjuvants, Growth Factors, and Immunorestoratives

Terry J. Fry and Crystal L. Mackall

SUMMARY

The molecular identification of a plethora of T-cell tumor antigens that can serve as targets for many human cancers, and the clinical development of techniques to administer tumor vaccines represent important advances toward the development of T-cell-specific immunotherapy for cancer. Despite this progress, current clinical results demonstrate that tumor vaccines, as single agents, are generally not potent enough to induce regression of existing tumors or long lasting enough to provide durable adjuvant benefit. Similarly, the full effectiveness of adoptive cellular therapies for cancer immunotherapy has not yet been realized because of difficulties in sustaining T-cells in vivo following adoptive transfer. Thus, the present challenge for the field of tumor immunology is to develop clinically applicable approaches for amplifying the T-cell-specific immunity induced by tumor vaccines and for augmenting survival of cells delivered in the context of adoptive therapies. The family of cytokines that signals through the common cytokine γ-chain (γ_c) demonstrates potent effects on T-cell development, expansion, and viability. Interleukin (IL)-2, a prototypic member of this family, has already demonstrated antitumor effects in some settings. However, recent studies have demonstrated that other members of the γ_c cytokine family possess characteristics that render them more favorable than IL-2 for amplifying T-cell-specific immunity toward tumors. IL-7, IL-15, and IL-21 have all shown promise in preclinical models of tumor immunotherapy. IL-7 is notable for its capacity to serve as an immunorestorative agent, as well as its ability to augment both CD4 and CD8 immune responses, with a particular capacity to amplify low-affinity, subdominant immune responses that are characteristically induced by tumor antigens. IL-15 provides potent survival and differentiation signals to both CD8 memory cells and natural-killer cells, features that are likely to be translatable in the context of both tumor vaccines and adoptive immunotherapy. IL-21 is less well studied than IL-7 or IL-15, but appears able to amplify responses to other cytokines, especially IL-15, thus further augmenting effector and memory cell expansion. Thus, a large amount of preclinical data suggest that integration of one or several new γ_c cytokines into immunotherapy regimens for cancer will play an important role in moving this field closer to clinical efficacy.

Key Words: IL-7; IL-15; IL-21; γ_c cytokines; T-cell homeostasis; adoptive immunotherapy; tumor vaccines; vaccine adjuvants.

From: *Cancer Drug Discovery and Development: Immunotherapy of Cancer*
Edited by: M. L. Disis © Humana Press Inc., Totowa, NJ

1. INTRODUCTION

Despite limited clinical success to date, there is continued optimism regarding the prospect of developing effective immunotherapy for cancer. This stems from advances at the basic science level, which have improved understanding of T-cell biology, and technological advances, which have provided new tools for clinical application. The insights into T-cell biology that pave the way for more effective cancer immunotherapy run the gamut from identification of a multitude of new tumor antigens to a better of understanding of T-cell co-stimulatory molecules and mechanisms of immune tolerance, to a more complete understanding of the factors that serve to maintain and/or disrupt T-cell homeostasis. The theoretical implications from all of this work continue to suggest that effective immunotherapy for cancer remains a realistic goal. However, despite the remarkable progress in bench research, major challenges remain in translating these tremendous insights to the clinic. New therapies must undergo stepwise preclinical development and iterative clinical testing to create regimens that can induce antitumor immunity that is potent and long lasting enough to clear established tumors and/or prevent tumor recurrence and specific enough to avoid autoimmunity.

Numerous clinical trials of tumor vaccines have demonstrated that measurable immune responses to a wide array of T-cell tumor antigens can be induced in most cancer patients, and that many different vaccine strategies, including genetic vectors, peptides, and dendritic cells (DCs), are effective at inducing measurable immune responses. Despite this progress, no tumor vaccine developed thus far has proved potent enough to reproducibly shrink established tumors and, whereas effectiveness in the adjuvant setting may ultimately be shown in some trials, it currently remains unproven. Thus, the consensus from these early trials is that tumor vaccines, as single agents, are unlikely to generate the robust immune responses required for immunotherapy of cancer (1). The next decade of work in tumor immunotherapy will seek to move beyond tumor antigen identification and testing of vaccines as single agents to the development of multimodality approaches that augment the strength and modulate the character of the immune responses induced by vaccination.

Cytokines are among the most promising agents available for potentiating weak immune responses induced by current tumor vaccines. As presented in Table 1, several cytokines are already approved for treatment in cancer patients, but most are aimed at improving supportive care and do not potentiate immunity *per se*. Interleukin (IL)-2 and interferon (IFN)-α2b are immunomodulatory cytokines with antitumor activity when used as single agents, but they are not active in the vast majority of cancer types, and the response rate to these agents remains low even in sensitive histologies. Further, whereas IL-2 can potentiate immune responses in some settings, a sizable body of evidence has demonstrated that, when compared with other cytokines in the same class, IL-2 is not especially well suited for enhancing T-cell immunity, because it predisposes to immune cell death and contributes to the induction of regulatory T-cells (2,3). Thus, the field of tumor immunology is awaiting anxiously the clinical availability of several new cytokines whose activity in preclinical models suggests that they will enhance immune responses toward tumor antigens. This chapter focuses on three cytokines currently under study that show promise for augmenting the effectiveness of T-cell and natural-killer (NK) cell-based immunotherapy for cancer: IL-7, IL-15, and IL-21. Like IL-2, signaling of each of these involves the common cytokine signaling γ-chain (γ_c) (Fig. 1), but as described in this chapter, each has unique properties that could be exploited in the context of cancer immunotherapy. We review basic biological properties of each agent and discuss the potential

Table 1
Cytokines in Cancer Therapy

	Primary activity	*Other potential uses*
FDA-approved		
GM-CSF	Ameliorates myelosuppression	Vaccine adjuvant
G-CSF/pegylated G-CSF	Ameliorates myelosuppression	Stem cell mobilization
Erythropoietin	Ameliorates anemia	
IL-11	Ameliorates thrombocytopenia	
KGF	Ameliorates mucositis after BMT	Thymic protection
IL-2	Antitumor activity: renal cell carcinoma, malignant melanoma	
IFN-α2b	Antitumor activity: renal cell carcinoma, malignant melanoma, hairy cell leukemia, chronic myelogenous leukemia	
In clinical trials		
TPO (c-Mpl ligand, MGDF)	Amelioration of thrombocytopenia	
IL-12	Antiangiogenic and antitumor effects when combined with IL-2	Vaccine adjuvant
Flt3 ligand	Dendritic cell expansion	Immunorestorative
IL-7	Immunorestorative	Vaccine adjuvant, adoptive therapy
Promise in preclinical studies		
IL-15	Vaccine adjuvant	Immunorestorative, adoptive therapy
IL-18	Antitumor effects when combined with IL-2, IL-12	Vaccine adjuvant
IL-21	Vaccine adjuvant, adoptive therapy	

FDA, Food and Drug Administration; GM-CSF, granulocyte-macrophage colony-stimulating factor; IL, interleukin; KGF, keratinocyte growth factor; BMT, bone marrow transplant; IFN, interferon; TPO, thrombopoietin; MGDF, megakaryocyte growth and development factor; Flt3, Fms-related tyrosine kinase 3 ligand.

for each to serve as a vaccine adjuvant, a growth factor in the context of adoptive immunotherapy, and/or an immunorestorative.

2. CYTOKINE BIOLOGY

2.1. Interleukin 7

2.1.1. IL-7 BIOLOGY

IL-7 was identified as a marrow stromal cell-derived growth factor that induced proliferation of developing B-cells. Subsequently, its critical and nonredundant role in lymphopoiesis established it as the quintessential lymphopoietic cytokine. IL-7 is necessary for T-cell development in both humans and mice, and although it is not necessary for B-cell development in humans, it likely plays an important role in human B-cell lymphopoiesis. IL-7 does not play a role in NK cell development. IL-7 exerts lymphopoietic effects

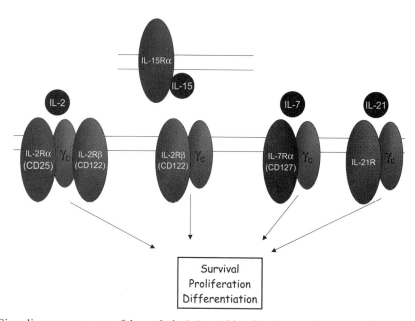

Fig. 1. Signaling components of the γ-chain (γ$_c$) cytokine family members currently under investigation for immunotherapy of cancer. The requisite components of the high-affinity interleukin (IL)-2 signaling complex are γ$_c$, shared with all members of this group; IL-2Rβ, shared with IL-15; and IL-2Rα, also known as CD25. Interaction between soluble IL-2 and this complex results in activation of a number of intracellular signaling molecules including Janus kinase/signal transduction activating transcription family members. IL-15 shares IL-2Rβ and γ$_c$ with IL-2, but is most commonly supplied as a cell associated cytokine, a feature that is unique amongst the γ$_c$ family. IL-7 signals through a γ$_c$ and IL-7Rα, which is shared with thymic stromal lymphopoietin but is not a member of the γ$_c$ family, as this chain is not involved in thymic stromal lymphopoietin signaling. IL-21 utilizes γ$_c$ in combination with the IL-21R chain, which is homologous to the IL-2Rβ chain. Other members of this family (IL-4 and IL-9) are not shown because they are not currently under investigation as therapeutic agents for cancer immunotherapy.

through multiple mechanisms including trophic effects mediated by modulation effects of B-cell leukemia 2 family members, proliferation of early thymocytes and developing B-cells, and direct modulation of T-cell receptor rearrangement. Importantly, IL-7 responsiveness during lymphoid development is tightly regulated in both B-cells and T-cells such that alterations in IL-7 availability or in IL-7 receptor expression can either increase or paradoxically diminish thymopoiesis, depending on the exact cell populations involved (reviewed in ref. *4*). In addition to the important role for IL-7 as a lymphopoietic cytokine, recent work has also shed light on critical roles for IL-7 in peripheral T-cell homeostasis (discussed in Subheading 2.1.2.).

The designation of IL-7 as an interleukin is a misnomer because it is generally not produced by white blood cells, but rather by stromal and parenchymal cells throughout the body including thymic epithelium and stromal cells in bone marrow, lymph nodes, spleen, and epithelial cells in the gut and nonlymphoid organs. Whereas some DCs and malignant B-cells have been reported to produce IL-7, marrow-derived populations contribute little to IL-7 production overall. IL-7 signals through a heterodimer comprised of γ$_c$ and IL-7Rα to induce an intracellular signaling cascade, that involves Janus kinase 1, Janus kinase 3, signal transduction activating transcription 5 and phosphoinositide-3 kinase activation.

Unlike receptors for most γ_c cytokines, which are not expressed on resting cells but are upregulated on activation, the IL-7R heterodimer is expressed on most resting lymphocytes, is downregulated following T-cell activation, then reexpressed on memory cell populations. Because IL-7 is produced by nonimmune cells in the absence of immune activation, is measurable in serum in healthy conditions, and because the IL-7R heterodimer is expressed on the vast majority of lymphocytes, IL-7 can be best conceptualized as a homeostatic cytokine whose signals are continuously available and play an important role in maintaining lymphocyte homeostasis.

2.1.2. IL-7 Is a Critical Modulator of Peripheral T-Cell Homeostasis

Thymopoiesis is critical for initial seeding of the peripheral T-cell pool and plays an important role in restoring T-cell populations following profound lymphocyte depletion. However, in the absence of a profound T-cell depleting event, peripheral T-cell populations are maintained throughout life through trophic signals supplied by major histocompatibility complex (MHC) and IL-7 for naïve cells and by IL-15 (independent of MHC) for memory CD8 cells (discussed in Subheading 2.2.1.) (5–7). Critical signals for maintenance of memory CD4 cells continue to be elucidated, but likely involve both MHC and IL-7 (8). In healthy hosts, cycling of naïve cells is infrequent, whereas cycling of memory cells is more significant, and together these processes serve to maintain, rather than expand, T-cell numbers. Importantly, however, T-cell cycling becomes exaggerated and modified in lymphopenic hosts, giving rise to an entity termed "homeostatic peripheral expansion" (HPE). HPE dramatically augments T-cell numbers and therefore serves as a primary pathway for immune reconstitution following T-cell depletion. The existence of HPE has been appreciated for more than 20 yr (9), but interest in HPE has blossomed recently because of new insights into its biology, and the prospect that exploiting HPE may prove effective in augmenting immune responses to cancer. HPE is composed of three distinct components: exaggerated responses to cognate antigen (10), exaggerated antigen-independent cycling of memory populations, and the induction of proliferative responses to low-affinity antigens that comprise both self-antigens and crossreactive environmental antigens (11–13). CD4+ lymphopenia in humans is associated with reciprocal rises in circulating IL-7 (14–16), and IL-7 plays a critical role in HPE because it is sufficient to sustain the exaggerated cycling of CD8+ memory cells (17,18) and is required absolutely for the proliferative responses of naïve cells to low-affinity antigen seen in this setting (19,20). Furthermore, as we discuss in more detail, supraphysiological levels of IL-7 augment responses to cognate antigen (21). Therefore, IL-7 appears to play a critical role in modulating the process termed HPE that serves to augment immune responses in lymphopenic hosts.

2.2. Interleukin 15

2.2.1. IL-15 Functions Largely as a Cell-Associated Cytokine

IL-15 was initially identified as a non-IL-2 growth factor that signaled through IL-2Rβ and γ_c (22–24). It is now appreciated that IL-15 has structural similarities to IL-2, but very distinct biological properties (2,25,26). Unlike IL-2, which is produced solely by activated T-cells, IL-15 is produced by many cell types, both bone marrow-derived and epithelial (27,28). At face value, IL-15 signaling in T-cells and NK cells appears to be similar to IL-2, because it signals through a trimeric receptor complex composed of γ_c chain, IL-2/IL-15Rβ, and a unique IL-15-specific receptor called IL-15Rα. Furthermore, like IL-2, IL-15 can bind and signal through the IL-2/IL-15βγ dimer, although it does so with a reduced affinity when compared with trimer binding. However, this description belies the true complexity of the biology, because unlike the IL-2 trimeric receptor complex (which is readily found on activated, IL-2-responsive T-cells), the IL-15 trimeric receptor complex is not present on most T- and NK cells that respond to IL-15. Furthermore, although mRNA for IL-15 is prevalent throughout the body (28), the protein itself is typically not found in normal body fluids or in the supernatant of activated lymphoid populations. These characteristics of IL-15 biology can now be explained by a model that holds that IL-15 largely functions as a cell-associated cytokine where it binds to IL-15Rα-expressing cells, which are represented by activated monocytes (29–32) and DCs (33). Recent evidence has also demonstrated that this process is most efficient if IL-15 is presented by the same cells in which it is produced (34). Therefore, IL-15 signaling most commonly proceeds from a cell-associated IL-15/IL-15Rα complex that signals T-cells or NK cells bearing the IL-2/IL-15βγ heterodimer. As activated and memory CD8 cells express high levels of IL-2/IL-15β, whereas resting CD8 cells do not, it is not surprising that IL-15 acts primarily on memory CD8 cells. Although this model appears to be the rule for IL-15 signaling, exceptions and unresolved questions remain. For instance, recent work demonstrated that trimeric IL-15 receptors might be biologically relevant, because during the evolution of a primary response to cognate antigen, a select few CD8[+] cells express the trimeric IL-15R complex, rendering these cells at a competitive advantage for IL-15 signaling that contributed to avidity maturation of the memory cell pool (35). In another model, IL-15 presentation "in trans" by colon carcinoma cells engineered to express IL-15Rα resulted in the induction of NK cell activity that improved immune surveillance (36), demonstrating that cell populations other than monocytes and DCs can present bioactive IL-15. Furthermore, although activated CD4 cells express IL-2/IL-15βγ, IL-15 signaling is significantly reduced in CD4 cells compared with CD8 cells, implying that other poorly understood elements contribute to IL-15 sensitivity. Finally, IL-15 can also signal mast cells through a receptor complex independent of IL-2/IL-15βγ that involves a unique receptor termed IL-15X (28). Despite these exceptions, it appears that IL-15 most prominently functions as a cytokine that is presented in trans by antigen-presenting cells to activated CD8[+] cells.

2.2.2. IL-15 Plays a Primary Role in CD8[+] Memory and NK Cell Homeostasis

As we have described, maintenance of memory cell populations in normal hosts involves antigen-independent cycling throughout life. In studies of T-cell-replete mice rendered IL-15 deficient, CD8[+] memory cells (but not CD4[+] memory cells) are essentially absent, a result that identifies IL-15 as a nonredundant factor for maintenance of CD8 memory cells in normal hosts (17,18). This absolute requirement for IL-15 for survival of memory T-cell populations, however, should not be confused with a requirement for IL-15 in the generation of memory cells. In fact, IL-15-deficient animals challenged with viral infections can readily clear the infection and generate a similar effector pool to normal mice (37). Rather, the critical role for IL-15 in memory cell homeostasis is at the level of maintenance of the memory pool (37), where it provides critical signals for both survival and cycling of CD8[+] memory cells (38,39). Although IL-7 cannot substitute for IL-15 in this regard in normal T-cell replete hosts, IL-7 can substitute for IL-15 in lymphopenic hosts where elevated IL-7 levels occur (40) or when IL-7 is overexpressed in T-cell-replete hosts (17). Thus, whereas basal levels of IL-7 are not sufficient to substitute for IL-15 in memory cell maintenance, supraphysiological levels can provide this effect.

IL-15 also plays critical roles in the development and maintenance of NK cells. Animals lacking IL-15 are nearly devoid of NK cells, and lack of IL-15 signaling is the cause for NK deficiency in humans lacking the γ_c receptor. In addition to an essential role in NK development, IL-15 also serves to maintain mature NK cell populations, because adoptively transferred NK cells do not survive in the absence of IL-15 signaling. Unlike memory CD8+ cells, wherein cycling is a critical component of population maintenance, mature NK cells have a relatively low cycling rate and proliferative potential. It is therefore not surprising that the primary effects of IL-15 in maintaining peripheral NK cell homeostasis is on prevention of programmed cell death as indicated by the fact that survival of NK cells in the absence of IL-15 can be rescued by constitutive expression of B-cell leukemia 2 *(41,42)*. Finally, IL-15 also is necessary for normal homeostasis of NK T-cells *(43)*. Thus, in normal hosts, basal levels of IL-15 play a central role in both NK development and maintenance and in maintenance of CD8+ memory T-cells and NK T-cells.

2.3. Interleukin 21

2.3.1. IL-21 Basic Biology

IL-21 is a new member of the γ_c cytokine family initially described in 2000 *(44,45)*. It is most homologous to IL-15, but also shares significant homology to IL-2 and IL-4. The gene for human IL-21 is located near the IL-2 and IL-15 genes on chromosome 4 *(46)*. Initial reports described signaling through a chimeric homodimer, but it is now clear that the physiological receptor for IL-21 is composed of a unique subunit designated IL-21R and γ_c *(47,48)*. IL-21R is most homologous to IL-2Rβ and IL-4Rβ, and is found on B-cells, CD4+ and CD8+ T-cells, and NK cells. Thus, the IL-21R complex is expressed on most mature lymphocyte populations. In contrast, production of IL-21 is restricted to activated CD4+ T-cells, preferentially T-helper (Th)2 cells *(49,50)*. In fact, similar transcription factors that control expression of the Th2 cytokines IL4, IL-5, and IL-13 also tightly control expression of IL-21. Thus, the evidence that IL-21 receptor is widely expressed on lymphocytes, but IL-21 production is restricted to activated CD4+ cells under the direction of Th2-type transcription factors leads to the conclusion that regulation of IL-21 signaling occurs at the level of cytokine availability.

As a recently identified cytokine, exact roles for IL-21 in immunity are still emerging. In general, IL-21 appears to play an important role in modulating responses of T-cells, NK cells, and B-cells to other cytokines and bridging adaptive and innate immunity, especially in the effector phase of the immune response. Importantly, the effects of IL-21 appears critically dependent on the context in which signaling occurs with both immune-enhancing and -limiting effects reported in different settings. IL-21 plays an important role in NK cell biology, enhancing the generation of human NK cells from CD34+ hematopoietic progenitors incubated with IL-15 and Fms-related tyrosine kinase 3 ligand *(46)*. In murine systems, the role for IL-21 in NK cell development has been less clear. On the one hand, mice lacking the γ_c have more severe defects in NK cells *(51)* than IL-15-deficient mice *(52)*, an effect that has been potentially attributed to loss of IL-21 signaling. However, there is no decrement in NK cell numbers in IL-21-deficient mice *(53)*. These data can be reconciled by the recent finding that, in both human and murine systems, IL-21 plays a complimentary role in NK cell development, contributing to the generation of a functional, mature NK profile in the presence of other cytokines, especially IL-15 *(54, 55)*. Similar complimentary effects of IL-21 are seen on mature NK cells, where IL-21 alone does not support growth and maintenance of NK cells, and in fact, has been shown to limit expansion and induce apoptosis of mature NK cells (53,56). However, in vitro exposure of NK cells to IL-21 with IL-2 or IL-15 or high levels of IL-21 in vivo enhances NK effector function. Thus, the dual effects of IL-21 on mature NK cells may serve to both amplify immunity early in an immune response, as well as playing a regulatory role by eventually downregulating responses in the later phases.

The effects of IL-21 on T-cell populations appear similarly complex, and as with NK cells, involve potentiation of effects mediated by other signals. IL-21 alone does not induce proliferation of T-cell populations; however proliferation of T-cells induced by other γ_c cytokines (especially IL-15 and to a lesser extent, IL-2 and IL-7), anti-CD3, or antigen is substantially enhanced in the presence of IL-21 (46,53,57,58). Although CD4 T-cells express IL-21R, the proliferative effects of IL-21 are most pronounced on the CD8 subset. With regard to CD4 populations, evidence that CD4 T-cells that have differentiated toward a Th2 functional profile preferentially secrete IL-21, and data showing that IL-21 inhibits differentiation of T helper precursor 1 cells into IFN-γ-producing Th1 cells could implicate IL-21 as a Th2-polarizing cytokine. However, in other reports, IL-21 actually induced expression of Th1-associated genes and IFN-γ production by T-cells (59,60), and IL-21 does not inhibit IFN-γ production by already differentiated Th1 cells (49). Thus, IL-21 likely does not conform to the standard Th1/Th2 paradigm. Finally, although IL-21's immunostimulatory effects on T-cells and NK cells suggest that this cytokine may prove useful for augmenting responses to tumor antigens, the maturation and activation of DC populations may be inhibited by IL-21, a feature that needs to be studied more carefully if IL-21 is to be used in the context of tumor vaccines.

As with T-cells and NK cells, the affect of IL-21 on mature B-cells depends on the nature of other signals provided. Proliferation of mature B-cells in response to anti-CD40 is enhanced by IL-21, but anti-immunoglobulin (Ig)M- and IL-4-mediated proliferation is inhibited (46), and IL-21 may induce apoptosis of resting and activated B-cells following these stimuli (61). Furthermore, mice deficient in IL-21 demonstrate increased IgE production and decreased IgG1 production in response to immunization (53,62,63). Thus, rather than being entirely a positive regulator of B-cell responses, IL-21 may be best conceptualized as a modulator of the B-cell responses with preferential enhancement of T-cell-dependent B-cell responses (64).

3. IL-7, IL-15, AND/OR IL-21 AS VACCINE ADJUVANTS

Although animals deficient in γ_c cytokines can generate effector cells in response to antigen, signaling by IL-7 and IL-15 plays important roles in the generation and maintenance of memory cell populations (65–69). Furthermore, because both IL-7 and IL-15 can co-stimulate for T-cell activation and provide potent survival signals for T-cells (5, 70,71), it is not surprising that supraphysiological doses of these agents can enhance the response to cognate antigen. IL-15 has been most well studied in this regard, with several studies demonstrating that IL-15 can increase the size of the effector and memory pool generated in response to infection or immunization (3,21,72–74). For instance, IL-15 enhances CD8+ T-cell immunity in mice infected with *Toxoplasma gondii* (74), IL-15 transgenic mice generate higher numbers of effectors following infection with *Listeria monocytogenes* (72), and therapy with either IL-7 or IL-15 improves survival of *Mycobacterium tuberculosis*-infected mice (73). Thus, IL-15 clearly enhances the immune response generated to intracellular pathogens, leading to increased eradication in the short term. Although augmentation of NK cell expansion and survival may contribute to these outcomes, some component of the effects are T-cell-mediated, because many studies have demonstrated that increased numbers of CD8$^+$ T-cell effectors are generated in response to infection or immunization when supraphysiological levels of IL-15 are available. Indeed, IL-15 therapy enhanced T-cell responses to DNA vaccines *(3,75)* and DC vaccines in mice *(21,76)* and to influenza and tetanus vaccines in rhesus macaques *(77)*. Remarkably, in three of these studies, IL-15 was directly compared with IL-2 as a vaccine adjuvant and in all studies, IL-15 proved to be superior *(3,21,77)*. Thus, it appears clear that IL-15 is superior to IL-2 as a vaccine adjuvant, although some synergistic effects were observed when the two agents were used together in a pleural tumor model *(78)* and in a melanoma model *(79)*.

In one study, evaluation of IL-15's relative effects on immunodominant and subdominant antigens demonstrated that IL-15 more potently augmented response to subdominant antigens when compared with dominant antigens, thus minimizing the effects of immunodominance hierarchies among antigens *(21)*. This is particularly pertinent for tumor antigens, which are generally weak antigens, and which may be better modeled by subdominant antigens. In addition to potent effects on the T-cell effector pool, two studies undertook careful analysis of IL-15's effects on the long-lived memory pool. In both, treatment with rhIL-15 at the time of immunization led to durable increases in the survival of the memory pool, an effect that remained long after the therapeutic levels IL-15 had cleared *(3, 21)*.

Although IL-7 is less well studied as an immune adjuvant, the available data demonstrate that it is also clearly capable of augmenting T-cell responses to cognate antigen, and therefore serving as a potential vaccine adjuvant. This was demonstrated in the *M. tuberculosis* model noted earlier *(73)*, as well as in a dendritic cell vaccine-based model *(21)*. Here, IL-7 was directly compared with IL-2 and IL-15 in terms of the quantity and quality of the effects induced. Both IL-7 and IL-15 augmented immunodominant CD8 responses to a similar degree; however, IL-7 had more-potent effects on CD4 effectors and more potently augmented the weak subdominant antigen, consistent with its known capacity to enhance responses to low affinity/weak antigens during homeostatic peripheral expansion. Similar to IL-15, IL-7 was significantly more effective than IL-2 overall, and provided even greater protection than IL-15 when animals were challenged with tumors bearing the immunizing antigens late following vaccination *(21)*. Furthermore, like IL-15, IL-7 therapy provided as a short course during vaccination provided long-term benefits for memory cell survival, which persisted long after the cytokines were discontinued. Thus, although limited data are available regarding IL-7's capacity to serve as an immune adjuvant, available data demonstrate that IL-7 is promising in this regard. IL-7's effects may be particularly important for targeting tumor antigens, which tend to have low-affinity interactions with T-cell receptors, which represent the type of antigenic responses that IL-7 is well poised to augment.

Although IL-21 is a more recently identified cytokine, there have been a number of studies to suggest that it as an attractive candidate as an adjuvant to immune-based therapies. In a number models of murine tumors genetically modified to secrete IL-21, improved outcome was observed *(80,81)*. As predicted by the understanding of the basic biology of IL-21, both CD8 and NK cell populations are critical for this effect. Interestingly, the presence of IL-21 at the tumor site also appears to recruit innate inflammatory cells, such as granulocytes, that also contribute to the response. Using a different approach, other investigators have utilized IL-21 plasmid injection to generate systemic levels of IL-21 not derived from the tumor. In one report using the B16 melanoma and the MCA205 fibrosarcoma, administration of an IL-21 plasmid alone resulted in improved tumor regression when compared with mice not receiving the cytokine plasmid (56). This effect was dependent on the presence of NK cells, with only a minimal contribution of CD8 T-cells. In a metastatic lymphoma model, gene transfer of IL-15 resulted in less metastatic foci but not in improved survival. However, the inclusion of an IL-21 plasmid resulted in regression of established tumors with survival in 60% of the mice (82). In this model, the combination of these cytokines resulted in enhanced NK and cytotoxic T-lymphocyte function, whereas IL-15 alone predominantly affected NK cell activity. Thus, the data available would strongly support the use of IL-21 as an adjuvant to tumor immunotherapy, in particular, when used in combination with other cytokines.

4. GROWTH FACTORS FOR ADOPTIVE IMMUNOTHERAPY

Advances in cell processing techniques, largely generated through clinical progress in bone marrow transplantation, have made the culture and expansion of large numbers of lymphocytes ex vivo now clinically feasible. However, two major hurdles remain before adoptive immunotherapy can fulfill its promise. First, the optimal conditions for growing lymphocytes and/or NK cells ex vivo need to be identified, and new therapies need to be developed that can enhance the viability of adoptively transferred cells in vivo following infusion. The capacity for IL-7, IL-15, and IL-21 to provide growth and survival signals to activated effector cells and to modulate effector cell differentiation suggests that the use of one or more of these agents during the ex vivo expansion phase or following adoptive cell infusion may improve the effectiveness of adoptively transferred cells.

A critical component of both IL-7 and IL-15's effects on lymphocytes is their capacity to serve as a "trophic" factor for mature T-cells via the inhibition of programmed cell death. Indeed, the addition of IL-7 to ex vivo lymphocyte cultures of expanding T-cell lines or clones improves cell yields (83,84), and IL-7 therapy provided to mice following adoptive transfer of human T-cells in a severe combined immunodeficiency mice with human skin grafts, peripheral blood leukocyte murine model improved the outcome following implantation of a colon carcinoma xenograft (85). Furthermore, recent studies demonstrating improved outcomes in both mice (86) and humans (87) following administration of T-cells to lymphopenic hosts when compared with the results of similar infusions in T-cell-replete hosts, indirectly implicate IL-7 in augmenting the efficacy of adoptive cell therapy, because elevated IL-7 levels are a key feature of the lymphopenic environment, where they play a critical role in augmenting T-cell proliferation.

IL-15 has also demonstrated promising effects in adoptive cell therapy models for cancer. For instance, antigen-primed effector cells cultured in the presence of IL-15 ex vivo were more potent than cells cultured in the absence of cytokines and were also more potent than cells culture with IL-2 in inducing regression of established tumors in a the murine *pmel* model (88). The authors hypothesized that the improved effectiveness of IL-15 in this setting was because of its capacity to differentiate fully effector cells into central memory populations, which appear to have more favorable survival and proliferative characteristics when compared with effector memory cells that were generated in the IL-2-based cultures. Similarly, in studies of tumor-reactive CD8[+] T-cells found in tumor draining lymph nodes, ex vivo culture of these cells with IL-15 led to further differentiation toward a central memory phenotype, directly implicating IL-15 in this process (89). Similar results have been observed using gene transduction of IL-15 into the adoptively transferred T-cells (90). Therefore, preclinical models using both IL-7 and IL-15 have demonstrated that either cytokine expands an effector T-cell population ex vivo that shows enhanced effectiveness against tumor following in vivo transfer when compared with effector cells generated in the absence of cytokines or in IL-2.

In addition to the potential use of IL-15 as a component of ex vivo culture conditions, the evidence that IL-15 therapy dramatically expands memory cells in vivo suggest that IL-15 administration therapy undertaken following adoptive transfer of activated effector cells is a promising therapeutic approach (21,91). Indeed, in the *pmel* experimental model wherein adoptive transfer of tumor antigen-primed T-cells was assessed for its capacity to eradicate established tumors, IL-15 therapy administered following the adoptive transfer of tumor-reactive CD8+ T-cells improved tumor regression (88). Using this same model, the combination of IL-21 with IL-15 substantially improved the response (57). In addition, IL-21 administered at 20 μg/d following injection of thymoma cells transfected with ovalbumin peptide and cotransfer of transgenic tumor reactive T-cells resulted in tumor regression and durable immunity (92). In this study, IL-21 was superior to IL-2 and IL-15 as an adjuvant to adoptive therapy at the doses used. Furthermore, IL-15 was superior to IL-2 in its ability to inhibit tumor growth in the *pmel* model (93), and expansion and cytotoxic function of lymphokine-activated killer cells expanded ex vivo was improved in the presence of IL-15 compared with IL-2 (94). Thus, preclinical studies provide compelling evidence for the potential of IL-15, IL-7, and IL-21 as a means to augment adoptive immunotherapy of T-cells.

NK cells are less proliferative than T-cells; however, recent work suggests that substantial numbers of NK cells for use in adoptive therapy may be generated either from bone marrow populations or from mature NK cells. As IL-15 is a growth and survival factor for both developing and mature NK cells, one would predict that combining IL-15 with NK cell-based therapies might improve outcome. Unlike the evidence that IL-15 is superior to IL-2 for the ex vivo expansion of T-cells, however, it remains unclear whether IL-2 or IL-15 is more potent at augmenting NK cell survival and/or expansion. Furthermore, IL-21 can also augment the generation and cytolytic potential of both murine and human NK cells from progenitors, especially in the presence of other cytokines, such as IL-2 and IL-15 (54,55). Thus, it is clear that IL-2, IL-15, and IL-21 all have substantial effects on NK cells, and it is likely that some combination of these factors will allow more optimal ex vivo expansion and in vivo survival of adoptively transferred NK cells; however, no clearly superior agent or combination has emerged thus far.

5. PROMISING IMMUNORESTORATIVES

The prospect of immunotherapy as a stand-alone treatment for cancer is intellectually attractive, but the evidence from murine models clearly demonstrates that immunotherapy is most effective when used in the setting of low tumor burdens. For many cancers that are under consideration for immunotherapy today, standard regimens that involve cytotoxic chemotherapy with or without radiation therapy induce substantial reductions in tumor burden, with recurrence being the major obstacle. Therefore, it is likely that immunotherapy will ultimately find its most useful application as an adjuvant to other treatment modalities for cancer. Furthermore, the emerging data demonstrating that lymphopenic hosts may be uniquely poised to generate more-potent responses to weak antigens than T-cell-replete hosts provides a further basis for the notion that integrating immunotherapy into existing standard cancer regimens may hold added promise. In this regard, the use of a cytokine capable of augmenting recovery of the immune system following immune-depleting therapy is particularly attractive.

IL-7 is a potent immunorestorative cytokine that improves the rate of recovery of T-cell populations following lymphodepletion. Although it was initially assumed that the primary effects of IL-7 on immune reconstitution would result from augmentation of thymopoiesis, it now appears that IL-7's immunorestorative effects occur mostly because of its ability to augment HPE. Indeed, when IL-7 is administered to normal, nonhuman primates, the percent of cycling cells in the blood increases dramatically (95), with the most profound changes in the naïve subset (96), indicating that IL-7 therapy itself can, to some extent, replicate the physiology responsible for HPE seen in lymphopenic hosts. Furthermore, despite the presumed physiological increase in IL-7 that occurs during T-cell depletion, treatment of both lymphopenic mice and lymphopenic primates with pharmacological doses of IL-7 results in more-rapid recovery of T-cell populations, suggesting that pharmacological doses of IL-7 administered to lymphopenic patients will result in added benefit, despite physiological elevations of IL-7 in this setting. Therefore, IL-7 is currently under development as an immunorestorative cytokine that is not only expected to augment specific immune responses as already described, but to also improve dramatically overall immune competence of lymphopenic hosts through a more rapid recovery of lymphocyte numbers. Importantly, it should be noted that although true increases in thymopoiesis induced by IL-7 are difficult to demonstrate, IL-7 can readily induce expansion of recent thymic emigrants that would be expected to actually diversify the available peripheral T-cell repertoire of lymphopenic hosts. Thus, one would predict that the administration of tumor vaccines under the influence of IL-7 in patients rendered lymphopenic by chemotherapy would lead to dramatic expansions of tumor-reactive T-cells as a result of the propensity for T-cell repertoires generated during the process of peripheral expansion to be oligoclonal and skewed toward dominant antigens provided by the vaccine (10), and as a result of the potent proliferative and survival effects rendered by the pharmacological levels of IL-7.

Although IL-15 is not known to provide thymopoietic effects or to augment survival of naïve T-cells or CD4 memory cells, IL-15 therapy would also be predicted to enhance recovery CD8 memory T-cells following T-cell depletion. Indeed, IL-15 therapy did increase recovery of memory T-cells and provided antileukemia effects in a murine model of allogeneic transplantation (97). Furthermore, IL-15's capacity to augment NK cell development and NK cell survival and expansion could provide beneficial effects when combined with cytolytic chemotherapy. Indeed, IL-15 plus cyclophosphamide improved outcome following bone marrow transplant through augmentation of NK cell numbers in a murine lymphoma model system (98). Thus, IL-15 therapy would be expected to augment recovery of NK cells, NK T-cells, and memory CD8$^+$ T-cell populations following dose-intensive chemotherapy or in the setting of bone marrow transplant and could provide important adjuvant benefits. Thus far, the immunorestorative properties of IL-21 have not been well studied.

6. CONCLUDING REMARKS

The γ_c cytokines represent a group of potent immunostimulator and immunomodulatory agents that have the potential to improve the effectiveness of immunotherapies for cancer (Fig. 2). Although IL-2 has been the most widely studied agent in this class, newer

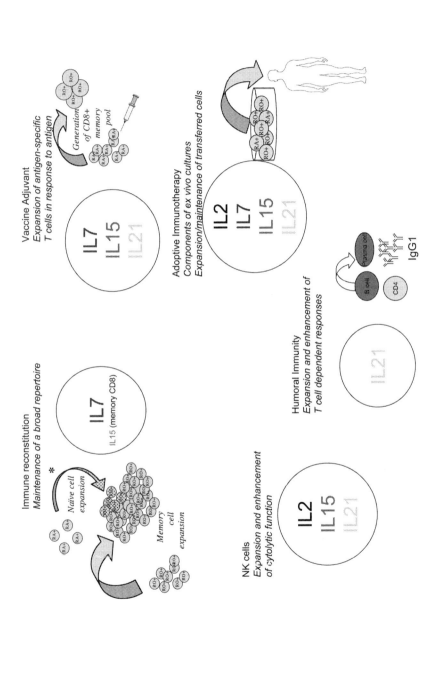

Fig. 2. Potential applications of the γ-chain (γ_c) cytokines for immunotherapy of cancer. All of the γ_c cytokines currently under consideration as therapeutic adjuvants have the potential to enhance the effects of adoptive immunotherapy by supporting the expansion and/or survival of T-cell populations in culture and following transfer. As adjuvants for antigen-specific vaccination targeting T-cell responses, interleukin (IL)-7 and IL-15 hold the most promise. IL-21 also has significant potential in this regard, but may be most potent in combination with IL-15 and/or IL-7. IL-2, IL-15, and IL-12 all have potent effects on natural-killer cell expansion and function. Among the cytokines under discussion, IL-21 is uniquely capable of augmenting humoral immune responses, in particular those that are dependent on T-cell help. IL-7 also has potent effects on immune reconstitution involving both CD4 and CD8 cells, whereas IL-15 also contributes to homeostasis of memory CD8 cells.

agents, such as IL-7, IL-15, and IL-21, show promise for the future. Whereas their effects on T-cell and NK cell development, proliferation, and survival are somewhat overlapping, each agent has unique characteristics that are potentially exploitable in the context of immunotherapy for cancer. IL-2 remains a potent agent for NK cell activation and expansion, but it is likely inferior to the other agents as a vaccine adjuvant. IL-7 is notable for its capacity to enhance vaccine responses, effectiveness of adoptively transferred cells, and its immunorestorative effects; however, IL-7 is not active on NK cell populations. IL-15 is a potent survival, proliferative, and differentiation factor for memory CD8$^+$ cells and is a potent growth and survival factor for NK cells. IL-21's properties are continuing to be elucidated, but it appears most notable for its capacity to synergize with other cytokines, especially IL-15 in augmenting CD8 and NK cell responses, as well as its capacity to enhance T-cell-dependent B-cell immunity. Among the new cytokines discussed, only IL-7 is in clinical trials; however, it is hoped that the promising preclinical data now available will serve as an impetus for clinical development of IL-15 and IL-21. Clearly, only through the study of these agents in carefully controlled human clinical trials will the ultimate usefulness of each agent in the context of immunotherapy for cancer be elucidated.

ACKNOWLEDGMENT

This research was supported by the Intramural Research Program of the National Institutes of Health, National Cancer Institute, and Center for Cancer Research.

REFERENCES

1. Rosenberg SA, Yang JC, Restifo NP. Cancer immunotherapy: moving beyond current vaccines. *Nat Med* 2004; 10:909–915.
2. Ku CC, Murakami M, Sakamoto A, Kappler J, Marrack P. Control of homeostasis of CD8+ memory T cells by opposing cytokines. *Science* 2000; 288:675–678.
3. Oh S, Berzofsky JA, Burke DS, Waldmann TA, Perera LP. Coadministration of HIV vaccine vectors with vaccinia viruses expressing IL-15 but not IL-2 induces long-lasting cellular immunity. *Proc Natl Acad Sci USA* 2003; 100:3392–3397.
4. Fry TJ, Mackall CL. The many faces of IL7: from lymphopoietic cytokine to modulator of peripheral T cell homeostasis. *J Immunol* 2005; 174:6571–6576.
5. Boise LH, Minn AJ, June CH, Lindsten T, Thompson CB. Growth factors can enhance lymphocyte survival without committing the cell to undergo cell division. *Proc Natl Acad Sci USA* 1995; 92:5491–5495.
6. Vella A, Teague TK, Ihle J, Kappler J, Marrack P. Interleukin 4 (IL-4) or IL-7 prevents the death of resting T cells: Stat 6 is probably not required for the effect of IL-4. *J Exp Med* 1997; 186:325–330.
7. Rathmell JC, Farkash EA, Gao W, Thompson CB. IL-7 enhances the survival and maintains the size of naive T cells. *J Immunol* 2001; 167:6869–6876.
8. Seddon B, Tomlinson P, Zamoyska R. Interleukin 7 and T cell receptor signals regulate homeostasis of CD4 memory cells. *Nat Immunol* 2003; 4:680–686.
9. Stutman O. Postthymic T cell development. *Immunol Rev* 1986; 91:159–194.
10. Mackall CL, Bare CV, Titus JA, Sharrow SO, Granger LA, Gress RE. Thymic-independent T cell regeneration occurs via antigen driven expansion of peripheral T cells resulting in a repertoire that is limited in diversity and prone to skewing. *J Immunol* 1996; 156:4609–4616.
11. Goldrath AW, Bevan MJ. Low-affinity ligands for the TCR drive proliferation of mature CD8+ T cells in lymphopenic hosts. *Immunity* 1999; 11:183–190.
12. Ernst B, Lee DS, Chang JM, Sprent J, Surh CD. The peptide ligands mediating positive selection in the thymus control T cell survival and homeostatic proliferation in the periphery. *Immunity* 1999; 11:173–181.
13. Viret C, Wong FS, Janeway CA Jr. Designing and maintaining the mature TCR repertoire: the continuum of self-peptide:self-MHC complex recognition. *Immunity* 1999; 10:559–568.
14. Fry TJ, Connick E, Falloon J, et al. A potential role for interleukin-7 in T-cell homeostasis. *Blood* 2001; 97:2983–2990.

15. Bolotin E, Annett G, Parkman R, Weinberg K. Serum levels of IL-7 in bone marrow transplant recipients: relationship to clinical characteristics and lymphocyte count. *Bone Marrow Transplant* 1999; 23: 783–788.
16. Napolitano LA, Grant RM, Deeks SG, et al. Increased production of IL-7 accompanies HIV-1-mediated T-cell depletion: implications for T-cell homeostasis. *Nat Med* 2001; 7:73–79.
17. Kieper WC, Tan JT, Bondi-Boyd B, et al. Overexpression of interleukin (IL)-7 leads to IL-15-independent generation of memory phenotype CD8+ T cells. *J Exp Med* 2002; 195:1533–1539.
18. Tan JT, Ernst B, Kieper WC, LeRoy E, Sprent J, Surh CD. Interleukin (IL)-15 and IL-7 jointly regulate homeostatic proliferation of memory phenotype CD8+ cells but are not required for memory phenotype CD4+ cells. *J Exp Med* 2002; 195:1523–1532.
19. Schluns KS, Kieper WC, Jameson SC, Lefrancois L. Interleukin-7 mediates the homeostasis of naive and memory CD8 T cells in vivo. *Nat Immunol* 2000; 1:426–432.
20. Tan JT, Dudl E, LeRoy E, et al. IL-7 is critical for homeostatic proliferation and survival of naive T cells. *Proc Natl Acad Sci USA* 2001; 98:8732–8737.
21. Melchionda F, Fry TJ, Milliron MJ, McKirdy MA, Tagaya Y, Mackall CL. Adjuvant IL7 or IL15 overcomes immunodominance and improves survival of the CD8+ memory cell pool. *J Clin Invest* 2005; 115: 1177–1187.
22. Bamford RN, Grant AJ, Burton JD, et al. The interleukin (IL) 2 receptor beta chain is shared by IL-2 and a cytokine, provisionally designated IL-T, that stimulates T-cell proliferation and the induction of lymphokine-activated killer cells. *Proc Natl Acad Sci USA* 1994; 91:4940–4944.
23. Burton JD, Bamford RN, Peters C, et al. A lymphokine, provisionally designated interleukin T and produced by a human adult T-cell leukemia line, stimulates T-cell proliferation and the induction of lymphokine-activated killer cells. *Proc Natl Acad Sci USA* 1994; 91:4935–4939.
24. Grabstein KH, Eisenman J, Shanebeck K, et al. Cloning of a T cell growth factor that interacts with the beta chain of the interleukin-2 receptor. *Science* 1994; 264:965–868.
25. Marks-Konczalik J, Dubois S, Losi JM, et al. IL-2-induced activation-induced cell death is inhibited in IL-15 transgenic mice. *Proc Natl Acad Sci USA* 2000; 97:11,445–11,4450.
26. Waldmann TA, Dubois S, Tagaya Y. Contrasting roles of IL-2 and IL-15 in the life and death of lymphocytes: implications for immunotherapy. *Immunity* 2001; 14:105–110.
27. Blauvelt A, Asada H, Klaus-Kovtun V, Altman DJ, Lucey DR, Katz SI. Interleukin-15 mRNA is expressed by human keratinocytes Langerhans cells, and blood-derived dendritic cells and is downregulated by ultraviolet B radiation. *J Invest Dermatol* 1996; 106:1047–1052.
28. Waldmann TA, Tagaya Y. The multifaceted regulation of interleukin-15 expression and the role of this cytokine in NK cell differentiation and host response to intracellular pathogens. *Annu Rev Immunol* 1999; 17:19–49.
29. Dubois S, Mariner J, Waldmann TA, Tagaya Y. IL-15Ralpha recycles and presents IL-15 In *trans* to neighboring cells. *Immunity* 2002; 17:537–547.
30. Lodolce JP, Burkett PR, Boone DL, Chien M, Ma A. T cell-independent interleukin 15Ralpha signals are required for bystander proliferation. *J Exp Med* 2001; 194:1187–1194.
31. Koka R, Burkett PR, Chien M, et al. Interleukin (IL)-15R[alpha]-deficient natural killer cells survive in normal but not IL-15R[alpha]-deficient mice. *J Exp Med* 2003; 197:977–984.
32. Burkett PR, Koka R, Chien M, Chai S, Boone DL, Ma A. Coordinate expression and *trans* presentation of interleukin (IL)-15Ralpha and IL-15 supports natural killer cell and memory CD8+ T cell homeostasis. *J Exp Med* 2004; 200:825–834.
33. Koka R, Burkett P, Chien M, Chai S, Boone DL, Ma A. Cutting edge: murine dendritic cells require IL-15R alpha to prime NK cells. *J Immunol* 2004; 173:3594–3598.
34. Sandau MM, Schluns KS, Lefrancois L, Jameson SC. Cutting edge: *trans*presentation of IL-15 by bone marrow-derived cells necessitates expression of IL-15 and IL-15R alpha by the same cells. *J Immunol* 2004; 173:6537–6541.
35. Oh S, Perera LP, Burke DS, Waldmann TA, Berzofsky JA. IL-15/IL-15Ralpha-mediated avidity maturation of memory CD8+ T cells. *Proc Natl Acad Sci USA* 2004; 101:15,154–15,159.
36. Kobayashi H, Dubois S, Sato N, et al. Role of trans-cellular IL-15 presentation in the activation of NK cell-mediated killing, which leads to enhanced tumor immunosurveillance. *Blood* 2005; 105:721–727.
37. Becker TC, Wherry EJ, Boone D, et al. Interleukin 15 is required for proliferative renewal of virus-specific memory CD8 T cells. *J Exp Med* 2002; 195:1541–1548.
38. Judge AD, Zhang X, Fujii H, Surh CD, Sprent J. Interleukin 15 controls both proliferation and survival of a subset of memory-phenotype CD8(+) T cells. *J Exp Med* 2002; 196:935–946.

39. Wu TS, Lee JM, Lai YG, et al. Reduced expression of Bcl-2 in CD8$^+$ T cells deficient in the IL-15 receptor alpha-chain. *J Immunol* 2002; 168:705–712.

40. Goldrath AW, Sivakumar PV, Glaccum M, et al. Cytokine requirements for acute and Basal homeostatic proliferation of naive and memory CD8+ T cells. *J Exp Med* 2002; 195:1515–1522.

41. Cooper MA, Bush JE, Fehniger TA, et al. In vivo evidence for a dependence on interleukin 15 for survival of natural killer cells. *Blood* 2002; 100:3633–3638.

42. Ranson T, Vosshenrich CA, Corcuff E, Richard O, Muller W, Di Santo JP. IL-15 is an essential mediator of peripheral NK-cell homeostasis. *Blood* 2003; 101:4887–4893.

43. Ranson T, Vosshenrich CA, Corcuff E, et al. IL-15 availability conditions homeostasis of peripheral natural killer T cells. *Proc Natl Acad Sci USA* 2003; 100:2663–2668.

44. Dumoutier L, Van Roost E, Colau D, Renauld JC. Human interleukin-10-related T cell-derived inducible factor: molecular cloning and functional characterization as an hepatocyte-stimulating factor. *Proc Natl Acad Sci USA* 2000; 97:10,144–10,149.

45. Ozaki K, Kikly K, Michalovich D, Young PR, Leonard WJ. Cloning of a type I cytokine receptor most related to the IL-2 receptor beta chain. *Proc Natl Acad Sci USA* 2000; 97:11,439–11,444.

46. Parrish-Novak J, Dillon SR, Nelson A, et al. Interleukin 21 and its receptor are involved in NK cell expansion and regulation of lymphocyte function. *Nature* 2000; 408:57–63.

47. Habib T, Senadheera S, Weinberg K, Kaushansky K. The common gamma chain (gamma c) is a required signaling component of the IL-21 receptor and supports IL-21-induced cell proliferation via JAK3. *Biochemistry* 2002; 41:8725–8731.

48. Asao H, Okuyama C, Kumaki S, et al. Cutting edge: the common gamma-chain is an indispensable subunit of the IL-21 receptor complex. *J Immunol* 2001; 167:1–5.

49. Wurster AL, Rodgers VL, Satoskar AR, et al. Interleukin 21 is a T helper (Th) cell 2 cytokine that specifically inhibits the differentiation of naive Th cells into interferon gamma-producing Th1 cells. *J Exp Med* 2002; 196:969–977.

50. Mehta DS, Wurster AL, Weinmann AS, Grusby MJ. NFATc2 and T-bet contribute to T-helper-cell-subset-specific regulation of IL-21 expression. *Proc Natl Acad Sci USA* 2005; 102:2016–2021.

51. DiSanto JP, Muller W, Guy-Grand D, Fischer A, Rajewsky K. Lymphoid development in mice with a targeted deletion of the interleukin 2 receptor gamma chain. *Proc Natl Acad Sci USA* 1995; 92:377–381.

52. Lodolce JP, Burkett PR, Koka RM, Boone DL, Ma A. Regulation of lymphoid homeostasis by interleukin-15. *Cytokine Growth Factor Rev* 2002; 13:429–439.

53. Kasaian MT, Whitters MJ, Carter LL, et al. IL-21 limits NK cell responses and promotes antigen-specific T cell activation: a mediator of the transition from innate to adaptive immunity. *Immunity* 2002; 16:559–569.

54. Sivori S, Cantoni C, Parolini S, et al. IL-21 induces both rapid maturation of human CD34+ cell precursors towards NK cells and acquisition of surface killer Ig-like receptors. *Eur J Immunol* 2003; 33:3439–3447.

55. Brady J, Hayakawa Y, Smyth MJ, Nutt SL. IL-21 induces the functional maturation of murine NK cells. *J Immunol* 2004; 172:2048–2058.

56. Wang G, Tschoi M, Spolski R, et al. In vivo antitumor activity of interleukin 21 mediated by natural killer cells. *Cancer Res* 2003; 63:9016–9022.

57. Zeng R, Spolski R, Finkelstein SE, et al. Synergy of IL-21 and IL-15 in regulating CD8+ T cell expansion and function. *J Exp Med* 2005; 201:139–148.

58. van Leeuwen EM, Gamadia LE, Baars PA, Remmerswaal EB, ten Berge IJ, van Lier RA. Proliferation requirements of cytomegalovirus-specific, effector-type human CD8+ T cells. *J Immunol* 2002; 169:5838–5843.

59. Strengell M, Matikainen S, Siren J, et al. IL-21 in synergy with IL-15 or IL-18 enhances IFN-gamma production in human NK and T cells. *J Immunol* 2003; 170:5464–5469.

60. Strengell M, Sareneva T, Foster D, Julkunen I, Matikainen S. IL-21 up-regulates the expression of genes associated with innate immunity and Th1 response. *J Immunol* 2002; 169:3600–3605.

61. Mehta DS, Wurster AL, Whitters MJ, Young DA, Collins M, Grusby MJ. IL-21 induces the apoptosis of resting and activated primary B-cells. *J Immunol* 2003; 170:4111–4118.

62. Ozaki K, Spolski R, Ettinger R, et al. Regulation of B cell differentiation and plasma cell generation by IL-21, a novel inducer of Blimp-1 and Bcl-6. *J Immunol* 2004; 173:5361–5371.

63. Ozaki K, Spolski R, Feng CG, et al. A critical role for IL-21 in regulating immunoglobulin production. *Science* 2002; 298:1630–1634.

64. Jin H, Carrio R, Yu A, Malek TR. Distinct activation signals determine whether IL-21 induces B cell costimulation, growth arrest, or Bim-dependent apoptosis. *J Immunol* 2004; 173:657–665.

65. Gett AV, Sallusto F, Lanzavecchia A, Geginat J. T cell fitness determined by signal strength. *Nat Immunol* 2003; 4:355–360.

66. Iezzi G, Karjalainen K, Lanzavecchia A. The duration of antigenic stimulation determines the fate of naive and effector T cells. *Immunity* 1998; 8:89–95.

67. Kaech SM, Tan JT, Wherry EJ, Konieczny BT, Surh CD, Ahmed R. Selective expression of the interleukin 7 receptor identifies effector CD8 T cells that give rise to long-lived memory cells. *Nat Immunol* 2003; 4:1191–1198.

68. Ku CC, Murakami M, Sakamoto A, Kappler J, Marrack P. Control of homeostasis of CD8+ memory T cells by opposing cytokines. *Science* 2000; 288:675–758.

69. Kaech SM, Wherry EJ, Ahmed R. Effector and memory T-cell differentiation: implications for vaccine development. *Nat Rev Immunol* 2002; 2:251–262.

70. Tan JT, Dudl E, LeRoy E, et al. IL-7 is critical for homeostatic proliferation and survival of naive T cells. *Proc Natl Acad Sci USA* 2001; 10:10.

71. Berard M, Brandt K, Bulfone-Paus S, Tough DF. IL-15 promotes the survival of naive and memory phenotype CD8+ T cells. *J Immunol* 2003; 170:5018–5026.

72. Yajima T, Nishimura H, Ishimitsu R, et al. Overexpression of IL-15 in vivo increases antigen-driven memory CD8+ T cells following a microbe exposure. *J Immunol* 2002; 168:1198–1203.

73. Maeurer MJ, Trinder P, Hommel G, et al. Interleukin-7 or interleukin-15 enhances survival of Mycobacterium tuberculosis-infected mice. *Infect Immun* 2000; 68:2962–2970.

74. Khan IA, Casciotti L. IL-15 prolongs the duration of CD8+ T cell-mediated immunity in mice infected with a vaccine strain of *Toxoplasma gondii. J Immunol* 1999; 163:4503–4509.

75. Xin KQ, Hamajima K, Sasaki S, et al. IL-15 expression plasmid enhances cell-mediated immunity induced by an HIV-1 DNA vaccine. *Vaccine* 1999; 17:858–866.

76. Rubinstein MP, Kadima AN, Salem ML, Nguyen CL, Gillanders WE, Cole DJ. Systemic administration of IL-15 augments the antigen-specific primary CD8+ T cell response following vaccination with peptide-pulsed dendritic cells. *J Immunol* 2002; 169:4928–4935.

77. Villinger F, Miller R, Mori K, et al. IL-15 is superior to IL-2 in the generation of long-lived antigen specific memory CD4 and CD8 T cells in rhesus macaques. *Vaccine* 2004; 22:3510–3521.

78. Kimura K, Nishimura H, Matsuzaki T, Yokokura T, Nimura Y, Yoshikai Y. Synergistic effect of interleukin-15 and interleukin-12 on antitumor activity in a murine malignant pleurisy model. *Cancer Immunol Immunother* 2000; 49:71–77.

79. Lasek W, Basak G, Switaj T, et al. Complete tumour regressions induced by vaccination with IL-12 gene-transduced tumour cells in combination with IL-15 in a melanoma model in mice. *Cancer Immunol Immunother* 2004; 53:363–372.

80. Di Carlo E, Comes A, Orengo AM, et al. IL-21 induces tumor rejection by specific CTL and IFN-gamma-dependent CXC chemokines in syngeneic mice. *J Immunol* 2004; 172:1540-1547.

81. Ma HL, Whitters MJ, Konz RF, et al. IL-21 activates both innate and adaptive immunity to generate potent antitumor responses that require perforin but are independent of IFN-gamma. *J Immunol* 2003; 171:608–615.

82. Kishida T, Asada H, Itokawa Y, et al. Interleukin (IL)-21 and IL-15 genetic transfer synergistically augments therapeutic antitumor immunity and promotes regression of metastatic lymphoma. *Mol Ther* 2003; 8:552–558.

83. Lynch DH, Namen AE, Miller RE. In vivo evaluation of the effects of interleukins 2, 4 and 7 on enhancing the immunotherapeutic efficacy of anti-tumor cytotoxic T lymphocytes. *Eur J Immunol* 1991; 21:2977–2985.

84. Wiryana P, Bui T, Faltynek CR, Ho RJ. Augmentation of cell-mediated immunotherapy against herpes simplex virus by interleukins: comparison of in vivo effects of IL-2 and IL-7 on adoptively transferred T cells. *Vaccine* 1997; 15:561–563.

85. Murphy WJ, Back TC, Conlon KC, et al. Antitumor effects of interleukin-7 and adoptive immunotherapy on human colon carcinoma xenografts. *J Clin Invest* 1993; 92:1918–1924.

86. Dummer W, Niethammer AG, Baccala R, et al. T cell homeostatic proliferation elicits effective antitumor autoimmunity. *J Clin Invest* 2002; 110:185–192.

87. Dudley ME, Wunderlich JR, Robbins PF, et al. Cancer regression and autoimmunity in patients after clonal repopulation with antitumor lymphocytes. *Science* 2002; 298:850–854.

88. Klebanoff CA, Finkelstein SE, Surman DR, et al. IL-15 enhances the in vivo antitumor activity of tumor-reactive CD8+ T cells. *Proc Natl Acad Sci USA* 2004; 101:1969–1974.

89. Anichini A, Scarito A, Molla A, Parmiani G, Mortarini R. Differentiation of CD8+ T cells from tumor-invaded and tumor-free lymph nodes of melanoma patients: role of common gamma-chain cytokines. *J Immunol* 2003; 171:2134–2141.

90. Brentjens RJ, Latouche JB, Santos E, et al. Eradication of systemic B-cell tumors by genetically targeted human T lymphocytes co-stimulated by CD80 and interleukin-15. *Nat Med* 2003; 9:279–286.

91. Zhang X, Sun S, Hwang I, Tough DF, Sprent J. Potent and selective stimulation of memory-phenotype CD8+ T cells in vivo by IL-15. *Immunity* 1998; 8:591–599.

92. Moroz A, Eppolito C, Li Q, Tao J, Clegg CH, Shrikant PA. IL-21 enhances and sustains CD8+ T cell responses to achieve durable tumor immunity: comparative evaluation of IL-2, IL-15, and IL-21. *J Immunol* 2004; 173:900–909.

93. Roychowdhury S, May KF Jr, Tzou KS, et al. Failed adoptive immunotherapy with tumor-specific T cells: reversal with low-dose interleukin 15 but not low-dose interleukin 2. *Cancer Res* 2004; 64:8062–8067.

94. Ozdemir O, Ravindranath Y, Savasan S. Mechanisms of superior anti-tumor cytotoxic response of interleukin 15-induced lymphokine-activated killer cells. *J Immunother* 2005; 28:44–52.

95. Fry TJ, Moniuszko M, Creekmore S, et al. IL-7 therapy dramatically alters peripheral T-cell homeostasis in normal and SIV-infected nonhuman primates. *Blood* 2003; 101:2294–2299.

96. Moniuszko M, Fry T, Tsai WP, et al. Recombinant interleukin-7 induces proliferation of naive macaque CD4+ and CD8+ T cells in vivo. *J Virol* 2004; 78:9740–9749.

97. Alpdogan O, Eng JM, Muriglan SJ, et al. Interleukin-15 enhances immune reconstitution after allogeneic bone marrow transplantation. *Blood* 2005; 105:865–873.

98. Evans R, Fuller JA, Christianson G, Krupke DM, Troutt AB. IL-15 mediates anti-tumor effects after cyclophosphamide injection of tumor-bearing mice and enhances adoptive immunotherapy: the potential role of NK cell subpopulations. *Cell Immunol* 1997; 179:66–73.

99. Katsanis E, Xu Z, Panoskaltsis-Mortari A, Weisdorf DJ, Widmer MB, Blazar BR. IL-15 administration following syngeneic bone marrow transplantation prolongs survival of lymphoma bearing mice. *Transplantation* 1996; 62:872–875.

23 The Therapeutic Use of Natural-Killer Cells in Hematological Malignancies

Sherif S. Farag and Michael A. Caligiuri

SUMMARY

The role of natural-killer (NK) cells in the treatment of hematological malignances has been investigated intensively during the past three decades. Until recently, the majority of research has focused on the use of in vitro or in vivo cytokine-expanded and -activated NK cells against autologous cancer cells, with generally disappointing results. The lack of observed efficacy of past attempts to harness the antitumor effect of NK cells can now be explained largely by inhibitory interactions between major histocompatibility complex class I molecules expressed on tumor cells and inhibitory receptors on NK cells. Better appreciation of how NK cells selectively recognize and kill target cells while sparing normal cells is evolving. Major families of cell surface receptors that inhibit and activate NK cells to lyse target cells have been characterized, including killer cell immunoglobulin-like receptors, C-type lectins, and natural cytotoxicity receptors. In addition, identification of NK cell receptor ligands and their expression on normal and transformed cells is becoming better elucidated. The improved understanding of NK cell receptor biology has paved the way for development of novel and rational clinical approaches to manipulating receptor–ligand interactions for immunotherapy.

Key Words: Natural-killer cells; immunotherapy; ADCC; transplantation.

1. INTRODUCTION

The role of immune cells in the treatment of hematological malignancies has been extensively investigated during the past two decades. The graft-vs-leukemia effect following allogeneic hematopoietic progenitor cell transplantation and donor lymphocyte infusion for relapsed leukemia has highlighted the significant potential of immunotherapy in chemotherapy-resistant malignancies. This effect, mediated largely by alloreactive T-lymphocytes recognizing minor or major histocompatibility complex (MHC) antigens shared by both neoplastic and normal cells, however, lacks specificity, resulting in severe graft-vs-host disease (GVHD) in many patients (*1*). Whereas a number of investigators

From: *Cancer Drug Discovery and Development: Immunotherapy of Cancer*
Edited by: M. L. Disis © Humana Press Inc., Totowa, NJ

have demonstrated the presence of tumor-specific T-lymphocytes in patients with cancer, success in harnessing the potential of these cells has been severely limited by the lack of knowledge of tumor-specific antigens in the vast majority of cases. As effectors of the innate immune response, however, natural-killer (NK) cells do not require recognition of tumor-specific antigen for killing target cells. Furthermore, NK cells have been shown to kill a large number of different tumor cells in vitro *(2–4)*, and their antitumor activity can be enhanced by clinically available cytokines, such as interleukin (IL)-2 and IL-12. As such, NK cells may have wider potential applicability in the treatment of malignancies. In this chapter, we review the potential role of NK cells in the treatment of human cancer, particularly the hematological malignancies.

2. NK CELLS

Human NK cells are critical cells of the innate immune system, and compose approx 10–15% of peripheral blood lymphocytes. They are identified by the surface expression of the neural cell adhesion molecule, CD56, and the lack of expression of CD3 *(5)*. Functionally, NK cells have the capacity for direct cytolytic activity against target cells (e.g., virus-infected cells or tumor cells) and are an important source of immunoregulatory cytokines (e.g., interferon [IFN]-γ, tumor necrosis factor [TNF]-α, TNF-β, IL-10, granulocyte macrophage-colony stimulating factor) *(6)*. In addition, NK cells can also mediate antibody-dependent cellular cytotoxicity (ADCC) via FcγRIII receptors (CD16) that bind to the Fc portion of immunoglobulin (Ig)G *(6)*.

The functional capacities of NK cells reside differentially in two distinct subsets defined by the extent of CD56 surface expression *(7,8)*. Approximately 90% of NK cells express low levels of CD56 (CD56^{dim}), and predominantly function in natural cytotoxicity and ADCC through high expression of CD16. The remaining subpopulation is CD56^{bright} and CD16^{dim}, and has predominantly an immunoregulatory role through the secretion of cytokines. In addition, CD56^{bright} NK cells constitutively express the high-affinity IL-2 receptor (IL-2R$\alpha\beta\gamma$) and expand in vitro and in vivo in response to low concentrations of IL-2 *(9,10)*, whereas resting CD56^{dim} NK cells express only the intermediate-affinity IL-2 receptor (IL-2R$\beta\gamma$), and proliferate weakly in response to IL-2 concentrations *(9,10)*. Although resting CD56^{bright} NK cells exhibit less cytotoxicity against NK-sensitive targets than CD56^{dim} cells, the former can exhibit similar or enhanced cytotoxicity against NK targets compared with CD56^{dim} cells after IL-2 activation *(12,13)*. The differences in response to IL-2 have important implications for the design of therapeutic cytokine schedules, as discussed under Heading 3.

Human NK cells arise from CD34$^+$ progenitor cells under the influence of cytokines produced by bone marrow stromal cells. The early-acting cytokines, FMS-related tyrosine kinase 3 ligand and c-kit ligand (stem cell factor [SCF]), stimulate CD34$^+$ NK cell progenitors to develop into intermediate precursors that are capable of responding to IL-15, which in turn induces terminal NK cell differentiation *(14)*. Significantly, whereas IL-15 is the physiological cytokine for the terminal differentiation of NK cells from precursor cells, IL-2 can substitute for its action in vivo and in vitro. The IL-15 receptor shares common signaling receptor subunits (β- and γ-chains) with that of IL-2, which together form the intermediate heterodimeric receptor complex, IL-2/15R$\beta\gamma$, upregulated by FMS-related tyrosine kinase 3 ligand and SCF *(15,16)*. However, IL-15 and IL-2 also utilize unique α-subunits, which confer high-affinity specific binding to their respective high-affinity receptors, IL-15Rαβγ and IL-2Rαβγ *(17)*. As discussed under Heading 3, this understanding has important implications for the therapeutic use of cytokines combinations, including IL-2 (or IL-15) with SCF for in vivo expansion of NK cells for the treatment of hematological malignancies.

3. EARLY STRATEGIES FOR NK CELL-BASED IMMUNOTHERAPY

Early studies attempting to harness the anti-tumor effects of NK cells focused on in vitro and/or in vivo expansion and activation of autologous NK cells through the use of IL-2. Initial trials involved infusion of high-dose IL-2, alone or in combination with ex vivo IL-2-activated lymphocytes or purer populations of activated NK cells, in the treatment of patients with acute leukemia *(18–22)*. In general, high-dose IL-2 ($8–18 \times 10^6$ IU/m^2) induced modest responses in acute myeloid leukemia (AML) patients, particularly those with low-disease burden, but with little demonstrable effect in patients with acute lymphoblastic leukemia *(23,24)*. Significant toxicity, however, has accompanied the use of high-dose IL-2, necessitating investigation of lower-dose schedules.

Early work by Caligiuri et al. demonstrated that low concentrations of IL-2 selectively expand CD56^{bright} NK cells, expressing IL-1Rαβγ *(9,11,25)*. In addition, the expanded CD56^{bright} NK cells demonstrated significant cytotoxicity against NK cell-resistant cells only on incubation in higher concentrations of IL-2 that saturate the intermediate-affinity receptors (IL-2βγ) *(9,11,25)*. Based on these observations, initial phase I/II trials showed that the schedule of recombinant human IL-2 (rhuIL-2) at 10^6 IU/m^2/d was found to consistently expand CD56^{bright} NK cells in vivo, with good tolerability in patients with human immunodeficiency virus infection and malignancy *(26,27)*. As an extension, a regimen of prolonged low-dose rhuIL-2 with intermittent intermediate-dose ($6–12 \times 10^6$ IU/m^2/ d for 3 d), rhuIL-2 pulsing was developed and found to be well tolerated following intensive chemotherapy in AML patients *(28)*. Other investigators have also demonstrated the improved tolerability of lower doses of IL-2 in patients with AML *(29)*. Similarly, rhuIL-2 has also been investigated in patients with active non-Hodgkin's lymphoma and Hodgkin's disease or to prevent progression following autologous bone marrow transplantation *(30,31)*.

Despite reduced toxicity with lower doses of IL-2, and consistent observations of a biological effect on NK cell expansion and activation in vivo, the efficacy of this strategy to harness antitumor activity of NK cells remains uncertain. A randomized trial of intermediate-dose rhuIL-2 (12×10^6 IU/m^2/d) in 130 acute leukemia patients in remission following autologous bone marrow transplantation has shown no benefit *(32)*. An interim analysis of a randomized trial by Cancer and Leukemia Group B (study 9420) comparing the schedule of low-dose IL-2 with intermediate-dose pulse IL-2 to observation following intensive induction and consolidation therapy in AML patients 60 yr of age or older has shown no benefit to IL-2 (R. Larson, personal communication). The results of phase II clinical trials using rhuIL-2 in patients with lymphoma have similarly been disappointing, and no randomized trials reported *(30,31,33–37)*. As discussed in the following section, recent understanding of the importance of activating and inhibitory receptors on the surface of NK cells in the recognition of target cells offers potential explanations for the limited efficacy of previous strategies to harness NK cells for treatment of malignancies and suggest novel directions for investigation.

4. TARGET CELL RECOGNITION BY NK CELLS:
IMPLICATIONS FOR IMMUNOTHERAPY

Although NK cells do not possess specific antigen receptors that recognize antigen in the context of MHC class I and II molecules, MHC class I molecules on target cells have long been known to modulate the function of NK cells. Early studies demonstrated that normal expression of MHC class I molecules by normal cells results in tolerance to lysis by autologous NK cells, whereas altered or downregulated MHC class I expression increases susceptibility to lysis *(38,39)*. Importantly, this inhibition is mediated by a number of inhibitory NK cells receptors that specifically recognize groups of classical (e.g., human leukocyte antigen [HLA]-A, -B, or -C) or nonclassical (e.g., HLA-E, -G) MHC class I molecules. Other evidence, however, indicates that MHC class I expression is not the only modulating influence. Indeed, expression of MHC class I molecules is not always necessary for protection from lysis by NK cells *(40)*, and inhibition by MHC class I is not always sufficient to prevent NK-mediated lysis *(41,42)*. It is now established that each NK cell expresses its own repertoire of activating and inhibitory receptors, and cytotoxicity is ultimately regulated by a balance of signals from these receptors that interact with MHC class I and class I-like molecules on target cells (Fig. 1). The principal inhibitory and activating NK cells receptors in humans are listed in Tables 1 and 2, respectively.

4.1. Paired Inhibitory and Activating Receptors

4.1.1. KILLER IG-LIKE RECEPTORS

The killer Ig-like receptors (KIRs) are the best-described family of paired inhibitory and activating receptors on human NK cells. Based on their structure, KIRs are classified according to the number of extracellular Ig-like domains and the lengths of their cytoplasmic tails (Fig. 2). Each set of paired activating and inhibitory KIR has an identical extracellular domain, and therefore, specifically binds to identical groups of MHC class I alleles. Differences in functional activity, however, reside in alternate intracellular motifs associated with the cytoplasmic tails. The long-tail receptors mediate an inhibitory signal via immunoreceptor tyrosine-based inhibition motifs in their cytoplasmic domains, whereas the short-tail receptors are associated with activating signals because of their association with adaptor proteins bearing immunoreceptor tyrosine-based activating motifs.

Of MHC class I molecules, HLA-C is the main ligand recognized by paired inhibitory and activating KIRs. KIR2DL1 (and its activating KIR2DS1counterpart) recognizes an epitope shared by group 1 HLA-C alleles characterized by asparagine at position 77 and lysine at position 80 in the α1 helix of the MHC molecule (i.e., Cw2, Cw4, Cw5, Cw6, Cw17, and Cw18) *(43,44)*. On the other hand, KIR2DL2 and KIR2DL3 (and the KIR2DS2-activating receptor) recognize an epitope shared by group 2 HLA-C alleles with serine-77 and aparagine-80 (i.e., Cw1, Cw3, Cw7, Cw8, Cw13, and Cw14) *(45)*. Other inhibitory KIRs, without activating counterparts, recognize epitopes shared by HLA-Bw4 (KIR3DL1) *(46,47)* and HLA-A3 and -A11 (KIR3DL2) alleles *(48)*, respectively. For many other KIRs, the ligands remain to be defined. Of note, however, the KIR repertoire is not all-inclusive for MHC class I allotypes *(49)*, with many HLA-A and -B alleles having no corresponding KIRs.

Phenotypically, the KIR repertoire of an individual's NK cells is determined by differential expression of *KIR* genes located in the leukocyte receptor cluster on chromosome 19p13.4 *(50)*. Two groups of KIR haplotypes, A and B, which differ qualitatively

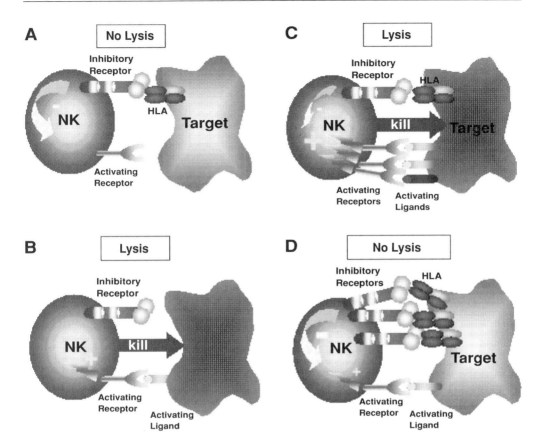

Fig. 1. Regulation of natural-killer (NK) cell response by activating and inhibitory receptors. Inhibitory receptors (e.g., inhibitory killer immunoglobulin-like receptors [KIRs], CD94/NKG2A) recognize and engage their ligands, major histocompatibility complex (MHC) class I molecules (human leukocyte antigens), on the surface of the target tumor cell, thereby initiating an inhibitory signal. Activating receptors (e.g. activating KIRs, CD94/NKG2C, NKG2D) bind ligands on the target cell surface and trigger NK cell activation and target cell lysis. **(A)** When inhibitory receptors engage human leukocyte antigens in the absence of an activating receptor–ligand interaction, a net negative signal is generated, resulting in no target cell lysis. **(B)** Conversely, when activating receptors engage their ligands on target cells in the absence of inhibitory receptor–ligand interaction a net activation signal is generated, resulting in target cell lysis. This scenario is likely operative in NK alloreactivity in the setting of KIR epitope mismatched transplantations (*see* Fig. 3). More-complex physiological scenarios are shown in **(C)** and **(D)**, with both inhibitory and activating receptor–ligand signals being generated when an NK cell interacts with a target cell. **(C)** Here, the activating receptor–ligand interactions predominate over weaker inhibitory receptor–ligand signals, with the net result being NK cell activation and target cell lysis. This may occur when activation receptors and ligands are upregulated, thereby amplifying the net activation signal to exceed the inhibitory signal. For example, the activating ligands *M*HC class *I* chain-related (MIC)A/B and UL-16 binding protein are expressed highly in stressed or transformed cells, thereby activating NKG2D/PI3K pathways that are not susceptible to inhibitory signals (*see* Subheading 4.2. for more details). Alternatively, when expression of self-MHC class I ligands is decreased in the setting of viral infection or transformation, the net signal may be positive also resulting in target cell lysis. **(D)** Here, inhibitory receptor–ligand interactions result in a net negative signal that prevents NK cell lysis of the target cell. This process may occur constantly as NK cells survey normal host tissues. Not shown is the scenario of absence of both inhibitory and activating signals that results in no NK cell activation. (Reprinted with permission from ref. *107*.)

Table 1
Human Inhibitory Natural-Killer Cell Receptors

Receptor	Ligand specificity
KIRs	
KIR2DL1 (CD158a)	Group 2 HLA-C Asn77Lys80 (w2, w4, w5, w6, and related alleles)
KIR2DL2 (CD158b)	Group 1 HLA-C Ser77Asn80 (w1, w3, w7, w8, and related alleles)
KIR2DL3 (CD158b)	Group 1 HLA-C Ser77Asn80 (w1, w3, w7, w8, and related alleles)
KIR2DL5	Unknown
KIR3DL1	HLA-Bw4
KIR3DL2	HLA-A3, -A11
KIR3DL7	Unknown
C-type lectin receptors	
CD94/NKG2A/B[a]	HLA-E (loaded with HLA-A,B,C,G leader peptides)
Ig-like transcripts	
ILT-2 (LIR-1)	Unknown
Others	
P75/AIRM	Unknown (sialic acid dependent)
IRp60	Unknown
LAIR-1	Ep-CAM

[a]NKG2A and NKG2B are splice transcripts.

KIRs, killer immunoglobulin-like receptors; HLA, human leukocyte antigen; Ig, immunoglobulin; Asn, asparagine; Lys, lysine; Ser, serine; ILT-2, Ig-like transcript 2; LIR-1, leukocyte immunoglobulin-like receptor 1; LAIR-1, leukocyte-associated Ig-like 1; Ep-CAM, epithelial cellular adhesion molecule.

(Reprinted with permission from ref. 107.)

and quantitatively in *KIR* gene content have been defined *(51,52)*. Group A haplotypes have extensive allelic polymorphisms but contain fewer *KIR* genes, with only *KIR2DS4* and *KIR2DL4* as activating receptor genes, whereas group B haplotypes are characterized by diverse combination of activating *KIR* genes *(52)*. As a result, there is extensive *KIR* genotypic diversity, which occurs at several levels.

4.1.2. C-Type Lectin Receptors

C-type lectin receptors exist as heterodimers that share a common subunit, CD94, linked to distinct glycoproteins encoded by *NKG2* gene family. The extracellular and cytoplasmic domains of the NKG2 molecules determine the functional specificity of the receptor, whereas the CD94 subunit lacks a cytoplasmic domain for intrinsic signal transduction *(53)*. The C-type lectin family of receptors is considerably less diverse than the KIR family. Only a single receptor of this family, CD94/NKG2A (and its splice variant NKG2B), is inhibitory, and analogous to KIR, possesses a long, intracytoplasmic tail containing immunoreceptor tyrosine-based inhibition motifs that mediate inhibitory signals. The other heterodimers of this family, CD94/NKG2C and CD94/NKG2E (and its splice variant NKG2H), are activating receptors and have only short cytoplasmic tails that associate with adaptor proteins bearing immunoreceptor tyrosine-based activating motifs. Both activating and inhibitory receptors recognize HLA-E, loaded with leader peptides derived from the signal sequences of classic class I MHC molecules HLA-A, -B and -C *(54,55)*, and in effect, sense overall MHC class I expression target cells. The *CD94* and *NKG2* genes are all closely linked on chromosome 12p12.3-p13.1, and are much less complex *(56,58)*.

Table 2
Human Activating Natural-Killer Cell Receptors

Receptor	Ligand specificity
MHC class I-specific	
KIRs	
KIR2DS1	Group 2 HLA-C Asn77Lys80 (w2, w4, w5, w6 and related alleles)
KIR2DS2	Group 1 HLA-C Ser77Asn80 (w1, w3, w7, w8 and related alleles)
KIR2DL4	HLA-G
KIR2DS4	Unknown
KIR2DS5	Unknown
KIR3DS1	Unknown
C-type lectin receptors	
CD94/NKG2C	HLA-E (loaded with HLA-A,B,C leader peptides)
CD94/NKG2E/H[a]	Unknown
Non-MHC class I-specific	
Natural cytotoxicity receptors	
NKp46	Unknown
NKp44	Unknown
NKp30	Unknown
C-type lectin receptor	
NKG2D	MICA, MICB
	ULBP-1, -2, -3
Other (coreceptors)	
CD16 (FcγRIII)	Fc of IgG
CD2	CD58 (LFA-3)
LFA-1	ICAM-1
2B4	CD48
NKp80	Unknown
CD69	Unknown
CD40 ligand	CD40

[a]NKG2E and NKG2H are splice variants.
MHC, major histocompatibility complex, MHC; HLA, human leukocyte antigen; KIR, killer immuno-globulin-like receptors; Asn, asparagine; Lys, lysine; Ser, serine; MIC-, MHC class I chain-related; ULBP, UL-16 binding protein; IgG, immunoglobulin G; LFA-1, lymphocyte function antigen 1; ICAM-1, intracellular adhesion molecule 1.
(Reprinted with permission from ref. 107.)

In a given individual, NK cells express different combinations of KIR and CD94/NKG2 receptors, with the receptor repertoire primarily determined by differential expression of *KIR* and *NKG2* genes, although a subtle modulatory effect by HLA genotype operates, particularly affecting the relative frequency of cells expressing particular KIRs (52, 58). The significance for the existence of paired inhibitory and activating receptors for MHC class I remains unclear. Under normal conditions, the signals mediated by the inhibitory KIR and CD94/NKG2 receptors override those from the activating counterparts, likely because of the lower affinity of the activating receptors to their ligands compared with that of the inhibitory receptors (59,60). However, only a minority of NK cells express both activating and inhibitory isoforms recognizing the same HLA allotypes (61,62). More commonly, NK cell clones expressing an activating receptor coexpress at least one

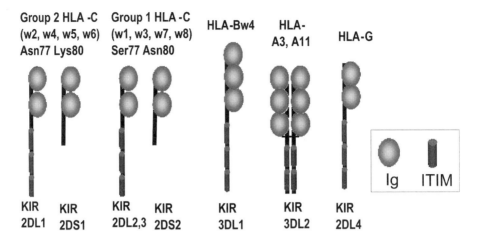

ITIM = immunoreceptor tyrosine inhibition motif

Fig. 2. Killer immunoglobulin-like receptors (KIRs). KIRs are classified according to the number of extracellular immunoglobulin-like domains and the lengths of their cytoplasmic tails. Each set of paired activating and inhibitory KIRs has an identical extracellular domain, and therefore, specifically binds to identical groups of major histocompatibility complex class I alleles. Differences in functional activity, however, reside in alternate intracellular motifs associated with the cytoplasmic tails. The long-tail receptors mediate an inhibitory signal via immunoreceptor tyrosine-based inhibition motifs in their cytoplasmic domains, whereas the short-tail receptors are associated with activating signals because of their association with adaptor proteins bearing immunoreceptor tyrosine-based activating motifs.

inhibitory receptor specific for a different HLA class I allele, which can be either a KIR or CD94/NKG2. The MHC class I-specific activating receptors may function to detect altered class I expression on cells.

4.2. Non-MHC Class I-Specific Activating Receptors

In addition to the activating KIR and CD94/NKG2 receptors, other activating receptors exist and are likely to play a more important role in mediating NK cell cytotoxicity against MHC class I deficient target cells. The best-characterized are the natural cytotoxicity receptors (NCRs) and NKG2D (63,64), which recognize non-MHC class I molecules on target cells. In addition, a number of activating receptors with no apparent specificity for MHC class I molecules have been reported, although many act as coactivators rather direct stimulators of NK cell function (63). Activating coreceptors include FcγRIII (CD16), CD2, 2B4, NKp80, CD69, lymphocyte function-associated antigen 1, and CD40 ligand, although their relative importance is interacting with NCRs and NKG2D are uncertain.

Three NCRs have been described on human NK cells, of which two, NKp46 and NKp30 (65,66), are constitutively expressed on all peripheral blood NK cells, whereas a third, NKp44, is expressed only on activated NK cells (67). Although the ligands for the NCRs remain poorly defined, the NCRs may be important in the recognition of virus-infected cells (68,69). Significantly, however, the NCRs have also been implicated in the recognition and lysis of a variety of tumor cells by NK cells (65,70–72), although differences in susceptibility suggests that tumor cells are likely to differ significantly in their expression of NCR ligands (72).

Table 3
Novel Natural-Killer Cell-Based Treatment Approaches

- IL-2 immunotherapy in subsets of patients whose tumors express high levels of activating NK cell receptor ligands and/or low levels of MHC class I molecules
- In vivo blockade of KIR-MHC class I molecule interactions using anti-KIR monoclonal antibodies to overcome NK cell inhibition
- Monoclonal antibodies directed at tumor cells to promote ADCC potential of NK cells
- Allogeneic alloreactive (KIR ligand-mismatched) NK cells
  - Haplotype mismatched hematopoietic stem cell transplantation
  - Mismatched unrelated donor hematopoietic stem cell transplantation

IL-2, interleukin-2; NK, natural-killer; MHC, major histocompatibility complex; KIR, killer immuno-globulin-like receptor; ADCC, antibody-dependent cellular cytotoxicity.

The NKG2D receptor is the best-characterized activating receptor, and is constitutively expressed by all NK cells. The ligands for the NKG2D receptor belong to two distinct families, the polymorphic MHC class I chain-related (MIC) peptides, MICA and MICB, and the human cytomegalovirus UL-16 binding proteins (ULBP)-1, -2, and -3 *(64,73,74)*. The ligands of NKG2D appear are either absent or expressed only in low density on normal tissues, but are induced or upregulated on target cells following stress and neoplastic transformation. Variable expression of NKG2D ligands has been demonstrated on a number of malignant cell lines, including leukemia cells *(72,75)*, and more recently in primary AML blasts *(28)*.

4.3. Implications for NK Cell Therapy

The appreciation of how NK cells recognize target cells has important implications for future NK cell-based therapy and offers a plausible explanation for the disappointing results observed previously with treatment aimed at in vivo-expanding and -activating autologous NK cells using IL-2 or other cytokines. It is likely that expression of MHC class I molecules by tumor cells results in an inhibitory influence on autologous NK cells expressing KIRs or CD94/NKG2A. Recent studies indicate that the expression of MHC class I molecules, however, may be normal in the vast majority of tumors, including AML and multiple myeloma *(76–78)*, suggesting that strategies that interfere with the interaction of MHC class I molecules with KIR or CD94/NKG2A receptors may results in greater efficacy. Alternatively, the use of allogeneic NK cells, where there is the possibility for mismatch between KIR receptors on donor NK cells and ligands on the patient's tumor cells, offers an additional therapeutic opportunity. Finally, the antitumor effect of NK cells may also be enhanced using monoclonal antibodies that interact with FcγR on NK cells (ADCC). Based on the improved understanding of NK cell receptor biology, a number of novel therapeutic approaches involving NK cells are currently under investigation (Table 3).

5. NOVEL STRATEGIES TO HARNESS THE ANTITUMOR EFFECTS OF NK CELLS

5.1. Identifying Patients Whose Tumor Cells Are Susceptible to NK Cell Lysis

As discussed, strategies that have used cytokines, such as IL-2, to in vivo or in vitro expand autologous NK cells in therapy of hematological malignancies have likely met with modest success because of the inhibitory effect of KIR-MHC class I interactions. Indeed, in vitro studies using fresh leukemic blasts have shown a strong inverse correlation between the numbers of MHC class I molecules expressed on blasts and NK cell-mediated lysis *(79)*. Furthermore, MHC class I expression may not be significantly altered on many neoplastic cells *(76–78)*. In spite of the negative results observed, however, it is still possible that subsets of patients will benefit from cytokine therapy directed at recruiting NK cells if their tumor cells express high levels of activating ligands whose activating signals can override the negative signals of MHC class I. Differences in NKG2D ligand expression by AML blasts have recently been demonstrated at both the RNA level *(28)* and surface expression (unpublished observations). It is hypothesized that patients whose leukemic cells express high levels of NKG2D ligands (and potentially NCR ligands) and/or low levels of MHC class I may be most susceptible to NK cell lysis. To test this hypothesis, we are currently correlating NKG2D ligand expression on AML blasts with relapse-free survival in patients treated with IL-2 to identify a potential subset of patients who may benefit from rhuIL-2. If this is confirmed, future studies should prospectively target such patients whose cancer cells are most susceptible to autologous NK cell lysis.

5.2. In Vivo Blockade of KIR-MHC Class I Molecules

KIR receptor interaction with MHC class I molecules on target cells appear to exert the most significant inhibitory effect on NK cells. Interference with this interaction using antibodies directed at either MHC class I molecules or KIRs could break tolerance and enhance cytotoxicity against cancer cells in vivo. In vitro studies have demonstrated that blocking MHC class I molecules by anti-HLA antibodies renders NK cell-resistant leukemic blasts susceptible to lysis *(79)*. The feasibility of such an approach in vivo was recently demonstrated in a mouse model, whereby treatment with F(ab')$_2$ anti-Ly49C (mouse counterpart of the human KIR) enhanced in vivo NK cell-mediated tumor activity and protected mice from leukemic death *(80)*. Significantly, treatment with F(ab')$_2$ anti-Ly49C did not result in significant pancytopenia because of killing of normal hematopoietic cells. Currently, antihuman KIR antibodies are being developed for therapeutic use and should provide an opportunity to test clinically this approach. Although not yet tested, it is possible that simultaneous blockade of CD94/NKG2A/B interactions with HLA-E might further increase antitumor activity.

5.3. Antibody-Dependent Cellular Cytotoxicity

ADCC is an important mechanism by which NK cells can kill target cells. The increasing availability of monoclonal antibodies (MAbs) has permitted the investigation of this therapeutic approach. Although multiple mechanisms have been proposed for the activity of MAbs, recent work has demonstrated that ADCC is an important mechanism in vivo *(81)*. For example, in a mouse xenograft human lymphoma model, FcγR knockout completely abrogated the response to rituximab *(81)*. In addition, the demonstration that response to rituximab is dependent on specific FcγRIIIa polymorphisms in non-Hodgkin's lymphoma patients supports the importance of ADCC in the in vivo activity of rituximab *(82)*. However, whereas NK cells are important effectors of ADCC, their ability to function in ADCC may be reduced in advanced malignancy *(83)*, possibly because of defective expression of NK cell-triggering receptors *(84)*. The reduced ADCC activity can be enhanced in vitro by cytokines, including IL-12, IFN-α, granulocyte macrophage-colony stimulating factor, IL-15, and IL-2 (85–91), and provides the rationale for the investigation of cytokine and MAb combination.

Phase I and II trials investigating the combination of rhuIL-2 and rituximab, using a variety of rhuIL-2 doses and schedules, are ongoing (92). If efficacy is confirmed, studies can be extended to the investigation of rhuIL-2 (or other cytokines that modulate FcγR-bearing immune cells) with other clinically available MAbs, including anti-CD22, Hu1D10, and alemtuzumab. The combination of rhuIL-12 and rituximab is also undergoing investigation (93). Of note, however, recent data in chronic lymphocytic leukemia suggest that ADCC may not be an important mechanism for the activity of rituximab in this disease (94), suggesting that combining cytokine with antibody may not be readily extrapolated to other diseases where an antibody shows single-agent activity. This is also illustrated by the modest activity of the combination of rhuIL-2 and HuM195 in patients with AML (95), in spite of the single-agent activity of HuM195 in relapsed patients with AML and the ability of the antibody to participate in ADCC (96). The success of harnessing the ADCC potential of NK cells may therefore be disease dependent and not simply a function of the availability of a MAb able to participate in ADCC.

As FcγR is essentially a coreceptor, it is likely that its effect is modulated by other NK cell receptors. However, the ability of activating (e.g., NKG2D or NCRs) and inhibitory (e.g., KIRs) NK cell receptors to modulate ADCC is currently unknown. It is possible that the reported variability in ADCC potential, and lack of correlation between CD20 density on lymphoma cells and the extent of rituximab-induced ADCC (97) may be because of modulation by MHC class I or NKG2D/NCR ligand expression on lymphoma cells. Investigation of this potentially important interaction has obvious implications for optimal therapeutic use of NK cells in the future, as blocking antibodies become available.

5.4. Allogeneic NK Cell Therapy

5.4.1. KIR Ligand Mismatching in Haplotype-Mismatched Transplants

As discussed in Subheading 5.3, the therapeutic use of autologous NK cell may be limited by inhibitory interactions of KIRs with MHC class I molecules, and may require antibody blockade of this interaction for optimal antitumor activity. The use of allogeneic NK cells, however, provides a readily available means of overcoming inhibitory interactions by the appropriate choice of donor and recipient pairs who are mismatched for KIR ligands. The utility of this approach has been best demonstrated in the setting of haplotype-mismatched hematopoietic stem cell transplantation. With KIR ligand mismatching between donor and recipient in the GVH direction, engrafting NK cells have been shown to exert an important antileukemic effect following T-cell-depleted, full haplotype-mismatched stem cell transplants (98). Following transplant, NK cells with a KIR repertoire identical to that of the donor rapidly reconstitute with a high-frequency-of-donor-vs-recipient alloreactive NK clones (98). In this setting (as shown in Fig. 3A), reconstituting donor NK cell clones do not recognize mismatched MHC class I ligands expressed on recipient leukemic cells and, therefore, the inhibitory effect on NK cells with the balance of signals favoring activation and killing of tumor cells. Where donor and recipient are KIR ligand-matched, in spite of being HLA-mismatched, no NK alloreactivity is demonstrable (see Fig. 3B). In a recent update from the University of Perugia of the clinical experience with haplotype-mismatched transplantation for patients with AML, the 5-yr risk of relapse was 79% in the absence of KIR ligand mismatching, as

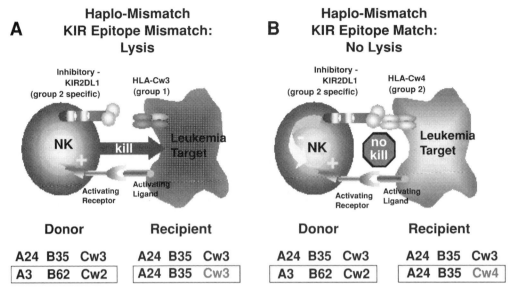

Fig. 3. Killer immunoglobulin-like receptor (KIR)-epitope mismatching in haplotype-mismatched stem cell transplantation. **(A)** In this example, donor and recipient are human leukocyte antigen (HLA) haplotype-mismatched and are KIR-epitope mismatched at the *HLA-C* locus. The donor NK cell clones expressing KIR2DL1 recognize and are inhibited by an epitope shared by the group 2 HLA-C alleles (HLA-Cw2, -Cw4, -Cw5, and -Cw6). The recipient's leukemic blasts express HLA-Cw3, a member of the group 1 HLA-C alleles, and are therefore not recognized by the donor's KIR2DL1, and activation of donor NK cell occurs with leukemic cell lysis. **(B)** Here, donor and recipient are haplotype-mismatched, but express HLA-C alleles of the same supertype group 2 (HLA-Cw2, -Cw4, -Cw5, and -Cw6). Therefore, donor NK cell clones expressing the inhibitory KIR2DL1 recognize a "self-epitope" (HLA-Cw4) on the recipient's cells with inhibition of lysis of leukemic blasts. KIR epitope mismatching exerts another level of graft alloreactivity and a potent graft-vs-leukemia effect. (Reprinted with permission from ref. *107*.)

compared to 17% where KIR ligand mismatch in the GVH direction existed ($p < 0.005$). The 5-yr survival for the KIR-mismatched group was 59% compared with 7% in KIR-matched patients ($p < 0.005$). KIR ligand incompatibility in the GVH direction was the only independent predictor of survival on multivariable analysis. Of note, however, an antileukemic effect of engrafted NK cells was not observed in patients with acute lymphoblastic leukemia where the tumor cells did not express the adhesion molecule lymphocyte function antigen 1 *(98)*, indicating that other molecules, in addition to KIR and their ligands, are also important. However, the possibility that the difference between acute lymphoblastic leukemia and AML blasts in their susceptibility to alloreactive NK cell-mediated killing might also be related to differences in expression of activating ligands has not been examined.

In spite of the antileukemic effect of alloreactive NK cells, KIR ligand mismatching in the T cell-depleted, haplotype-mismatched setting was not associated with GVHD *(98,99)*. Although this observation may be explained by differences in expression of activating ligands between hematopoietic and nonhematopoietic cells, evidence also exists for a direct effect of alloreactive NK cells on host antigen-presenting cells *(99)*, which are known to be important in the pathogenesis of GVHD *(100)*. In a mouse model, the infusion of high numbers of purified alloreactive NK cells into lethally irradiated mice not only failed to produce GVHD, but also actually prevented it by killing host antigen-presenting cells. Furthermore, the infusion of alloreactive NK cells permitted the safe add-back of 20 times the lethal dose of allogeneic T-cells *(99)*. Finally, infusion of alloreactive NK cells in nonlethally irradiated mice also facilitated engraftment, suggesting that engraftment of MHC disparate bone marrow following reduced-intensity regimens may be promoted by alloreactive NK cells. These findings provide rationale for the use of alloreactive NK cells as part of the preparative regimen in nonmyeloablative transplants, which may extend this approach to older and more medically frail patients, as well as permit the infusion of greater numbers of T-cells in the graft to improve posttransplant immune function. In addition, adoptive infusion of alloreactive NK cells posttransplant may improve immune function and may prevent or treat relapse in high-risk patients. Clinical trials to test prospectively these hypotheses are awaited.

5.4.2. KIR Ligand Mismatching in Unrelated Donor Transplantation

A similar opportunity to mismatch for KIR ligands also exists in the unrelated donor transplant setting. Whereas no prospective studies have been conducted, retrospective analyses of large data sets have yielded conflicting results as to the potential benefit of this approach. In a study that compared the outcome of 20 KIR ligand-mismatched unrelated donor transplants to that of 110 transplants where incompatibility was not present, significantly superior 4.5-yr disease-free survival (87 vs 39%, $p = 0.0007$) and overall survival (87 vs 48%, $p = 0.006$) were observed for KIR-mismatched transplants *(101)*. This effect was most pronounced in patients with myeloid malignancies, and was largely related to a reduced risk of relapse rather than a reduction in acute GVHD. In the latter study, in vivo T-cell depletion with antithymocyte globulin was uniformly used, but post-transplant immunosuppression with cyclosporine and methotrexate was used. A beneficial effect of KIR ligand mismatching has not been demonstrated in larger studies. A retrospective analysis of 175 mismatched unrelated donor transplants did not demonstrate any beneficial effect of KIR ligand incompatibility in the GVH direction with respect to the risks of severe GVHD, relapse, or overall survival *(102)*. Indeed, an increase in the risk of acute GVHD was reported in another larger study *(103)*. Furthermore, in a large study of over 1700 unrelated donor transplants mismatched at HLA-B and/or -C for myeloid malignancies, reported by the KIR study Group of the Center for International Blood and Marrow Transplant Research, KIR ligand incompatibility in the GVH direction was associated with an increased risk of grade II–IV acute GVHD, extensive chronic GVHD, treatment-related mortality, and shorter leukemia-free survival and overall survival compared to HLA-matched transplants *(104)*. The adverse effect of KIR ligand incompatibility was not apparent in ex vivo T-cell-depleted transplants, although the number of T-cell-depleted transplants was too small to reach definitive conclusions.

The reasons for the differences in results between studies are not entirely clear; however, it is likely that peritransplant conditions under which KIR epitope mismatching results in NK cell alloreactivity are important. In all the latter studies in unrelated donor transplants, it is unknown if the transplant conditions resulted in emergence of alloreactive clones posttransplant, as these were not assayed. The lack of T-cell depletion, use of post-transplant immunosuppression, and/or the occurrence of GVHD and other complications may possibly have adversely affected NK cell development. Recent data suggest that KIR reconstitution posttransplant is significantly diminished following T-cell-replete compared with T-cell-depleted transplants *(105)*, and that the lack of T-cell depletion may favor the development of activating KIRs on NK cells posttransplant *(106)*, which may, in turn, adversely affect outcome by increasing the risk of GVHD. The significance of the peritransplant conditions on the development of alloreactive NK cells and their receptor repertoire requires further investigation. It is possible that a beneficial effect of KIR ligand mismatching in unrelated donor transplants will be observed if transplants are performed under similar conditions as those previously reported for haplotype-mismatched transplants, where a beneficial effect of KIR ligand incompatibility was observed.

6. CONCLUSIONS

The antileukemic activity of NK cells remains a potentially powerful tool for the immunotherapy of hematological malignancies, as well as other cancers. The optimal use of NK cells in the treatment, however, will depend on careful consideration of NK cell receptor mechanisms in target cell recognition. Novel directions exploiting the ADCC potential of autologous NK cells using combinations of cytokines to expand efficiently NK cells in vivo for use with tumor-specific MAbs are currently under investigation. A particularly exciting approach will be the use of antibodies to block inhibitory interactions of autologous NK cells with tumor cells. Such antibodies are currently under development for clinical use, and the next few years should allow a better appreciation of the feasibility and efficacy of this approach. Manipulation of alloreactive NK cells in the mismatched transplant setting may permit safer and more effective application of the procedure to a greater number of patients who may benefit from this approach. Whereas most investigations to date have focused on KIR receptors on NK cells, it is likely that better appreciation of activating ligand expression on target cells will lead to better patient and disease selection for NK cell-based immunotherapy. The success and limitation of the approaches discussed in this chapter are likely be defined in the coming decade.

REFERENCES

1. Horowitz MM, Gale RP, Sondel PM, et al Graft-versus-leukemia reactions after bone marrow transplantation. *Blood* 1990; 75:555–562.
2. Allavena P, Damia G, Colombo T, et al. Lymphokine-activated killer (LAK) and monocyte-mediated cytotoxicity on tumor cell lines resistant to antitumor agents. *Cell Immunol* 1989; 120:250–258.
3. Landay AL, Zarcone D, Grossi CE, et al. Relationship between target cell cycle and susceptibility to natural killer lysis. *Cancer Res* 1987; 47:2767–2670.
4. Oshimi K, Oshimi Y, Akutsu M, et al. Cytotoxicity of interleukin 2-activated lymphocytes for leukemia and lymphoma cells. *Blood* 1986; 68:938–948.
5. Robertson MJ, Ritz J. Biology and clinical relevance of human natural killer cells. *Blood* 1990; 76: 2421–2438.
6. Trinchieri G. Biology of natural killer cells. *Adv Immunol* 1989; 47:187–376.
7. Cooper MA, Fehniger TA, Caligiuri MA. The biology of human natural killer-cell subsets. *Trends Immunol* 2001; 22:633–640.
8. Cooper MA, Fehniger TA, Turner SC, et al. Human natural killer cells: a unique innate immunoregulatory role for the CD56(bright) subset. *Blood* 2001; 97:3146–3151.
9. Caligiuri MA, Zmuidzinas A, Manley TJ, et al. Functional consequences of interleukin 2 receptor expression on resting human lymphocytes. Identification of a novel natural killer cell subset with high affinity receptors. *J Exp Med* 1990; 171:1509–1526.
10. Baume DM, Robertson MJ, Levine H, et al. Differential responses to interleukin 2 define functionally distinct subsets of human natural killer cells. *Eur J Immunol* 1992; 22:1–6.
11. Caligiuri MA, Murray C, Robertson MJ, et al. Selective modulation of human natural killer cells in vivo after prolonged infusion of low dose recombinant interleukin 2. *J Clin Invest* 1993; 91:123–132.

12. Nagler A, Lanier LL, Phillips JH. Constitutive expression of high affinity interleukin 2 receptors on human CD16-natural killer cells in vivo. *J Exp Med* 1990; 171:1527–1533.

13. Robertson MJ, Soiffer RJ, Wolf SF, et al. Response of human natural killer (NK) cells to NK cell stimulatory factor (NKSF): cytolytic activity and proliferation of NK cells are differentially regulated by NKSF. *J Exp Med* 1992; 175:779–788.

14. Mrozek E, Anderson P, Caligiuri MA. Role of interleukin-15 in the development of human CD56+ natural killer cells from CD34+ hematopoietic progenitor cells. *Blood* 1996; 87:2632–2640.

15. Fehniger TA, Caligiuri MA. Ontogeny and expansion of human natural killer cells: clinical implications. *Int Rev Immunol* 2001; 20:503–534.

16. Fehniger TA, Caligiuri MA. Interleukin 15: biology and relevance to human disease. *Blood* 2001; 9: 14–32.

17. Fehniger TA, Cooper MA, Caligiuri MA. Interleukin-2 and interleukin-15: immunotherapy for cancer. *Cytokine Growth Factor Rev* 2002; 13:169–183.

18. Lim SH, Newland AC, Kelsey S, et al. Continuous intravenous infusion of high-dose recombinant interleukin-2 for acute myeloid leukaemia—a phase II study. *Cancer Immunol Immunother* 1992; 34: 337–342.

19. Maraninchi D, Vey N, Viens P, et al. A phase II study of interleukin-2 in 49 patients with relapsed or refractory acute leukemia. *Leuk Lymphoma* 1998; 31:343–349.

20. Meloni G, Foa R, Vignetti M, et al. Interleukin-2 may induce prolonged remissions in advanced acute myelogenous leukemia. *Blood* 1994; 84:2158–2163.

21. Meloni G, Vignetti M, Andrizzi C, et al. Interleukin-2 for the treatment of advanced acute myelogenous leukemia patients with limited disease: updated experience with 20 cases. *Leuk Lymphoma* 1996; 21: 429–435.

22. Olive D, Chambost H, Sainty D, et al. Modifications of leukemic blast cells induced by in vivo high-dose recombinant interleukin-2. *Leukemia* 1994; 8:1230–1235.

23. Foa R, Meloni G, Tosti S, et al. Treatment of residual disease in acute leukemia patients with recombinant interleukin 2 (IL2): clinical and biological findings. *Bone Marrow Transplant* 1990; 6:98–102.

24. Meloni G, Vignetti M, Pogliani E, et al. Interleukin-2 therapy in relapsed acute myelogenous leukemia. *Cancer J Sci Am* 1997; 3:S43–S47.

25. Caligiuri MA, Murray C, Soiffer RJ, et al. Extended continuous infusion low-dose recombinant interleukin-2 in advanced cancer: prolonged immunomodulation without significant toxicity. *J Clin Oncol* 1991; 9:2110–2119.

26. Bernstein ZP, Porter MM, Gould M, et al. Prolonged administration of low-dose interleukin-2 in human immunodeficiency virus-associated malignancy results in selective expansion of innate immune effectors without significant clinical toxicity. *Blood* 1995; 86:3287–3294.

27. Bernstein ZP, Khatri V, Poiesz B, et al. Phase I/II study of daily subcutaneous (sc) low dose interleukin-2 (IL-2) in AIDS-associated lymphomas (AIDS-NHL). *Blood* 1998; 92:625a.

28. Farag SS, George SL, Lee EJ, et al. Postremission therapy with low-dose interleukin 2 with or without intermediate pulse dose interleukin 2 therapy is well tolerated in elderly patients with acute myeloid leukemia: Cancer and Leukemia Group B study 9420. Clin *Cancer Res* 2002; 8: 2812–2819.

29. Cortes JE, Kantarjian HM, O'Brien S, et al. A pilot study of interleukin-2 for adult patients with acute myelogenous leukemia in first complete remission. *Cancer* 1999; 85:1506–1513.

30. Gisselbrecht C, Maraninchi D, Pico JL, et al. Interleukin-2 treatment in lymphoma: a phase II multicenter study *Blood* 1994; 83:2081–2085.

31. Duggan DB, Santarelli MT, Zamkoff K, et al. A phase II study of recombinant interleukin-2 with or without recombinant interferon-beta in non-Hodgkin's lymphoma. A study of the Cancer and Leukemia Group B. *J Immunother* 1992; 12:115–122.

32. Blaise D, Attal M, Reiffers J, et al. Randomized study of recombinant interleukin-2 after autologous bone marrow transplantation for acute leukemia in first complete remission. *Eur Cytokine Netw* 2000; 11:91–98.

33. Gonzalez-Barca E, Granena A, Fernandez-Sevilla A, et al. Low-dose subcutaneous interleukin-2 in patients with minimal residual lymphoid neoplasm disease. *Eur J Haematol* 1999; 62:231–238.

34. Raspadori D, Lauria F, Ventura MA, et al. Low doses of rIL2 after autologous bone marrow transplantation induce a "prolonged" immunostimulation of NK compartment in high-grade non-Hodgkin's lymphomas. *Ann Hematol* 1995; 71:175–191.

35. Vey N, Blaise D, Tiberghien P, et al. A pilot study of autologous bone marrow transplantation followed by recombinant interleukin-2 in malignant lymphomas. *Leuk Lymphoma* 1996; 21:107–114.

36. Lauria F, Raspadori D, Ventura MA, et al. Immunologic and clinical modifications following low-dose subcutaneous administration of rIL-2 in non-Hodgkin's lymphoma patients after autologous bone marrow transplantation. *Bone Marrow Transplant* 1996; 18:79–85.

37. van Besien K, Margolin K, Champlin R, et al. Activity of interleukin-2 in non-Hodgkin's lymphoma following transplantation of interleukin-2-activated autologous bone marrow or stem cells. *Cancer J Sci Am* 1997; 3:S54–S58.

38. Storkus WJ, Alexander J, Payne JA, et al. Reversal of natural killing susceptibility in target cells expressing transfected class I HLA genes. *Proc Natl Acad Sci USA* 1989; 86:2361–2364.

39. Shimizu Y, DeMars R. Demonstration by class I gene transfer that reduced susceptibility of human cells to natural killer cell-mediated lysis is inversely correlated with HLA class I antigen expression. *Eur J Immunol* 1989; 19:447–451.

40. Zijlstra M, Auchincloss H Jr, Loring JM, et al. Skin graft rejection by beta 2-microglobulin-deficient mice. *J Exp Med* 1992; 175: 885–893.

41. Malnati MS, Lusso P, Ciccone E, et al. Recognition of virus-infected cells by natural killer cell clones is controlled by polymorphic target cell elements. *J Exp Med* 1993; 178: 961–969.

42. Moretta A, Bottino C, Pende D, et al. Identification of four subsets of human CD3-CD16+ natural killer (NK) cells by the expression of clonally distributed functional surface molecules: correlation between subset assignment of NK clones and ability to mediate specific alloantigen recognition. *J Exp Med* 1990; 172:1589–1598.

43. Mandelboim O, Reyburn HT, Vales-Gomez M, et al. Protection from lysis by natural killer cells of group 1 and 2 specificity is mediated by residue 80 in human histocompatibility leukocyte antigen C alleles and also occurs with empty major histocompatibility complex molecules. *J Exp Med* 1996; 184:913–922.

44. Biassoni R, Falco M, Cambiaggi A, et al. Amino acid substitutions can influence the natural killer (NK)-mediated recognition of HLA-C molecules. Role of serine-77 and lysine-80 in the target cell protection from lysis mediated by "group 2" or "group 1" NK clones. *J Exp Med* 1995; 182:605–609.

45. Winter CC, Gumperz JE, Parham P, et al. Direct binding and functional transfer of NK cell inhibitory receptors reveal novel patterns of HLA-C allotype recognition. *J Immunol* 1998; 161:571–577.

46. Rojo S, Wagtmann N, Long EO. Binding of a soluble p70 killer cell inhibitory receptor to HLA-B*5101: requirement for all three p70 immunoglobulin domains. *Eur J Immunol* 1997; 27:568–571.

47. Gumperz JE, Barber LD, Valiante NM, et al. Conserved and variable residues within the Bw4 motif of HLA-B make separable contributions to recognition by the NKB1 killer cell-inhibitory receptor. *J Immunol* 1997; 158:5237–5241.

48. Dohring C, Scheidegger D, Samaridis J, et al. A human killer inhibitory receptor specific for HLA-A1,2. *J Immunol* 1996; 156:3098–3101.

49. Lanier LL. Activating and inhibitory NK cell receptors. *Adv Exp Med Biol* 1998; 452:13–18.

50. Wilson MJ, Torkar M, Trowsdale J. Genomic organization of a human killer cell inhibitory receptor gene. *Tissue Antigens* 1997; 49:574–579.

51. Vilches C, Parham P. KIR: diverse, rapidly evolving receptors of innate and adaptive immunity. *Annu Rev Immunol* 2002; 20:217–251.

52. Shilling HG, Guethlein LA, Cheng NW, et al. Allelic polymorphism synergizes with variable gene content to individualize human KIR genotype. *J Immunol* 2002; 168:2307–2315.

53. Chang C, Rodriguez A, Carretero M, et al. Molecular characterization of human CD94: a type II membrane glycoprotein related to the C-type lectin superfamily. *Eur J Immunol* 1995; 25:2433–2437.

54. Braud VM, Allan DS, O'Callaghan CA, et al. HLA-E binds to natural killer cell receptors CD94/NKG2A, B and C. *Nature* 1998; 391:795–799.

55. Borrego F, Ulbrecht M, Weiss EH, et al. Recognition of human histocompatibility leukocyte antigen (HLA)-E complexed with HLA class I signal sequence-derived peptides by CD94/NKG2 confers protection from natural killer cell-mediated lysis. *J Exp Med* 1998; 187:813–818.

56. Glienke J, Sobanov Y, Brostjan C, et al. The genomic organization of NKG2C, E, F, and D receptor genes in the human natural killer gene complex. *Immunogenetics* 1998; 48:163–173.

57. Sobanov Y, Glienke J, Brostjan C, et al. Linkage of the NKG2 and CD94 receptor genes to D12S77 in the human natural killer gene complex. *Immunogenetics* 1999; 49:99–105.

58. Shilling HG, McQueen KL, Cheng NW, et al. Reconstitution of NK cell receptor repertoire following HLA-matched hematopoietic cell transplantation. *Blood* 2003; 101:3730–3740.

59. Vales-Gomez M, Reyburn HT, Mandelboim M, et al. Kinetics of interaction of HLA-C ligands with natural killer cell inhibitory receptors. *Immunity* 1998; 9:337–344.

60. Vales-Gomez M, Reyburn HT, Erskine RA, et al. Kinetics and peptide dependency of the binding of the inhibitory NK receptor CD94/NKG2-A and the activating receptor CD94/NKG2-C to HLA-E. *EMBO J* 1999; 18:4250–4260.

61. Valiante NM, Uhrberg M, Shilling HG, et al Functionally and structurally distinct NK cell receptor repertoires in the peripheral blood of two human donors. *Immunity* 1997; 7:739–751.

62. Uhrberg M, Valiante NM, Shum BP, et al. Human diversity in killer cell inhibitory receptor genes. *Immunity* 1997; 7:753–763.

63. Moretta A, Bottino C, Vitale M, et al. Activating receptors and coreceptors involved in human natural killer cell-mediated cytolysis. *Annu Rev Immunol* 2001; 19:197–223.

64. Bauer S, Groh V, Wu J, et al. Activation of NK cells and T cells by NKG2D, a receptor for stress-inducible MICA [*see* comment]. *Science* 1999; 285:727–729.

65. Pende D, Parolini S, Pessino A, et al. Identification and molecular characterization of NKp30, a novel triggering receptor involved in natural cytotoxicity mediated by human natural killer cells. *J Exp Med* 1999; 190:1505–1516.

66. Sivori S, Vitale M, Morelli L, et al. p46, a novel natural killer cell-specific surface molecule that mediates cell activation. *J Exp Med* 1997; 186:1129–1136.

67. Vitale M, Bottino C, Sivori S, et al. NKp44, a novel triggering surface molecule specifically expressed by activated natural killer cells, is involved in non-major histocompatibility complex-restricted tumor cell lysis. *J Exp Med* 1998; 187:2065–2072.

68. Arnon TI, Lev M, Katz G, et al. Recognition of viral hemagglutinins by NKp44 but not by NKp30. *Eur J Immunol* 2001; 31:2680–2689.

69. Mandelboim O, Lieberman N, Lev M, et al. Recognition of haemagglutinins on virus-infected cells by NKp46 activates lysis by human NK cells. *Nature* 2001; 409:1055–1060.

70. Cantoni C, Bottino C, Vitale M, et al. NKp44, a triggering receptor involved in tumor cell lysis by activated human natural killer cells, is a novel member of the immunoglobulin superfamily. *J Exp Med* 1999; 189:787–796.

71. Pessino A, Sivori S, Bottino C, et al. Molecular cloning of NKp46: a novel member of the immunoglobulin superfamily involved in triggering of natural cytotoxicity. *J Exp Med* 1998; 188:953–960.

72. Pende D, Cantoni C, Rivera P, et al. Role of NKG2D in tumor cell lysis mediated by human NK cells: cooperation with natural cytotoxicity receptors and capability of recognizing tumors of nonepithelial origin. *Eur J Immunol* 2001; 31:1076–1086.

73. Bahram S. MIC genes: from genetics to biology. *Adv Immunol* 2000; 76:1–60.

74. Sutherland CL, Chalupny NJ, Schooley K, et al. UL16-binding proteins, novel MHC class I-related proteins, bind to NKG2D and activate multiple signaling pathways in primary NK cells. *J Immunol* 2002; 168:671–679.

75. Groh V, Rhinehart R, Randolph-Habecker J, et al. Costimulation of CD8alphabeta T cells by NKG2D via engagement by MIC induced on virus-infected cells. *Nat Immunol* 2001; 2:255–260.

76. Wetzler M, Baer MR, Stewart SJ, et al. HLA class I antigen cell surface expression is preserved on acute myeloid leukemia blasts at diagnosis and at relapse. *Leukemia* 2001; 15:128–133.

77. Frohn C, Hoppner M, Schlenke P, et al. Anti-myeloma activity of natural killer lymphocytes. *Br J Haematol* 2002; 119:660–664.

78. Igarashi T, Srinivasan R, Wynberg J, et al. Generation of alloreactive NK cells with selective cytotoxicity to melanoma and renal cell carcinoma based on KIR-ligand incompatibility. *Blood* 2002; 100:73a.

79. Handgretinger R, Lang P, Schumm M, et al. Immuological aspects of haploidentical stem cell transplantation. *Ann NY Acad Sci* 2001; 938:340–357.

80. Koh CY, Blazar BR, George T, et al. Augmentation of antitumor effects by NK cell inhibitory receptor blockade in vitro and in vivo. *Blood* 2001; 97:3132–3137.

81. Clynes RA, Towers TL, Presta LG, et al. Inhibitory Fc receptors modulate in vivo cytoxicity against tumor targets. *Nat Med* 2000; 6:443–446.

82. Cartron G, Dacheux L, Salles G, et al. Therapeutic activity of humanized anti-CD20 monoclonal antibody and polymorphism in IgG Fc receptor FcgammaRIIIa gene. *Blood* 2002; 99:754–758.

83. Kono K, Takahashi A, Ichihara F, et al. Impaired antibody-dependent cellular cytotoxicity mediated by herceptin in patients with gastric cancer. *Cancer Res* 2002; 62:5813–5817.

84. Costello RT, Sivori S, Marcenaro E, et al. Defective expression and function of natural killer cell-triggering receptors in patients with acute myeloid leukemia. *Blood* 2002; 99:3661–3667.

85. Dabholkar M, Tatake R, Amin K, et al. Modulation of natural killer and antibody-dependent cellular cytotoxicity by interferon and interleukin-2 in chronic myeloid leukemia patients in remission. *Oncology* 1989; 46:123–137.

86. Hank JA, Robinson RR, Surfus J, et al. Augmentation of antibody dependent cell-mediated cytotoxicity following in vivo therapy with recombinant interleukin 2. *Cancer Res* 1990; 50:5234–5239.

87. Masucci G, Ragnhammar P, Wersall P, et al. Granulocyte-monocyte colony-stimulating-factor augments the interleukin-2-induced cytotoxic activity of human lymphocytes in the absence and presence of mouse or chimeric monoclonal antibodies (mAb 17-1A). *Cancer Immunol Immunother* 1990; 31:231–235.

88. Carson WE, Giri JG, Lindemann MJ, et al. Interleukin (IL) 15 is a novel cytokine that activates human natural killer cells via components of the IL-2 receptor. *J Exp Med* 1994; 180:1395–1403.

89. Carson WE, Parihar R, Lindemann MJ, et al. Interleukin-2 enhances the natural killer cell response to Herceptin-coated Her2/neu-positive breast cancer cells. *Eur J Immunol* 2001; 31:3016–3025.

90. Nguyen QH, Roberts RL, Ank BJ, et al. Interleukin (IL)-15 enhances antibody-dependent cellular cytotoxicity and natural killer activity in neonatal cells. *Cell Immunol* 1998; 185:83–92.

91. Friedberg JW, Neuberg D, Gribben JG, et al. Combination immunotherapy with rituximab and interleukin 2 in patients with relapsed or refractory follicular non-Hodgkin's lymphoma. *Br J Haematol* 2002; 117:828–834.

92. Morgensztern D, Wolin M, Rosenblatt J. Interleukin-2 and rituximab in lymphoma: rationale and current trials. *Biol Ther Lymphoma* 2002; 5:12–14.

93. Ansell SM, Witzig TE, Kurtin PJ, et al. Phase 1 study of interleukin-12 in combination with rituximab in patients with B-cell non-Hodgkin lymphoma. *Blood* 2002; 99:67–74.

94. Farag SS, Flinn I, Lehman T, et al. FcgammaRIIIa an FcgammaIIa polymorphisms do not predict response to rituximab in B-cell chronic lymphocytic leukemia. *Blood* 2004; 103:1472–1474.

95. Kossman SE, Scheinberg DA, Jurcic JG, et al. A phase I trial of humanized monoclonal antibody HuM195 (anti-CD33) with low-dose interleukin 2 in acute myelogenous leukemia. *Clin Cancer Res* 1999; 5:2748–2755.

96. Caron PC, Co MS, Bull MK, et al. Biological and immunological features of humanized M195 (anti-CD33) monoclonal antibodies. *Cancer Res* 1992; 52:6761–6767.

97. Weng W, Levy R. Rituximab-induced antibody-dependent cellular cytotoxicity (ADCC) in follicular non-Hodgkin's lymphoma. *Blood* 2002; 100:157a.

98. Ruggeri L, Capanni M, Casucci M, et al. Role of natural killer cell alloreactivity in HLA-mismatched hematopoietic stem cell transplantation. *Blood* 1999; 94:333–339.

99. Ruggeri L, Capanni M, Urbani E, et al. Effectiveness of donor natural killer call alloreactivity in mismatched hematopoietic transplants. *Science* 2002; 295:2097–3100.

100. Shlomchik WD, Couzens MS, Tang CB, et al. Prevention of graft versus host disease by inactivation of host antigen-presenting cells. *Science* 1999; 285:412–415.

101. Geibel S, Locatelli F, Maccario R, et al. Survival advantage with KIR ligand incompatibility in unrelated donor transplantation. *Blood* 2003; 102:814–819.

102. Davies SM, Ruggeri L, DeFor T, et al. Evaluation of KIR ligand incompatibility in mismatched unrelated donor hematopoietic transplants. Killer immunoglobulin-like receptor. *Blood* 2002; 100:3825–3827.

103. Morishima Y, Yabe T, Inoko H, et al. Clinical significance of killer Ig-like receptor (KIR) on acute GVHD, rejection, and leukemia relapse in patients transplanted non-T cell depleted marrow from unrelated donors; roles of inhibitory KIR epitope matching and activating KIR genotype. *Blood* 2003; 102:153a.

104. Farag SS, Bacigalupo A, Dupont B, et al. The effect of killer immunoglobulin-like receptor (KIR) ligand incompatibility on outcome of unrelated donor bone marrow transplantation. *Blood* 2004; 104:127a.

105. Miller JS, Xiao F, McCullar V, et al. NK cell killer immunoglobulin receptor reconstitution is diminished in recipients of unrelated donor transplants who receive unmanipulated (T-cell replete) marrow grafts. *Blood* 2003; 102:726a.

106. Gagne K, Brizard G, Gueglio B, et al. Relevance of KIR gene polymorphisms in *Bone Marrow Transplant*ation outcome. *Hum Immunol* 2002; 63:27–280.

107. Farag SS, Fehniger TA, Ruggeri L, Velardi A, Caligiuri MA. Natural killer cell receptors: new biology and insights into the graft-versus-leukemia effect. *Blood* 2002; 100:1935–1947.

24 Antibody Therapy for Solid Tumors

*Cristina I. Truica, Dorinda Rouch,
and Carlos L. Arteaga*

SUMMARY

Over the last several years the use of monoclonal antibody (MAb) therapy for the treatment of human malignancy has advanced from experimental therapy to standard of care for some malignancies. The success of MAb therapy stems not only from the ability to humanize the antibody, thus, decreasing the inherent immunogenicity of the approach but also from targeting appropriate proteins. Human cancers associated with the overexpression of particular growth factor receptors such as HER-2/neu, epidermal growth factor receptor, and vascular endothelial growth factor, have been impacted by commercially available antibodies. This review focuses on the mechanisms of action and clinical benefit of MAb therapy against common growth factor receptors.

Key Words: Monoclonal antibody; EGFR; HER-2/neu; VEGF; growth factor receptors.

1. INTRODUCTION

For almost a century, scientists and physicians have toiled with the idea of using antibodies for the treatment of tumors. The first breakthrough came in the 1950s, when administration of pooled sera to cancer patients was noted to induce tumor regression. However, the development of antibodies for therapeutic use continued to be hampered by the limited availability of pooled sera for clinical trials, and because the immune system of the patients treated did not recognize cancer cells as foreign. In the 1970s, a tremendous boost came from the discovery of hybridoma technology (as described by Kohler and Milstein) that allowed for massive production of monoclonal antibodies (MAbs) against tumor cells. The first antibodies were completely murine, obtained from mice exposed to specific human tumor antigens. Murine antibodies were frequently associated with allergic reactions and the development of neutralizing antibodies, or human antimurine antibodies.

During the 1980s, advances in DNA recombinant technology allowed for the engineering of chimeric or completely humanized antibodies by replacing most of the structure of the antibody with human immunoglobulin (Ig)G. Chimeric antibodies retain the murine variable regions, whereas in humanized antibodies, only the hypervariable regions are murine. This reduced the antigenicity of the antibodies and essentially eliminated the problem of neutralization, while also giving a better toxicity profile and longer half-life.

From: *Cancer Drug Discovery and Development: Immunotherapy of Cancer*
Edited by: M. L. Disis © Humana Press Inc., Totowa, NJ

Further progress in the development of therapeutic antibodies for the treatment of solid tumors came from the identification of better targets on the cancer cells. The ideal molecular target is (1) essential for cancer pathogenesis and/or tumor progression and viability, (2) not essential for host organ function, (3) stably and homogenously expressed by tumor cells and minimally expressed by normal host tissues, and (4) found in minimal quantity in soluble form to avoid rapid clearance. The target should also correlate with clinical outcome, and its inhibition should lead to a clinical response in patients. In addition, it is becoming increasingly recognized that the success of targeted therapy relies on the ability to measure reproducibly the target in clinical samples and on the ability to select the patients based on the presence of the specified target *(1)*.

2. ANTIBODIES AGAINST THE EPIDERMAL GROWTH FACTOR FAMILY

The epidermal growth factor receptor (EGFR) family of transmembrane tyrosine kinases regulates intracellular signal transduction pathways that control normal cell growth and differentiation. They belong to the type I receptor tyrosine kinase family and consist of four members: ErbB1 (EGFR or HER-1), ErbB2 (HER-2/*neu*), ErbB3 (HER-3), and ErbB4 (HER-4). All four receptors have three different domains: an N-terminal extracellular domain that recognizes and binds ligands to activate the receptor, the transmembrane domain that spans the cellular membrane only once, and the C-terminal portion that houses the tyrosine kinase and regulatory phosphorylation sites. ErbB-3 has impaired tyrosine kinase activity (reviewed in refs. *2* and *3*).

An ErbB receptor is activated when a peptide ligand binds to its extracellular domain. The ligands that bind to ErbB-1 include EGF, transforming growth factor-α, amphiregulin, epiregulin, betacellulin, and heparin-binding EGF-like growth factor. The ligands for ErbB-3 include neuroregulin (NRG)-1/heregulin isoforms and NRG-α and -β. The ligands for ErbB-4 include NRG-1/heregulin isoforms, NRG-2α and -β, NRG-3, NRG-4, heparin-binding EGF-like growth factor, betacellulin, and epiregulin *(4)*. There is no known ligand for ErbB2.

Once the ligand binds the receptor, dimerization must occur in order for the tyrosine kinase to be active. The receptors can pair with receptors of the same type (homodimerization) or of another type (heterodimerization). All combinations of heterodimers have been identified, but the three most frequent heterodimers include ErbB-2/ErbB-3, ErbB-2/ErbB4, and Erb-B1/ErbB-4. ErbB-2 seems to be the preferred dimerization partner for the other three ErbB receptors *(5)*. By forming heterodimers, the lack of ligand for ErbB-2 and impaired tyrosine kinase of ErbB-3 can be overcome. Interestingly, ErbB-2/ErbB-3 heterodimers are the most potent in inducing mitogenesis and cell transformation *(6)*.

The ErbB receptors and their ligands, in particular ErbB-1 and ErbB-2, are often overexpressed in human carcinomas. The overexpression and/or gene amplification of ErbB receptors, coupled or not with ligand overexpression, until recently have been thought the only mechanisms by which these signaling systems increase tumorigenicity and cancer progression. However, three recent studies by Paez et al. *(7)*, Lynch et al. *(8)*, and Pao et al. *(9)* have identified somatic mutations in the *EGFR* gene in patients with non-small cell lung cancer (NSCLC) that had durable clinical responses to the EGFR small-molecule tyrosine kinase inhibitors gefitinib and erlotinib. The mutations were either short, in-frame deletions or substitutions clustered around the region encoding the adenosine triphosphate-binding pocket of the receptor's tyrosine kinase domain. The striking association with a durable clinical response after therapy with EGFR tyrosine kinase inhibitors strongly suggests that these are "gain-of-function" mutations that represent a functional marker of EGFR dependence in NSCLC.

2.1. Anti-HER-2 Antibodies: Trastuzumab (Herceptin)

The *ErbB-2* gene is overexpressed in approx 25% of human breast carcinomas *(10,11)*. When the gene is amplified, a greater number of ErbB-2 receptors are expressed on the cell surface. This may lead to constitutive homodimerization of ErbB-2, rendering it constitutively active. In addition, the presence of ErbB-2 in a heterodimer appears to increase its affinity for ligand binding and decrease the internalization of the heterodimer–ligand complex, thus increasing the length of signaling from the complex *(5,12)*. In vitro, this corresponds to an increase in DNA synthesis, increase in angiogenesis *(13)*, increase in cell growth rate, and an increase in tumorigenicity and metastatic potential *(14)*. In vivo, studies have shown that patients whose tumors overexpress ErbB-2 have a decreased survival and resistance to chemotherapy *(10)*.

Because ErbB-2 is overexpressed in some breast cancer cells, and overexpression of the gene leads to increased tumorigenicity, it became a logical target for antineoplastic therapy. A humanized MAb (trastuzumab) to HER-2 was engineered from a cloned human IgG1 and the antigen binding residues of the murine MAb 4D5 *(15)*. Trastuzumab was first shown to be effective in breast cancer cell lines that overexpressed ErbB-2 *(16)*. In addition, it was effective in animal models. Proposed mechanisms of action include HER-2 downregulation, prevention of heterodimer formation, induction of the Cdk inhibitor p27 and G_1 arrest, prevention of HER-2 cleavage, inhibition of angiogenesis, and induction of host immune response, among others (reviewed in ref. *17*).

Hudziak et al. showed that treating cells with *HER-2* gene amplification with a MAb against the extracellular portion of HER-2 leads to downregulation of the receptor *(18)*. Drebin et al. showed that exposure of neuoncogene-transformed cells to a MAb similar to herceptin decreases both the cell surface and total cellular HER-2 receptor *(19)*. In addition, the cells treated with these antibodies reverted to a nontransformed phenotype. MAbs to ErbB-2 were also found to lead to accelerated endocytic degradation and downregulation of the receptor, and to inhibit heterodimerization with other receptors of the EGFR family. The heterodimers that are formed in the presence of the monoclonal antibody are unstable, and have increased rates of ligand dissociation *(20)*.

In HER-2-overexpressing cells, traztuzumab has increases the number of cells G_1 and decreases the numbers undergoing S phase. The antibody does not affect cell lines expressing low levels of the HER-2 protein or single copies of the *HER-2* gene *(16,21)*. Intriguingly, MAbs to ErbB-2/*neu* have also been shown to decrease vascular endothelial growth factor (VEGF) production. For example, cells transformed by ErbB-2 exposed to a neutralizing monoclonal antibody to ErbB-2 had a dose-depended decrease in VEGF expression. Similar decreases in VEGF expression and decreases in tumor blood vessel counts were seen in vivo *(13)*. Finally, trastuzumab can induce antibody-dependent cell-mediated cytotoxicity (ADCC) against cells that overexpress HER-2. This trastuzumab-dependent ADCC occurs primarily through NK cells and monocytes *(22)*.

Whereas the above mechanisms of action of MAbs to ErbB-2 have been demonstrated in vitro, one recent study has evaluated the effects of trastuzumab in vivo in humans. The study, by Gennari et al. included 11 patients with HER-2-positive metastatic breast cancer who received treatment with trastuzumab for 4 wk *(23)*. The primary tumor was subsequently removed after treatment and analyzed. No tumor had downmodulation of HER-2 or changes in vessel diameter. On the other hand, there was a strong infiltration of lymphoid cells in all cases, with a higher *in situ* infiltration of lymphocytes in patients with complete or partial remissions. These data suggest that ADCC may play a role in the mechanism of action of trastuzumab in vivo.

In 1998, the Food and Drug Administration (FDA) approved trastuzumab for use in women with metastatic breast cancer whose tumors overexpress HER-2/*neu*. Currently, two methods are being used for the detection of HER-2/*neu* expression. The first is by immunohistochemistry (IHC), which detects the overexpression of the HER-2/*neu* gene product *(24)*. The second is fluorescence *in situ* hybridization (FISH), which detects HER-2/*neu* gene amplification. Both tests can be performed on paraffin-embedded tissue. Whereas there is some controversy regarding the consistency of results when IHC is used, IHC is less expensive than FISH, and has been shown to have a high level of correlation with FISH in the evaluation of HER2/*neu* status in breast cancers *(25)*. (Most practitioners obtain a FISH study only if the IHC score is 2+.)

Single-agent trastuzumab is usually administered as a loading dose of 4 mg/kg intravenously, followed by 2 mg/kg weekly. However, given its long half-life (approx 28 d), an alternative schedule has been evaluated, with a loading dose of 8 mg/kg, followed by 6 mg/kg every 3 wk. The latter schedule of every 3-wk trastuzumab has been evaluated in combination with paclitaxel, and has been shown safe and well tolerated *(26)*. The most common side effects of trastuzumab given weekly or every 3 wk are infusion-related. These may occur in up to 40% of patients and include fever and chills. Most reactions are mild and can be controlled with acetaminophen and diphenhydramine, but anaphylaxis has been reported. Trastuzumab has also been associated with cardiac toxicity. The risk factors for trastuzumab-induced cardiotoxicity include previous concomitant treatment with anthracyclines, age greater than 50 yr, previous cardiac disease, and a history of hyperlipidemia. The incidence of congestive heart failure may be as high as 28% in patients receiving trastuzumab in combination with anthracyclines, compared with 3.6% in patients receiving trastuzumab alone *(27)*. Based on this increased incidence of congestive heart failure, left ventricular function should be evaluated in patients before and during treatment with trastuzumab.

The efficacy of trastuzumab as monotherapy was evaluated in 222 women with HER-2/*neu*-overexpressing metastatic breast cancer that progressed after previous chemotherapy. The patients had up to two previous chemotherapy regimens. The objective response rate of single-agent trastuzumab was 15%, and the median duration of response was 9.1 mo, with a median survival of 13 mo *(28)*. When used as single agent in the first-line treatment of HER-2-overexpressing metastatic breast cancer, an objective response rate of 35% was seen in those patients whose tumors had 3+ overexpression of HER-2 by IHC *(29)*.

Trastuzumab has been also studied in combination with cytotoxic chemotherapy. In a randomized phase III trial comparing chemotherapy alone or chemotherapy plus trastuzumab as the initial treatment in women with HER-2-positive metastatic breast cancer, trastuzumab was found to increase the clinical benefit of chemotherapy. Specifically, 281 women were assigned to receive an anthracycline (doxorubicin or epirubicin) plus cyclophosphamide, with or without trastuzumab, if they had no previous anthracycline therapy, or a taxane, with or without trastuzumab, if they had adjuvant therapy with an anthracycline. The addition of trastuzumab to chemotherapy was associated with a longer time to disease progression (7.4 vs 4.6 mo; $p < 0.001$), higher rate of objective response (50 vs 32%; $p < 0.001$), a longer duration of response (median 9.1 vs 6.1 mo; $p < 0.001$), a lower rate of death at 1 yr (22% vs 33%; $p > 0.008$), and a longer survival (median survival 25.1 vs 20.3 mo; $p > 0.046$). There was a higher incidence of cardiotoxicity when trastuzumab was used with adriamycin and cytoxan (30).

Whereas the above study assessed trastuzumab in combination with adriamycin and cytoxan or paclitaxel, preclinical studies have indicated that the antibody may be synergistic with other chemotherapeutic agents, such as carboplatin, cyclophosphamide, docetaxel, and vinorelbine (31). Pegram et al. conducted two open-label, multicenter phase II studies combining docetaxel, carboplatin or cisplatin, and trastuzumab in women with HER-2-overexpressing metastatic breast cancer. An overall response rate of 79% was seen in the group receiving the combination containing cisplatin, and an overall response rate of 58% in the group receiving the combination containing carboplatin (32). Trastuzumab in combination with vinorelbine was studied in patients with HER-2-overexpressing metastatic breast cancer in a multicenter phase II trial. Fifty-four women were enrolled, and an overall response rate of 68% was observed (33).

In the neoadjuvant setting, trastuzumab has been evaluated in combination with docetaxel in a small number of patients with locally advanced HER-2-overexpressing breast cancer. Patients were given weekly trastuzumab alone for 3 wk, and then docetaxel given every 3 wk for four cycles was added to the weekly trastuzumab. Patients underwent surgery, followed by four cycles of doxorubicin/cyclophosphamide) without trastuzumab, followed by weekly trastuzumab for a year. Seventeen of 22 patients had an objective clinical response, and 2 of the 22 had decreased cardiac function (34). Currently, several major cooperative groups are evaluating the role of trastuzumab in the adjuvant setting.

Whereas trastuzumab is approved for use in breast cancer, it has also been used in other malignancies that overexpress HER-2. For example, the combination of trastuzumab and carboplatin and paclitaxel has been studied in patients with advanced NSCLC. Although the number of patients was small, the patients who had HER-2 overexpression of 3+ did better as compared with the historical controls (35). A phase II study performed in men with hormone refractory metastatic prostate cancer showed little benefit of single-agent trastuzumab (36). Phase II studies are underway investigating the use of trastuzumab in metastatic pancreatic, colon, and esophageal malignancies.

2.2. Anti-EGFR Antibodies

EGFR was the first HER family member to be described. It is expressed by normal epithelial cells and most carcinomas. Whereas in normal cells the expression of EGFR is in the range of 40,000–100,000 receptors per cell, in certain tumors (for example, head and neck and NSCLC, EGF) receptors can be as high as 2×10^6 per cell. Overexpression of EGFR using a plethora of FDA-unapproved methods has been reported in NSCLC, head and neck, breast, renal cell, ovarian, and colon cancers, as well as in bladder and pancreatic cancers and central nervous system gliomas (37).

Several MAbs are currently undergoing clinical investigation including IMC-C225, ABX-EGF, EMD 7200, hR3, and ICR62. All these antibodies bind to EGFR and competitively inhibit ligand binding, thereby preventing the activation of the receptor tyrosine kinase. Inhibition of EGFR activity leads to cell cycle arrest in G_1, potentiates apoptosis, inhibits angiogenesis by decreasing the tumor-cell production of angiogenic growth factors, and inhibits tumor cell invasion and metastasis by inhibiting the expression and activity of several matrix metalloproteinases. In addition, these antibodies markedly augment the antitumor effects of chemotherapy and radiation therapy a property that has been successfully exploited in clinical trials (reviewed in refs. *38* and *39*).

2.2.1. IMC-C225

IMC-C225 (Cetuximab, Erbitux; ImClone Systems and Bristol-Myers Squibb, New York, NY) is a chimeric antibody, having a human IgG1 and a murine variable region *(40)*. It is the first MAb that binds specifically and with high affinity to the extracellular domain of HER-1. This binding blocks ligand-induced activation of the receptor tyrosine kinase activity and subsequent downstream signaling activity, as well as receptor internalization. Cetuximab has mostly a cytostatic effect in vitro by blocking cell cycle progression at G_1 and inhibiting proliferation. It also increases the expression of proapoptotic proteins, decreases the expression of antiapoptotic proteins, inhibits angiogenesis via decreasing VEGF, interleukin-8, basic fibroblast growth factor, and it may also enhance the immunological effector cell activity.

2.2.1.1. Cetuximab in Colorectal Cancer. In colorectal xenograft models Cetuximab activity was potentiated by coadministration with irinotecan (Camptosar) and complete tumor growth inhibition was seen only with the combination of Cetuximab and irinotecan. The initial phase II study in colorectal cancer evaluated the combination of Cetuximab and irinotecan. The study enrolled 120 patients with EGFR-positive ($\geq$1+ by IHC) metastatic disease that had progressive disease on irinotecan or shortly after; a small number of patients also had stable disease while treated with irinotecan. The response rate was 22.5% in the irinotecan-refractory cohort and 44% in the cohort that had previously stable disease on irinotecan. The most common side effect was a folliculitis-type rash, and there was a trend in favor of better survival in patients that developed rash as compared with those who did not *(41)*.

Cetuximab was also studied as single agent in patients with EGFR-positive colorectal cancer after failure of an irinotecan-containing regimen. The phase II study conducted by Saltz et al. *(42)* enrolled 57 patients with metastatic colorectal cancer and used Cetuximab with a loading dose of 400 mg/m^2 intravenously for 2 h, followed by weekly 250 mg/m^2. Partial responses were seen in 10.5% of patients, and 35% had either a minor response or stable disease that lasted for at least 12 wk from the date of treatment initiation. The most common adverse reactions were an acne-like skin rash predominantly on the upper face and torso, and asthenia. Grade 3 allergic reactions requiring discontinuation of study treatment were seen in 3.5% of patients. In this study, the response rate did not correlate with either the percentage of positive cells or the intensity of EGFR expression.

A comparison between Cetuximab monotherapy and the combination of Cetuximab and irinotecan in irinotecan-refractory colorectal cancer showed that the combination led to a significantly higher response than the monotherapy. This large phase III study enrolled 329 patients from 11 different countries *(43)*. All tumors were required to be EGFR-positive by IHC performed at a central location. To be eligible, patients had to have received one of several prespecified irinotecan-containing regimens for at least 6 wk with documented disease progression that was verified by an independent review committee. Patients were randomized to receive either Cetuximab alone or Cetuximab with irinotecan. The response rate in the combination-therapy group (irinotecan-Cetuximab) was 23%, significantly higher than in the monotherapy group (10.8%). The median time to progression was also longer in the combination chemotherapy arm (4.1 mo) as compared with the Cetuximab monotherapy arm (1.5 mo), but the difference in median overall survival was not statistically significant (8.6 mo in the combination arm vs 6.0 mo in the single-agent arm, $p = 0.48$). Whereas the patients in the combination therapy arm experienced more-frequent adverse events, these events were similar in frequency and severity to the expected toxicity from irinotecan alone, suggesting that Cetuximab did not worsen the irinotecan-induced toxicity. In addition, no overall differences in safety and efficacy were observed between elderly patients ($\geq$65 yr of age) and younger patients. This pivotal study led to the approval by the FDA of Cetuximab used in combination with irinotecan for the treatment of EGFR-expressing metastatic colorectal carcinoma after progression on irinotecan-based chemotherapy. In addition, Cetuximab administered as single agent is indicated for the treatment of EGFR-expressing metastatic colorectal carcinoma in patients who are intolerant to irinotecan-based chemotherapy. The most common adverse reactions were an acnelike skin rash predominantly on the upper face and torso (1%), infusion reactions (3.5% of patients experienced grade 3 allergic reactions requiring drug discontinuation), asthenia (grades 3 or 4 in 10%) fever (5%), dehydration, and interstitial lung disease (<0.5%). Currently, Cetuximab is been studied as part of first-line therapy against metastatic colorectal cancer.

2.2.1.2. Cetuximab in Lung Cancer. The addition of Cetuximab to standard chemotherapy has also been studied in untreated metastatic NSCLC. A randomized phase II study comparing standard cisplatinum and Navelbine to the same agents in combination with Cetuximab showed that the addition of Cetuximab led to a higher response rate (53% with the combination vs 26% with chemotherapy alone) and a higher rate of disease control (93 vs 77%, respectively) *(44)*.

In patients with relapsed NSCLC, treatment with docetaxel can lead to a response rate ranging from 7.8 to 8.9%. In a promising study, the combination of docetaxel every 3 wk with concurrent weekly Cetuximab the response rate was 28%, and nearly 66% of patients had stable disease, suggesting again that the addition of Cetuximab to chemotherapy may improve the efficacy of the chemotherapy agents *(45)*. The activity of single-agent Cetuximab has not been investigated in NSCLC. Also unexplored is the potential synergy between Cetuximab and radiation in NSCLC and the use of Cetuximab as radiation sensitizer in locally advanced NSCLC.

2.2.1.3. Cetuximab in Head and Neck Cancer. EGFR expression is detected in 90% of head and neck cancers and is associated with a more aggressive clinical course. Preclinical data support synergistic antitumor activity with the combination of Cetuximab and cisplatin or radiation in head and neck cancer cell lines and xenograft models. Based on these data, Cetuximab has been studied in combination with radiotherapy in treatment naïve patients with locally advanced squamous cell carcinoma of the head and neck, with promising results *(46)*. The combination of Cetuximab and cisplatin has been compared with cisplatin and placebo in patients with metastatic and/or recurrent squamous cell cancer of the head and neck in a study lead by the Eastern Cooperative Oncology Group study that recently finished accrual.

2.2.2. EMD 7200

EMD 7200 (Matuzumab) is a humanized IgG1 MAb against the extracellular domain of EGFR. Dose-limiting toxicities include headache and fever, whereas follicular rash is the most common adverse event at doses used in clinical trials. In one study *(47)*, skin and tumor biopsies taken before and after treatment showed a decrease in phosphorylated

EGFR and mitogen-activated protein kinase treatment, confirming a downstream effect resulting from receptor blockade.

2.2.3. ABX-EGF

ABX-EGF (Panitumumab) is a fully humanized IgG2 MAb against EGFR, developed using the XenoMouse technology. In phase I studies, no hypersensitivity reactions were seen, and no dose-limiting toxicities at dosages predicted to achieve receptor saturation. When used as single agent in metastatic colorectal cancer after failure of fluoropyrimidines, irinotecan, and/or oxalipatin, partial responses were seen in 10% of patients and 55% of patients had stable disease *(48)*. Unlike Cetuximab and EMD 7200, which (because of their IgG1 backbones) can participate in ADCC, ABX-EGF (having an IgG2 backbone) cannot engage ADCC.

3. ANTI-VEGF ANTIBODIES

A crucial step in the growth of tumors and their subsequent metastases is the development of new blood vessels, or angiogenesis. This is achieved mainly through the induction of new blood vessels, but also through the co-opting of existing blood vessels. Angiogenesis is regulated by a vast array of factors produced by the tumor, the surrounding tissue, and by the tumor-infiltrating macrophages and fibroblasts. Some of these factors are proangiogenic, whereas others are antiangiogenic. The majority of the proangiogenic factors act as ligands for endothelial cell surface receptors. VEGF-A, originally described as a vascular permeability factor, is one of the most important proangiogenic molecules and the best characterized member of the VEGF–platelet derived growth factor superfamily. Other family members include VEGF-B, -C, -D, -E and placenta-derived growth factor. VEGF expression is increased in the majority of cancers, such as colorectal cancer, liver, lung cancer, kidney, bladder, thyroid, and breast cancer *(49,50)*.

VEGF exerts its action through its binding to two tyrosine kinase receptors on endothelial cells, VEGF-1 and VEGF-2. VEGF-2 provides the major contribution to angiogenesis, whereas VEGF-1 serves as a decoy, modulating the availability of ligand to VEGFR-2. The receptors contain seven extracellular domains, a transmembrane domain, and a cytoplasmic tyrosine kinase domain and share 44% homology with each other. The binding of VEGF to the endothelial receptors triggers the phosphorylation of adaptors and signal transducers *(51)*. The result is a powerful mitogenic signal for the endothelial cells, increased vascular permeability, and upregulation of antiapoptotic proteins, such as B-cell lymphoma 2. The VEGF-driven signal can be interrupted at several levels: through antibodies directed against VEGF itself, antibodies directed against the VEGF receptors, by soluble extracellular domains of the VEGF receptors that effectively trap the available VEGF, by small molecules that interfere either with VEGF binding or with receptor signaling, or by ribozymes that degrade VEGF receptor RNA.

Whereas most of these methods are currently being explored for clinical use, the inhibition of VEGF itself using a MAb was the first to show effectiveness and is already approved for use in colorectal cancer. The antibody bevacizumab (Avastin™; Genentech, South San Francisco, CA) is a recombinant humanized monoclonal IgG-derived from the murine antibody A.4.6.1. In initial laboratory studies, the antibody had a potent inhibitory effect on several tumor cell lines injected in nude mice, but no effect on the same cell lines in vitro. A recent elegant study showed that administration of the anti-VEGF antibody to patients with colorectal cancer results in decreased tumor perfusion, decreased microvascular density, decreased interstitial fluid pressure, and vascular volume, supporting the hypothesis that the antibody is acting through the inhibition of angiogenesis *(52)*.

Based on promising data from phase II studies combining bevacizumab with 5-fluoro-uracil/leucovorin in first-line chemotherapy for patients with colorectal cancer, a phase III study was designed to compare standard chemotherapy with bolus irinotecan/5-FU/LV, with or without bevacizumab. The randomized double-blind placebo-controlled study enrolled 813 patients with previously untreated metastatic colorectal cancer. The addition of bevacizumab led to an increase in median duration of survival of 4.7 mo, increased the progression-free survival from a median of 6.2 –10.6 mo, the overall response rate from 34.8 to 44.8%, and the median duration of response from 7.1 to 10.4 mo *(53)*. Whereas in phase I and II trials hemorrhage, thromboembolism, proteinuria, and hypertension were identified as bevacizumab-related adverse events, the phase III study showed that only the incidence of hypertension was higher among the patients receiving bevacizumab. In addition, six cases (1.5%) of gastrointestinal perforation were seen in the bevacizumab group and none in the placebo group.

Bevacizumab is also being investigated in the treatment of lung cancer, where a number of studies have shown a correlation between VEGF expression, microvessel density correlates, and poor prognosis. The combination of carboplatinum and paclitaxel with or without bevacizumab is currently in phase III studies in patients with advanced, metastatic, or recurrent NSCLC.

Both hereditary and the majority of sporadic renal cell contain mutations in the von Hippel-Lindau tumor suppressor gene. Because von Hippel-Lindau is the ubiquitin ligase for the transcription factor hypoxia-inducible factor 1α, these mutations result in constitutive activation of hypoxia-inducible factor 1α and, in turn, enhanced transcription VEGF, tumor growth factor-α, and platelet-derived growth factor *(54)*, implying clearly that renal cell cancer is a promising target for anti-VEGF therapy. A prospective double-blind placebo-controlled study compared low-dose (3 mg/kg every 2 wk) and high-dose (10 mg/kg every 2 wk) bevacizumab to placebo in patients with metastatic renal cell cancer. An interim analysis showed a significant prolongation of the median time to progression in the high-dose antibody group compared with the placebo group (4.8 compared with 2.5 mo, $p < 0.001$). The response rate was 10% in the high-dose bevacizumab group, with no responses in the placebo arm *(55)*. Although there was no difference in the overall survival between treatment arms, this may have been confounded by the crossover from the placebo arm to the antibody treatment arm after disease progression. Based on these results, bevacizumab is now investigated in a phase III study in combination with interferon in metastatic renal cell cancer.

Bevacizumab is also being explored in the treatment of prostate cancer, gynecological cancers, head and neck cancer, pancreatic cancer, and hematological malignancies *(56)*.

4. ANTIBODIES AGAINST EPITHELIAL ANTIGENS

4.1. CD17-1A

CD17-1A (Edrecolomab, Pannorex) is an antigen overexpressed by many epithelial tumors and plays a role in epithelial cell adhesion. The antibody against CD19-1A, Edrecolomab is a murine IG2A MAb that induces ADCC, complement-mediated cytolysis, induces an anti-idiotypic network, and directly inhibits the growth of tumor cells in vivo.

Edrecolomab was studied in Europe in a randomized placebo-controlled study in the adjuvant treatment of patients with resected Dukes' C stage III colon adenocarcinoma. Patients randomized to receive the MAb after surgery had a 32% reduction in mortality rate and a 23% reduction in recurrence rate at median follow-up of 7 yr compared with the patients who received placebo. The treatment was well tolerated, with the most prominent side effects being malaise, low-grade fever and chills, diarrhea, and allergic reactions (57). The antibody is currently being evaluated in a study that randomizes patients to either 5-fluorouracil-based adjuvant chemotherapy or chemotherapy in combination with CD17-1A.

ACKNOWLEDGMENTS

Supported in part by R01 CA80195 (CLA), Breast Cancer Specialized Program of Research Excellence (SPORE) Grant P50 CA98131, and Vanderbilt-Ingram Cancer Center Support Grant P30 CA68485.

REFERENCES

1. Harris M. Monoclonal antibodies as therapeutic agents for cancer. *Lancet Oncol* 2004; 5:292–302.
2. Holbro T, Hynes NE. ErbB receptors: directing key signaling networks throughout life. *Annu Rev Pharmacol Toxicol* 2004; 44:195–217.
3. Yarden Y, Sliwkowski MX. Untangling the ErbB signalling network. *Nat Rev Mol Cell Biol* 2001; 2: 127–137.
4. Normanno N, Bianco C, De Luca A, Salomon DS. The role of EGF-related peptides in tumor growth. *Front Biosci* 2001; 6:D685–D707.
5. Graus-Porta D, Beerli RR, Daly JM, Hynes NE. ErbB-2, the preferred heterodimerization partner of all ErbB receptors, is a mediator of lateral signaling. *EMBO J* 1997; 16:1647–1655.
6. Holbro T, Beerli RR, Maurer F, Koziczak M, Barbas CF III, Hynes NE. The ErbB2/ErbB3 heterodimer functions as an oncogenic unit: ErbB2 requires ErbB3 to drive breast tumor cell proliferation. *Proc Natl Acad Sci USA* 2003; 100:8933–8938.
7. Paez JG, Janne PA, Lee JC, et al. EGFR mutations in lung cancer: correlation with clinical response to gefitinib therapy. *Science* 2004; 304:1497–1500.
8. Lynch TJ, Bell DW, Sordella R, et al. Activating mutations in the epidermal growth factor receptor underlying responsiveness of non-small-cell lung cancer to gefitinib. *N Engl J Med* 2004; 350:2129–2139.
9. Pao W, Miller V, Zakowski M, et al. EGF receptor gene mutations are common in lung cancers from "never smokers" and are associated with sensitivity of tumors to gefitinib and erlotinib. *Proc Natl Acad Sci USA* 2004; 101:13,306–13,311.
10. Slamon DJ, Godolphin W, Jones LA, et al. Studies of the HER-2/*neu* proto-oncogene in human breast and ovarian cancer. *Science* 1989; 244: 707–712.
11. Slamon DJ, Clark GM, Wong SG, Levin WJ, Ullrich A, McGuire WL. Human breast cancer: correlation of relapse and survival with amplification of the HER-2/*neu* oncogene. *Science* 1987; 235:177–182.
12. Sliwkowski MX, Schaefer G, Akita RW, et al. Coexpression of erbB2 and erbB3 proteins reconstitutes a high affinity receptor for heregulin. *J Biol Chem* 1994; 269:14,661–14,665.
13. Petit AM, Rak J, Hung MC, et al. Neutralizing antibodies against epidermal growth factor and ErbB-2/*neu* receptor tyrosine kinases down-regulate vascular endothelial growth factor production by tumor cells in vitro and in vivo: angiogenic implications for signal transduction therapy of solid tumors. *Am J Pathol* 1997; 151:1523–1530.
14. Benz CC, Scott GK, Sarup JC, et al. Estrogen-dependent, tamoxifen-resistant tumorigenic growth of MCF-7 cells transfected with HER2/*neu*. *Breast Cancer Res Treat* 1993; 24:85–95.
15. Carter P, Presta L, Gorman CM, et al. Humanization of an anti-p185HER2 antibody for human cancer therapy. *Proc Natl Acad Sci USA* 1992; 89:4285–4289.
16. Lewis GD, Figari I, Fendly B, et al. Differential responses of human tumor cell lines to anti-p185HER2 monoclonal antibodies. *Cancer Immunol Immunother* 1993; 37:255–263.

17. Arteaga CL. Trastuzumab, an appropriate first-line single-agent therapy for HER2-overexpressing metastatic breast cancer. *Breast Cancer Res* 2002; 5:96–100.

18. Hudziak RM, Lewis GD, Winget M, Fendly BM, Shepard HM, Ullrich A. p185HER2 monoclonal antibody has antiproliferative effects in vitro and sensitizes human breast tumor cells to tumor necrosis factor. *Mol Cell Biol* 1989; 9:1165–1172.

19. Drebin JA, Link VC, Stern DF, Weinberg RA, Greene MI. Down-modulation of an oncogene protein product and reversion of the transformed phenotype by monoclonal antibodies. *Cell* 1985; 41:697–706.

20. Klapper LN, Waterman H, Sela M, Yarden Y. Tumor-inhibitory antibodies to HER-2/ErbB-2 may act by recruiting c-Cbl and enhancing ubiquitination of HER-2. *Cancer Res* 2000; 60:3384–3388.

21. Yakes FM, Chinratanalab W, Ritter CA, King W, Seelig S, Arteaga CL. Herceptin-induced inhibition of phosphatidylinositol-3 kinase and Akt Is required for antibody-mediated effects on p27, cyclin D1, and antitumor action. *Cancer Res* 2002; 62:4132–4141.

22. Clynes RA, Towers TL, Presta LG, Ravetch JV. Inhibitory Fc receptors modulate in vivo cytoxicity against tumor targets. *Nat Med* 2000; 6:443–446.

23. Gennari R, Menard S, Fagnoni F, et al. Pilot study of the mechanism of action of preoperative trastuzumab in patients with primary operable breast tumors overexpressing HER2. *Clinical Cancer Res* 2004; 10: 5650–5655.

24. Mass R. The role of HER-2 expression in predicting response to therapy in breast cancer. *Semin Oncol* 2000; 27:46–52; discussion 92–100.

25. Jacobs TW, Gown AM, Yaziji H, Barnes MJ, Schnitt SJ. Comparison of fluorescence in situ hybridization and immunohistochemistry for the evaluation of HER-2/*neu* in breast cancer. *J Clin Oncol* 1999; 17:1974–1982.

26. Leyland-Jones B, Gelmon K, Ayoub JP, et al. Pharmacokinetics, safety, and efficacy of trastuzumab administered every three weeks in combination with paclitaxel. *J Clin Oncol* 2003; 21:3965–3971.

27. Suter TM, Cook-Bruns N, Barton C. Cardiotoxicity associated with trastuzumab (Herceptin) therapy in the treatment of metastatic breast cancer. *Breast* 2004; 13:173–183.

28. Cobleigh MA, Vogel CL, Tripathy D, et al. Multinational study of the efficacy and safety of humanized anti-HER2 monoclonal antibody in women who have HER2-overexpressing metastatic breast cancer that has progressed after chemotherapy for metastatic disease. *J Clin Oncol* 1999; 17:2639–2648.

29. Vogel CL, Cobleigh MA, Tripathy D, et al. Efficacy and safety of trastuzumab as a single agent in first-line treatment of HER2-overexpressing metastatic breast cancer. *J Clin Oncol* 2002; 20:719–726.

30. Slamon DJ, Leyland-Jones B, Shak S, et al. Use of chemotherapy plus a monoclonal antibody against HER2 for metastatic breast cancer that overexpresses HER2. *N Engl J Med* 2001; 344:783–792.

31. Pegram MD, Konecny GE, O'Callaghan C, Beryt M, Pietras R, Slamon DJ. Rational combinations of trastuzumab with chemotherapeutic drugs used in the treatment of breast cancer. *J Natl Cancer Inst* 2004; 96:739–749.

32. Pegram MD, Pienkowski T, Northfelt DW, et al. Results of two open-label, multicenter phase II studies of docetaxel, platinum salts, and trastuzumab in HER2-positive advanced breast cancer. *J Natl Cancer Inst* 2004; 96:759–769.

33. Burstein HJ, Harris LN, Marcom PK, et al. Trastuzumab and vinorelbine as first-line therapy for HER2-overexpressing metastatic breast cancer: multicenter phase II trial with clinical outcomes, analysis of serum tumor markers as predictive factors, and cardiac surveillance algorithm. *J Clin Oncol* 2003; 21:2889–2895.

34. Van Pelt AE, Mohsin S, Elledge RM, et al. Neoadjuvant trastuzumab and docetaxel in breast cancer: preliminary results. *Clin Breast Cancer* 2003; 4:348–353.

35. Langer CJ, Stephenson P, Thor A, Vangel M, Johnson DH. Trastuzumab in the treatment of advanced non-small-cell lung cancer: is there a role? Focus on Eastern Cooperative Oncology Group study 2598. *J Clin Oncol* 2004; 22:1180–1187.

36. Ziada A, Barqawi A, Glode LM, et al. The use of trastuzumab in the treatment of hormone refractory prostate cancer; phase II trial. *Prostate* 2004; 60:332–337.

37. Salomon DS, Brandt R, Ciardiello F, Normanno N. Epidermal growth factor-related peptides and their receptors in human malignancies. *Crit Rev Oncol Hematol* 1995; 19:183–232.

38. Arteaga CL, Baselga J. Clinical trial design and end points for epidermal growth factor receptor-targeted therapies: implications for drug development and practice. *Clin Cancer Res* 2003; 9:1579–1589.

39. Arteaga CL. ErbB-targeted therapeutic approaches in human cancer. *Exp Cell Res* 2003; 284:122–130.

40. Goldstein NI, Prewett M, Zuklys K, Rockwell P, Mendelsohn J. Biological efficacy of a chimeric antibody to the epidermal growth factor receptor in a human tumor xenograft model. *Clin Cancer Res* 1995; 1:1311–1318.

41. Saltz L, Rubin M, Hochster H, et al. Cetuximab (IMC-225) plus irinotecan (CPT-11) is active in CPT-11-refractory colorectal cancer that expresses epidermal growth factor receptors. *Proc Am Soc Clin Oncol* 2001; 20:3a.

42. Saltz L, Meropol NJ, Loehrer PJ, Waksal H, Needle MN, Mayer RJ. Single agent IMC-C225 (Erbitux) has activity in CPT-11-refractory colorectal cancer (CRC) that expresses the epidermal growth factor receptor (EGFR). *Proc Am Soc Clin Oncol* 2002; 21:127a.

43. Cunningham D, Humblet Y, Siena S, et al. Cetuximab monotherapy and cetuximab plus Irinotecan in Irinotecan-refractory Metastatic Colorectal Cancer. *N Engl J Med* 2004; 351:337–345.

44. Gatzemeieer U, Rosell R, Ramlau R, et al. Cetuximab (c225) in combination with cisplatin/vinorelbine vs. cisplatin/vinorelbine alone in the first-line treatment of patients with epidermal growth factor receptor positive advanced non-small cell lung cancer. *Proc Am Soc Clin Oncol* 2003; 22:642.

45. Kim ES, Mauer Am, Tran HT, et al. A Phase II study of cetuximab, an epidermal growth factor receptor (EGFR) blocking antibody, in combination with docetaxel in chemotherapy refractory/resistant patients with advanced non-small cell lung cancer. *Proc Am Soc Clin Oncol* 2003; 22:642.

46. Robert F, Ezekiel MP, Spencer SA, et al. Phase I study of an anti-epidermal growth factor receptor antibody cetuximab in combination with radiation therapy in patients with advanced head and neck cancer. *J Clin Oncol* 2001; 19:3234–3243.

47. Tabernero J, Rojo F, Jimenez E, et al. A phase I pharmacokinetic (PK) and serial tumor and skin pharmacodynamic (PD) study of weekly, every 2 weeks or every 3 weeks 1-hour (h) infusion EMD72000, an humanized monoclonal anti-epidermal growth factor receptor (EGFR) antibody, in patients (pt) with advanced tumors. *Proc Am Soc Clin Oncol* 2003; 22:192.

48. Lynch DH, Yang XD. Therapeutic potential of ABX-EGF: a fully human anti-epidermal growth factor receptor monoclonal antibody for cancer treatment. *Semin Oncol* 2002; 29:47–50.

49. Carmeliet P. Angiogenesis in health and disease. *Nat Med* 2003; 9:653–660.

50. Ferrara N. VEGF and the quest for tumour angiogenesis factors. *Nat Rev Cancer* 2002; 2:795–803.

51. Ferrara N. Vascular endothelial growth factor: basic science and clinical progress. *Endocr Rev* 2004; 25:581–611.

52. Willett CG, Boucher Y, di Tomaso E, et al. Direct evidence that the VEGF-specific antibody bevacizumab has antivascular effects in human rectal cancer. *Nat Med* 2004; 10:145–147.

53. Hurwitz H, Fehrenbacher L, Novotny W, et al. Bevacizumab plus irinotecan, fluorouracil, and leucovorin for metastatic colorectal cancer. *N Engl J Med* 2004; 350:2335–2342.

54. George DJ, Kaelin WG Jr. The von Hippel-Lindau protein, vascular endothelial growth factor, and kidney cancer. *N Engl J Med* 2003; 349:419–421.

55. Yang JC, Haworth L, Sherry RM, et al. A randomized trial of bevacizumab, an anti-vascular endothelial growth factor antibody, for metastatic renal cancer. *N Engl J Med* 2003; 349:427–434.

56. Chen HX. Expanding the clinical development of bevacizumab. *Oncologist* 2003; 9(Suppl 1):27–35.

57. Riethmuller G, Holz E, Schlimok G, et al. Monoclonal antibody therapy for resected Dukes' C colorectal cancer: seven-year outcome of a multicenter randomized trial. *J Clin Oncol* 1998; 16:1788–1794.

Antibody Therapy
for Non-Hodgkin's Lymphoma

Stephen M. Ansell and Thomas E. Witzig

SUMMARY

Monoclonal antibodies have made a significant impact on the treatment of non-Hodgkin's lymphoma (NHL), and there has been a dramatic increase in clinical data regarding their use. The anti-CD20 antibody, rituximab, has shown substantial single-agent activity in both indolent and aggressive B-cell lymphomas. Rituximab is now standard therapy in relapsed indolent NHL, and it is the front-line treatment in combination with cyclophosphamide/doxorubicin/vincristine/prednisone chemotherapy for patients with large B-cell lymphoma. Combinations of rituximab with other cytotoxic agents or cytokines are currently being explored in a number of different studies, and some of these combinations show promise for the future. Other antibodies directed at different targets on lymphoma cells, such as epratuzumab, apolizumab, alemtuzumab, and galiximab, have also shown clinical activity in early trials. The radioconjugated anti-CD20 antibodies [90]yttrium ibritumomab tiuxetan and [131]iodine tositumomab also have significant clinical activity in low-grade B-cell NHL, and the former has demonstrated superior complete response rates when compared with rituximab. The challenge for the future will be to determine the place of each antibody in the treatment of NHL.

Key Words: Monoclonal antibody; non-Hodgkin's lymphoma; rituximab; radioimmunotherapy.

1. INTRODUCTION

Non-Hodgkin's lymphoma (NHL) is the fifth most common type of cancer in the United States, and the incidence of lymphoma is increasing (1). Currently, approximately half of all patients with aggressive lymphomas may be cured with cytotoxic therapy; however, most indolent lymphomas remain incurable with current therapy. New therapies are needed to treat patients with NHL more effectively.

Significant advances in technology and in the manufacture of monoclonal antibodies (MAbs) have allowed these agents to be developed for clinical use in patients with NHL. Research over the last 20 yr has focused on the development of antibodies directed at targets on lymphoma cells and has established that MAb therapy of NHL is safe and effective. This chapter highlights the MAbs currently in development and clinical use for patients with NHL, and discusses the mechanisms of action of these agents, as well as the results of clinical trials using these antibodies in patients with lymphoma.

From: *Cancer Drug Discovery and Development: Immunotherapy of Cancer*
Edited by: M. L. Disis © Humana Press Inc., Totowa, NJ

2. RITUXIMAB

Rituximab is a chimeric murine/human MAb that binds specifically to the antigen CD20 located on pre-B- and mature B-lymphocytes *(2,3)*. It is composed of human immunoglobulin G1 and κ-constant regions and variable antigen recognition sites from the murine CD20 MAb IDEC-2B8 *(4)*. CD20 is expressed on more than 90% of B-cell NHL *(5)*, and is not found on hematopoietic stem cells, normal plasma cells, or other normal tissues *(6)*. Studies suggest that CD20 acts as a calcium channel and plays a role in B-cell activation, proliferation, and differentiation. Furthermore, CD20 is a good target for monoclonal antibody therapy, as it is not internalized. The Fab domain of rituximab binds to the CD20 antigen on B-lymphocytes, and the Fc domain recruits immune effector functions to mediate lysis of the B-cell *(4)*.

2.1. Mechanisms of Action

The major reason for selecting CD20 as an appropriate target in NHL was the fact that the antigen is expressed at high levels on malignant cells and is not downregulated after antibody binding. In vitro, rituximab induces apoptosis *(7,8)*, complement-dependent cytotoxicity *(9,10)*, and antibody-dependent cellular cytotoxicity (ADCC) *(11,12)* in malignant B-cell lines. Most data suggest that the predominant effector mechanism is ADCC, with a minor role for complement. The efficacy of rituximab has been shown to require mononuclear cells as effector cells for ADCC *(4,9)*. Recent data have suggested that monocytes are the dominant effector cells for B-cell depletion *(13)*, but neutrophils have also been shown to function as effector cells in ADCC induced by rituximab *(11–14)*.

In some, but not all, lymphoma cell lines evaluated, rituximab binding to CD20 can lead to apoptosis. Currently, there is no consensus as to the precise pathways that are most important, nor the degree to which this mechanism contributes to the clinical response of lymphoma to rituximab *(7,8)*. Whereas the exact role of the transmembrane CD20 molecule is not known, it is involved in B-cell differentiation and activation *(6,15)*. CD20 can act as a calcium channel *(16)*, either directly or by binding to, or activating, a calcium channel. Binding by rituximab, especially if crosslinked, initiates a cascade of intracellular signals including the activation of c-Jun NH_2-terminal protein kinase, extracellular signal-regulated kinase, and p38 mitogen-activated protein kinase *(17)*. These signals may play a role, at least in part, in rituximab-mediated cell killing. Rituximab-mediated apoptosis is thought to be a consequence of caspase 3 activation *(18)*, whereas the fatty acid synthase ligand/fatty acid synthase death pathway does not appear to be necessary. The role of B-cell lymphoma (bcl)-2-dependent pathways remains unclear. A recent study found that rituximab binding led to a decrease in bcl-2 expression and sensitization to chemotherapy acting via mitochondrial pathways *(19)*. This was shown to be because of downregulation of interleukin (IL)-10, resulting in decreased activation of signal transduction activating transcription 3 through an IL-10/IL-10R autocrine loop. In contrast, others have shown that bcl-2-expressing, as well as bcl-2-nonexpressing cell lines, were equally sensitive to anti-CD20 apoptosis *(7)*, with no significant alterations in bcl-2 levels seen after anti-CD20 treatment.

Intracellular signal transduction may be dependent on the density of CD20, as well as the clustering of CD20, and the amount of antibody present *(8)*. After CD20 is bound, it rapidly redistributes into a cell membrane fraction called a lipid raft *(20, 21)*, which may aid in signal activation through the Src family tyrosine kinases. These membrane changes may be long-lived, and is one of several potential explanations for late responses to antibody therapy.

A variety of effector cell populations including monocytes/macrophages, natural-killer (NK) cells, and activated granulocytes mediate rituximab-directed cell lysis. Depletion of select effector cell populations including monocytes, NK cells, and granulocytes in animal models decreases the efficacy of rituximab therapy *(22)*. Additionally, ADCC is regulated by the selective use of specific Fcγ receptors (FcγR). The antitumor effect is enhanced in mice lacking inhibitory Fcγ RII2B receptors, whereas the antitumor effect is totally absent in mice lacking the FcγR subunit responsible for sending the activation signal to the immune effector cell *(23)*. A clinical correlative analysis of low-affinity FcγRIII CD16 genetic polymorphisms in rituximab-treated patients demonstrated that those who were homozygous for the higher-affinity allele of CD16 had significantly higher clinical response rates to rituximab than did subjects that were heterozygotes or homozygous for the lower-affinity allele *(24)*. These data suggest that ADCC is a significant mechanism of action for MAbs, such as rituximab.

There has been substantial but conflicting evidence regarding the role of complement-mediated cytotoxicity in the antitumor effect of rituximab. In vitro, the expression of the complement inhibitory proteins on the target cell correlated with complement-mediated lysis *(9,10)*. This effect was important for the action of rituximab, but was not shown to be important for the action of B1, another anti-CD20 antibody *(25)*. Furthermore, in an animal model, rituximab was shown to have antitumor effects in wild-type mice, but not in syngeneic knockout mice lacking C1q, a critical component of the complement pathway, suggesting that an intact complement pathway is necessary for antitumor activity of rituximab *(26)*. Conversely, the expression of inhibitory molecules on cells from patient biopsy specimens does not reliably predict for clinical responses to rituximab *(27)*. At this time, the role of complement in the antitumor activity of rituximab remains unclear.

2.2. Clinical Use of Rituximab

Rituximab has become an established component of therapy for patients with B-cell NHL because of clinically significant antitumor effects, as well as its ease of administration. In the initial phase I study of rituximab, patients with previously treated B-cell NHL received weekly infusions for 4 wk. The treatment was well tolerated, and approximately half of the patients responded to therapy, the majority of which were partial responses *(28,29)*. No immunological responses to rituximab, such as human antichimeric antibody responses, were noted. These observations were confirmed in a phase II trial of patients with low-grade or follicular NHL *(30)*. Patients treated in this study had a 48% overall response rate (ORR) with a median duration of response of 11.6 mo. The main toxicity was infusion-related reactions, with few other toxicities noted. Depletion of B-cells from the peripheral blood was not associated with significant hypogammaglobulinemia or infections.

In the phase I trial, no true maximum-tolerated dose was reached because of lack of toxicity, so the dose and schedule were selected somewhat empirically and based on the amount of available antibody for use in the trial. Thus, higher doses, more frequent administration, additional doses, and administration earlier in the disease course are issues currently being investigated. Owing to its efficacy and tolerability in relapsed NHL, trials of rituximab as induction therapy have been performed, and initial results suggest higher responses than in relapsed patients *(31,32)*. There have been two studies that enrolled previously untreated, advanced-stage follicular NHL patients, and treated them with a standard course of rituximab without maintenance. Colombat et al. found an ORR of 73%, with 27% of patients achieving a complete response (CR) or unconfirmed CR *(31)*. Witzig et al. treated 36 patients with the same schedule and found a 72% ORR with 36% CR *(33)*. In a similar study by Hainsworth et al. *(33)*, responding patients or those with stable disease at 6-mo intervals received subsequent courses of rituximab for up to 2 yr. The eventual ORR was 65%, with 27% CRs, and the 1- and 2-yr progression-free survival rates were 69 and 67%, respectively *(32,34)*. The high response rate in chemotherapy-naïve patients observed in these studies should be interpreted cautiously because of potential issues, such as patient selection and the long-term implications on time to progression and time to next chemotherapy, are not yet known. However, these results strongly support the inclusion of rituximab as upfront therapy in a comparative randomized trial. A recently activated cooperative group randomized study will compare retreatment with rituximab to a rituximab maintenance strategy in previously untreated patients.

Other studies have evaluated the duration of rituximab therapy. In a single-arm phase II study utilizing eight weekly doses of rituximab, an ORR of 57% was observed *(35)*. The median duration of response in this study was 13.4+ mo. In the phase II study by Hainsworth et al. *(34)*, subjects who had not progressed after an initial 4-wk course of rituximab received additional 4-wk courses of rituximab at 6-mo intervals for up to 2-yr. As outlined, the results from this trial are also promising. It appears, therefore, that additional doses or prolonged administration of rituximab results in higher response rates and longer durations of response than those seen with the weekly-for-4-wk dosing schedule. This is supported by the results of a recently published randomized study comparing no further treatment after four weekly doses of rituximab to prolonged rituximab administration (375 mg/m^2 every 2 mo for four times). At a median follow-up of 35 mo, the median event-free survival was 12 mo in the no-further-treatment arm vs 23 mo in the prolonged-treatment arm ($p = 0.02$) *(36)*.

Synergy between rituximab and chemotherapy drugs in vitro has led to clinical trials exploring rituximab combined with cytotoxic agents in both indolent and aggressive non-Hodgkin's lymphomas. Czuczman et al. treated patients with relapsed or refractory low-grade or follicular lymphoma patients with rituximab and cyclophosphamide, doxorubicin, vincristine, and prednisone (CHOP), and found an ORR of 95% with CR rate of 55% *(37)*. Toxicity was similar to that seen with CHOP alone. The median progression-free survival was not reached with a median follow-up of 65 mo. The combination of CHOP and rituximab has also been examined in trials involving patients with previously untreated aggressive NHL. In a phase II study, patients with previously untreated diffuse large cell and follicular large cell lymphoma were treated with six cycles of rituximab in combination with CHOP chemotherapy *(38)*. The ORR was 94 and 93% of patients who achieved partial response or CR remained in remission with a median follow up of 26 mo.

Two phase III studies have been conducted comparing CHOP plus rituximab (R-CHOP) to CHOP alone in elderly patients with aggressive B-cell NHL. In a French multicenter (Groupe d'Etude des Lymphomes de l'Adulte [GELA]) study, R-CHOP was superior to CHOP alone with respect to CR rate (75 vs 63%), progression during treatment (9 vs 22%), and 2-yr overall survival (70 vs 57%) *(39)*. A similar North American intergroup study comparing R-CHOP to CHOP was recently reported *(40)*. Although the administration of rituximab differed from the GELA study, the results from the intergroup study supported the findings of the GELA study.

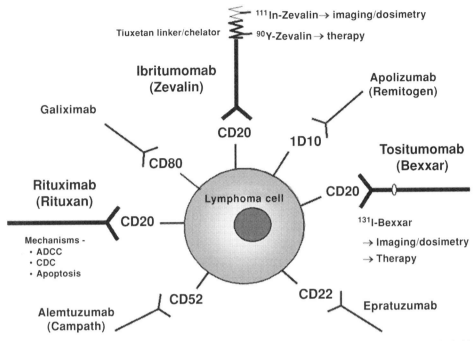

Fig. 1. Current monoclonal antibody therapy in the treatment of patients with non-Hodgkin's lymphoma.

In view of the fact that ADCC plays a significant role in the activity of rituximab, agents that can activate immune effector cells are being given to improve the efficacy of rituximab therapy. In a phase II study of rituximab and interferon-α2a, the response rate to rituximab plus interferon was approximately the same (45%) as other studies of rituximab alone, but the duration of response was longer (22.3 mo) *(41)*. A second study using this combination showed similar results with an ORR of 70% and a median duration of remission of 19 mo *(42)*. IL-2 in combination with rituximab has been shown to be well tolerated, and resulted in increased numbers of effector cells *(43)*. The combination of rituximab and IL-12 upregulated interferon-γ and IP-10 (CXCL10) expression and increased NK cell lytic activity *(44)*. Studies evaluating immunostimulatory cytosine–phosphate–guanine-oligodeoxynucleotides showed that they activate monocytes and NK cells, and induce production of both type 1 interferon and IL-12 *(45)*. cytosine–phosphate–guanine-oligodeoxynucleotides also induce upregulation of CD20 by primary malignant B-cells *(46)*, making the combination of this agent and rituximab a promising approach.

Multiple other agents are currently being combined with rituximab for a variety of B-cell diseases. It is becoming clear that rituximab can improve the response rate to therapy and may lead to improved long term clinical outcomes particularly in patients with large B-cell lymphoma *(39,40)*.

3. OTHER MAbs IN THE THERAPY OF LYMPHOMA

Rituximab has served as the prototype in the development of MAb therapy of NHL. However, other MAb directed at different antigens expressed on lymphoma cells are currently being evaluated in clinical trials (Fig. 1).

3.1. Epratuzumab

This humanized monoclonal antibody binds to CD22, a surface antigen that is B-cell-restricted and is expressed by greater than 80% of B-cell malignancies *(47)*. CD22 is rapidly internalized when bound, and can be reexpressed on the cell membrane after modulation. In an initial phase I/II clinical trial, epratuzumab was safely administered weekly for 4 wk to subjects with CD22-expressing B-cell malignancies *(48)*. Eighteen percent of patients treated achieved an objective response, including three complete responses. All responses were in patients with follicular NHL. A preliminary evaluation of the combination of epratuzumab and rituximab in B-cell NHL has yielded encouraging findings *(49)*. The combination therapy was well tolerated, with infusion-related toxicities comparable to those seen with antibody monotherapy. Objective responses were demonstrated in the majority of patients (66% of follicular patients), and the number of patients achieving a CR or unconfirmed CR (60% in follicular patients) appeared to be greater than that expected with rituximab alone *(50)*. Furthermore, a recent pilot study has also shown that epratuzumab can be safely combined with rituximab and CHOP chemotherapy and the combination appeared effective *(51)*. However, whether epratuzumab/rituximab-CHOP is superior to R-CHOP will require further comparative clinical trials.

3.2. Apolizumab

Apolizumab (Hu1D10) is a humanized human leukocyte antigen-DR-specific antibody that targets the 1D10 antigen on NHL cells. The expression of this class II antigen is not limited to B-cells, and expression of 1D10 on malignant B-cells is present in approx 50% of lymphoma cases. Binding of class II molecules by apolizumab can induce rapid apoptosis mediated by a pathway that appears to be different from that mediated by other antibodies *(52)*. In a phase I dose-escalation study, increased toxicity was seen at higher dose levels, and pharmacokinetic studies demonstrated marked intersubject variability in the clearance of apolizumab. Interestingly, responses in rituximab-refractory follicular lymphoma patients were seen. In addition, the median time to response was more than 100 d, which is longer than that seen typically with rituximab *(53)*. Serum from one responding patient contained autologous antilymphoma immunoglobulin (Ig)G, suggesting this patient may have developed an active humoral anti-lymphoma immune response *(54)*. These studies suggest a possible unique mechanism of action for this antibody. However, the subsequent phase II study failed to confirm the responses seen in the phase I trial *(55)*, and further studies will be necessary to confirm the efficacy of this antibody.

3.3. Alemtuzumab

The utility of this MAb targeting CD52 on lymphoma cells has been limited because of decreased penetration into nodal sites of disease, low response rates, and infectious complications. In an initial study, 14% of patients with B-cell lymphomas achieved a partial remission. Opportunistic infections were diagnosed in 14% of patients and 18% of patients had bacterial septicemia. Death related to infectious complications occurred in 6% of patients treated *(56)*. In a second study, 2 of the 16 patients with nonbulky NHL achieved a CR, and one patient achieved a partial response. One of two patients with minimal residual NHL achieved a molecular CR. Because of excessive infectious complications observed in the study, the trial was terminated early *(57)*. At this time, the role of alemtuzumab in the treatment of NHL is uncertain.

3.4. Galiximab

CD80 has also recently been identified as a target for MAb therapy. In addition to direct apoptosis, ADCC, and complement activation, galiximab may also alter the interaction between malignant B-cell and host T-cells by blocking the interaction between CD80 and its ligands, CD28 and CTLA4. The preliminary clinical evaluation of this MAb in patients with lymphoma suggests that it can be safely administered, and has some clinical activity (58).

3.5. Anti-CD30 Antibodies

Two anti-CD30 antibodies are currently being developed for use in anaplastic large cell lymphoma and other CD30-positive lymphomas, such as Hodgkin's lymphoma. MDX-060, a fully human MAb, and SGN-30, a chimeric antibody, have recently completed their phase I studies and are currently in phase II trials. In the initial trials, both agents were well tolerated, and clinical responses to both antibodies were seen primarily in patients with anaplastic large cell lymphoma (59,60).

4. RADIOIMMUNOTHERAPY FOR LYMPHOMA

Radioimmunotherapy (RIT) involves the linking of a radionuclide to an antibody to form a radioimmunoconjugate (RIC). In RIT, the goal is to attach a radionuclide with high energy but with a short path length to the antibody. This will focus the radiation on the tumor, while sparing the effects of radiotherapy on the nearby normal tissue. The RIC kills tumor cells by the direct effects of the antibody, as well as the effects of ionizing radiation. For effective RIT, several components are required: a suitable antigenic target that is highly expressed on tumor cells, a MAb, a radionuclide to attach to the antibody that is readily available and can be handled by the local nuclear medicine facility, and properly trained personnel to administer the RIC. When choosing an antibody for RIT, it is desirable to target those antigens that are expressed on tumor cells but not normal cells, to avoid toxicity to normal organs.

Although there are many radionuclides that can be used for RIT, ^{131}Iodine (^{131}I) and ^{90}Yttrium (^{90}Y) have been the ones used most commonly to date. The target antigen has been CD20 in most cases. During the last 15 yr, phase I, II, and III trials have been performed with single-agent ^{131}I tositumomab (Bexxar) or ^{90}Y-ibritumomab tiuxetan (Zevalin). These trials enrolled patients with relapsed disease and adequate bone marrow function with less than 25% marrow involvement with NHL. The results showed a high ORR with an acceptable toxicity profile, and ^{90}Y-ibritumomab tiuxetan was approved by the FDA in 2002 and ^{131}I tositumomab in 2003. Both agents are now available commercially in the United States.

Initial studies involving use of myeloablative and nonmyeloablative doses of ^{131}I tositumomab, an anti-CD20 antibody conjugated with ^{131}I, were done and showed that this agent could be safely administered (61,62). Trials evaluating ibritumomab tiuxetan, a murine anti-CD20 antibody conjugated with the radioisotope ^{90}Y (63,64) have demonstrated an ORR and CR rate that was higher than would be expected with rituximab alone, but with durations of response that were similar to those seen with the unlabeled antibody. There has been no normal organ toxicity other than reversible myelosuppression, which occurs approx 6 wk from the dose of the RIC and lasts several weeks. In a randomized trial comparing ^{90}Y ibritumomab tiuxetan to rituximab alone, the ORR was 80% with ^{90}Y ibritumomab tiuxetan and 56% with rituximab, with 30 and 16% CR rates, respectively *(65)*. A comparative study of ^{131}I tositumomab and ^{90}Y ibritumomab tiuxetan is being planned.

The current studies with RIT are evaluating the agents in sequence with chemotherapy and stem cell transplantation. There are several phase I/II trials using Bexxar and Zevalin with high-dose chemotherapy and stem cell support that are ongoing. Other studies evaluating RIT in combination with chemotherapy are being performed. A trial of previously untreated, advanced-stage follicular lymphoma treated with CHOP, followed 4–8 wk later by ^{131}I tositumomab reported an ORR of 90%, with 67% CRs and a 2-yr progression-free survival estimate of 81% *(66)*. Because of the significant results seen with ^{90}Y ibritumomab tiuxetan and ^{131}I tositumomab in clinical trials, radiolabeled MAbs targeting molecules other than CD20 are also in development *(67–69)*. Future studies will need to focus on the safety and efficacy of using these agents early in the disease course and evaluate the utility of administering multiple doses of RIT.

Myelosuppression associated with these agents has raised concerns about the feasibility and toxicity associated with subsequent therapy administered to patients with progressive disease. Recent publications, however, have suggested that response rates and toxicity associated with subsequent treatments appear no different to that seen after other chemotherapy regimens *(70,71)*. It should be noted that these were retrospective analyses and this issue will require further prospective study.

5. CONCLUSION

As we look to the future, the challenge will be to determine the place of each antibody in the treatment of NHL. Future studies will need to focus on using the various MAbs in combination with each other and with chemotherapy to take advantage of their unique targets and possible different mechanisms of action. We will also need to develop a rational approach to the use of MAbs based on their efficacy in lymphoma patients, potential long-term toxicities, as well as the financial constraints of the heath care system.

REFERENCES

1. Greenlee RT, Hill-Harmon MB, Murray T, Thun M. Cancer statistics, 2001. *CA Cancer J Clin* 2001; 51: 15–36.
2. Valentine MA, Meier KE, Rossie S, Clark EA. Phosphorylation of the CD20 phosphoprotein in resting B lymphocytes. *J Biol Chem* 1989; 264:11,282–11,287.
3. Einfeld DA, Brown JP, Valentine MA, Clark EA, Ledbetter JA. Molecular cloning of the human B cell CD20 receptor predicts a hydrophobic protein with multiple transmembrane domains. *EMBO J* 1988; 7: 711–717.
4. Reff ME, Carner K, Chambers KS, et al. Depletion of B cells in vivo by a chimeric mouse human monoclonal antibody to CD20. *Blood* 1994; 83:435–445.
5. Anderson KC, Bates MP, Slaughenhoupt B, Schlossman SF, Nadler LM. Expression of human B cell-associated antigens on leukemias and lymphomas: A model of human B cell differentiation. *Blood* 1984; 63:1424–1433.
6. Tedder TF, Boyd AW, Freedman AS, Nadler LM, Schlossman SFl. The B cell surface molecule B1 is functionally linked with B cell activation and differentiation. *J Immunol* 1985; 135:973–979.
7. Shan D, Ledbetter JA, Press OW. Signaling events involved in anti-CD20-induced apoptosis of malignant human B cells. *Cancer Immunol Immunother* 2000; 48:673–683.
8. Hofmeister JK, Cooney D, Coggeshall KM. Clustered CD20 induced apoptosis: Src-family kinase, the proximal regulator of tyrosine phosphorylation calcium influx and caspase 3-dependent apoptosis. *Blood Cell Mol Dis* 2000; 26:133–143.

9. Golay J, Zaffaroni L, Vaccari T, et al. Biologic response of B lymphoma cells to anti-CD20 monoclonal antibody rituximab in vitro: CD55 and CD59 regulate complement-mediated cell lysis. *Blood* 2000; 95: 3900–3908.

10. Harjunpaa A, Junnikkala S, Meri S. Rituximab (anti-CD20) therapy of B cell lymphomas: direct complement killing is superior to cellular effector mechanisms. Scand *J Immunol* 2000; 51:634–641.

11. Wurflein D, Dechant M, Stockmeyer B, et al. Evaluating antibodies for their capacity to induce cell-mediated lysis of malignant B cells. *Cancer Res* 1998; 58:3051–3058.

12. Elsasser D, Valerius T, Repp R, et al. HLA class II as potential target antigen on malignant B cells for therapy with bispecific antibodies in combination with granulocyte colony-stimulating factor. *Blood* 1996; 87:3803–3812.

13. Uchida J, Hamaguchi Y, Oliver JA, et al. The innate mononuclear phagocyte network depletes B lymphocytes through Fc receptor-dependent mechanisms during anti-CD20 antibody immunotherapy. *J Exp Med* 2004; 199:1659–1669.

14. Hernandez-Ilizaliturri FJ, Jupudy V, Ostberg J, et al. Neutrophils contribute to the biological antitumor activity of rituximab in a non-Hodgkin's lymphoma severe combined immunodeficiency mouse model. *Clin Cancer Res* 2003; 9(Pt 1):5866–5873.

15. Golay JT, Clark EA, Beverley PC. The CD20 (Bp35) antigen is involved in activation of B cells from the G0 to the G1 phase of the cell cycle. *J Immunol* 1985; 135:3795–3801.

16. Bubien JK, Zhou LJ, Bell PD, Frizzell RA, Tedder TF. Transfection of the CD20 cell surface molecule into ectopic cell types generates a Ca2+ conductance found constitutively in B lymphocytes. *J Cell Biol* 1993; 121:1121–1132.

17. Pedersen IM, Buhl AM, Klausen P, Geisler CH, Jurlander J. The chimeric anti-CD20 antibody rituximab induces apoptosis in B-cell chronic lymphocytic leukemia cells through a p38 mitogen activated protein-kinase-dependent mechanism. *Blood* 2002; 99:1314–1319.

18. Byrd JC, Kitada S, Flinn IW, et al. The mechanism of tumor cell clearance by rituximab in vivo in patients with B-cell chronic lymphocytic leukemia: evidence of caspase activation and apoptosis induction. *Blood* 2002; 99:1038–1043.

19. Alas S, Ng CP, Bonavida B. Rituximab modifies the cisplatin-mitochondrial signaling pathway, resulting in apoptosis in cisplatin-resistant non-Hodgkin's lymphoma. *Clin Cancer Res* 2002; 8:836–845.

20. Deans JP, Li H, Polyak MJ. CD20-mediated apoptosis: signalling through lipid rafts. *Immunology* 2002; 107:176–182.

21. Petrie RJ, Deans JP. Colocalization of the B cell receptor and CD20 followed by activation-dependent dissociation in distinct lipid rafts. *J Immunol* 2002; 169:2886–2891.

22. van Ojik HH, Bevaart L, Dahle CE, et al. CpG-A and B oligodeoxynucleotides enhance the efficacy of antibody therapy by activating different effector cell populations. *Cancer Res* 2003; 63:5595–5600.

23. Clynes RA, Towers TL, Presta LG, Ravetch JV. Inhibitory Fc receptors modulate in vivo cytoxicity against tumor targets. *Nat Med* 2000; 6:443–446.

24. Cartron G, Dacheux L, Salles G, et al. Therapeutic activity of humanized anti-CD20 monoclonal antibody and polymorphism in IgG Fc receptor FcgammaRIIIa gene. *Blood* 2002; 99:754–758.

25. Cragg MS, Morgan SM, Chan HT, et al. Complement-mediated lysis by anti-CD20 mAb correlates with segregation into lipid rafts. *Blood* 2003; 101:1045–1052.

26. Di Gaetano N, Cittera E, Nota R, et al. Complement activation determines the therapeutic activity of rituximab in vivo. *J Immunol* 2003; 171:1581–1587.

27. Weng WK, Levy R. Expression of complement inhibitors CD46, CD55, and CD59 on tumor cells does not predict clinical outcome after rituximab treatment in follicular non-Hodgkin's lymphoma. *Blood* 2001; 98:1352–1357.

28. Maloney DG, Grillo-Lopez AJ, White CA, et al. IDEC-C2B8 (Rituximab) anti-CD20 monoclonal antibody therapy patients with relapsed low-grade non-Hodgkin's lymphoma. *Blood* 1997; 90:2188–2195.

29. Maloney DG, Grillo-Lopez AJ, Bodkin DJ, et al. IDEC-C2B8: results of a phase I multiple-dose trial in patients with relapsed non-Hodgkin's lymphoma. *J Clin Oncol* 1997; 15:3266–3274.

30. McLaughlin P, Grillo-Lopez AJ, Link BK, et al. Rituximab chimeric anti-CD20 monoclonal antibody therapy for relapsed indolent lymphoma: half of patients respond to a four-dose treatment program. *J Clin Oncol* 1998; 16:2825–2833.

31. Colombat P, Salles G, Brousse N, et al. Rituximab (anti-CD20 monoclonal antibody) as single first-line therapy for patients with follicular lymphoma with a low tumor burden: clinical and molecular evaluation. *Blood* 2001; 97:101–106.

32. Hainsworth JD, Litchy S, Burris HA III, et al. Rituximab as first-line and maintenance therapy for patients with indolent non-hodgkin's lymphoma. *J Clin Oncol* 2002; 20:4261–4267.

33. Witzig TE, Vukov AM, Habermann TM, et al. Rituximab therapy for patients with newly diagnosed, advanced-stage follicular grade I non-Hodgkin's lymphoma: a Phase II trial in the North Central Cancer Treatment Group. *J Clin Oncol* 2005; 23:1056–1058.

34. Hainsworth JD. First-line and maintenance treatment with rituximab for patients with indolent non-Hodgkin's lymphoma. *Semin Oncol* 2003; 30(Suppl 2):9–15.

35. Piro LD, White CA, Grillo-Lopez AJ, et al. Extended Rituximab (anti-CD20 monoclonal antibody) therapy for relapsed or refractory low-grade or follicular non-Hodgkin's lymphoma. *Ann Oncol* 1999; 10: 655–661.

36. Ghielmini M, Schmitz SF, Cogliatti SB, et al. Prolonged treatment with rituximab in patients with follicular lymphoma significantly increases event-free survival and response duration compared with the standard weekly × 4 schedule. *Blood* 2004; 103:4416–4423.

37. Czuczman MS, Grillo-Lopez AJ, White CA, et al. Treatment of patients with low-grade B-cell lymphoma with the combination of chimeric anti-CD20 monoclonal antibody and CHOP chemotherapy. *J Clin Oncol* 1999; 17:268–276.

38. Vose JM, Link BK, Grossbard ML, et al. Phase II study of rituximab in combination with chop chemotherapy in patients with previously untreated, aggressive non-Hodgkin's lymphoma. *J Clin Oncol* 2001; 19: 389–397.

39. Coiffier B, Lepage E, Briere J, et al. CHOP chemotherapy plus rituximab compared with CHOP alone in elderly patients with diffuse large-B-cell lymphoma. *N Engl J Med* 2002; 346:235–242.

40. Habermann TM, Weller EA, Morrison VA, et al. Phase III trial of rituximab-CHOP (R-CHOP) vs. CHOP with a second randomization to maintenance rituximab (MR) or observation in patients 60 years of age and older with diffuse large B-cell lymphoma (DLBCL). *Blood* 2003; 102:248(abstract no. 870).

41. Davis TA, Maloney DG, Czerwinski DK, Liles TM, Levy R. Anti-idiotype antibodies can induce long-term complete remissions in non-Hodgkin's lymphoma without eradicating the malignant clone. *Blood* 1998; 92:1184–1190.

42. Sacchi S, Federico M, Vitolo U, et al. GISL. Clinical activity and safety of combination immunotherapy with IFN-alpha 2a and Rituximab in patients with relapsed low grade non-Hodgkin's lymphoma. *Haematologica* 2001; 86:951–958.

43. Friedberg JW, Neuberg D, Gribben JG, et al. Combination immunotherapy with rituximab and interleukin 2 in patients with relapsed or refractory follicular non-Hodgkin's lymphoma. *Br J Haematol* 2002; 117:828–834.

44. Ansell SM, Witzig TE, Kurtin PJ, et al. Phase 1 study of interleukin-12 in combination with rituximab in patients with B-cell non-Hodgkin lymphoma. *Blood* 2002; 99:67–74.

45. Jahrsdorfer B, Weiner GJ. Immunostimulatory CpG oligodeoxynucleotides and antibody therapy of cancer. *Semin Oncol* 2003; 30:476–482.

46. Jahrsdorfer B, Hartmann G, Racila E, et al. CpG DNA increases primary malignant B cell expression of costimulatory molecules and target antigens. *J Leukoc Biol* 2001; 69:81–88.

47. Leung SO, Goldenberg DM, Dion AS, et al. Construction and characterization of a humanized, internalizing, B-cell (CD22)-specific, leukemia/lymphoma antibody, LL2. *Mol Immunol* 1995; 32:1413–1427.

48. Leonard JP, Coleman M, Ketas JC, et al. Phase I/II trial of epratuzumab (humanized anti-CD22 antibody) in indolent non-Hodgkin's lymphoma. *J Clin Oncol* 2003; 21(16):3051–3059.

49. Leonard JP, Coleman M, Matthews JC, et al. Epratuzumab (Anti-CD22) and rituximab (anti-CD20) combination immunotherapy for non-Hodgkin's lymphoma: preliminary response data. *Proc Am Soc Clin Oncol* 2002; 21:1060a.

50. Coleman M, Goldenberg DM, Siegel AB, et al. Epratuzumab: targeting B-cell malignancies through CD22. *Clin Cancer Res* 2003; 9:39,915–39,945.

51. Micallef INM, Kahl B, Gayko U, et al. A pilot study of epratuzumab and rituximab in combination with CHOP chemotherapy (ER-CHOP) in previously untreated patients with diffuse large B-cell lymphoma (DLBCL). *Proc Am Soc Hematol* 2003.

52. Bains SK, Mone A, Yun Tso J, et al. Mitochondria control of cell death induced by anti-HLA-DR antibodies. *Leukemia* 2003; 17:1357–1365.

53. Link BK, Wang H, Byrd JC, et al. Phase I study of Hu1D10 monoclonal antibody in patients with B-cell lymphoma. *Proc Am Soc Clin Oncol* 2001; 20:284a.

54. Link BK, Wang H, Byrd JC, et al. Prolonged clinical responses in patients with follicular lymphoma treated on a Phase I trial of the anti-hla-dr monoclonal antibody Remitogen[a] (Hu1D10). *Proc Am Soc Hematol* 2001; 98:244b.

55. Link BK, Kahl B, Czuczman M, et al. A Phase II study of Remitogen™ (Hu1D10), a humanized monoclonal antibody in patients with relapsed or refractory follicular, small lymphocytic, or marginal zone/MALT B-cell lymphoma. *Proc Am Soc Hematol* 2001; 98:2540.

56. Lundin J, Osterborg A, Brittinger G, et al. CAMPATH-1H monoclonal antibody in therapy for previously treated low-grade non-Hodgkin's lymphomas: a phase II multicenter study. European Study Group of CAMPATH-1H treatment in low-grade non-Hodgkin's lymphoma. *J Clin Oncol* 1998; 16:3257–3263.

57. Khorana A, Bunn P, McLaughlin P, Vose J, Stewart C, Czuczman MS. A phase II multicenter study of CAMPATH-1H antibody in previously treated patients with nonbulky non-Hodgkin's lymphoma. *Leuk Lymphoma* 2001; 41:77–87.

58. Younes A, Hariharan K, Allen RS, Leigh BR. Initial trials of anti-CD80 monoclonal antibody (Galiximab) therapy for patients with relapsed or refractory follicular lymphoma. *Clin Lymphoma* 2003; 3:257–259.

59. Ansell S, Byrd J, Horwitz S, et al. Phase I/II study of a fully human anti-CD30 monoclonal antibody (MDX-060) in Hodgkin's disease (HD) and anaplastic large cell lymphoma (ALCL). *Blood* 2003; 102: 181a.

60. Bartlett NL, Bernstein SH, Leonard JP, et al. Safety, antitumor activity and pharmacokinetics of six weekly doses of SGN-30 (anti-CD30 monoclonal antibody) in patients with refractory or recurrent CD30+ hematologic malignancies. *Blood* 2003; 102:647a.

61. Kaminski MS, Zasadny KR, Francis IR, et al. Iodine-131-anti-B1 radioimmunotherapy for B-cell lymphoma. *J Clin Oncol* 1996; 14:1974–1981.

62. Liu SY, Eary JF, Petersdorf SH, et al. Follow-up of relapsed B-cell lymphoma patients treated with iodine-131-labeled anti-CD20 antibody and autologous stem-cell rescue. *J Clin Oncol* 1998; 16:3270–3278.

63. Witzig TE, White CA, Wiseman GA, et al. Phase I/II trial of IDEC-Y2B8 radioimmunotherapy for treatment of relapsed or refractory CD20(+) B-cell non-Hodgkin's lymphoma. *J Clin Oncol* 1999; 17:3793–3803.

64. Witzig TE, White CA, Gordon LI, et al. Safety of yttrium-90 ibritumomab tiuxetan radioimmunotherapy for relapsed low-grade, follicular, or transformed non-Hodgkin's lymphoma. *J Clin Oncol* 2003; 21: 1263–1270.

65. Witzig TE, Gordon LI, Cabanillas F, et al. Randomized controlled trial of yttrium-90-labeled ibritumomab tiuxetan radioimmunotherapy versus rituximab immunotherapy for patients with relapsed or refractory low-grade, follicular, or transformed B-cell non-Hodgkin's lymphoma. *J Clin Oncol* 2002; 20:2453–2463.

66. Press OW, Unger JM, Braziel RM, et al. A phase 2 trial of CHOP chemotherapy followed by tositumomab/iodine I 131 tositumomab for previously untreated follicular non-Hodgkin's lymphoma: Southwest Oncology Group Protocol S9911. *Blood* 2003; 102:1606–1612.

67. Vose JM, Colcher D, Gobar L, et al. Phase I/II trial of multiple dose [131]Iodine-MAb LL2 (CD22) in patients with recurrent non-Hodgkin's lymphoma. *Leuk Lymphoma* 2000; 3:91–101.

68. Denardo GL, Lamborn KR, Goldstein DS, Kroger LA, Denardo SJ. Increased survival associated with radiolabeled Lym-1 therapy for non-Hodgkin's lymphoma and chronic lymphocytic leukemia. *Cancer* 1997; 80:2706–2711.

69. Postema EJ, Raemaekers JM, Oyen WJ, et al. Final results of a phase I radioimmunotherapy trial using (186)Re-epratuzumab for the treatment of patients with non-Hodgkin's lymphoma. *Clin Cancer Res* 2003; 9(10 Pt 2):3995S–4002S.

70. Schilder RJ, Witzig TE, Gordon L, et al. 90Y ibritumomab tiuxetan (Zevalin˙) radioimmunotherapy does not preclude effective delivery of subsequent therapy for lymphoma. *Proc Am Soc Clin Oncol* 2002; 21:267a.

71. Ansell SM, Ristow KM, Habermann TM, Wiseman GA, Witzig TE. Subsequent chemotherapy regimens are well tolerated after radioimmunotherapy with yttrium-90 ibritumomab tiuxetan for non-Hodgkin's lymphoma. *J Clin Oncol* 2002; 20:3885–3890.

.

26 Approaches to In Vivo Imaging of Cancer Immunotherapy

George A. Vielhauer, Bond Almand,
Mary L. Disis, David A. Mankoff,
and Keith L. Knutson

SUMMARY

Advancements in our understanding of the immune system have ushered in a new era of immune-based therapeutic strategies to treat and prevent cancer. However, the success of refining and clinical testing of these novel therapeutic strategies has required the development of new ways to monitor tumor and immune responses for a number of reasons. First, in vitro measures of the immune response are limited, and do not reflect important immune events that occur in vivo. Second, commonly used tumor response criteria may not be indicative of therapeutic activity. Lastly, typical approaches to defining the dose of a drug to treat cancer are not applicable to immune-based cancers. These problems have led to the development of newer monitoring strategies including a wide variety of whole-body imaging approaches. Imaging can provide insight into the actions of immune-based therapies that ordinarily would not be possible, and will likely result in enhanced decision making as to what strategies should, or should not be, moved into advanced clinical testing. In this chapter, a number of imaging techniques are discussed as well as their application to the development, understanding, and clinical monitoring of immune-based therapies.

Key Words: Imaging; PET; MRI; immunotherapy; vaccines; T-cells; immunity; CT.

1. INTRODUCTION

New paradigms in the treatment of cancer have emerged over the past decade because of improved capabilities for identifying molecular cancer targets and the production of therapeutics directed at those targets. These novel targeted therapies include cancer vaccines, antiangiogenics, tyrosine kinase inhibitors, T-cell therapy, proteasome inhibitors, and monoclonal antibodies (MAbs). A major obstacle preventing the successful development and clinical translation of target therapies is the lack of appropriate measures of therapeutic effectiveness of the drug. Novel in vivo imaging techniques have been developed in recent years that can be used as markers to improve assessing therapeutic and clinical outcome. The three major problems that novel imaging techniques can overcome are

From: *Cancer Drug Discovery and Development: Immunotherapy of Cancer*
Edited by: M. L. Disis © Humana Press Inc., Totowa, NJ

1. The inability of commonly used tumor size measurement strategies (e.g., the Response Evaluation Criteria in Solid Tumors standard) to measure slow or cytostatic responses.
2. The inability of assessment strategies to detect altered tumor phenotype that can be induced by targeted therapies.
3. The inadequacy of toxicity-based dosing for early clinical trials of immune-based approaches.

In clinical trials of cytotoxic antitumor drugs, the standard platform for assessing the clinical response of existing, as well as novel therapeutic strategies, is the Response Evaluation Criteria in Solid Tumors standard. This platform was specifically designed for rapid-acting drugs that can induce significant tumor responses within a matter of weeks. However, this approach is not well suited for treatments that do not result in an appreciable change in tumor size or where such changes occur slowly. To accurately evaluate certain targeted therapeutics, especially with respect to novel immunotherapies, more immediate and sensitive modalities are required to evaluate individual patient responses, enabling accurate prediction of efficacy and outcome.

Acquired resistance may be because of out growth of tumors that have undergone phenotypic changes because of exposure to the targeted therapies. For example, animal studies have shown that cytostatic immune-based approaches targeting single antigens (e.g., Herceptin, rituximab) can generate antigen-low or antigen-negative variants (1). An important question arising from these scenarios is how should we detect the outgrowth of antigen-loss variants, and if they are detected, what would be the best course of action? Would it be wise to continue therapy, discontinue therapy and risk the reemergence of the antigen-expressing phenotype, or would it be best to add another targeted therapy to combat the tumor that has emerged despite therapy?

Several newer targeted therapies have remarkable safety profiles. A typical approach to assess the appropriate dosing in early-phase clinical trials of cancer cytotoxic agents is to increase the dose until dose-limiting toxicity is attained. Immune-based targeted therapies, for example, are relatively safe, and increasing the dose to a toxic level may not be possible and if so, it may not be useful for defining the most immunogenic dose. In this case, the most appropriate marker for assessing maximum and potentially therapeutic activity would be evaluating an immune parameter, such as the recruitment of T-cells to malignant tissues. In addition, patient heterogeneity may require increasing or decreasing doses to attain the desired level of activity.

Problems such as those summarized have required us to consider developing alternative strategies to act as surrogates of therapeutic success. Novel imaging strategies represent one avenue for developing surrogates of drug action or clinical responses. A variety of imaging techniques—some old, some new, and some revitalized—are currently available for determining the answers to many of the questions related to the activities of novel targeted therapies. In this chapter, we review the major imaging modalities and how their strengths can be applied to the monitoring of targeted immune-based approaches for cancer treatment.

2. IMAGING MODALITIES

2.1. Magnetic Resonance Imaging

Magnetic resonance imaging (MRI) uses strong magnetic fields to align the unpaired nuclear spins or magnetic dipoles, such as hydrogen atoms in water (2). Radiofrequency pulses are applied, causing a "flip" in the spin state of hydrogen nuclei into an excited state. Subsequent relaxation of the spin results in the hydrogen nuclei realigning with the principal magnetic field to emit electromagnetic signals that can be detected and quantified. The use of contrast agents (e.g., gadolinium or iron oxide) modulates the local magnetic properties of tissue, leading to signal changes associated with contrast accumulation. A significant advantage of MRI over some other techniques such as optical imaging and ultrasound is that signal strength and spatial resolution are depth invariant *(3)*. MRI allows for much higher spatial resolution for structural imaging than optical techniques and avoids the need for ionizing radiation as in computed tomography (CT) and single-photon emission computed tomography (SPECT)/positron-emission tomography (PET). The major limitations of MRI, with respect to molecular imaging, include relatively long imaging times (up to hours) and the need for relatively high and potentially toxic levels of contrast reagents *(4)*. Some contrast agents are bulky, and may encounter barriers to delivery from the blood stream to the target tissues. Recently, a variety of MRI techniques and contrast reagents has been developed with the potential to assess cellular and tissue functional properties. For example, MRI applications can assess tissue blood volume, blood flow, perfusion, and the permeability of capillaries that are macroscopic indicators of the physiological status of the vasculature *(5)*. More recently, enzyme-activated magnetic resonance contrast reagents have been developed that can report on the metabolic and physiological status of an organ or tissue *(6)*. Included in this group are intracellular calcium *(7)*, pH *(8)*, and pO_2 *(9,10)* reporters that could potentially be used for several purposes including detection of angiogenesis and intracellular signal transduction.

2.2. Ultrasound

Clinical ultrasound imaging is the most common imaging modality used in the world *(11)*. Advantages of ultrasound are its safety, portability, and high spatial resolution (40–500 µm) *(12)*. Ultrasound imaging uses high-frequency sound waves that are reflected from the body's fluid and tissues. A transducer records the reflections to produce an image. Clinically, ultrasound has typically been used for assessing organ perfusion, as well as anatomical characterization. Contrast agents (e.g., lipid microsomes or microbubbles) have been developed that can enhance the reflection or echo of sound waves improving image resolution. These microbubbles are composed of a gas (usually air or perfluorocarbon) surrounded by a lipid monolayer (solubilizing agent) and are less than 10 µm in diameter, allowing them to cross capillary beds. Microbubbles can also have protein ligands or antibodies incorporated into their lipid surface to be directed at specific cellular targets (c.g., adhesion proteins or growth factor receptors) *(12)*. For example, microbubbles in experimental models have demonstrated active targeting of endothelial cell receptors and adhesion proteins, such as α_v-integrins and P selectin, respectively *(13,14)*. As opposed to other contrast agents, they cannot leave the vasculature, thus limiting their utility. A drawback of ultrasound is that it is limited by the tissue depth, and is primarily more useful for superficial imaging. Imaging deep tissues causes an attenuation of the sound wave echo, resulting in a lack of signal and subsequent image. There have been recent efforts at making ultrasound quantitative for research purposes, including the development of an approach called second harmonic, or stimulated acoustic, emission imaging *(15)*. This technique picks up the second resonant frequency that is specific for microbubbles and not detectable from other tissues. The utility of this technique to detect quantitatively parametric changes has been recently demonstrated by Mauer and colleagues in a study of intracellular adhesion molecule 1 expression in the spinal cord and brain in the experimental autoimmune encephalitis (EAE) model. They demonstrated that changes in intracellular adhesion molecule 1 expression could be detected using acoustic emission imaging in animals receiving corticosteroids as treatment *(16)*.

2.3. Computed Tomography

CT is a type of X-ray imaging regularly used to observe anatomy using contrast, such as the lungs. Images are obtained as specimen tissues differentially absorb X-rays that are passed through a body. Unlike ultrasound, there is no limit to the depth of penetration, and resolution can be as good as 10 μm for micro-CT imagers *(17,18)*. CT obtains three-dimensional (volumetric) data by rotating a source and detector around the specimen or by rotating the specimen within a stationary detector. Like MRI, CT uses contrast agents to examine the vascularity of tissue and enhance contrast to delineate structures, such as the intestines. Some of the more commonly used contrast reagents are iodine and barium. The potential for toxicity or physiological interference caused by these agents is high, because they must be used at relatively high concentrations. This restricts CT's potential as a molecular imaging tool. CT is also currently used in combination with PET to provide combined anatomical and biochemical information.

2.4. Positron-Emission Tomography

PET involves the imaging of detected annihilation γ-photons that are released when radionuclides (^{18}F, ^{11}C, and ^{15}O) release positrons that undergo annihilation with electrons. PET has a theoretical spatial resolution limit of 1–2 mm, with no limit to depth of penetration. A significant advantage is that PET requires only nanogram amounts of molecular probe to make an image, making PET and other nuclear methods true tracer imaging *(19,20)*. Human imaging devices can achieve practical spatial resolution as low as 4–5 mm, whereas dedicated small-animal imaging devices can approach a physical limit of 1–2 mm. Positron-emitting isotopes include more "biological" nuclei such as carbon and fluorine, and therefore can be used to synthesize radioactive imaging probes that can closely mimic native biochemicals. ^{18}F is used to synthesize 2-[^{18}F]-fluoro-2-deoxy-D-glucose (FDG), which can be used to measure glucose metabolism. Similarly, ^{11}C can be incorporated into methionine, choline, or thymidine to measure protein metabolism, membrane biosynthesis, or DNA synthesis rates, respectively *(21)*. Because all isotopes result in release of two γ-rays of the same energy, injecting two probes of different isotopes to measure two separate parameters simultaneously will not allow PET detectors to distinguish them. Thus, to investigate multiple molecular events, each probe must be injected independently, allowing for the decay of the first probe before the second is administered. Another major drawback of PET imaging is that there is a significant lack of anatomic detail. The development of PET–CT that combines PET with the anatomic detail provided by CT is underway, and may be an important tool for both clinical practice and biological research *(22)*.

2.5. Single-Photon Emission Computed Tomography

SPECT is a radionuclide imaging method similar in concept to PET. SPECT imaging utilizes single-photon γ-emitting radioisotopes, e.g., ^{99m}technetium (^{99m}Tc), ^{111}indium (^{111}In), and ^{131}iodine (^{131}I), producing low-energy γ-rays that interact with sodium iodide crystals that can be imaged by positron-sensitive radiation detectors, often called γ-cameras.

By rotating the camera around the subject and acquiring images at different angles, the radiopharmaceutical distribution generates tomographic images with of reconstruction algorithms similar to PET *(23)*. Because isotopes with the aid of different photon energies can be distinguished, SPECT allows for imaging of more than one radiopharmaceutical at the same time. Unlike PET, however, SPECT detectors need physical collimation to form an image, introducing a trade-off between resolution and sensitivity that limits image quality. Quantification of radiopharmaceutical concentration is less accurate in SPECT than in PET, and most SPECT isotopes (e.g., ^{99m}Tc) are not native to biological systems, limiting the design of the probes.

2.6. Optical Imaging

Optical molecular imaging capable of producing physiological images by generating visible light can also be utilized for whole-body imaging *(24)*. This type of optical imaging is termed bioluminescent imaging (BLI). The most common detector system for this application is based on charge-coupled device cameras. BLI utilizes the expression of transgenes, such as luciferase enzyme, from glowing species (e.g., algae or fireflies) that produce a wide spectrum of visible light wavelengths when contacted with oxygen and enzyme substrate in a given specimen *(25)*. BLI has been used for infections, tumors, and explicit gene expression patterns in whole-body live rodents *(26)*. Several advantages of this application include the virtual lack of background noise (resulting in detection of very low signals), the ability to image multiple anesthetized animals at once, ease of operation and inexpensiveness, as well as short acquisition times. BLI has high detection sensitivity. In laboratory rodents, BLI is capable of imaging tumors in as few as 1000 cells compared with current clinical oncology imaging that has a tumor detection limit of 500,000 cells *(27)*. The major shortcomings of this modality begin with the efficiency of light transmission through an opaque animal, which depends largely on the tissue type and scattering of light. Skin and muscle have the highest transmission but are comparatively wavelength dependent, whereas highly perfused organs, such as the liver and spleen, have low transmission because of absorption of light by oxyhemoglobin and deoxyhemoglobin *(20)*. It is estimated from in vitro studies that the overall reduction of BLI signal is approx 10-fold for every centimeter of tissue depth, enabling only reliable images to be obtained 2 cm below the surface, with exact variation depending on tissue type *(20,28)*. A second limitation is that the images are two-dimensional and lack depth information. Rotating charge-coupled device cameras would alleviate this disadvantage and allow for volumetric imaging, but this technology has yet to be designed. The most important limitation is the lack of an equivalent imaging modality for humans, preventing its translation to clinical use.

Another recent optical approach is quantum dots (QDs) that are metal or semiconductor nanoparticles ranging from 2 to 6 nm. QDs have unique size-tunable optical and electrical properties. These nanoparticles emit a multicolor fluorescence signal that is detected by an optical imager. Functional QDs have been covalently bioconjugated to biological molecules (10–15 nm in size), such as peptides, antibodies, small ligands, and nucleic acids, for use as probes by in vivo microscopy *(29–32)*. Disadvantages include a restricted volume of distribution to the vasculature that prevents penetration of the endothelium, excretion into the urine, and nonspecific clearance by reticuloendothelial cells (e.g., dendritic cells [DCs] and macrophages), which decreases their bioavailability *(33)*. QDs have recently been used to image human prostate tumors in mice following injection of a QD-conjugated antibody against the prostate-specific membrane antigen *(34)*. In this case, the tumor vasculature is leaky enough to permit labeling of the tumor cells with the antibody. Overall, low cost and ease of use make optical imaging methods attractive for imaging animal models. However, limited penetration depth makes optical imaging less applicable to human studies outside of tissues close to epithelial surfaces.

3. PREDICTION AND EVALUATION OF RESPONSE TO THERAPY USING IN VIVO IMAGING

Imaging tumors to predict or assess therapeutic response can be advantageous for a number of reasons. Predicting whether there will be a response is critical for patient care, because therapeutic strategies often require long courses of treatment to stabilize or cause regression of disease. Imaging before or early in the course of disease can also be useful for adjusting treatment to reflect inherent patient heterogeneity. Many of the novel imaging technologies that have been developed to detect and stage cancers are being modified and improved to be useful in quantifying tumor phenotype or response to therapy. Probes are now available that can directly evaluate intratumoral events related to immune-based therapy, including apoptosis, metabolic changes in tumor, changes in the tumor microenvironment (e.g., blood flow), and changes in the tumor phenotype.

3.1. Apoptosis

Apoptosis, or programmed cell death, can be induced by several immune-based approaches including MAb (e.g., anti-CD22), cytokine (e.g., tumor necrosis factor-related apoptosis-inducing ligand), and T-cell therapy, all of which have been shown to, or are postulated to, induce apoptosis in vivo *(35–37)*. One of the earliest hallmarks of the induction of the apoptosis cascade is the fast externalization of phosphatidylserine (PS) from the intracellular to the extracellular side of the cell membrane *(38)*. Annexin V is a calcium-dependent, phospholipid-binding protein that rapidly recognizes external PS and has been used extensively to identify apoptotic cells *(39)*. Annexin V can be labeled for in vivo imaging detection by a number of different methods including ^{99m}Tc for SPECT, ^{124}I or ^{18}fluorine (^{18}F) for PET, and Alexa Flour 488 for optical imaging *(40,41)*. Figure 1 shows how ^{99m}Tc-annexin labels apoptosis of lymphoma immediately following treatment with an apoptosis inducer *(42)*. The minimal cell mass required for successful detection of apoptosis varies with the in vivo imaging technique, but studies indicate that some methods have high resolution. For example, heart transplant rejection studies have demonstrated evidence of apoptosis in less than 10% of cells when performing annexin imaging *(43,44)*. Cordiero and colleagues demonstrated the capability of real-time optical imaging of single-nerve cell apoptosis in retinal degeneration *(45)*. One limitation of Annexin V imaging is its specificity. Cells dying of necrosis may also be labeled, because the intracellular PS will become available for binding once the cell membrane ruptures. Thus, it is probable in tumor masses that it will be difficult to distinguish between apoptosis or necrosis. Nonetheless, if the outcome of therapy is cell death, this may not be an important issue.

Another hallmark of apoptosis is the activation of a family of cysteine-containing aspartate-specific proteases called the caspases *(46)*. Radiolabeled caspase substrates and inhibitors are being developed as more-specific apoptotic detectors compared to PS imaging, where necrotic cells can contribute to the cell death signals *(38)*. Several optical imaging

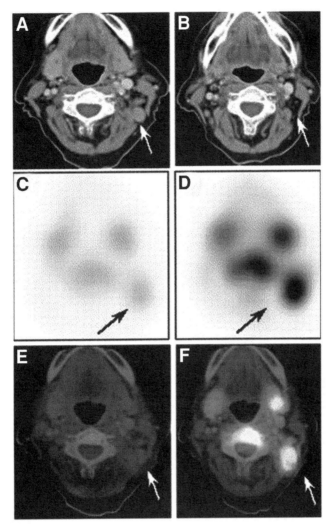

Fig. 1. Folicular non-Hodgkin's lymphoma in 60-yr-old women with enlarged lymph nodes in the neck on the left side, level III. Baseline computed tomography (CT) scan (**A**) demonstrates enlarged lymph nodes, with complete response on the follow up CT scan (**B**) performed 1 mo after the start of radiotherapy (white arrows). Single-photon emission computed tomography before (**C**) and early after (**D**) the start of radiotherapy show increase of ^{99m}technetium–Annexin V uptake from weak to intense (black arrows). Fusion single-photon emission computed tomography/CT images (**E,F**) allows precise localization and grading of increased tracer uptake in the tumor (white arrows), salivary gland, and the cervical bone marrow. (Adapted with permission from ref. *42*.)

approaches are being examined for suitability in detecting caspase activation in vivo. Peptide substrates of caspase 1 linked to a near-infrared-fluorescent probe have been used in living animals to detect apoptosis *(47)*. Similar strategies are also being developed that use fluorescent resonance energy transfer combined with substrates of caspases *(48)*. Caspase inhibitors have also been examined but may not be useful substrates because of sensitivity issues. For example, benzyloxycarbonyl-Val-Ala-DL-Asp(*O*-methyl)-fluoro-methyl ketone, a pancaspase inhibitor, has been examined as a potential imaging agent in the form of [^{131}I] benzyloxycarbonyl-Val-Ala-DL-Asp(*O*-methyl)-fluoromethyl ketone by Haberkorn and colleagues *(49)*. Whereas they could detect changes in binding of the radioligand following the induction of apoptosis, the changes were only twofold. Caspase substrates, therefore, may be a more attractive option, because continued activity of the caspases can lead to accumulation of radioactive metabolites *(38)*. This would serve as an amplification of the tracer signal, improving target to background ratio.

3.1.1. Tumor Proliferation

Proliferation is a hallmark observation of tumors and is more specific for tumors than glycolysis (discussed in Subheading 3.3.) that is also associated with inflammation and tissue healing. One of the most commonly used approaches to image proliferation in the tumor is with PET imaging following injection of ^{11}carbon (^{11}C)-thymidine, a tracer that is chemically identical to native thymidine. ^{11}C-thymidine can be directly incorporated into DNA, and imaging it in tumors may be useful for predicting responses to therapy as has been previously shown by Shields and colleagues *(50)*. In that study, five patients with small cell lung cancer or high-grade sarcoma were monitored for response to therapy using ^{11}C-thymidine PET imaging before and after a single cycle of chemotherapy. PET imaging showed an early response to successful treatment. Three patients who ultimately had a complete response to therapy demonstrated 100% declines in thymidine flux, whereas a patient with a partial response had a 40% reduction. The remaining patient, however, had neither a response to therapy nor a reduction in thymidine incorporation. Imaging of proliferation will likely be a useful strategy for several immunotherapy modalities, such as MAb therapies, because unlike chemotherapy, antibodies can act by inhibiting growth signaling (e.g., trastuzumab) with or without altering tumor metabolism. Our laboratory has tested this approach in combination with cellular metabolism tracers for monitoring responses to therapy. Figure 2 shows murine ex vivo data that indicate that the assessment of cellular proliferation using labeled thymidine and intratumoral metabolism using labeled deoxyglucose may provide a quantitative approach to monitor cancer patients undergoing MAb therapy. In that experiment, *neu*-transgenic mice (a mouse model of HER-2/*neu* breast cancer) with breast tumors were treated with a *neu*-specific MAb or control vehicle beginning on day 12 and subsequently tested for tumor size, proliferation, and metabolism. The therapy resulted in disease stabilization as shown in Fig. 2A. Proliferation and metabolism (discussed in Subheading 3.3.) were assessed using ^{3}H-deoxyglucose and ^{14}C-thymidine, respectively. As shown, treatment was associated with both decreased metabolism and proliferation, suggesting that imaging these parameters may be useful for detecting or predicting response to antibody-based therapies (Fig. 2B). The use of ^{11}C-thymidine, however, has been problematic because of its extensive metabolism, resulting in the labeling of other cellular molecules. Thus, other nonmetabolizable analogs of thymidine are being developed *(51)*. For example, 3'deoxy-3'-[^{18}F]fluorothymidine (FLT) has recently been shown to be useful for evaluating tumor proliferation. The imaged signal obtained with FLT correlates with in vitro measures of proliferation that were performed on biopsy specimens *(52)*. Future studies will determine whether FLT can be used to monitor response to therapy.

Compared with metabolism, measuring proliferation in vivo may have a greater advantage for use in adoptive cellular therapy strategies, because any decrease in metabolism following adoptive transfer of immune cells may be masked by the contribution to the metabolism signal by the infiltrating immune cells *(37)*. Alternatively, given that many

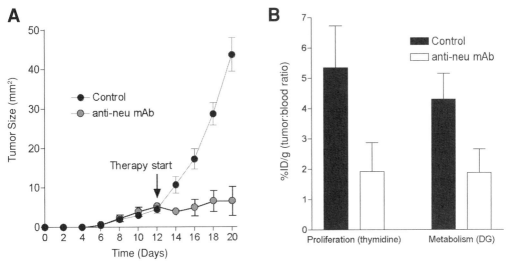

Fig. 2. Tumors treated with monoclonal antibody therapy demonstrate reduced glycolysis and proliferation. Tumor-bearing *neu*-transgenic mice were treated with control vehicle (control) or *neu*-specific antibody. **(A)** Tumor measurements over the course of therapy. **(B)** Before removal of tumor, radiotracers specific for glycolysis and DNA synthesis were injected. Tumors uptake of radiotopes was evaluated by scintillation. (Note that tumors have reduced proliferation and metabolism in treated animals.)

immune-based approaches are cytostatic, the imaging of proliferation may be more appropriate because cytostatic agents may not necessarily affect glycolysis.

3.2. Perfusion and Angiogenesis

All tumors are dependent on perfusion for growth *(53)*. Tumors release angiogenesis-inducing factors that result in the growth of new capillary blood vessels. In the absence of angiogenesis, tumor growth remains microscopic and cannot migrate through the body via the circulatory system *(53)*. Based on these tumor characteristics, many strategies in immunotherapy rely on targeting the tumor vasculature and angiogenesis to prevent further tumor growth. This is accomplished either passively with antibodies or through the induction of antivascular T-cells with vaccines or T-cell infusions *(54,55)*. The affect of antivascular or antiangiogenic therapies may not be observable at the macroscopic tumor level for many months, and therefore, it is critical to ascertain whether an effect is occurring as a results of treatment *(56)*. Although many approaches to monitoring perfusion and angiogenesis are being developed, at the forefront are novel in vivo imaging techniques *(57)*.

Vascular endothelial growth factor (VEGF) is an angiogenic factor produced by most tumors and results in neovascular growth by activating VEGF receptors (VEGF-R) found on several tissues. VEGF induces hyperpermeability of the tumor vasculature, an important property that occurs during angiogenesis that can be imaged in vivo. Blocking the effects of VEGF either with anti-VEGF or anti-VEGF-R antibodies can result in rapid decreases in vascular permeability that can be imaged. Morgan and colleagues studied whether a specific type of MRI, called dynamic contrast-enhanced MRI, could be used as a surrogate marker for an antitumor effect of a VEGF-R tyrosine kinase inhibitor,

PTK787/ZK 222584 *(58).* Twenty-six patients had dynamic contrast-enhanced MRI done before therapy, on day 2, and at the end of each 28-d cycle. Tumor permeability and vascularity were assessed by calculating the bidirectional transfer constant. Patients were given varying doses of the drug, ranging from 50 to 2000 mg once daily. Results showed that PTK787/ZK 222584 caused a statistically significant reduction in tumor vascular permeability and that the reduction was dose-dependent (Fig. 3). There was also a significant relationship between reduction in permeability and disease response. This was an important study, because it demonstrated the utility of MRI imaging of vascular permeability as a surrogate for the therapeutic efficacy of a targeted drug. Imaging early in therapy may assist clinicians in altering doses to achieve the desired affect.

Other imaging strategies can also be used to directly detect blood flow into a tumor that could be useful for monitoring responses to immune approaches aimed at directly destroying the tumor vasculature. The positron emitter ^{15}O has been used extensively to produce $H_2^{15}O$ to evaluate blood flow through tumor tissues using PET imaging *(59).* PET offers rigorous quantification, and studies have shown that quantitative changes in tumor blood flow predict therapy response and disease recurrence in some settings *(60).* Lodge and colleagues developed a parametric imaging approach that gave better image quality and quantitative accuracy that could possibly lead to a broader use of PET analysis of blood flow to monitor responses to therapy *(61).* ^{99m}Tc-sestamibi, a radiopharmaceutical developed for myocardial perfusion that may also indicate tumor blood flow, has also been shown to be predictive of response and survival when applied to treatment monitoring *(62).* In another approach, Kiessling and colleagues developed a CT-based technique that images the vasculature with exquisite detail *(63).* This unique approach, called volumetric CT, produces three-dimensional imaging (Fig. 4). The technique is able to define the fine intricate vessel structure in the tumor and peritumor areas and can image vessels as small as 50 μm.

Strategies that monitor specific vascular or vascular-related molecules are also being developed. For example, endostatin has been labeled with ^{99m}Tc to help understand antiangiogenic therapy using SPECT *(64).* Endostatin, discovered approx 5 yr ago, is an inhibitor of angiogenesis, and an endostatin-radionuclide conjugate could assist in predicting which patients would respond directly to endostatin treatment *(64).* Similar approaches are also being taken to develop PET imaging agents that detect the expression of cell adhesion integrins involved in angiogenesis *(65).*

3.3. Tumor Metabolism

Like proliferation, increased glycolysis is also a hallmark of cancer and is the basis for the increasing use of ^{18}FDG PET imaging in clinical cancer care *(19).* FDG is transported into the cell and phosphorylated in parallel to glucose, but is not further metabolized. Phosphorylated FDG is trapped within the cells and therefore, the amount of FDG retention in tissues reflects the glucose metabolic rate. Whereas the most common use of ^{18}FDG PET imaging in clinical practice is for cancer staging, recent chemotherapy studies have shown that it can accurately predict therapeutic responses *(19,66–68).* For example, Smith and colleagues tested whether ^{18}FDG PET could predict the pathologic response of breast cancer to primary chemotherapy *(68).* In a cohort of 31 patients, they observed that the mean reduction in uptake of ^{18}FDG after the first pulse of imaging chemotherapy was significantly greater in patients who had a complete or partial pathological response. ^{18}FDG PET had the ability to predict a complete pathological response with a sensitivity of 90% and

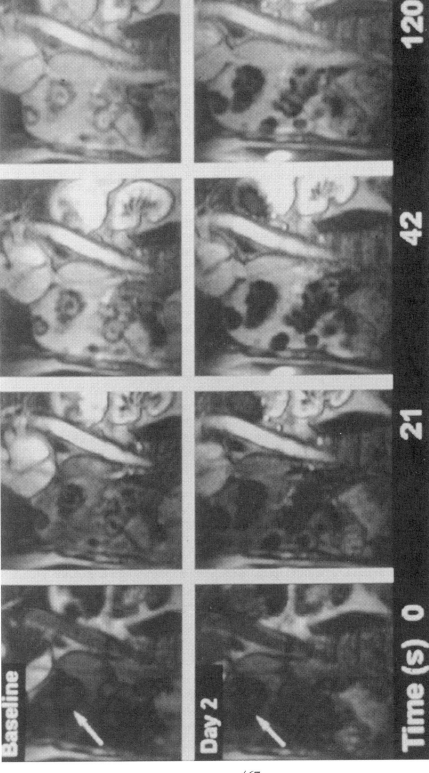

Fig. 3. Reduction of blood flow in a liver metastasis. A liver metastasis is shown at baseline and on day 2 after a dose of PTK787/ZK 222584, a vascular endothelial growth factor receptor tyrosine kinase inhibitor. The sequential images show the tumor (indicated by arrow) at different time points after contrast bolus. Blood flow into the tumor is shown as whitening. (Note that following the administration of the drug, vascular permeability is reduced.) (Adapted with permission from ref. 58.)

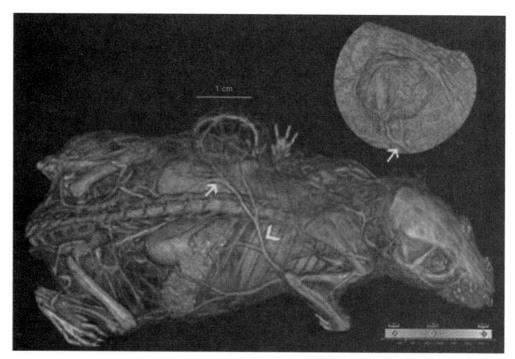

Fig. 4. Three-dimensional (3D) visualization showing volumetric computed tomography angiography of a tumor-bearing nude mouse, and detailed image of the tumor after magnification (top right). The 3D angiography of the whole mouse gives a concise overview of the vascular system, including larger subcutaneous vessels of the skin. Dilatation of subcutaneous vessels (arrow on whole-body visualization), which interact with the tumor tissue, is clearly visible. One large vessel can be tracked from the tumor to the contralateral side of the mouse (arrowhead). The magnification of the tumor shows the increase of vessel density around the tumor and visualizes vessels infiltrating the tumor (arrow on detailed visualization), showing dilatation and an irregular course as typical morphological criteria of malignant tumor vessels. (Adapted with permission from ref. *63*.)

a specificity of 74% *(68)*. These results indicate that glycolytic metabolism may be an effective way of predicting whether there will likely be a response to therapy.

3.4. Phenotype Analysis and Antigen Loss

Sophisticated advances in scientific technology, such as phenotypic and genotypic characterization of many tumor types, have led to an increase in the number of cellular targets that have been discovered and characterized. This has led to a parallel increase in the number of targeted therapies are being developed. To ensure rapid development of these new targeted therapies, prescreening of patients will be required for target expression before or following therapy to ensure that patients still retain target expression. The traditional approach is to identify targets by using biopsy and in vitro assessment of target expression (e.g., HER-2/*neu*, estrogen receptor). However, as is the case with many metastatic cancers, this is not always feasible because of inaccessibility of the tumor tissue. Noninvasive in vivo imaging techniques can assist in assessing the phenotype of the tumor and ultimately aid in therapy design and monitoring.

Behr and colleagues studied whether pretherapeutic immunoscintigraphy with radiolabeled Herceptin could predict the therapeutic efficacy and toxicity of Herceptin therapy in breast cancer patients. Ten patients with HER-2/*neu*-overexpressing metastatic breast cancer underwent daily SPECT following the injection of 5 mCi of ^{111}In-DPTA-trastuzumab for a total of seven scans *(69)*. The patients were then treated for 6 mo with Herceptin. Although the study number was small, it was observed that the six patients who had good tumor targeting of the radioconjugate also had good responses to therapy, whereas the four patients who did not have good localization did not respond. These results suggest that phenotyping the metastatic lesions first may indicate whether therapy will be effective. In addition to a correlation with the clinical response, the investigators also observed that SPECT might also be useful for predicting toxicity. It is well-known that Herceptin therapy is associated with cardiotoxicity in a subset of patients. They observed that the two patients that had cardiac uptake of the drug also experienced cardiac toxicity. These results clearly show the value of using in vivo imaging to assess the responses in patients with advanced disease that is not ordinarily amendable to biopsy sampling.

An alternative approach that may be useful if antibodies are not available was recently developed by Groot-Wassink and colleagues, who described a novel method that permits the imaging of transcriptional activities of genes *(70)*. Promoter fragments from either the RNA or the catalytic protein components of the telomerase genes were used to drive expression of the sodium iodide symporter/PET reporter. The reporters are then placed into adenoviruses and subsequently injected into tumor-bearing animals. Expression of the constructs occurs only in the tumors where telomerase gene transcription rates are abnormally high.

4. IMAGING IMMUNITY IN VIVO

In addition to understanding the qualities of the tumors, it is also necessary to understand the dynamics of the immune response in vivo. A number of strategies have emerged over the past 5 yr that permits the imaging of both endogenous immunity and that which is applied exogenously.

4.1. Imaging Endogenous Immune Effectors

The imaging of antigen- or tissue-specific immunity that is generated endogenously can be used to answer a number of questions related to immune therapy, such as whether there is an expansion of the appropriate immune effector subset and whether there is significant localization to tumor tissue. The major problem with identifying immune effectors that are generated endogenously is that they can be unavailable for labeling techniques (i.e., transfection) that can only be applied to cells when they are removed from the body. This is particularly problematic when the goal is to assess the localization and biodistribution of antigen specific T-cells, which may be of low abundance.

Macrophage accumulation can be indicative of an inflammatory response. A property of macrophages that can be exploited for imaging studies is their ability to engulf particulates. Ultrasmall superparamagnetic iron oxide is a contrast reagent that can detect macrophage accumulation *(71)*. Deloire and colleagues showed that during immunotherapy of EAE with anti-very late antigen-4 (VLA)-4 antibody, macrophage recruitment into lesions cancer be monitored with ultrasmall superparamagnetic iron oxide *(72)*. Anti-VLA-4 antibody therapy, currently in phase III clinical trials for multiple sclerosis, blocks extravasation of T-cells into the brain. A central question in the study by Deloire and colleagues was whether treatment with anti-VLA-4 antibody reduced macrophage and T-cell recruitment to the brain tissue. Endogenous T-cell infiltration was examined with immunohistochemistry. Those animals that failed to develop disease did not have T-cell infiltration into the central nervous system, but still had macrophage infiltration, clearly showing that macrophage accumulation was, alone, not sufficient to mediate EAE alone. Other studies have shown the MRI can also be used to track macrophages to the central nervous system *(73)*.

The imaging of endogenous antigen-specific T-cells is in the hypothetical realm currently because of the lack of appropriate highly selective in vivo labeling methodologies. Imaging of endogenous antigen-specific T-cells will likely require the use of any number of current technologies available for in vitro detection. One strategy, which has been investigated extensively in vitro, is the use of major histocompatibility complex (MHC) class I and class II monomers or multimers. The best-characterized multimers are tetramers that are highly specific probes that bind with high specificity to the T-cell receptor. They consist of MHC molecules complexed to antigen-derived peptides. The complexes are stabilized by tetramerization of four peptide-bound MHC molecules. Tetramers have successfully been labeled with optical probes, such as fluorescent imaging probes, and have been successfully used to study specific T-cell populations in vitro. It is possible that technologies for labeling with other imaging reagents, such as radionuclides, could be developed, followed by testing to examine how long tetramers survive in the systemic circulation and whether the capabilities exist for localization in tumor tissues. Other types of MHC multimers are also being developed that may be effective as imaging agents, such as dimers. Rather than four, the dimers have only two peptide-bound MHC molecules. Recent studies suggest that dimers may be stable enough in vivo to be useful for imaging. For example, Masteller and colleagues produced dimers specific for diabetogenic T-cells, which could be infused into mice to protect against diabetes *(74)*. Moore and colleagues recently described a nanoparticle technology that can incorporate through an avidin and biotin interaction up to eight peptide-bound MHC monomers *(75)*. These nanoparticles consist of superparamagnetic iron oxide, making them useful for MRI. The peptide in this study was the NRP-V7 peptide recognized by diabetogenic CD8 T-cells derived from nonobese diabetic/severe combined immunodeficient mice. The peptide was bound to MHC class I monomers that were subsequently absorbed onto the particles. The final nanoparticle was used to label CD8 T-cells that were subsequently transferred into the mice to monitor for inflammation in the pancreatic islets (Fig. 5). It is unknown if the nanoparticle could be used to label antigen-specific T-cells in vivo, but a significant advantage of this approach is that the localization of eight monomers on the nanoparticle increases the avidity and may improve the detection of low-avidity T-cells. This attribute is particularly attractive for the detection of tumor-antigen-specific T-cells, because it is anticipated that a high frequency of these T-cells will have moderate to low affinities if the population was subject to central tolerizing mechanisms in the thymus.

The in vivo imaging of DCs is an emerging technology that could greatly facilitate our understanding of DC mobilization and particularly antigen presentation. It could potentially improve our understanding of adjuvant action and ways to improve immunization. Typically, the method of choice to monitor whether or not an antigen is processed and presented is by measuring the T-cell response ex vivo. Unfortunately, this method is fraught with problems. First, T-cells require co-stimulation that may not have any correlation with the ability of the DC to process and present antigen. Second, T-cell assays are highly variable and lack sensitivity in unfractionated T-cell populations. Over the last decade, several techniques have been developed to produce probes that specifically recognize

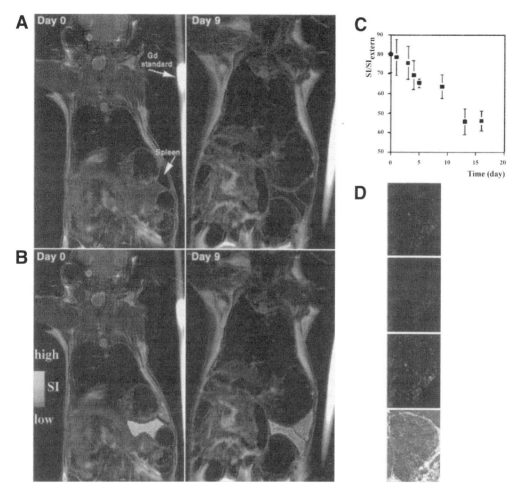

Fig. 5. (A) In vivo imaging of pancreatic infiltration of CD8+ T-cells labeled with crosslinked iron oxide nanoparticles (CLIO)-NRP-V7 and adoptively transferred into 5-wk-old nonobese diabetic severe combined immunodeficient mice. **(B)** Color-encoded signal intensity of the spleen and tail of the pancreas. **(C)** The decrease of the signal intensity from day 0 to day 16 in the pancreas (outlined in red) is owing to the accumulation of CLIO-NRP-V7-labeled CD8+ T-cells. **(D)** Dual-channel fluorescence microscopy of the excised pancreas after the 16th day of magnetic resonance imaging. Green channel shows the presence of CLIO-NRP-V7-labeled cells in the islet; staining with anti-CD8-PE antibodies (red channel) confirmed the presence of transferred cells. Superimposition of two images shows that CLIO-NRP-V7-labeled cells were also positive for CD8+ T-cell markers. Histological hematoxylin and eosin stain of the same islet (consecutive section) shows the infiltration of mononuclear cells in the islet. Magnification ×20. (Adapted with permission from ref. *75*.)

human leukocyte antigen (HLA) class I antigen/tumor antigen–peptide complexes present on DCs. Antibodies (single-chain variable fragments) have been produced that can recognize several MHC-bound human tumor antigen-derived peptides such as the HLA-A1-melanoma-associated antigen $1_{161-169}$ *(76)*, HLA-A2-gp100$_{154-162, 209-217, 280-288}$ *(77)*, and HLA-A2-telomerase catalytic subunit$_{540-548, 865-973}$ *(78)* complexes. Labeling of these antibodies will likely provide additional insight into the realm of antigen presentation in vivo that until recently has remained obscure.

4.2. Imaging-Infused Effectors

Effectors isolated for ex vivo manipulation can be labeled with a variety of imaging agents. In addition to the MRI nanoparticle technology already described, other ex vivo labeling techniques have been developed, including SPECT, MRI, BLI, and PET. ^{111}In oxine has been used for nonspecific cell labeling for SPECT imaging and is commonly used clinically as an approach to image infection. Meidenbauer and colleagues used ^{111}In oxine to label a Melan A peptide-specific T-cell line for tracking cells following infusion in patients with melanoma and observed that the infused T-cells could localize to metastatic tumor deposits *(79)*. Because of its relatively long half-life of approx 3 d, ^{111}In oxine is useful for studying T-cell distribution over several hours to days.

Adonai and colleagues recently developed a labeling technology using ^{64}Cu that has a half-life of 12.7 h *(80)*. The delivery system they developed is ^{64}Cu-pyruvaldehyde-*bis* (N^4-methylthiosemicarbazone) that complexes and shuttles the copper into the cell. Once inside the cell, the copper ion is released from the complex and trapped within the cell. MicroPET studies of T-cell trafficking using ^{64}Cu-pyruvaldehyde-*bis*(N^4-methylthiosemicarbazone) have shown that T-cells can be tracked for up to 36 h following transfer. This is significant, because in the initial phase of T-cell therapy the infused T-cells are often retained in lungs for several hours. Thus, to accurately monitor distribution many additional hours are required to fully determine whether the immune effectors will localize to malignant or diseased tissues.

MRI contrast reagents have also been developed that can make them useful for tracking T-cells. Highly derivatized, crosslinked iron oxide nanoparticles (CLIO-HD), was recently developed that can be used to efficiently label T-cells. Kirscher used CLIO-HD to make the discovery that serial infusion of T-cells results in better penetration of T-cells into the tumor. The signal produced by CLIO-HD was high resolution and could be measured over several days *(81)*.

Reporter gene marking has recently emerged as a technique that is useful for studying not only in vivo trafficking, but also functional changes associated with infused immune effectors. Several of the imaging platforms that are currently available have been adapted for gene-marking studies including bioluminescence *(82)* and PET imaging *(83)*. Edinger and colleagues produced a retroviral construct containing the luciferase enzyme that was transfected into antitumor NKT-cells, which, following infusion, could be tracked *(82)*. They observed that during the first day, the NKT-cells were largely localized to the lung, followed by distribution to the liver on day 2, and finally, establishing in the tumor tissue for at least 12 d (Fig. 6). Similarly, bioluminescent imaging has been used to track antigen-specific CD4 T-cells to sites of inflammation in a collagen-induced arthritis model *(84)*.

The herpes simplex virus *(HSV)*-thymidine kinase *(TK)* gene, transfected into T-cells, has been used with PET imaging to reveal localization of T-cell to tumor sites *(83)*. The utility of HSV-TK lies in its ability, unlike that of endogenous TK, to phosphoylate thymidine analogues that can be accumulated and trapped within the T-cells. Dubey and colleagues were able to image, using PET, the localization of tumor antigen-specific T-cells in tumor-bearing nude mice *(83)*. In that study, immunogen-sensitized splenic T-cells were retrovirally transfected with HSV-TK and infused into tumor-bearing mice. The tumor-specific T-cells were then visualized in vivo, by injecting 9-(4-[^{18}F]fluoro-3-(hydroxymethylbutyl) guanine, which becomes phosphorylated and trapped in the HSV-TK-expressing cells. This study resulted in a number of important findings such as demonstrating that antigen-specific T-cells home specifically to antigen-positive tumors only. It could be envisioned

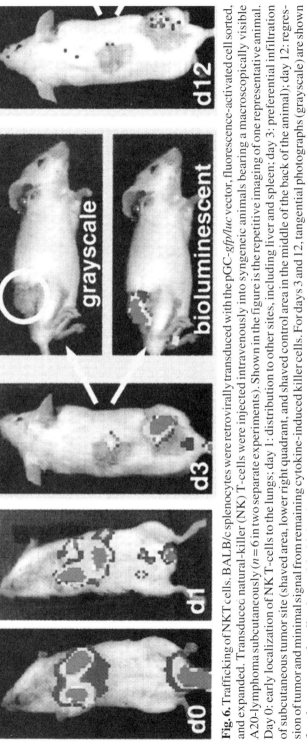

Fig. 6. Trafficking of NKT cells. BALB/c splenocytes were retrovirally transduced with the pGC-*gfp/luc* vector, fluorescence-activated cell sorted, and expanded. Transduced natural-killer (NK) T-cells were injected intravenously into syngeneic animals bearing a macroscopically visible A20-lymphoma subcutaneously (*n* = 6 in two separate experiments). Shown in the figure is the repetitive imaging of one representative animal. Day 0: early localization of NK T-cells to the lungs; day 1: distribution to other sites, including liver and spleen; day 3: preferential infiltration of subcutaneous tumor site (shaved area, lower right quadrant, and shaved control area in the middle of the back of the animal); day 12: regression of tumor and minimal signal from remaining cytokine-induced killer cells. For days 3 and 12, tangential photographs (grayscale) are shown for a better tumor localization and the bioluminescent overlay (bioluminescence) for cytokine-induced killer cell localization. (Adapted with permission from ref. *80*.)

473

that the *HSV-TK* gene could be inserted downstream of a promoter that is only expressed on activation of T-cells that would allow for imaging only at sites able to induce functional changes in T-cells. Overall, in recent years, many strategies have permitted imaging of immune effectors that can lead to improved understanding of immune-based therapies. Although the number of studies of imaging of immune-based therapies is limited, the few studies that have been accomplished have revealed striking in vivo biology that will ultimately pave the way for the more rapid advancement of immunotherapies.

5. CONCLUSION

Over the last several years, the tremendous advances in imaging technology has begun to permit investigators and clinicians to answer important question that would not have been possible using standard in vitro approaches to monitoring responses to immunotherapy. For example, conducting consecutive measurements of the immune response in vivo is now feasible. These improved technologies are reshaping how we can develop drugs. The older paradigms of drug development, such as defining the dose-limiting toxicity or measuring regression early in the course of treatment, do not apply. Imaging is providing us with the ability to define surrogates of tumor responses to therapy. Imaging will also be a valuable tool following drug development when there is a need for early assessments of responses to therapies in order to maximize therapeutic benefit and outcome. Given the plethora of current techniques, in the future it is likely that for each immune-based modality there will be an adequate, feasible, and accurate method to monitor responses and provide customized therapeutics to the cancer patient.

ACKNOWLEDGMENTS

The authors thank Marsha Weese for expert editorial assistance. This work was supported by NIH grants K01-CA100764 (KLK), R01-CA72064 (DAM), and R01-CA85374 (MLD).

REFERENCES

1. Knutson KL, Almand B, Dang Y, Disis ML. *Neu* antigen-negative variants can be generated after *neu*-specific antibody therapy in *neu* transgenic mice. *Cancer Res* 2004; 64:1146–1151.
2. Funovics MA, Kapeller B, Hoeller C, et al. MR imaging of the her2/*neu* and 9.2.27 tumor antigens using immunospecific contrast agents. *Magn Reson Imaging* 2004; 22:843–850.
3. Jacobs RE, Cherry SR. Complementary emerging techniques: high-resolution PET and MRI. *Curr Opin Neurobiol* 2001; 11:621–629.
4. Bulte JW, Duncan ID, Frank JA. In vivo magnetic resonance tracking of magnetically labeled cells after transplantation. *J Cereb Blood Flow Metab* 2002; 22:899–907.
5. Brasch RC, Li KC, Husband JE, et al. In vivo monitoring of tumor angiogenesis with MR imaging. *Acad Radiol* 2000; 7:812–823.
6. Meade TJ, Taylor AK, Bull SR. New magnetic resonance contrast agents as biochemical reporters. *Curr Opin Neurobiol* 2003; 13:597–602.
7. Li WH, Parigi G, Fragai M, Luchinat C, Meade TJ. Mechanistic studies of a calcium-dependent MRI contrast agent. *Inorg Chem* 2002; 41:4018–4024.
8. Lowe MP, Parker D, Reany O, et al. pH-dependent modulation of relaxivity and luminescence in macrocyclic gadolinium and europium complexes based on reversible intramolecular sulfonamide ligation. *J Am Chem Soc* 2001; 123:7601–7609.
9. Thulborn KR, Waterton JC, Matthews PM, Radda GK. Oxygenation dependence of the transverse relaxation time of water protons in whole blood at high field. *Biochim Biophys Acta* 1982; 714:265–270.
10. Ogawa S, Tank DW, Menon R, et al. Intrinsic signal changes accompanying sensory stimulation: functional brain mapping with magnetic resonance imaging. *Proc Natl Acad Sci USA* 1992; 89:5951–5955.
11. Goldberg BB. International arena of ultrasound education. *J Ultrasound Med* 2003; 22:549–551.

12. Schirner M, Menrad A, Stephens A, Frenzel T, Hauff P, Licha K. Molecular imaging of tumor angiogenesis. *Ann NY Acad Sci* 2004; 1014:67–75.

13. Lindner JR, Song J, Christiansen J, Klibanov AL, Xu F, Ley K. Ultrasound assessment of inflammation and renal tissue injury with microbubbles targeted to P-selectin. *Circulation* 2001; 104:2107–2112.

14. Leong-Poi H, Christiansen J, Klibanov AL, Kaul S, Lindner JR. Noninvasive assessment of angiogenesis by ultrasound and microbubbles targeted to alpha(v)-integrins. *Circulation* 2003; 107:455–460.

15. Calliada F, Campani R, Bottinelli O, Bozzini A, Sommaruga MG. Ultrasound contrast agents: basic principles. *Eur J Radiol* 1998; 27(Suppl 2):S157–S660.

16. Maurer M, Linker R, Hauff HP, et al. Imaging of ICAM-1 in experimental encephalomyelitis (EAE) with a specific ultrasound contrast agent. *J Neurol* 2002; 249(Suppl 1):I/57.

17. Hildebrandt IJ, Gambhir SS. Molecular imaging applications for immunology. *Clin Immunol* 2004; 111:210–224.

18. Ritman EL. Micro-computed tomography-current status and developments. *Annu Rev Biomed Eng* 2004; 6:185–208.

19. Mankoff DA, Bellon JR. Positron-emission tomographic imaging of cancer: glucose metabolism and beyond. *Semin Radiat Oncol* 2001; 11:16–27.

20. Massoud TF, Gambhir SS. Molecular imaging in living subjects: seeing fundamental biological processes in a new light. *Genes Dev* 2003; 17:545–580.

21. Krohn KA, Mankoff DA, Eary JF. Imaging cellular proliferation as a measure of response to therapy. *J Clin Pharmacol* 2001; Suppl:96S–103S.

22. Alessio AM, Kinahan PE, Cheng PM, Vesselle H, Karp JS. PET/CT scanner instrumentation, challenges, and solutions. *Radiol Clin North Am* 2004; 42:1017–1032, vii.

23. Jaszczak RJ, Coleman RE. Single photon emission computed tomography (SPECT). Principles and instrumentation. *Invest Radiol* 1985; 20:897–910.

24. Contag PR, Olomu IN, Stevenson DK, Contag CH. Bioluminescent indicators in living mammals. *Nat Med* 1998; 4:245–247.

25. Furlow B. Molecular imaging of cancer: the basics. *Radiol Technol* 2003; 74:486–497; quiz 498–500.

26. Contag CH, Jenkins D, Contag PR, Negrin RS. Use of reporter genes for optical measurements of neoplastic disease in vivo. *Neoplasia* 2000; 2:41–52.

27. Edinger M, Sweeney TJ, Tucker AA, Olomu AB, Negrin RS, Contag CH. Noninvasive assessment of tumor cell proliferation in animal models. *Neoplasia* 1999; 1:303–310.

28. Contag CH, Contag PR, Mullins JI, Spilman SD, Stevenson DK, Benaron DA. Photonic detection of bacterial pathogens in living hosts. *Mol Microbiol* 1995; 18:593–603.

29. Gerion D, Parak WJ, Williams SC, Zanchet D, Micheel CM, Alivisatos AP. Sorting fluorescent nanocrystals with DNA. *J Am Chem Soc* 2002; 124:7070–7074.

30. Larson DR, Zipfel WR, Williams RM, et al. Water-soluble quantum dots for multiphoton fluorescence imaging in vivo. *Science* 2003; 300:1434–1436.

31. Rosenthal SJ, Tomlinson I, Adkins EM, et al. Targeting cell surface receptors with ligand-conjugated nanocrystals. *J Am Chem Soc* 2002; 124:4586–4594.

32. Wu X, Liu H, Liu J, et al. Immunofluorescent labeling of cancer marker Her2 and other cellular targets with semiconductor quantum dots. *Nat Biotechnol* 2003; 21:41–46.

33. Kim S, Lim YT, Soltesz EG, et al. Near-infrared fluorescent type II quantum dots for sentinel lymph node mapping. *Nat Biotechnol* 2004; 22:93–97.

34. Gao X, Cui Y, Levenson RM, Chung LW, Nie S. In vivo cancer targeting and imaging with semiconductor quantum dots. *Nat Biotechnol* 2004; 22:969–976.

35. Cesano A, Gayko U. CD22 as a target of passive immunotherapy. *Semin Oncol* 2003; 30:253–257.

36. Kelley SK, Ashkenazi A. Targeting death receptors in cancer with Apo2L/TRAIL. *Curr Opin Pharmacol* 2004; 4:333–339.

37. Knutson KL, Almand B, Mankoff DA, Schiffman K, Disis ML. Adoptive T-cell therapy for the treatment of solid tumours. *Expert Opin Biol Ther* 2002; 2:55–66.

38. Lahorte CM, Vanderheyden JL, Steinmetz N, Van de Wiele C, Dierckx RA, Slegers G. Apoptosis-detecting radioligands: current state of the art and future perspectives. *Eur J Nucl Med Mol Imaging* 2004; 31:887–919.

39. Allen RT, Hunter WJ 3rd, Agrawal DK. Morphological and biochemical characterization and analysis of apoptosis. *J Pharmacol Toxicol Methods* 1997; 37:215–228.

40. Hofstra L, Liem IH, Dumont EA, et al. Visualisation of cell death in vivo in patients with acute myocardial infarction. *Lancet* 2000; 356:209–212.

41. Hofstra L, Dumont EA, Thimister PW, et al. In vivo detection of apoptosis in an intracardiac tumor. *JAMA* 2001; 285:1841–1842.
42. Kartachova M, Haas RL, Valdes Olmos RA, Hoebers FJ, Van Zandwijk N, Verheij M. In vivo imaging of apoptosis by (99m)Tc-Annexin V scintigraphy: visual analysis in relation to treatment response. *Radiother Oncol* 2004; 72:333–339.
43. Vriens PW, Blankenberg FG, Stoot JH, et al. The use of technetium Tc 99m annexin V for in vivo imaging of apoptosis during cardiac allograft rejection. *J Thorac Cardiovasc Surg* 1998; 116:844–853.
44. Blankenberg F, Narula J, Strauss HW. In vivo detection of apoptotic cell death: a necessary measurement for evaluating therapy for myocarditis, ischemia, and heart failure. *J Nucl Cardiol* 1999; 6: 531–539.
45. Cordeiro MF, Guo L, Luong V, et al. Real-time imaging of single nerve cell apoptosis in retinal neurodegeneration. *Proc Natl Acad Sci USA* 2004; 101:13,352–13,356.
46. Dotto GP, Silke J. More than cell death: caspases and caspase inhibitors on the move. *Dev Cell* 2004; 7:2–3.
47. Messerli SM, Prabhakar S, Tang Y, et al. A novel method for imaging apoptosis using a caspase-1 near-infrared fluorescent probe. *Neoplasia* 2004; 6:95–105.
48. Zhang Y, Haskins C, Lopez-Cruzan M, Zhang J, Centonze VE, Herman B. Detection of mitochondrial caspase activity in real time in situ in live cells. *Microsc Microanal* 2004; 10:442–448.
49. Haberkorn U, Kinscherf R, Krammer PH, Mier W, Eisenhut M. Investigation of a potential scintigraphic marker of apoptosis: radioiodinated Z-Val-Ala-DL-Asp(*O*-methyl)-fluoromethyl ketone. *Nucl Med Biol* 2001; 28:793–798.
50. Shields AF, Mankoff DA, Link JM, et al. Carbon-11-thymidine and FDG to measure therapy response. *J Nucl Med* 1998; 39:1757–1762.
51. Eubank WB, Mankoff DA. Current and future uses of positron emission tomography in breast cancer imaging. *Semin Nucl Med* 2004; 34:224–240.
52. Vesselle H, Grierson J, Muzi M, et al. In vivo validation of 3'deoxy-3'-[(18)F]fluorothymidine ([(18) F]FLT) as a proliferation imaging tracer in humans: correlation of [(18)F]FLT uptake by positron emission tomography with Ki-67 immunohistochemistry and flow cytometry in human lung tumors. *Clin Cancer Res* 2002; 8:3315–3323.
53. Folkman J. Role of angiogenesis in tumor growth and metastasis. *Semin Oncol* 2002; 29:15–18.
54. Zondor SD, Medina PJ. Bevacizumab: an angiogenesis inhibitor with efficacy in colorectal and other malignancies. *Ann Pharmacother* 2004; 38:1258–1264.
55. Liu JY, Wei YQ, Yang L, et al. Immunotherapy of tumors with vaccine based on quail homologous vascular endothelial growth factor receptor-2. *Blood* 2003; 102:1815–1823.
56. Kerbel R, Folkman J. Clinical translation of angiogenesis inhibitors. *Nat Rev Cancer* 2002; 2:727–739.
57. Sinusas AJ. Imaging of angiogenesis. *J Nucl Cardiol* 2004; 11:617–633.
58. Morgan B, Thomas AL, Drevs J, et al. Dynamic contrast-enhanced magnetic resonance imaging as a biomarker for the pharmacological response of PTK787/ZK 222584, an inhibitor of the vascular endothelial growth factor receptor tyrosine kinases, in patients with advanced colorectal cancer and liver metastases: results from two phase I studies. *J Clin Oncol* 2003; 21:3955–3964.
59. Laking GR, Price PM. Positron emission tomographic imaging of angiogenesis and vascular function. *Br J Radiol* 2003; 76(Suppl 1):S50–S59.
60. Mankoff DA, Dunnwald LK, Gralow JR, et al. Changes in blood flow and metabolism in locally advanced breast cancer treated with neoadjuvant chemotherapy. *J Nucl Med* 2003; 44:1806–1814.
61. Lodge MA, Carson RE, Carrasquillo JA, Whatley M, Libutti SK, Bacharach SL. Parametric images of blood flow in oncology PET studies using [^{15}O]water. *J Nucl Med* 2000; 41:1784–1792.
62. Mankoff DA, Dunnwald LK, Gralow JR, et al. [Tc-99m]-sestamibi uptake and washout in locally advanced breast cancer are correlated with tumor blood flow. *Nucl Med Biol* 2002; 29:719–727.
63. Kiessling F, Greschus S, Lichy MP, et al. Volumetric computed tomography (VCT): a new technology for noninvasive, high-resolution monitoring of tumor angiogenesis. *Nat Med* 2004; 10:1133–1138.
64. Barthel H. Endostatin imaging to help understanding of antiangiogenic drugs. *Lancet Oncol* 2002; 3: 520.
65. Chen X, Park R, Shahinian AH, et al. ^{18}F-labeled RGD peptide: initial evaluation for imaging brain tumor angiogenesis. *Nucl Med Biol* 2004; 31:179–189.
66. Wahl RL, Zasadny K, Helvie M, Hutchins GD, Weber B, Cody R. Metabolic monitoring of breast cancer chemohormonotherapy using positron emission tomography: initial evaluation. *J Clin Oncol* 1993; 11:2101–2111.

67. Jansson T, Westlin JE, Ahlstrom H, Lilja A, Langstrom B, Bergh J. Positron emission tomography studies in patients with locally advanced and/or metastatic breast cancer: a method for early therapy evaluation? *J Clin Oncol* 1995; 13:1470–1477.
68. Smith IC, Welch AE, Hutcheon AW, et al. Positron emission tomography using [(18)F]-fluorodeoxy-D-glucose to predict the pathologic response of breast cancer to primary chemotherapy. *J Clin Oncol* 2000; 18:1676–1688.
69. Behr TM, Behe M, Angerstein C, et al. Does pretherapeutic immunoscintigraphy allow for diagnostic predictions with respect to the toxicity and therapeutic efficacy of cold immunotherapy with trastuzumab (Herceptin)? *J Nucl Med* 2000; 41:73(abstract no 287).
70. Groot-Wassink T, Aboagye EO, Wang Y, Lemoine NR, Keith WN, Vassaux G. Noninvasive imaging of the transcriptional activities of human telomerase promoter fragments in mice. *Cancer Res* 2004; 64: 4906–4911.
71. Raynal I, Prigent P, Peyramaure S, Najid A, Rebuzzi C, Corot C. Macrophage endocytosis of superparamagnetic iron oxide nanoparticles: mechanisms and comparison of ferumoxides and ferumoxtran-10. *Invest Radiol* 2004; 39:56–63.
72. Deloire MS, Touil T, Brochet B, Dousset V, Caille JM, Petry KG. Macrophage brain infiltration in experimental autoimmune encephalomyelitis is not completely compromised by suppressed T-cell invasion: in vivo magnetic resonance imaging illustration in effective anti-VLA-4 antibody treatment. *Mult Scler* 2004; 10:540–548.
73. Stoll G, Wesemeier C, Gold R, Solymosi L, Toyka KV, Bendszus M. In vivo monitoring of macrophage infiltration in experimental autoimmune neuritis by magnetic resonance imaging. *J Neuroimmunol* 2004; 149:142–146.
74. Masteller EL, Warner MR, Ferlin W, et al. Peptide–MHC class II dimers as therapeutics to modulate antigen-specific T-cell responses in autoimmune diabetes. *J Immunol* 2003; 171:5587–5595.
75. Moore A, Grimm J, Han B, Santamaria P. Tracking the recruitment of diabetogenic CD8+ T-cells to the pancreas in real time. *Diabetes* 2004; 53:1459–1466.
76. Chames P, Hufton SE, Coulie PG, Uchanska-Ziegler B, Hoogenboom HR. Direct selection of a human antibody fragment directed against the tumor T-cell epitope HLA-A1-MAGE-A1 from a nonimmunized phage-Fab library. *Proc Natl Acad Sci USA* 2000; 97:7969–7974.
77. Denkberg G, Cohen CJ, Lev A, Chames P, Hoogenboom HR, Reiter Y. Direct visualization of distinct T cell epitopes derived from a melanoma tumor-associated antigen by using human recombinant antibodies with MHC-restricted T cell receptor-like specificity. *Proc Natl Acad Sci USA* 2002; 99:9421–9426.
78. Lev A, Denkberg G, Cohen CJ, et al. Isolation and characterization of human recombinant antibodies endowed with the antigen-specific, major histocompatibility complex-restricted specificity of T cells directed toward the widely expressed tumor T-cell epitopes of the telomerase catalytic subunit. *Cancer Res* 2002; 62:3184–3194.
79. Meidenbauer N, Marienhagen J, Laumer M, et al. Survival and tumor localization of adoptively transferred Melan-A-specific T cells in melanoma patients. *J Immunol* 2003; 170:2161–2169.
80. Adonai N, Nguyen KN, Walsh J, et al. Ex vivo cell labeling with ^{64}Cu-pyruvaldehyde-bis(N^4-methylthiosemicarbazone) for imaging cell trafficking in mice with positron-emission tomography. *Proc Natl Acad Sci USA* 2002; 99:3030–3035.
81. Kircher MF, Allport JR, Graves EE, et al. In vivo high resolution three-dimensional imaging of antigen-specific cytotoxic T-lymphocyte trafficking to tumors. *Cancer Res* 2003; 63:6838–6846.
82. Edinger M, Cao YA, Verneris MR, Bachmann MH, Contag CH, Negrin RS. Revealing lymphoma growth and the efficacy of immune cell therapies using in vivo bioluminescence imaging. *Blood* 2003; 101:640–648.
83. Dubey P, Su H, Adonai N, et al. Quantitative imaging of the T cell antitumor response by positron-emission tomography. *Proc Natl Acad Sci USA* 2003; 100:1232–1237.
84. Nakajima A, Seroogy CM, Sandora MR, et al. Antigen-specific T cell-mediated gene therapy in collagen-induced arthritis. *J Clin Invest* 2001; 107:1293–1301.

27

Design Issues for Early-Stage Clinical Trials for Cancer Vaccines

Gina R. Petroni

SUMMARY

The development of cancer vaccines provides a challenge to the accepted methods for the design of early-stage clinical trials, which were developed primarily with chemotherapeutic agents in mind. Although the ultimate goals are the same, there are inherent differences between vaccine therapies and chemotherapeutic regimens in the frequency and nature of adverse events, and more importantly, in the measures used to determine therapeutic benefit. This chapter describes the ways in which these differences may necessitate alternative approaches for the design of vaccine trials.

Key Words: Clinical trial; vaccine trial end points; ranking and selection; bivariate designs.

1. OVERVIEW: SIMILARITIES AND DIFFERENCES WITH TRADITIONAL PHASE I AND II CHEMOTHERAPEUTIC TRIALS

The designation of a trial into a "phase" classification has been widely accepted, especially in the field of cancer research, where early development was centered on therapeutic cytotoxic drugs. As discussed by Piantadosi *(1)*, this terminology does not necessarily lend itself to all applications. This is often true for vaccine studies.

The principal belief that drives the design of a traditional phase I chemotherapeutic trial is that higher doses have greater antitumor activity and therefore, will be more efficacious. With this underlying assumption, the goal of a traditional phase I trial is to determine the maximum tolerated dose, and the designs are based on observed proportions of subjects experiencing dose limiting adverse events. In contrast, many cancer vaccines are considered intrinsically safe, and higher doses do not necessarily result in the greater immune response *(2)*. It is assumed that increased immune response will ultimately be an indicator for increased efficacy. In this scenario, the design is based on determining the dose, often referred to as the "optimal biological dose," which results in the greatest proportion of subjects experiencing a predefined measure of immune response. Even so, one must still consider the rate of adverse events among the various dose levels under investigation, and if results from previous work, such as preclinical or previous trials invalidate the safety assumption, then traditional design strategies may be appropriate.

From: *Cancer Drug Discovery and Development: Immunotherapy of Cancer*
Edited by: M. L. Disis © Humana Press Inc., Totowa, NJ

The goals of traditional phase II chemotherapeutic and vaccine trials are similar: to find preliminary evidence that the treatment(s) may be efficacious. It is the choice of end points that differs and as such drives the design. An accepted end point for chemotherapeutic trials has often been to assess antitumor activity by measuring the amount of tumor shrinkage (e.g., complete or partial response). For vaccine trials, often the end point of interest is a measure of biologic activity or immune response. Hence, the traditional phase I and II chemotherapeutic design terminology does not have a one-to-one correspondence for vaccine trials.

There is a broad range of design strategies that can be used in the design of early phase chemotherapeutic trials (3), and these strategies are appropriate for many but not all vaccine studies. This chapter describes the issues involved in identifying an appropriate design for a vaccine trial.

2. VACCINE TRIAL STUDY END POINTS

All early-phase vaccine development trials must assess safety. Generally, a treatment is considered safe as long as the proportion of subjects experiencing unacceptable adverse events is low. The definition of an unacceptable adverse event is protocol-specific, and is often based on specified grades of adverse events as described by the National Cancer Institute common terminology criteria (i.e., Common Terminology Criteria for Adverse Events). Early-phase designs should include some predefined monitoring of safety, even if the underlying assumption of the study is that the vaccines under investigation are inherently safe.

Study-specific immunological end points provide the investigator with a measure of biological activity and are important for all early phase trials. It is assumed, although not known, that increased immune response is beneficial clinically; therefore, demonstration of association may be a central goal of the study. Clear definitions of how the immune response parameters are measured must be provided. Common end points include the assessment of differences, fold changes, and threshold measures, with or without adjustment for background and relative to negative controls. Simon et al. (2) suggest that the variability of the proposed end point be included in the protocol. Specifically, the following three sources should be incorporated: variability among assay results within the same specimen, variability among the specimens from the same individual over time, and variability among subjects.

Clinical end points, such as measures of tumor shrinkage of bulky disease or time to progression, are more generalizable; however, they may not be appropriate for many vaccine trials. The vaccine may not be expected to cause tumor shrinkage, but it may be hoped to cause disease stabilization. Time to progression can provide a measure of disease stabilization, but only if there are good data that can be viewed as a valid historical control (2). Without the requirement of bulky disease, vaccine trials may include a more wide-ranging or nonstandard study population, which makes comparisons to historical control data problematic.

3. GENERAL DESIGN STRATEGIES

3.1. Phase I

"Traditional" escalation designs (3) treat a small number of subjects at prespecified dose levels. Cohorts of subjects, usually three, are treated at the starting dose, and subjects are accrued to the next higher dose if, and only if, the stopping guideline is not met. Stopping guidelines provide decision rules to determine where the next cohort of subjects should be treated and are based on the number of subjects treated at each dose level that have experienced a dose-limiting adverse event (DLT). Common guidelines are to escalate to the next higher dose if none of the three patients experience a DLT, accrue and additional cohort of subjects to the current dose if one of three subjects experience a DLT, and stop accrual permanently to the current dose if two or more subjects experience a DLT. When DLTs are observed, then accrual to the dose level where the adverse events occurred or the level below it is expanded to allow additional cohorts of subjects to be treated to determine better the maximum-tolerated dose (MTD). With this type of design, the MTD is defined (commonly) as the highest dose where fewer than two out of six subjects experienced a DLT. Cohort sizes and decision rules may vary depending on subject availability, the definition of DLT and determination of other study end points. Although the design is simple to follow, it provides a conservative approach to determining the MTD.

Continual reassessment (4) or *modified continual reassessment methods (5,6)* were developed initially to reduce the number of subjects treated at ineffective doses using designs such as the traditional method. Their use in vaccine studies would be limited when all doses under study are assumed safe. With a safety end point, the methods would put most subjects at the highest dose, which may not be near the optimal dose.

Accelerated titration designs (7) were developed to allow for intrasubject escalation of doses with decision rules being dependent on disease status, and whether or not the subject experienced a DLT. In vaccine studies, it is important to obtain preliminary data to support and define the potential association between biological activity and clinical response. This may be difficult to obtain with an intrasubject escalation design. As with the continual reassessment, use of accelerated titration designs in vaccine studies would be limited when all doses under study are assumed safe.

3.2. Phase II

Multistaged designs for a single end point are applicable if data exist from a previous trial that indicates the regimen has been shown to be safe and worthy of further investigation. These designs are described in a hypothesis-testing format and allow for at least one interim analysis of the data. The sample size and stopping guidelines depend on the null (H_0) and alternative (H_a) hypotheses that the investigator wishes to test. H_0 identifies a result that would indicate that the treatment is not worthy of further study, whereas H_a specifies a result that would indicate that the treatment is worthy of further study (i.e., clinically relevant). Commonly employed designs, such as those proposed by Simon (8) and Fleming (9), can be used when the end point of interest is a dichotomous measure of tumor shrinkage, a reduction in a known biological marker, or an accepted measure of immune response.

Ranking and selection designs are used to select the most promising treatment from a fixed number of regimens based on a single end point. They can be based on a continuous measure of the end point or a dichotomous measure. These designs do not provide a formal comparison among the treatments and should not be viewed as a substitute for a comparative trial. These designs are useful in studying a particular vaccine regimen and slight modifications to the current vaccine (e.g., the addition of new peptides) are being considered. Here, subjects are randomized among two or more vaccine regimens. When immune response is defined as a dichotomous outcome (subject does or does not experience an immune response), and if any treatment has a true immune response rate δ-percentage points higher (e.g., $\delta = 20\%$) than any of the others, then that regimen should be selected for further study. With a ranking and selection design, the most promising regimen is chosen with high probability (e.g., 90%) if a treatment is truly better than the others by the predefined difference, δ.

One-sample time-to-event designs can be used to assess time to progression as compared with historical control data. The design requires an assumed form for time to progression and is often set up in the hypothesis-testing format. The goal would be to collect preliminary data to support that the vaccine caused disease stabilization and therefore, a longer time to progression. If historical control data are the basis for the choice of H_0, then the same study population is required for the current study. For vaccine studies, it may be more appropriate to target study populations that have the strongest immune system, which would include subjects without clinical evidence of disease. Comparison with historical control data is problematic, unless the historical control data is based on subjects treated at the same institution in previous studies with the same eligibility criteria in the period before the current study.

Multisample time-to-event designs can be used to compare time to progression among subjects receiving the vaccines(s) and a control group receiving standard treatment. Subjects are randomized to a group, and the goal is to establish preliminary comparative data to support moving forward to a definitive phase III comparative trial. In this setting a hypothesis-testing format is used with a higher type I error rate (i.e., 10%). Simon et. al. *(2)* have referred to these designs as "phase 2.5 trials."

3.3. Phase I/II

Dose-finding and efficacy trade-off designs (10,11) endeavor to determine the dose that satisfies both safety and efficacy requirements. With these designs, the number of accrued subjects needs to be large enough to provide reliable estimates of safety and efficacy end points. In designs such as Thall and Cook's *(11)*, one can reasonably replace immune response with efficacy. This model accommodates biological agents where the effect may go up, and then the plateau goes down at higher doses. In this setting, dose finding will be dependent on a response measurement that can be assessed in a limited amount of time.

3.4. Hybrid Designs

Bivariate designs incorporate two variables (end points) formally into the decision rules for a study. Often they are used to allow for at least one interim look at the data (two-staged design). Designs that incorporate two variables *(12–16)* provide the framework that can be used in the setting of assessing a single-arm trial with a dichotomous immune response end point, while also considering observed adverse event rates. The goal is to stop the trial early if there is evidence that the immune response rate is lower than would be acceptable to warrant further investigation, or if an unacceptable adverse event rate is observed. Assume both immune response and adverse events are defined as dichotomous measures. For example, a subject with be classified as having an immune response if he or she experience at least a threefold increase over baseline in a study-specific immune parameter, and a subject will be considered to have had a DLT if he or she experience any unexpected treatment-related grade 4 or higher adverse event as defined by the National

Cancer Institute Common Terminology Criteria for Adverse Events. The study should be designed to stop at the first interim analysis if there is evidence that the immune response rate is less than 50%, and that the DTL rate is greater than 25%. With these designs, one suspends accrual early only if there is evidence for poor outcomes; otherwise, accrual continues. Other paired parameters, such as clinical response and immune response, could be used, and the methods of Conaway and Petroni *(12,14)*, and Thall et al. *(15,16)* can be extended to more than one interim look.

Modified-dose escalation designs can be used to assess safety while collecting preliminary results on biological response. They can be a combination of a traditional phase I trial and a ranking and selection design. It is assumed that a monotonic increasing order exists among the dose levels under study. Here, although the vaccine may be assumed to be safe, regulatory bodies may insist on a conservative setup procedure before letting the investigator proceed with a randomized ranking and selection type design. In this situation, accrual to the study can occur in two phases. In the initial phase, a fixed cohort size of subjects (e.g., three) can be accrued in a sequential order to increasing doses, and accrual to the next higher dose level will not occur until the previous cohort has been assessed for DLT. After the initial accrual phase, if no subjects experience a dose-limiting adverse event, then subjects will be randomized until each open dose level has accrued an additional fixed cohort size of subjects. If no DLTs are observed (or a limit may be set, e.g., fewer than 33%), this randomization process can continue until the required number subjects have been accrued as required by a ranking and selection design. If, contrary to expectations, an unacceptable number of DLTs are observed in the initial phase, then the design would require that additional subjects be accrued in the traditional sequential manner.

3.5. Examples

3.5.1. BIVARIATE

Assume we are testing a multipeptide-based vaccine where safety is assumed but not known. The primary immune response parameter is a dichotomous measure where a subject is considered to have a positive immune response if the subject experiences a fivefold response compared with baseline to any peptide. Adverse events will be classified as meeting a DLT definition or not. Data about immune response, overall or for each peptide under investigation, are either limited or nonexistent in this subject population. Therefore, the null and alternative overall immune response rates are chosen to define levels of activity that would be considered "not interesting" or "worthy of further study," respectively. Specifically, for this vaccine regimen, a design that differentiates between a positive immune response rate of 5 and 30%, and a DLT rate of 5 and 25% will be used. We are interested in testing the following H_o and H_a; H_o: $p_r \leq 5\%$ or $p_t \geq 25\%$ vs H_a: $p_r > 5\%$ and $p_t < 25\%$, where p_r denotes the unknown overall positive immune response rate, and p_t denotes the unknown DLT rate for the vaccine regimen. The sample size and stopping rules for the study are based on having sufficient power at a particular point in the alternative region. Specifically, we are interested in the point at which the DLT rate is 5% and the immune response rate is 30%.

For the first stage of the study, accrue six subjects. The period between registration and a minimum of 1-wk postadministration of the third vaccine will be used to guide the decisions rules for toxicity assessment. At the end of the first monitoring stage, accrual to the study will be suspended until it is possible to assess whether stopping criteria have

Table 1
Decision Rules

Decision rule, if number subjects with:	End of stage 1, n = 6; go to stage 2 if both:	End of stage 2, n = 6 + 9 = 15; at final analysis reject H_o if both:
Positive immune response	≥0 (0%)	≥3 (20%)
DLT	≤1 (17%)	≤2 (13%)

H_o, null hypothesis; DLT, dose-limiting adverse event.

Table 2
Example of a Modified-Dose Escalation Design

		Three groups		Two groups	
Smallest rate	Largest rate	Minimum sample size per group for P = 0.90	Probability for n = 31 per group	Minimum sample size per group for P = 0.90	Probability for n = 31 per group
0.3	0.5	30	0.91	20	0.95
0.4	0.6	31	0.90	21	0.94
0.5	0.7	30	0.91	20	0.95
0.6	0.8	26	0.93	18	0.96
0.7	0.9	20	0.96	13	0.98

been met. Use the rules in Table 1 to determine whether accrual will continue to the second stage. If the observed DLT rate is low, then accrue an additional nine eligible subjects (a total of eligible 15) to the study.

The rules were found by exact enumeration with an assumed odds ratio of one *(12)*. With this design, if the true overall positive immune response rate is 5% or the true toxicity rate is 25%, then the probability of rejecting H_o is 0.01. If the true overall positive immune response rate is 30% and the true toxicity rate is 5% then the probability of rejecting H_o is 0.825. If the true overall positive immune response and toxicity rates are, such that, either $p_r ≤ 5\%$ (i.e., insufficient evidence of immune activity) or $p_t ≥ 25\%$ (i.e., too toxic) then the probability of rejecting H_o (i.e., declare that the treatment warrants further investigation) is no more than 0.214.

3.5.2. Modified-Dose Escalation Designs

Assume safety criteria are satisfied for the "standard" vaccine and the additional vaccines under investigation. The study is designed to select the best treatment worthy of further investigation in single-factor Bernoulli response experiments using the ranking and selection procedure, B_{SH}, *(17)*. With this design, the treatment with the highest positive immune response rate over a specified period will be considered for further investigation. Sample size is established to ensure that if the difference between the immune response rates is at least δ = 20%, then the higher sample will be selected with high probability, P. The choice of P is arbitrary. For this study, we set P ≥ 0.90 to select the best treatment whenever δ ≥ 0.20. Preliminary data from previous studies indicate an 80% (95% confidence interval, 44 to 97%) response rate to the standard vaccine. For sample size determination, we will use the limits of a 95% confidence interval to estimate the maximum expected response rate of interest. Shown in the Table 2 is the value of *p* for fixed

$\delta = 0.20$ over the range of expected response rates, with $n = 31$ per dose, assuming selection between two or three dose levels. Accrual of 31 eligible subjects per regimen, regardless of selecting between two or three, satisfies the minimum criteria of $P \geq 0.90$.

REFERENCES

1. Piantadosi S. *Clinical Trials, a Methodologic Perspective*. New York: Wiley. 1997.
2. Simon RM, Steinberg SM, Hamilton M, et al. Clinical trial designs for the early clinical development of therapeutic cancer vaccines. *J Clin Oncol* 2001; 19:1848–1854.
3. Crowley J, ed., *Handbook of Statistics in Clinical Oncology*. New York: Marcel Dekker. 2001.
4. O'Quigley J, Pepe M, Fisher L. Continual reassessment method: a practical design for phase I clinical trials in cancer. *Biometrics* 1990; 46:33–48.
5. Faries D. Practical modifications of the continual reassessment method for phase I clinical trials. *J Biopharm Stat* 1994; 4:147–164.
6. Moller S. An extension of the continual reassessment methods using preliminary up-and-down design in a dose finding study in cancer patients in order to investigate a greater ranges of doses. *Stat Med* 1995; 14:911–922.
7. Simon RM, Freidlin B, Rubinstein LV, Arbuck SG, Collins J, Christian MC. Accelerated titration designs for phase I clinical trials in oncology. *J Nat Cancer Inst* 1997; 89:1138–1147.
8. Simon R. Optimal two-stage designs for phase II clinical trials. *Controlled Clin Trials* 1989; 10:1–10.
9. Fleming TR. One-sample multiple testing procedures for phase II clinical trials. *Biometrics* 1982; 38:143–151.
10. Thall PF, Russell KT. A strategy for dose-finding and safety monitoring based on efficacy and adverse outcomes in phase I/II clinical trials. *Biometrics* 1998; 54:251–264.
11. Thall PF, Cook JD. Dose-finding based on efficacy-toxicity trade-offs. *Biometrics* 2004; 60:684–693.
12. Conaway MR, Petroni GR. Bivariate sequential designs for phase II trials. *Biometrics* 1995; 51:656–664.
13. Bryant J, Day R. Incorporating toxicity considerations into the design of two-stage phase II clinical trials. *Biometrics* 1995; 51:1372–1383.
14. Conaway MR, Petroni GR. Designs for phase II trials allowing for trade-off between response and toxicity. *Biometrics* 1996; 52:1375–1386.
15. Thall PF, Simon RM, Estey EH. Bayesian sequential monitoring designs for single-arm clinical trials with multiple outcomes. *Stat Med* 1995; 14:357–379.
16. Thall PF, Simon RM, Estey EH. New statistical strategy for monitoring safety and efficacy in single-arm clinical trials. *J Clin Oncol* 1996; 14:296–303.
17. Bechhofer RE, Santer TJ, Goldsman DM. *Design and Analysis of Experiments for Statistical Selection, Screening and Multiple Comparisons*. New York: John Wiley. 1995.

28

Monoclonal Antibody Therapy of Cancer

Hossein Borghaei,
Matthew K. Robinson,
and Louis M. Weiner

SUMMARY

Treatment of cancer has dramatically changed in recent years. Some of this change is because of the introduction of monoclonal antibodies into clinical practice. The exact mechanism of action of the clinically relevant antibodies remains unknown. This chapter provides an overview of the science and techniques used in the construction of these antibodies in addition to a brief review of some of the available clinical data.

Key Words: Monoclonal antibody; cancer; immunoconjugate; immunotoxin; antibody-dependent cellular cytotoxicity.

1. INTRODUCTION

Monoclonal antibody (MAb) therapy has emerged as an increasingly important modality in cancer therapy. Antibody-based therapeutics have shown efficacy alone and as components of effective therapies for an increasing number of human malignancies. Unconjugated antibodies directed against the B-cell idiotype *(1)*, CD20 *(2,3)*, and CD22 *(4)* exhibit significant utility in the therapy of lymphomas, and one anti-CD20 antibody has become a widely used, Food and Drug Administration (FDA)-approved agent, with potential applications to other malignancies as well. Radioimmunoconjugates directed against CD20 exhibit significant antitumor activity *(5,6)*, and two such agents have entered standard clinical practice for lymphoma therapy. An anti-CD52 antibody that efficiently mediates complement fixation has been approved for use in chemotherapy-refractory chronic lymphocytic leukemia *(7)*. An immunoconjugate consisting of an anti-CD33 antibody and calicheamicin has been approved for use in refractory acute myeloid leukemia *(8)*. Immunotoxins consisting of recombinant antibody fragments and catalytic toxins also demonstrate antitumor activity *(9)*. An unconjugated anti-HER2/*neu* antibody is widely used alone and in combination with chemotherapy agents in breast cancer *(10–12)*. Antibodies directed against the extracellular domain of the epidermal growth factor receptor

From: *Cancer Drug Discovery and Development: Immunotherapy of Cancer*
Edited by: M. L. Disis © Humana Press Inc., Totowa, NJ

(EGFR) exhibit activity in advanced cancer *(13,14)*. Antibodies that inhibit T-cell activation by blocking the function of the cytotoxic T-lymphocyte-associated protein 4 co-receptor on T-cells exhibit preclinical promise *(15)* and are undergoing clinical evaluation. An antibody that blocks vascular endothelial growth factor (VEGF)-promoted angiogenesis improves survival in colorectal cancer patients undergoing chemotherapy.

Antibodies may mediate antitumor effects by employing a variety of effector mechanisms, such as antibody-directed cellular cytotoxicity (ADCC), but the exact mechanism of action of many of these clinically active antibodies remain unknown.

The development of hybridoma technology by Kohler and Milstein *(16)* led to the speculation that MAbs would provide a "magic bullet" for the treatment of diseases, such as cancer. However, despite the high degree of specificity and the high affinity that MAbs can exhibit for their target antigens, development of antibody-based therapeutics for the treatment of cancer has proven to be more complex than originally envisioned.

Initial MAbs used in clinical trials were murine in origin and it became clear early on that patients developed human anti-mouse antibody responses against the therapeutic agents that limited both efficacy of the MAb by rapidly clearing it from the body and the number of times the therapy could be administered. In addition, murine MAbs inconsistently elicit responses in human effector cells. Methods to reduce the immunogenicity and boost effector function of MAbs by creating chimeric (variable regions transferred onto the human Fc region) or humanized (complementarity-determining regions grafted onto a human antibody) versions of the MAb are now routine and almost all of the MAbs currently approved by the US FDA are either chimeric or humanized MAbs.

This chapter reviews some of the latest developments in the field of antibody generation and provide an overview of the some of the possible mechanisms of action for the recently approved MAbs.

2. AN IDEAL ANTIBODY

Although there is no evidence that the ideal antibody has been prepared, a discussion of the properties of a desirable antibody might be helpful in understanding various issues related to the production and engineering of these molecules. An ideal antibody would be specific against one target. The targeted antigen would only be expressed on malignant cells and not normal tissue, thus limiting the side effects from treatment. The interaction of the antibody with the target on the cell surface would lead to the killing of the targeted cells by one or more of several mechanisms:

1. Inducing apoptosis.
2. Inducing ADCC.
3. Inducing complement-directed cytotoxicity.
4. Attracting immune effector cells to the site of the tumor.
5. Delivery of toxic payload (radioactive or toxins) to the affected cells.

The antibody should not be immunogenic and should (preferably) be fully human. There should not be a need for repeated administration of the agent. However, if needed there should not be an impediment to the repeated treatment with this antibody.

3. BASIC STRUCTURE

Antibodies, also known as immunoglobulins (Igs), are among the most critical components of the immune system. They are capable of recognizing a wide array of antigens and interacting with and activating a number of host effector cells and systems. The antibody molecule consists of two light and two heavy chains linked by disulfide bonds *(17)*. Heavy and light chains are encoded by separate genes. The variable region (variable-heavy [V_H] and variable-light [V_L]), which is responsible for antigen binding, is located at the amino terminus of the heavy and light chains. The constant (C) region is the part of the molecule that is responsible for its effector function. A flexible hinge region holds the antibody together and facilitates antigen binding and some effector functions. All antibodies contain carbohydrates in the C region of their heavy chains. The presence of this carbohydrate is thought to be critical for the effector functions of the antibodies. Digestion of IgG with papain results in two Fab fragments that are capable of antigen binding and an Fc domain that is responsible for antibody dependent cellular cytotoxicity and other effector functions *(17)*.

Five different classes of antibodies are recognized based on the differences in the C regions of their heavy chains. These are IgG, IgM, IgA, IgD, and IgE. In humans IgD, IgE, and IgG are present as monomeric structures with molecular weights in the 150–190 kDa range. IgA is a dimeric structure, and IgM is a pentameric structure. IgGs are further subdivided into four subclasses, IgG1 through IgG4. IgA is also subdivided into IgA1 and IgA2 subclasses. The isotype of the heavy chain determines the ability of the antibody to participate in ADCC, activate the complement cascade, and be transported across the placenta *(17)*. The isotype of the light chain does not play a role in its effector function *(18)*.

4. MURINE MAbs

The normal physiological response to the presence of an antigen is the production of polyclonal antibodies with different variable regions or the same variable region associated with different C regions. The heterogeneity of this immune response poses safety concerns that limit the application of polyclonal antibodies *(18)*.

Hybridoma technology has led to the ability to produce antibodies that are the products of a single antibody-producing cell and have a single variable region associated with one C region *(16)*. The hybridoma cell line, once developed, can be grown in vitro or in vivo indefinitely to ensure a constant supply of MAb. These antibodies tend to be highly specific with a high affinity, but have short half-lives in humans, leading to a need for frequent dose administration to maintain a therapeutic level *(18)*. Also, the human immune system recognizes the mouse MAb as a foreign protein, thus leading to the formation of human anti-mouse antibodies, which further decreases the circulating half-life of these antibodies, and can lead to severe allergic reactions *(19,20)*.

5. CHIMERIC AND HUMANIZED ANTIBODIES

In order to overcome problems associated with the administration of murine MAbs, mouse–human chimeric antibodies are produced by genetically fusing the mouse variable domain to human constant domains. The anti-CD20 MAb rituximab is an example of a chimeric antibody widely used in the treatment of non-Hodgkin's lymphoma *(21)*.

Although chimeric antibodies possess reduced immunogenicity, they can elicit human anti-chimeric antibody responses. To address this issue, the complementary determining regions within the variable regions, which are responsible for antigen binding, have been transferred to a human Ig backbone, thereby creating humanized antibodies *(22)*. Trastuzumab (Herceptin™) is an example of a humanized MAb commonly used in the treatment of patients with metastatic breast cancers that overexpress the HER2/*neu* antigen *(23)*.

6. BISPECIFIC ANTIBODIES

Antibodies are in general monospecific. They usually recognize only one epitope in an antigen. It is, however, possible to engineer antibodies that recognize two separate antigens and to have two binding specificities. Bispecific antibodies can be prepared by the fusion of two hybridomas (quadroma) secreting antibodies of different specificities or by chemical modifications *(24)*. It is also possible to create bispecific single-chain antibodies (scFv) that consist of two distinct binding units comprised of V_H chains fused to V_L chains via amino acid spacers. Chemical modification is considered to be inefficient and can result in damage to the binding site. In a quadroma only a small fraction of antibodies can be expected to be the desired antibody, whereas bispecific scFvs lack the desired effector functions of other antibodies. Another approach, as shown by Coloma and Morrison *(25)*, is to fuse a specific scFv after the hinge or at the carboxy terminus of another antibody with a different specificity. This fusion protein would have two different specificities and maintain some effector function of an Ig molecule along with a longer half-life and Fc receptor binding.

Bispecific antibodies are used to bring effector cells to particular targets via one of their binding sites and could be beneficial in recruiting immune cells to the disease site (i.e., cancer cells). Several bispecific antibodies have been tested in phase I and II trials. 2B1 is specific for HER2/*neu* and FcγRIII (Fc γ-receptor on NK cells and neutrophils) *(26)*. MDX-210 is a chemically conjugated hetero F(ab)'2 fragment specific for HER2/*neu* and FcγRI (the Fc γ-receptor expressed by monocytes, macrophages, and activated granulocytes). MDX-210 has shown some clinical activity in advanced stage cancer patients refractory to conventional treatments *(27–29)*.

7. PHAGE DISPLAY TECHNOLOGY
AND SINGLE-CHAIN ANTIBODIES

The utility of MAbs as therapeutic agents has led to extensive research and development of new technologies to engineer antibodies. Although the use of hybridoma technology continues, the recognized limitations of the murine antibodies generated by this approach has sparked an interest in the development of additional methodologies to generate human antibodies with binding specificities against targets of interest. Phage display technology represents one such approach *(30,31)*. scFvs are engineered antibody fragments comprised solely of the antigen-binding domains (V_H and V_L chains) of IgGs fused into a single polypeptide by the addition of a short, flexible linker sequence. These molecules possess the antigen-binding specificity of intact IgGs and have been used to create human scFv phage libraries *(31)*. Creation of such libraries is carried out by amplifying the entire complement of V_H and V_L chains of antibodies from multiple naïve or immunized donors. The V_H and V_L domains are then randomly fused into full-length scFvs and displayed on the surface of filamentous phage. The process of isolating variable domains from multiple donors and randomly fusing the heavy and light chains acts to increase the repertoire of binding specificities over that which is theoretically possible for any single individual. Such libraries can contain up to 10^7 individual V_H and V_L fragments that when randomly combined, can theoretically give rise to more than of 10^{14} unique scFvs. The vast repertoire of binding specificities, when combined with the inherent biology of the phage system, allows for more rapid and extensive screening against target antigens than is possible with standard hybridoma technology.

8. IMPROVING MAbs

Advances in antibody engineering have led to the development of novel molecular frameworks based on scFv building blocks and allowed tailoring of the physical and pharmacokinetic properties of the antibody fragments. In turn, this has allowed the identification of many physical properties that impact on the ability of these molecules to target solid tumors. Molecular size is one such determinant. The lack of draining lymphatics in solid tumor leads to high interstitial pressure and a net outward gradient from the center of the tumor that acts to slow the diffusion of proteins into tumor and at least in part is responsible for the nonuniform distribution of IgGs seen in tumors *(32,33)*. Models and experimental data *(34)* suggest that the interstitial pressure differentially inhibits larger molecules, such as IgG, and can be more readily overcome by smaller molecules, such as scFvs (26 kDa vs 150 kDa for IgG). However, the residence time of proteins in blood is inversely correlated with their molecular size. Molecules smaller than approx 65 kDa are rapidly cleared by first-pass renal clearance. Therefore, smaller antibody-based fragments that exhibit more rapid tumor penetration are also more rapidly cleared both from the tumor and systemically *(35,36)*. Despite the benefit to tumor penetration, the rapid clearance of small molecules limits the concentration to which the fragments can accumulate in the tumor and may ultimately affect the types of applications amenable to small antibody-based fragments. Such applications may be imaging or therapeutic strategies involving toxic payloads (e.g., radioimmunotherapy) where high tumor:organ ratios are required to increase efficacy and patient safety.

The overall tumor targeting of antibody fragments can be increased by slowing the dissociation of antibody–antigen complexes once they have formed in the tumor. This can be accomplished by either increasing the intrinsic affinity of the antibody for its target *(37)* or by increasing the valency of the molecules to impart an avidity effect to the binding *(38,39)*. Using scFvs specific for the HER2 tumor antigen and tumor xenograft models, Adams and colleagues *(38)* showed that a minimum affinity of between 10^{-7} and 10^{-8} is required for tumor targeting and that increased affinity correlated with increased retention to affinities of 10^{-9}. Interestingly, scFvs with affinities above 10^{-9} showed no increase in tumor retention and, in fact, scFvs with very high affinities (10^{-11}) exhibited a marked decrease in tumor targeting *(40)*.

Numerous molecular frameworks that increase the valency of scFv-based antibody fragments have been described in the literature. One such structure that has proven to successfully increase tumor targeting is the dimeric scFv [(scFv')$_2$]. This structure can be created either as a single polypeptide by incorporating a carboxy-terminal cysteine residue that links two scFvs via a disulfide bridge. The anti-HER2 741F8 (scFv')$_2$ has been reported to increase tumor retention compared with both the monomeric 741F8 scFv' and a (scFv')$_2$ comprised of the anti-HER2 scFv' and an irrelevant scFv' *(38,41)*. A second structure that has proven successful is the diabody. Diabodies are formed by forcing interchain pairing of V_H and V_L domains through shortening the peptide linker that separates the V_H and V_L domains of an scFv. The resulting noncovalent dimer structure had been shown to be capable of bivalent binding to antigens and possess improved tumor targeting as compared with monomeric scFvs *(42)*. Both (scFv')$_2$ and diabodies are small enough to be cleared through first-pass renal clearance and therefore show rapid systemic clearance. Larger bivalent molecules with slower clearance rates have also been described *(43,44)*. The inherent nature of the CH3 domain of an IgG to homodimerize has been utilized to create one such molecule. The minibody is created by fusion of scFv to the CH3 domain of an IgG with the resulting dimeric molecule having a molecular weight (~80 kDa) higher than the renal threshold. Work with the cT84.66 anti-carcinoembryonic antigen minibody has shown it to have slower clearance kinetics than either the scFv of diabody form of the molecule. Radioiodinated minibody also displays better tumor uptake than the diabody: 20.5 vs 4.5% ID/g at 18 h post-injection *(45)*. This in part exemplifies the interplay between variables, such as clearance rate and valency and their effect on targeting. Structures have been taken one step further by fusing scFvs not only to the CH3 but rather to a CH2–CH3 domain. The intact Fc domain of these molecules not only results in dimer formation, but has the additional benefit of being able to marshal the immune system by interacting with Fc receptors present on effector cells.

9. CLINICAL APPLICATIONS

9.1. Unconjugated Antibodies

9.1.1. RITUXIMAB

Rituximab is the first MAb to be approved by the FDA for use in human malignancy *(46,47)*. The testing and evaluation of the chimeric anti-CD20 antibody, rituximab, demonstrated impressive clinical responses. Rituximab is a chimeric MAb, and multiple doses can be safely administered. In vitro studies have demonstrated multiple mechanisms by which anti-CD20 antibodies lead to cell death *(48)*. In the phase I study to determine the maximum tolerated dose, patients with relapsed low-grade and intermediate/high-grade non-Hodgkin's lymphoma received four weekly infusions of rituximab *(47)*. Thrombocytopenia and B-cell lymphocytopenia were observed. The lymphocytopenia persisted for 3–6 mo. Six of 18 patients, all of whom had low-grade lymphomas, demonstrated partial responses (33%). Phase II studies using the maximum tolerated dose, 375 mg/m^2, confirmed the efficacy of this therapy, demonstrating 46 and 48% response rates in two separate studies *(2,49)*. Although phase I testing had not suggested significant activity in intermediate/high-grade lymphomas, a phase II trial evaluated rituximab in relapsing or refractory diffuse, large B-cell lymphoma, mantle cell lymphoma, or other intermediate- or high-grade B-cell non-Hodgkin's lymphomas *(50)*. The study randomized 54 patients to either eight weekly treatments of 375 mg/m^2 of intravenous rituximab or 375 mg/m^2 in week 1 followed by seven weekly intravenous infusions of 500 mg/m^2. Five complete responses and 12 partial responses were observed for an overall response rate of 31%; there was no evidence of superiority of either treatment regimen. Patients with refractory disease and those with histologies other than diffuse large B-cell lymphoma appeared to have lower response rates.

Rituximab has been tested in conjunction with chemotherapy *(51)*. Preclinical data show that this antibody can sensitize chemotherapy-resistant cell lines to the cytotoxic effects of chemotherapy *(52)*. Forty patients with low-grade or follicular B-cell non-Hodgkin's lymphoma were enrolled in the study. Thirty-five patients received all six planned cycles of CHOP every 21 d, with six infusions of rituximab at a dose of 375 mg/m^2 given before, during, and after chemotherapy. Three patients did not complete treatment owing to intercurrent infections ($n = 2$) and patient choice ($n = 1$), and two patients were withdrawn from the study prior to therapy. The overall response rate was 95% (38/40), with 55% complete responses and 40% partial responses. Fewer complete responses were noted in patients with bulky disease. Median response duration and time to progression had not been reached after 29 mo of follow-up. Seven of eight patients who had initially been positive for the bcl-2 translocation became negative for the translocation by polymerase chain reaction assay after therapy; this has not been seen with CHOP chemotherapy alone *(53)*. A preliminary analysis of a randomized study in elderly patients with diffuse large-cell lymphoma comparing standard CHOP chemotherapy to CHOP with rituximab demonstrated a 76% complete response rate in the combination arm compared with 60% complete response rate in the chemotherapy arm without significant differences in toxicity between the two groups *(50)*. Furthermore, the addition of rituximab prolonged event-free survival and overall survival.

In some patients with circulating blood tumor cells, rituximab therapy has induced an infusion-related syndrome characterized by fever, rigors, thrombocytopenia, tumor lysis, bronchospasm, and hypoxemia, requiring discontinuation of the antibody infusion. Symptoms typically resolve with supportive care and patients may continue further therapy without sequelae *(54)*. Circulating CD20-positive cells, including lymphoma cells, may affect the efficacy of rituximab. Peak levels of circulating antibody inversely correlate with pretreatment B-cell counts, as well as the bulk of tumor *(55,56)*. Greater numbers of peripheral lymphocytes and/or tumor bulk serve as an antigen sink, removing antibodies from the circulation. For patients with bulky disease, a higher antibody dose or a greater number of cycles may be warranted because patients with lower serum rituximab concentrations have had statistically significant lower response rates. A dosage of eight cycles of weekly rituximab has been used safely in low-grade and follicular non-Hodgkin's lymphoma *(57)*. The efficacy of rituximab in chronic lymphocytic leukemia is clearly affected by lower circulative levels of the antibody. Initial studies revealed a 20% response rate. Chronic lymphocytic leukemia has lower antigen density than many lymphomas that express CD20, and the cells circulate, acting as an antigen sink. A dose-escalation study demonstrated a clear dose–response relationship *(58)*.

9.1.2. CAMPATH-1

The CAMPATH-1 antibody has specificity for CD52, a glycopeptide that is highly expressed on T- and B-lymphocytes. It has been tested as a therapeutic agent for chronic lymphocytic and promyelocytic leukemias, as well as other non-Hodgkin's lymphomas, and as a means to deplete T-cells from allogeneic transplant grafts. Half of the patients with fludarabine-resistant chronic lymphocytic leukemia or B-prolymphocytic leukemia exhibited clinical responses to CAMPATH-1 *(59)*. A larger phase II study reported a 42% response rate in patients with relapsed or refractory chronic lymphocytic leukemia, but at the cost of an increase in opportunistic infections and septicemia. CAMPATH-1 has also been evaluated as first-line therapy for patients with chronic lymphocytic leukemia. All patients responded with loss of peripheral blood malignant lymphocytes. However, patients with involvement of lymph nodes and/or spleen were less likely to respond completely. There was evidence of reactivation of cytomegalovirus infections. Subcutaneous administration of the antibody was found to be safe and effective. A humanized version of the antibody (CAMPATH-1H) has been extensively tested.

In a phase II, multicenter study of CAMPATH-1H in previously treated patients with low-grade non-Hodgkin's lymphomas, 50 patients with relapsed or refractory disease were treated with 30 mg of CAMPATH-1H three times weekly for up to 12 wk *(60)*. Infection, anemia, and thrombocytopenia were common, and myocardial infarction occurred in one patient with a prior history of angina and congestive heart failure. The overall response rate was 20% (16% partial response, 4% complete response). Responses were short in duration, with a median time to progression of 4 mo. Patients with mycosis fungoides responded more frequently and had a longer time to progression (10 mo) than did patients with low-grade non-Hodgkin's lymphoma (4 mo). Treatment was associated with reactivation of herpes simplex, oral candidiasis, *pneumocystis carinii* pneumonia, cytomegalovirus pneumonitis, pulmonary aspergillosis, disseminated tuberculosis, and seven cases of pneumonia and septicemia.

9.2. Solid Tumor Antigens

9.2.1. HERCEPTIN

HER-2/*neu* (c-erbB-2), a member of the EGFR family, has been targeted for antibody therapy because it is overexpressed on 25% of breast cancers, as well as other adenocarcinomas of the ovary, prostate, lung, and gastrointestinal tract. Trastuzumab *(23,61)*, also known as Herceptin, and rhuMAb HER2, is a humanized antibody derived from 4D5, a murine MAb that recognizes an epitope on the extracellular domain of HER-2/*neu*. A phase II trial in women with metastatic breast cancer reported an objective response rate of 11.6%, with responses seen in the liver, mediastinum, lymph nodes, and chest wall. Patients received 10 or more treatments with the antibody, and none developed an antibody response against trastuzumab. In a second phase II study, 222 women with metastatic breast cancer were treated with 2 mg/kg of trastuzumab weekly, with an objective response rate of 16% *(23)*. The median response duration was 9.1 mo, with a median overall survival of 13 mo, both of which are superior to outcomes reported for second-line chemotherapy in metastatic disease. In each of these trials, about 30% of the patients had stable disease lasting more than 5 mo. Overexpression of HER-2/*neu* associated with gene amplification correlates with a clinical response to trastuzumab. Earlier studies utilized variable criteria to define HER2 positivity that may account for the differences in the response rates *(62)*.

A large, randomized phase III trial evaluating cytotoxic chemotherapy alone and with trastuzumab has shown the efficacy of combination therapy *(63)*. Patients receiving initial therapy for metastatic breast cancer were treated with cyclophosphamide plus doxorubicin or epirubicin, or with paclitaxel if they had received an anthracycline in the adjuvant setting. Patients were randomized to receive this chemotherapy alone or in combination with weekly antibody therapy. Response rates for combination therapy with an anthracycline regimen increased from 43 to 52% with the addition of trastuzumab. Using paclitaxel, response rates increased from 16 to 42% with the addition of trastuzumab. In addition, there was evidence that the addition of trastuzumab to chemotherapy improved survival at one year by 16% *(64)* and improved survival at 29 mo by 25% *(65)*. Myocardial dysfunction was observed more frequently in patients receiving doxorubicin or epirubicin when trastuzumab was added. Therefore, trastuzumab is not recommended in combination with anthracyclines.

Based on these clinical trial results, trastuzumab was approved by the FDA to treat women with metastatic breast cancer with HER-2/*neu* overexpression, given either alone or in combination with paclitaxel. Herceptin also has activity in combination with other chemotherapeutic agents *(66,67)*. In addition, breast cancer patients with lymph node involvement whose cancers overexpress HER-2/*neu* are candidates for participation in a randomized phase III trial evaluating standard adjuvant chemotherapy with or without trastuzumab. Recent interim analysis of this study has led to its early closure since a significant improvement in disease free survival of patient in the Herceptin arm has been observed (oral presentation, ASCO 2005).

Herceptin has been a success story in breast cancer therapy. However, despite the overexpression of Her2/*neu* in other solid tumors, such as non-small-cell lung cancer, to date, no significant clinical benefit has been seen in patients with diseases other than breast cancer treated with Herceptin.

9.3. Epidermal Growth Factor Receptor

EGFR is a widely expressed glycoprotein. It has three main domains: the extracellular domain is the ligand-binding portion of the molecule. It can bind to a number of regulatory factors, such as EGF and transforming growth factor-α, leading to EGFR dimerization and autophosphorylation. The hydrophobic transmembrane portion connects the extra and intracellular portions together. The cytoplasmic domain contains the tyrosine kinase catalytic activity component, which responds to receptor autophosphorylation by increasing the tyrosine kinase activity *(68)*. This, in turn, leads to phosphorylation of other tyrosine motifs and activation of a number of intracellular signaling pathways, such as phosphatidylinositol-3 kinase and Akt, which result in cellular proliferation, differentiation, transformation, and antiapoptotic functions.

The possible role of EGFR overexpression in tumor growth and development is best studied in colorectal cancers *(68)*. It is generally accepted that that EGFR overexpression is found in 65–70% of colorectal carcinomas *(69)*, although there is heterogeneity in tumor biopsies examined and the lack of a uniform method of evaluating levels of EGFR. The available anti-EGFR MAbs bind to the EGFR and block the binding of the ligand to the receptor and prevent downstream events. Cetuximab (C225) is a chimeric MAb directed against the extracellular domain of the EGFR. ABX-EGF is a fully human IgG2 MAb against EGFR. This antibody is generated through the Xenomouse transgenic strain that lacks functional mouse Ig genes, but has human Ig genes instead *(68)*. Clinical trials with this antibody are ongoing. Both of these antibodies are capable of inhibiting the growth of EGFR-expressing cell lines in vitro and in vivo *(70,71)*. Cetuximab is capable of enhancing the antitumor effects of chemotherapy and radiation therapy in preclinical and clinical studies. This agent has been used either alone or in combination with radiotherapy or various chemotherapeutic agents primarily in patients with head and neck or colorectal cancers. The most common side effect seen with this agent is acne in the form of a rash and occasional allergic reactions. In a phase II study of 120 patients with EGFR-positive colorectal tumors who were refractory to fluorouacil or irinotecan, the combination of cetuximab and irinotecan had a response rate of 22.5% *(72)*. A subsequent phase II trial of single-agent cetuximab in irinotecan refractory patients showed a partial response rate of 9% with 37% of patients having either minor responses or stable disease *(73)*. A subsequent randomized, phase III trial involving 329 patients with EGFR-positive irinotecan refractory colorectal cancers was conducted. Patients were randomized to receive cetuximab (400 mg/m^2 loading dose followed by 250 mg/m^2 weekly) plus irinotecan or cetuximab alone. There was a significantly higher response rate (22.9 vs 10.8%) and median time to progression in the combination arm *(74)*. Cetuximab has been approved by the FDA for the treatment of advanced or refractory colorectal cancers in conjunction with irinotecan.

Colorectal cancer patients with EGFR-negative tumors also seem to have the potential to respond to cetuximab-based therapies. It appears that EGFR analysis by current immunohistochemistry techniques does have predictive value *(75)*.

9.4. Vascular Endothelial Growth Factor

VEGF is produced by many cancers to stimulate the growth of new blood vessels, and in some studies, its expression at tumor sites is correlated with the risk for metastases. Molecules, such as VEGF, that are selectively expressed in the tissue matrix surrounding the tumor are potentially important targets for antibody therapy. VEGF, which resides in the vasculature that feeds tumor cell, is the first anti-angiogenic target to be exploited. Bevacizumab is a humanized MAb that blocks binding of the VEGF to its receptor on vascular endothelium. A phase I clinical study of bevacizumab tested doses of 0.1–10 mg/kg infused on days 1, 28, 35, and 42 *(76)*. No severe toxicities were found. At doses of 3–10 mg/kg, increases in systolic and diastolic blood pressure of greater than 10 mmHg were noted during therapy *(76)*, and subsequent studies have confirmed that hypertension is a toxicity of this agent *(77)*. Two patients receiving 3 mg/kg experienced bleeding into their tumors. One patient with hepatocellular carcinoma bled into a previously undiagnosed brain metastasis. Another patient with an extremity sarcoma and lung metastases bled into the extremity mass and experienced hemoptysis.

In a phase II study of bevacizumab combined with carboplatin and paclitaxel in patients with non-small-cell lung cancer, 6 of 66 patients developed pulmonary hemorrhage, 4 of whom died *(78)*. Patients with squamous cell lung cancers and tumors with evidence of cavitation or squamous cell histology appeared to be at higher risk of hemoptysis.

In a randomized trial involving 813 patients with previously untreated metastatic colorectal cancer, 402 patients received irinotecan, bolus fluorouracil, and leucovorin (IFL) plus bevacizumab (5 mg/kg of body weight every 2 wk) and 411 received IFL plus placebo *(79)*. The median survival was 20.3 mo in the chemotherapy plus antibody arm vs 15.6 mo in the placebo arm. The overall response rates were also higher in the antibody treated arm (44.8 and 34.8%, $p = 0.004$). The most common side effect was grade 3 hypertension during treatment with IFL plus bevacizumab (11 vs 2.3%) but was easily managed. This study has lead to the FDA approval of bevacizumab for the treatment of patients with metastatic colorectal cancer.

10. IMMUNOTOXINS

MAbs that are not capable of directly eliciting antitumor effects, either by altering signal transduction or directing immune system cells, can still be effective against tumors by delivering cytotoxic payloads. MAbs have been employed to deliver a wide variety of agents including chemotherapeutic drugs, toxins, radioisotopes, and cytokines *(80)*. Immunotoxins are antibodies or antibody fragments that are conjugated to a toxin and are designed to deliver the toxin to the cell surface *(81)*. The therapeutic goal is to deliver the toxin to the surface of the cancer cells via antibody binding to a target, and after internalization of the toxin, causing cell death. The clinical benefit is more likely if the antigen is expressed only on cancer cells and not on vital tissue. The more potent the toxin is, the smaller the number of immunotoxin molecules needed to achieve a therapeutic benefit. Toxins can be derived from plants or bacteria. They can be small molecules, such as calicheamicins *(81)*, or toxins, such as the *pseudomonas (82)* or diphtheria toxin *(83)*. Mylotarg, an anti-CD33 MAb conjugated to calicheamicin, is an immunotoxin approved for use in patients with recurrent or refractory acute myelogenous leukemia *(8)*.

Recombinant immunotoxins are produced in bacterial expression systems from gene fusions that combine antibody DNA fragments with toxin domain coding sequences *(84)*. Once expressed, the hybrid protein has to be chemically modified to be properly folded and activated. The antibody must be able to recognize the target as expressed on the surface of cancer cells, antibody-binding of the target must lead to the internalization of the toxin. The target should ideally be absent from the normal cells and should not be shed. The Fv portion of an antibody can be used instead of the whole antibody as the binding capacity is retained through this fragment. This small fragment can potentially increase tumor penetration.

These toxic agents are very potent due to their catalytic nature, which allows as few as one toxin molecule to kill a cell. The most commonly utilized toxins are derived from plants (e.g., ricin) or micro-organisms (e.g., *pseudomonas*). In constructing an immunotoxin, the toxin's natural translocation domain is replaced by an antibody in order to limit its internalization to cells that express the target antigen. Additional modifications, such as the endoplasmic reticulum retention sequence, KDEL, have been incorporated to facilitate the transfer of the toxin from the endosomal compartment to the cytoplasm of the target cell *(85)*. Immunotoxins have demonstrated significant antitumor effects in preclinical models. For example, Kreitman et al. have reported complete regressions of human Burkitt's lymphoma xenografts in mice that were treated with a recombinant anti-CD22 immunotoxin, RFB4(dsFv)-PE38, at relevant doses based on those tolerated by cynomolgus monkeys *(86)*. However, in clinical trials, the use of immunotoxins has been associated with unacceptable neurotoxicity *(87)* and life-threatening vascular leak syndrome *(88)*.

11. RADIOIMMUNOCONJUGATES

So far, two radioimmunoconjugates have been approved for use in clinical practice by the FDA, Zevalin™ (ibritumomab) and Bexxar™ (tositumomab). Both of these agents are approved for use in patients with recurrent or refractory non-Hodgkin's lymphoma.

Zevalin is an Yttrium-90 (Y-90) labeled anti-CD20 MAb that has demonstrated effectiveness for the treatment of non-Hodgkin's lymphoma. In clinical trials, the overall response rate of lymphoma patients treated with Zevalin was 67% (25% complete responses and 41% partial responses). Patients with low-grade disease exhibited an even better overall response rate of 82% (27% complete responses and 56% partial responses) *(89)*. Significantly, therapeutic efficacy was seen even in the presence of bulky disease and splenomegaly. The β particles emitted by Y-90 and iodine-131 have a moderate linear energy transfer on the order of approx 0.2 keV/μm, therefore requiring up to thousands of "hits" to kill a cell *(90)*. This is balanced by their long mean track length (approx 4000 μm for Y-90). This broad field of impact leads to a "crossfire" effect that can kill tumor cells that lack the targeted antigen or lie beyond the diffusion radius of the radioimmunoconjugate. The importance of these long track-length effects is balanced by the exciting results obtained with the iodine 131 anti-CD20 immunoconjugate, tositumumab (Bexxar regimen), which has yielded similar degrees of efficacy. Indeed, treatment with this agent has yielded very impressive rates of response and prolonged durations of complete remission in patients with favorable, low-grade indolent lymphoma when used as initial therapy *(91)*.

Although the use of radioimmunotherapy has proven useful in the treatment of patients with lymphomas, patients with solid tumors have not benefited from this approach. This could be related to either lack of tumor penetration or incomplete tumor targeting with currently available antibody constructs.

Targeting the vascular endothelium as a means of interrupting the tumor blood supply with antibodies against specific tumor endothelial markers is an approach that is being investigated. Targeting the angiogenic pathway might prove beneficial in treatment of solid tumors. Radio labeled antibodies directed against tumor related vasculature could provide additional "killing" by directing radiation to the tumor.

12. PRETARGETED THERAPY

Multistep, pretargeted immunotherapy strategies have been developed to take advantage of the specificity of antibody-based targeting without subjecting the host to the potentially considerable toxic side effects associated with the systemic delivery of an active chemotherapeutic drug or the relatively slow delivery of a radioimmunoconjugate. In pretargeted antibody therapy, an antibody–enzyme or antibody–ligand conjugate is administered and allowed to localize in the tumor. After it has cleared from the circulation and normal tissues, or has been actively removed through the use of a clearing agent, a cytotoxic agent is administered that can only be activated or retained by the pretargeted antibody in the tumor. In this manner, the cytotoxic effects are further focused on the tumor.

13. CONCLUSIONS

Antibodies have become widely used, standard treatments for a number of important cancers. Although the use of immunoconjugates has lagged behind the use of unconjugated antibodies that mediate ADCC or directly perturbed signaling, recent advances in antibody engineering and in the tailored use of immunoconjugates to treat lymphoma provide compelling evidence that substantial gains can be expected in the next few years.

ACKNOWLEDGMENT

Supported by CA50633 (LMW), CA06927, the Frank Strick Foundation, the Bernard A. and Rebecca S. Bernard Foundation, and an appropriation from the Commonwealth of Pennsylvania.

REFERENCES

1. Miller RA, Maloney DG, Warnke R, Levy R. Treatment of B-cell lymphoma with monoclonal anti-idiotype antibody. *N Engl J Med* 1982; 306:517–522.
2. McLaughlin P, Grillo-Lopez AJ, Link BK, et al. Rituximab chimeric anti-CD20 monoclonal antibody therapy for relapsed indolent lymphoma: half of patients respond to a four-dose treatment program. *J Clin Oncol* 1998; 16:2825–2833.
3. Coiffier B. Rituximab in combination with CHOP improves survival in elderly patients with aggressive non-Hodgkin's lymphoma. *Semin Oncol* 2002; 29(2 Suppl 6):18–22.
4. Leonard JP, Link BK. Immunotherapy of non-Hodgkin's lymphoma with hLL2 (epratuzumab, an anti-CD22 monoclonal antibody) and Hu1D10 (apolizumab). *Semin Oncol* 2002; 29(1 Suppl 2):81–86.
5. Witzig TE, Gordon LI, Cabanillas F, et al. Randomized controlled trial of yttrium-90-labeled ibritumomab tiuxetan radioimmunotherapy versus rituximab immunotherapy for patients with relapsed or refractory low-grade, follicular, or transformed B-cell non-Hodgkin's lymphoma. *J Clin Oncol* 2002; 20: 2453–2463.

6. Kaminski MS, Estes J, Zasadny KR, et al. Radioimmunotherapy with iodine (131)I tositumomab for relapsed or refractory B-cell non-Hodgkin lymphoma: updated results and long-term follow-up of the University of Michigan experience. *Blood* 2000; 96:1259–1266.

7. Lundin J, Kimby E, Bjorkholm M, et al. Phase II trial of subcutaneous anti-CD52 monoclonal antibody alemtuzumab (Campath-1H) as first-line treatment for patients with B-cell chronic lymphocytic leukemia (B-CLL). *Blood* 2002; 100:768–773.

8. Sievers EL, Appelbaum FR, Spielberger RT, et al. Selective ablation of acute myeloid leukemia using antibody-targeted chemotherapy: a phase I study of an anti-CD33 calicheamicin immunoconjugate. *Blood* 1999; 93:3678–3684.

9. Kreitman RJ, Wilson WH, Bergeron K, et al. Efficacy of the anti-CD22 recombinant immunotoxin BL22 in chemotherapy-resistant hairy-cell leukemia. *N Engl J Med* 2001; 345:241–247.

10. Cobleigh MA, Vogel CL, Tripathy D, et al. Multinational study of the efficacy and safety of humanized anti-HER2 monoclonal antibody in women who have HER2-overexpressing metastatic breast cancer that has progressed after chemotherapy for metastatic disease. *J Clin Oncol* 1999; 17:2639–2648.

11. Vogel CL, Cobleigh MA, Tripathy D, et al. Efficacy and safety of trastuzumab as a single agent in first-line treatment of HER2-overexpressing metastatic breast cancer. *J Clin Oncol* 2002; 20:719–726.

12. Slamon DJ, Leyland-Jones B, Shak S, et al. Use of chemotherapy plus a monoclonal antibody against HER2 for metastatic breast cancer that overexpresses HER2. *N Engl J Med* 2001; 344:783–792.

13. Robert F, Ezekiel MP, Spencer SA, et al. Phase I study of anti-epidermal growth factor receptor antibody cetuximab in combination with radiation therapy in patients with advanced head and neck cancer. *J Clin Oncol* 2001; 19:3234–3243.

14. Figlin RA, Belldegrun AS, Crawford J, et al. ABX-EGF, a fully human anti-epidermal growth factor receptor (EGFR) monoclonal antibody (mAb) in patients with advanced cancer: phase 1 clinical results (Abstract). *Proceedings ASCO* 2002; 21:35.

15. Egen JG, Kuhns MS, Allison JP. CTLA-4: new insights into its biological function and use in tumor immunotherapy. *Nat Immunol* 2002; 3:611–618.

16. Kohler G, Milstein C. Continuous cultures of fused cells secreting antibody of predefined specificity. *Nature* 1975; 256:495–497.

17. Janeway C, Travers, P., Walport, M., Shlomchik, M. The generation of lymphocyte antigen receptors. 5th ed. New York: Garland Publishing; 2001.

18. Penichet M, Morrison, S. Design and engineering human forms of monoclonal antibodies. *Drug Dev Res* 2004; 61:121–136.

19. Abramowicz D, Crusiaux A, Goldman M. Anaphylactic shock after retreatment with OKT3 monoclonal antibody. *N Engl J Med* 1992; 327:736.

20. Bajorin DF, Chapman PB, Wong GY, et al. Treatment with high dose mouse monoclonal (anti-GD3) antibody R24 in patients with metastatic melanoma. *Melanoma Res* 1992; 2:355–362.

21. Czuczman M, Grillo-Lopez A, White C, et al. Treatment of patients with low-grade B-cell lymphoma with the combination of chimeric anti-CD20 monoclonal antibody and CHOP chemotherapy. *J Clin Oncol* 1999; 17:268–276.

22. Wright A, Shin SU, Morrison SL. Genetically engineered antibodies: progress and prospects. *Crit Rev Immunol* 1992; 12:125–168.

23. Cobleigh M, Vogel C, Tripathy D, et al. Multinational study of the efficacy and safety of humanized anti-HER2 monoclonal antibody in women who have HER2-overexpressing metastatic breast cancer that has progressed after chemotherapy for metastatic disease. *J Clin Oncol* 1999; 17:2639–2648.

24. Carter P. Improving the efficacy of antibody-based cancer therapies. *Nat Rev Cancer* 2001; 1:118–129.

25. Coloma MJ, Morrison SL. Design and production of novel tetravalent bispecific antibodies. *Nat Biotechnol* 1997; 15:159–163.

26. Weiner LM, Clark JI, Ring DB, Alpaugh RK. Clinical development of 2B1, a bispecific murine monoclonal antibody targeting c-erbB-2 and Fc gamma RIII. *J Hematother* 1995; 4:453–456.

27. Lewis LD, Cole BF, Wallace PK, et al. Pharmacokinetic-pharmacodynamic relationships of the bispecific antibody MDX-H210 when administered in combination with interferon gamma: a multiple-dose phase-I study in patients with advanced cancer which overexpresses HER-2/neu. *J Immunol Methods* 2001; 248:149–165.

28. James ND, Atherton PJ, Jones J, Howie AJ, Tchekmedyian S, Curnow RT. A phase II study of the bispecific antibody MDX-H210 (anti-HER2 x CD64) with GM-CSF in HER2+ advanced prostate cancer. *Br J Cancer* 2001; 85:152–156.

29. Valone FH, Kaufman PA, Guyre PM, et al. Phase Ia/Ib trial of bispecific antibody MDX-210 in patients with advanced breast or ovarian cancer that overexpresses the proto-oncogene HER-2/neu. *J Clin Oncol* 1995; 13:2281–2292.

30. Hoogenboom HR, Chames P. Natural and designer binding sites made by phage display technology. *Immunol Today* 2000; 21:371–378.

31. Sheets MD, Amersdorfer P, Finnern R, et al. Efficient construction of a large nonimmune phage antibody library: the production of high-affinity human single-chain antibodies to protein antigens. *Proc Natl Acad Sci USA* 1998; 95:6157–6162.

32. Jain RK, Baxter LT. Mechanisms of heterogeneous distribution of monoclonal antibodies and other macromolecules in tumors: significance of elevated interstitial pressure. *Cancer Res* 1988; 48:7022–7032.

33. Jain RK. Physiological barriers to delivery of monoclonal antibodies and other macromolecules in tumors. *Cancer Res* 1990; 50(Suppl 3):814s–819s.

34. Yokota T, Milenic DE, Whitlow M, Schlom J. Rapid tumor penetration of a single-chain Fv and comparison with other immunoglobulin forms. *Cancer Res* 1992; 52:3402–3408.

35. Milenic DE, Yokota T, Filpula DR, et al. Construction, binding properties, metabolism, and tumor targeting of a single-chain Fv derived from the pancarcinoma monoclonal antibody CC49. *Cancer Res* 1991; 51:6363–6371.

36. Pavlinkova G, Beresford GW, Booth BJ, Batra SK, Colcher D. Pharmacokinetics and biodistribution of engineered single-chain antibody constructs of MAb CC49 in colon carcinoma xenografts. *JNucl Med* 1999; 40:1536–1546.

37. Adams GP, Schier R, Marshall K, et al. Increased affinity leads to improved selective tumor delivery of single-chain Fv antibodies. *Cancer Res* 1998; 58:485–490.

38. Adams GP, McCartney JE, Tai M-S, et al. Highly specific *in vivo* tumor targeting by monovalent and divalent forms of 741F8 anti-c-erbB-2 single-chain Fv. *Cancer Res* 1993; 53:4026–4034.

39. Tai MS, McCartney JE, Adams GP, et al. Targeting c-erbB-2 expressing tumors using single-chain Fv monomers and dimers. *Cancer Res* 1995; 55:5983s–5989s.

40. Adams GP, Schier R, McCall AM, et al. High affinity restricts the localization and tumor penetration of single-chain Fv antibody molecules. *Cancer Res* 2001; 61:4750–4755.

41. Adams GP, McCartney JE, Wolf EJ, et al. Influence of avidity on the tumor retention of monospecific and bispecific anti-c-erbB-2 single-chain Fv dimers. *Proc Amer Assoc Cancer Res* 1996; 37:472.

42. Adams GP, Schier R, McCall AM, et al. Prolonged in vivo tumour retention of a human diabody targeting the extracellular domain of human HER2/neu. *Br J Cancer* 1998; 77:1405–1412.

43. Hu S, Shively L, Raubitschek A, et al. Minibody: A novel engineered anti-carcinoembryonic antigen antibody fragment (single-chain Fv-CH3) which exhibits rapid, high-level targeting of xenografts. *Cancer Res* 1996; 56:3055–3061.

44. Powers DB, Amersdorfer P, Poul M-A, et al. Expression of single-chain Fv-Fc fusions in Pichia pastoris. *J Immunol Methods* 2001; 251:123–135.

45. Sundaresan G, Yazaki PJ, Shively JE, et al. 124I-labeled engineered anti-CEA minibodies and diabodies allow high-contrast, antigen-specific small-animal PET imaging of xenografts in athymic mice. *J Nucl Med* 2003; 44:1962–1969.

46. Maloney DG, Grillo-Lopez AJ, Bodkin DJ, et al. IDEC-C2B8: results of a phase I multiple-dose trial in patients with relapsed non-Hodgkin's lymphoma. *J Clin Oncol* 1997; 15:3266–3274.

47. Maloney DG, Grillo-Lopez AJ, White CA, et al. IDEC-C2B8 (Rituximab) anti-CD20 monoclonal anti-body therapy in patients with relapsed low-grade non-Hodgkin's lymphoma. *Blood* 1997; 90:2188–2195.

48. Shan D, Ledbetter JA, Press OW. Signaling events involved in anti-CD20-induced apoptosis of malignant human B cells. *Cancer Immunol Immunother* 2000; 48:673–683.

49. Berinstein NL, Grillo-Lopez AJ, White CA, et al. Association of serum Rituximab (IDEC-C2B8) concentration and anti-tumor response in the treatment of recurrent low-grade or follicular non-Hodgkin's lymphoma. *Ann Oncol* 1998; 9:995–1001.

50. Coiffier B, Haioun C, Ketterer N, et al. Rituximab (anti-CD20 monoclonal antibody) for the treatment of patients with relapsing or refractory aggressive lymphoma: a multicenter phase II study. *Blood* 1998; 92:1927–1932.

51. Czuczman MS, Grillo-Lopez AJ, White CA, et al. Treatment of patients with low-grade B-cell lymphoma with the combination of chimeric anti-CD20 monoclonal antibody and CHOP chemotherapy. *J Clin Oncol* 1999; 17:268–276.

52. Demidem A, Lam T, Alas S, Hariharan K, Hanna N, Bonavida B. Chimeric anti-CD20 (IDEC-C2B8) monoclonal antibody sensitizes a B cell lymphoma cell line to cell killing by cytotoxic drugs. *Cancer Biother Radiopharm* 1997; 12:177–186.

53. Gribben JG, Freedman A, Woo SD, et al. All advanced stage non-Hodgkin's lymphomas with a polymerase chain reaction amplifiable breakpoint of bcl-2 have residual cells containing the bcl-2 rearrangement at evaluation and after treatment. *Blood* 1991; 78:3275–3280.

54. Byrd JC, Waselenko JK, Maneatis TJ, et al. Rituximab therapy in hematologic malignancy patients with circulating blood tumor cells: association with increased infusion-related side effects and rapid blood tumor clearance. *J Clin Oncol* 1999; 17:791–795.

55. McLaughlin P, Grillo-Lopez A, Link B, et al. Rituximab chimeric anti-CD20 monoclonal antibody therapy for relapsed indolent lymphoma: half of patients respond to a four-dose treatment program. *J Clin Oncol* 1998; 16:2825–2833.

56. Berinstein N, Grillo-Lopez A, White C, et al. Association of serum Rituximab (IDEC-C2B8) concentration and anti-tumor response in the treatment of recurrent low-grade or follicular non-Hodgkin's lymphoma. *Ann Oncol* 1988; 9:995–1001.

57. Piro L, White C, Grillo-Lopez A, et al. Extended rituximab (anti-CD20 monoclonal antibody) therapy for relapsed or refractory low-grade or follicular non-Hodgkin's lymphoma. *Ann Oncol* 1999; 10:619–621.

58. Keating M, O'Brien S. High-dose rituximab therapy in chronic lymphocytic leukemia. *Semin Oncol* 2000; 27(6 Suppl 12):86–90.

59. Bowen A, Zomas A, Emmett E, Matutes E, Dyer M, Catovsky D. Subcutaneous CAMPATH-1H in fludarabine-resistant/relapsed chronic lymphocytic and B-prolymphocytic leukaemia. *Br J Haematol* 1997; 96:617–619.

60. Lundin J, Osterborg A, Brittinger G, et al. CAMPATH-1H monoclonal antibody in therapy for previously treated low-grade non-Hodgkin's lymphomas: a phase II multicenter study. European Study Group of CAMPATH-1H Treatment in Low-Grade Non-Hodgkin's Lymphoma. *J Clin Oncol* 1998; 16:3257–3263.

61. Baselga J, Tripathy D, Mendelsohn J, et al. Phase II study of weekly intravenous recombinant humanized anti-p185HER2 monoclonal antibody in patients with HER2/neu-overexpressing metastatic breast cancer. *J Clin Oncol* 1996; 14:737–744.

62. von Mehren M, Adams GP, Weiner LM. Monoclonal antibody therapy for cancer. *Annu Rev Med* 2003; 54:343–369.

63. Slamon D, Leyland-Jones B, Shak S, et al. Use of chemotherapy plus a monoclonal antibody against HER2 for metastatic breast cancer that overexpresses HER2. *N Engl J Med* 2001; 344:783–792.

64. Norton L, Slamon D, Leyland-Jones B. Overall survival (OS) advantage to simultaneous chemotherapy (CRx) plus the humanized anti-HER2 monoclonal antibody Herceptin® (H) in HER2-everexpressing (HER2+) metastatic breast cancer (MBC). In: *Proc Amer Soc Clin Oncol* 1999; 18:127a.

65. Baselga J. Clinical Trials of Herceptin® (trastuzumab). *Eur J Cancer* 2001; 37(Suppl1):S18–S24.

66. Burstein HJ, Kuter I, Campos SM, et al. Clinical activity of trastuzumab and vinorelbine in women with HER2-overexpressing metastatic breast cancer. *J Clin Oncol* 2001; 19:2722–2730.

67. Pegram M, Lipton A, Hayes D, et al. Phase II study of receptor-enhanced chemosensitivity using recombinant humanized anti-p185her2/neu monoclonal antibody plus cisplatin in patients with HER2/neu-overexpressing metastatic breast cancer refractory to chemotherapy treatment. *J Clin Oncol* 1998; 16: 2659–2671.

68. Lockhart C, Berlin JD. The epidermal growth factor receptor as a target for colorectal cancer therapy. *Semin Oncol* 2005; 32:52–60.

69. Messa C, Russo F, Caruso MG, Di Leo A. EGF, TGF-alpha, and EGF-R in human colorectal adenocarcinoma. *Acta Oncol* 1998; 37:285–289.

70. Baselga J. The EGFR as a target for anticancer therapy—focus on cetuximab. *Eur J Cancer* 2001; 37 (Suppl 4):S16–S22.

71. Yang XD, Jia XC, Corvalan JR, Wang P, Davis CG. Development of ABX-EGF, a fully human anti-EGF receptor monoclonal antibody, for cancer therapy. *Crit Rev Oncol Hematol* 2001; 38:17–23.

72. Saltz L, Rubin M, Hochster H. Cetuximab (IMC-C225) plus irinotecan (CPT-11) is active in CPT-11 refractory colorectal cancer (CRC) that expresses epidermal growth factor receptor (EGFR). *Proc Amer Soc Clin Oncol* 2001; 20:7.

73. Saltz LB, Meropol NJ, Loehrer PJ, Sr., Needle MN, Kopit J, Mayer RJ. Phase II trial of cetuximab in patients with refractory colorectal cancer that expresses the epidermal growth factor receptor. *J Clin Oncol* 2004; 22:1201–1208.

74. Cunningham D, Humblet Y, Siena S, et al. Cetuximab monotherapy and cetuximab plus irinotecan in irinotecan-refractory metastatic colorectal cancer. *N Engl J Med* 2004; 351:337–345.
75. Chung KY, Shia J, Kemeny NE, et al. Cetuximab shows activity in colorectal cancer patients with tumors that do not express the epidermal growth factor receptor by immunohistochemistry. *J Clin Oncol* 2005; 23:1803–1810.
76. Gordon MS, Margolin K, Talpaz M, et al. Phase I safety and pharmacokinetic study of recombinant human anti-vascular endothelial growth factor in patients with advanced cancer. *J Clin Oncol* 2001; 19:843–850.
77. Cobleigh MA, Langmuir VK, Sledge GW, et al. A phase I/II dose-escalation trial of bevacizumab in previously treated metastatic breast cancer. *Semin Oncol* 2003; 30(5 Suppl 16):117–124.
78. Johnson DH, Fehrenbacher L, Novotny WF, et al. Randomized phase II trial comparing bevacizumab plus carboplatin and paclitaxel with carboplatin and paclitaxel alone in previously untreated locally advanced or metastatic non-small-cell lung cancer. *J Clin Oncol* 2004; 22:2184–2191.
79. Hurwitz H, Fehrenbacher L, Novotny W, et al. Bevacizumab plus irinotecan, fluorouracil, and leucovorin for metastatic colorectal cancer. *N Engl J Med* 2004; 350:2335–2342.
80. Allen TM. Ligand-targeted therapeutics in anti-cancer therapy. *Nat Rev Cancer* 2002; 2:750–763.
81. Presta LG. Engineering antibodies for therapy. *Curr Pharm Biotechnol* 2002; 3:237–256.
82. Tur MK, Sasse S, Stocker M, et al. An anti-GD2 single chain Fv selected by phage display and fused to Pseudomonas exotoxin A develops specific cytotoxic activity against neuroblastoma derived cell lines. *Int J Mol Med* 2001; 8:579–584.
83. LeMaistre CF, Saleh MN, Kuzel TM, et al. Phase I trial of a ligand fusion-protein (DAB389IL-2) in lymphomas expressing the receptor for interleukin-2. *Blood* 1998; 91:399–405.
84. FitzGerald DJ, Kreitman R, Wilson W, Squires D, Pastan I. Recombinant immunotoxins for treating cancer. *Int J Med Microbiol* 2004; 293:577–582.
85. Kreitman RJ, Pastan I. Importance of the glutamate residue of KDEL in increasing the cytotoxicity of Pseudomonas exotoxin derivatives and for increased binding to the KDEL receptor. *Biochem J* 1995; 307:29–37.
86. Kreitman RJ, Wang QC, FitzGerald DJ, Pastan I. Complete regression of human B-cell lymphoma xenografts in mice treated with recombinant anti-CD22 immunotoxin RFB4(dsFv)-PE38 at doses tolerated by cynomolgus monkeys. *Int J Cancer* 1999; 81:148–155.
87. Pai LH, Bookman MA, Ozols RF, et al. Clinical evaluation of intraperitoneal Pseudomonas exotoxin immunoconjugate OVB3-PE in patients with ovarian cancer. *J Clin Oncol* 1991; 9:2095–2103.
88. Baluna R, Vitetta ES. Vascular leak syndrome: a side effect of immunotherapy. *Immunopharmacology* 1997; 37:117–132.
89. Witzig TE, White CA, Wiseman GA, et al. Phase I/II trial of IDEC-Y2B8 radioimmunotherapy for treatment of relapsed or refractory CD20(+) B-cell non-Hodgkin's lymphoma. *J Clin Oncol* 1999; 17: 3793–3803.
90. McDevitt MR, Sgouros G, Finn RD, et al. Radioimmunotherapy with alpha-emitting nuclides. *Eur J Nucl Med* 1998; 25:1341–1351.
91. Kaminski MS, Tuck M, Estes J, et al. 131I-tositumomab therapy as initial treatment for follicular lymphoma. *N Engl J Med* 2005; 352:441–449.

Index